Walsh and Hoyt's

Clinical
Neuro-Ophthalmology
The Essentials

W9-BVS-012

RE
725
.W3
2016
c.3

Walsh and Hoyt's
Clinical Neuro-Ophthalmology
The Essentials

Third Edition

Neil R. Miller, MD

Professor of Ophthalmology, Neurology, and Neurosurgery
Frank B. Walsh Professor of Neuro-Ophthalmology
Director, Neuro-Ophthalmology and Orbit Units
Wilmer Eye Institute
Johns Hopkins Hospital
Baltimore, Maryland

Prem S. Subramanian, MD

Associate Professor of Neuro-Ophthalmology
Wilmer Eye Institute
Johns Hopkins Hospital
Baltimore, Maryland

Vivek R. Patel, MD

Wilmer Eye Institute
Johns Hopkins Hospital
Baltimore, Maryland

Illinois College of Optometry Library
3241 South Michigan Avenue
Chicago, IL 60616
312-949-7160

 Wolters Kluwer

Philadelphia • Baltimore • New York • London
Buenos Aires • Hong Kong • Sydney • Tokyo

Acquisitions Editor: Kel MacGowan
Senior Product Development Editor: Emilie Moyer
Editorial Assistant: Diane Solomon
Marketing Manager: Stephanie Kindlick
Production Project Manager: David Orzechowski
Design Coordinator: Holly McLaughlin
Art Director/Media: Freddie Patane
Manufacturing Coordinator: Beth Welsh
Prepress Vendor: Aptara, Inc.

3rd edition

Copyright © 2016 Wolters Kluwer

2nd edition Copyright © 2008 Wolters Kluwer Health/Lippincott Williams & Wilkins. 1st edition Copyright © 1999 Williams & Wilkins. All rights reserved. This book is protected by copyright. No part of this book may be reproduced or transmitted in any form or by any means, including as photocopies or scanned-in or other electronic copies, or utilized by any information storage and retrieval system without written permission from the copyright owner, except for brief quotations embodied in critical articles and reviews. Materials appearing in this book prepared by individuals as part of their official duties as U.S. government employees are not covered by the above-mentioned copyright. To request permission, please contact Wolters Kluwer at Two Commerce Square, 2001 Market Street, Philadelphia, PA 19103, via email at permissions@lww.com, or via our website at lww.com (products and services).

9 8 7 6 5 4 3 2 1

Printed in China

978-1-4511-9447-0
1-45119-447-1
Library of Congress Cataloging-in-Publication Data
available upon request

This work is provided "as is," and the publisher disclaims any and all warranties, express or implied, including any warranties as to accuracy, comprehensiveness, or currency of the content of this work.

This work is no substitute for individual patient assessment based upon healthcare professionals' examination of each patient and consideration of, among other things, age, weight, gender, current or prior medical conditions, medication history, laboratory data and other factors unique to the patient. The publisher does not provide medical advice or guidance and this work is merely a reference tool. Healthcare professionals, and not the publisher, are solely responsible for the use of this work including all medical judgments and for any resulting diagnosis and treatments.

Given continuous, rapid advances in medical science and health information, independent professional verification of medical diagnoses, indications, appropriate pharmaceutical selections and dosages, and treatment options should be made and healthcare professionals should consult a variety of sources. When prescribing medication, healthcare professionals are advised to consult the product information sheet (the manufacturer's package insert) accompanying each drug to verify, among other things, conditions of use, warnings and side effects and identify any changes in dosage schedule or contraindications, particularly if the medication to be administered is new, infrequently used or has a narrow therapeutic range. To the maximum extent permitted under applicable law, no responsibility is assumed by the publisher for any injury and/or damage to persons or property, as a matter of products liability, negligence law or otherwise, or from any reference to or use by any person of this work.

LWW.com

CCS0615

To Our Patients: Past, Present, and Future

RE
6335
U.S.N.12

This third edition of *Walsh and Hoyt's Clinical Neuro-Ophthalmology: The Essentials*, is borne from the same need that motivated the development of its 1st edition 15 years ago—to provide a thorough, yet much more concise complement to the 3-volume sixth edition of the comprehensive parent text, *Walsh and Hoyt's Clinical Neuro-Ophthalmology*. We are encouraged by the extent to which our readers have embraced the first two editions; however, we felt that given the tremendous advances that have occurred over the past decade, it was time for an updated, refined version while preserving its brevity and readability. In particular, we have emphasized the role of modern imaging techniques such as OCT, high resolution CT/MRI, and multifocal ERG in patients with known and presumed neuro-ophthalmologic disorders. Diagrams and tables have been enhanced wherever possible, and the vast majority of photos are now in color. Coverage of complex eye movement disorders has been greatly enriched by the inclusion of videos available online.

In this new edition, we have incorporated new information, both text and illustrations, within the pre-existing organization and content of its predecessors. Five sections—the afferent and efferent visual systems, disorders of the pupil, disorders of the eyelids, and non-organic disorders—provide the framework for 23 chapters. As we recognize that the way in which we acquire information is constantly evolving and that the speed with which information changes also is increasing, we have not included any references but trust that the reader interested in more detailed information will find it online. Nevertheless, we believe that there continues to be a need for knowledge of the fundamentals of neuro-ophthalmology, allowing the reader to integrate more effectively this knowledge with information acquired from the multitude of sources available.

We sincerely hope we have accomplished our goal of enhancing our readers' understanding and appreciation of the fascinating world of neuro-ophthalmology.

CONTENTS

SECTION I   THE AFFERENT VISUAL SYSTEM

1   Examination of the Visual Sensory System 1
2   Anatomy and Physiology of the Retina and Optic Nerve 33
3   Congenital Anomalies of the Optic Disc 61
4   Topical Diagnosis of Acquired Optic Nerve Disorders 91
5   Papilledema 109
6   Optic Neuritis 130
7   Ischemic Optic Neuropathies 145
8   Compressive and Infiltrative Optic Neuropathies 161
9   Traumatic Optic Neuropathies 179
10   Toxic and Deficiency Optic Neuropathies 186
11   Hereditary Optic Neuropathies 195
12   Topical Diagnosis of Optic Chiasmal and Retrochiasmal Lesions . . . 209
13   Central Disorders of Visual Function 242

SECTION II   THE PUPIL

14   Examination of the Pupils and Accommodation 261
15   Disorders of Pupillary Function and Accommodation 271

SECTION III   THE EFFERENT SYSTEM

16   Examination of Ocular Motility and Alignment 299
17   Supranuclear and Internuclear Ocular Motor Disorders 310
18   Nuclear and Infranuclear Ocular Motility Disorders 341
19   Disorders of Neuromuscular Transmission 372
20   Myopathies of Neuro-ophthalmologic Significance 386
21   Nystagmus and Related Ocular Motility Disorders 402

SECTION IV   EYELID

22   Normal and Abnormal Eyelid Function 423

SECTION V   NONORGANIC DISEASE

23   Neuro-Ophthalmologic Manifestations of Nonorganic Disease 451

Appendix: Video List 465
Index 467

Examination of the Visual Sensory System

History
Clinical Office Examination
 Visual Acuity
 Contrast Sensitivity
 Stereoacuity
 Color Vision
 Visual Field Examination
 Pupillary Examination
 Brightness Comparison
 Photostress Recovery Test
 Cranial Nerves, External Examination, Anterior
  Segment Examination, and Exophthalmometry
 Fundus Examination
Ancillary Testing
 Ocular Imaging
 Electrophysiologic Testing

Despite continuous advances in neuroimaging and other new techniques, the examination of the afferent visual sensory system is still the core of the neuro-ophthalmologic examination. This chapter describes the most common subjective and objective testing parameters used in the afferent visual system examination.

Evaluation of the afferent system begins with a thorough medical history, followed by an ophthalmologic examination, including assessment of best-corrected or at least pinhole visual acuity at distance and near, color vision, visual fields, anterior segments (including the media), vitreous, intraocular pressure (IOP), and appearance of the optic discs, retinas (especially the macula), and retinal vessels. At the completion of the examination, one should have an idea as to the structure involved in the patient's visual sensory difficulties or at least have a differential diagnosis. If the diagnosis remains unclear, a number of ancillary tests are available, including ocular imaging and electrophysiologic procedures, that should lead to the correct diagnosis.

History

A thorough history is one of the most important parts of the examination because it determines the initial strategy for differential diagnostic evaluation. For example, it is essential to establish if the visual loss is monocular or binocular; if its location is central, peripheral, altitudinal, or hemianopic; and if the onset of the loss is gradual, sudden, or intermittent.

It also is important to ask about photopsias (visual phenomena such as flashing black squares, flashes of lights, or showers of sparks) distortions in vision (metamorphopsia or micropsia), and positive scotomas. A positive scotoma is one that is seen by the patient, like the purple spot that is often seen after a flash bulb goes off, whereas a negative scotoma refers to a nonseeing area of the visual field. Metamorphopsia, micropsia, and positive scotomas often occur in patients with maculopathies, whereas photopsias may be present in patients with retinal disease, optic nerve dysfunction, or cerebral dysfunction from migraine and other disorders.

Clinical Office Examination

Clinical evaluation of the afferent visual system for each eye incorporates the items described below, all of which can be performed in the office. The first goal for the neuro-ophthalmology examination is to determine if the visual loss is caused by a disorder anterior to the retina (ocular media), in the retina, in the optic nerve, in the optic chiasm, in the retrochiasmal pathways, or is nonorganic. The second goal is to establish a differential and working diagnosis. By examining various parameters of afferent visual function, the examiner frequently can determine the anatomic site of the afferent system abnormality and the most probable cause or causes.

Visual Acuity

The most common measurement of visual function in a clinical setting is visual acuity. It is the primary method of assessing the integrity of the optics of the eye and the neural mechanisms subserving the fovea. Visual acuity is used to monitor central visual function in patients, is an essential part of clinical refraction procedures, and is important to the patient for reading, face recognition, and other tasks involving fine visual detail. Visual acuity is specified in terms of the visual angle subtended by the finest spatial detail that can be identified by the observer. The physical size of an object and its distance from the observer determines its visual angle.

The most common form of reporting visual acuity is the "Snellen notation," consisting of a fraction in which the numerator is the testing distance (20 ft or 6 m) and the denominator is the distance at which

a "normal" observer is able to read the letter. The standard of 20/20 for "normal" vision was developed more than 100 years ago, and with today's high-contrast eye charts and better light sources, most normal persons under the age of 50 can be corrected to better than 20/20.

The measurement of visual acuity in special populations (e.g., young children and physically challenged persons) is not always possible with a standard letter chart (Fig. 1.1). Testing of central visual function of

Figure 1.1 Objects used to test vision. A: An example of a standard eye chart for testing distance visual acuity. B: A "tumbling" E that can be used to assess acuity in children, illiterate individuals, and patients who are cognitively impaired. Note that the E can be turned around, so that it resembles a "W" or an "M." C: Allen cards. These cards, designed by Dr. Henry Allen, can be used to test acuity in children and adults who have not yet learned, do not know, or, for neurologic reasons, have forgotten their letters.

infants begins with an assessment of how well the infant fixes and follows the examiner's face, a small toy, or other objects of interest. For older children, the "Tumbling E Cube" can be used for visual acuity testing. This cube is a white block with black E letters of different sizes on each of its sides. By rotating the cube, an individual E can be presented in four different orientations to test the patient's ability to distinguish the direction of the E. The cube can be placed at various distances from the patient, and different-sized E targets can be evaluated to make a determination of visual acuity. The Tumbling E Cube thus relies on a child's ability to orient the hand according to the direction of the E. For older children, the "E game" can be performed using a projected "E" acuity chart. The "HOTV" test involves matching each test letter to one of four letters (H, O, T, or V) printed on a card held by the child. Some visual acuity tests use pictures or symbols. These may be more reliable than the HOTV test. The most popular of the picture visual acuity tests are the Allen Cards that are available as hand-held picture cards or projected images. The objects include an easily identifiable birthday cake, a bird, a house, and a car (although one older card has a picture of a rotary telephone that most children have never seen!).

"Preferential-looking" techniques, ocular motor responses such as optokinetic nystagmus, and electrophysiologic measures such as the visual-evoked potential (VEP) can be used to estimate visual acuity (see below). In addition, a number of eye charts and behavior test procedures can be used to assess visual acuity in nonverbal or physically challenged patients.

Visual acuity measurements in children present special problems, in part because the child wants to do well and please the examiner. It is therefore important for the examiner to ensure that the nontested eye is properly occluded to avoid peeking. The examiner must work quickly, may need to use more than one procedure to establish visual acuity capabilities, and should provide continuous positive feedback to the child to maintain cooperation.

In patients suspected of having nonorganic visual loss, several additional methods of assessing visual acuity may be useful. These are discussed in Chapter 23.

In normal observers, visual acuity is highest for the foveal region and decreases rapidly with increasing visual field eccentricity. In many instances, central visual field loss and reduced visual acuity appear to be closely related; however, visual acuity can also be reduced when there is generalized depression of the central visual field. In such instances, a central scotoma is not present. There also are several conditions for which the visual field may be at or near normal sensitivity, but visual acuity may be dramatically reduced. These conditions include refractive errors,

corneal surface irregularities, cataract, retinal edema or serous detachment, and amblyopia.

Contrast Sensitivity

Visual acuity defines the smallest spatial detail that can be resolved for high-contrast stimuli, but it does not specify the responses of the visual system to objects of different sizes and contrasts. However, one also can assess afferent visual function by looking at the behavior of the visual system at **threshold** contrast levels.

A number of factors influence the measurement of contrast sensitivity, including background adaptation luminance, stimulus size, visual field eccentricity, pupil size, temporal characteristics, stimulus orientation, and various optical factors such as defocus, dioptric blur, diffusive blur, and astigmatism. From a neuro-ophthalmologic standpoint, measurement of contrast sensitivity can reveal subtle deficits in patients with a variety of optic neuropathies as well as in other neurologic conditions such as Alzheimer disease and Parkinson disease.

In general, assessment of contrast sensitivity is clinically useful for detecting early or subtle visual loss (especially when visual acuity is normal), making comparisons between the two eyes, and for monitoring the progression of or improvement in visual function. Assessing contrast sensitivity also may be helpful in predicting the performance for various daily tasks, such as the identification of distant objects, reading highway signs and books, recognizing faces, and mobility. Thus, it may be useful not only for revealing subtle visual deficits associated with ocular and neuro-ophthalmologic disorders but also for identifying problems that a patient is likely to encounter during daily activities.

Contrast sensitivity may be measured in several different ways. One method is the Pelli–Robson chart (Fig. 1.2), consisting of letters of a fixed size that vary in contrast. Each line consists of six letters, with the three left-most and three right-most letters having the same amount of contrast. The patient reads the chart in a manner similar to a standard visual acuity chart, and the minimum contrast at which the letters can be detected is recorded. This method of testing contrast sensitivity is highly reproducible and is capable of detecting disturbances in visual function that are not evident with standard visual acuity testing.

Contrast sensitivity can also be measured with Low-Contrast Sloan Letter Charts. These charts have gray letters of progressively smaller size on a white background (Fig. 1.3); each chart in the set corresponds to a different level of contrast, ranging from high (100%, about the same contrast as standard visual acuity charts) to medium (5%) to low (1.25%, 0.6%) contrast levels. Patients are asked to read each of the four charts at 2 m distance under consistent lighting while wearing their

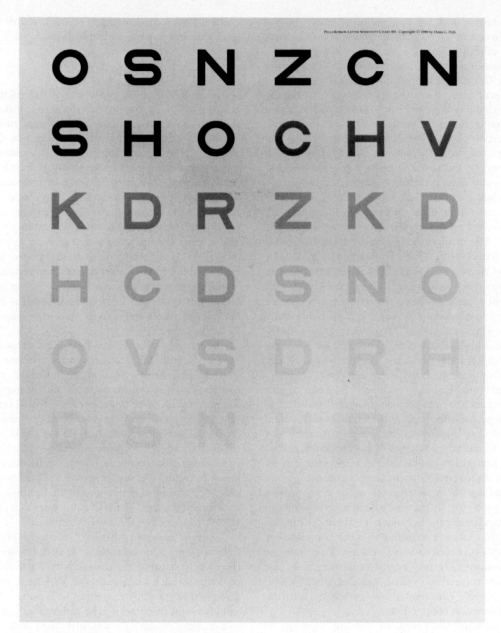

Figure 1.2 The Pelli–Robson contrast sensitivity chart.

usual distance refractive correction. The charts are readily available and provide a practical, quantitative, and standardized method of visual function assessment. They have proven particularly useful in identifying subtle visual dysfunction in patients with a history of recovered optic neuritis as well as in patients with multiple sclerosis but without any other evidence of optic nerve dysfunction.

Stereoacuity

Stereoacuity requires good visual acuity in both eyes and normal cortical development. As such, stereoacuity can be helpful in establishing if a patient has visual loss from congenital amblyopia or monofixation syndrome, as well as verifying the extent of any monocular visual acuity loss. Using the Titmus or Randot Stereo Testers, stereoacuity in normal observers with good binocular function and visual acuity should be at least 40 seconds of arc or better when both eyes have 20/20 visual acuity.

Color Vision

From a clinical diagnostic standpoint, it is important to distinguish if a color vision deficiency is congenital

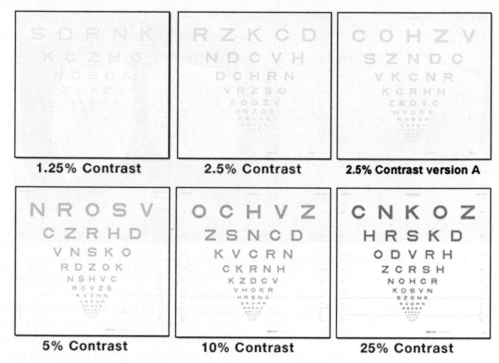

Figure 1.3 Sloan low-contrast letters. Note varying amounts of contrast.

or acquired. Congenital color vision deficits usually are easy to classify using standard clinical color vision tests because color discrimination is impaired for a specific region of the visual spectrum, and the deficits are long-standing, stable, symmetric in the two eyes, and unassociated with other visual symptoms or complaints. In patients with acquired color vision loss, however, color discrimination may be impaired throughout the visual spectrum or along a specific axis, and the deficits may be mild or severe, of sudden or insidious onset, symmetric or asymmetric, and often associated with other visual symptoms or complaints. In acquired color vision deficiencies, tritan (blue) and blue-yellow deficiencies most often are associated with diseases affecting the photoreceptors and the outer plexiform layer, whereas red-green deficiencies most often are associated with diseases affecting the optic nerve and posterior visual pathways. Some notable exceptions include glaucoma, dominant hereditary optic atrophy, and chronic papilledema, that may demonstrate blue-yellow deficits, and Stargardt and Best disease, that often produce red-green deficits. Optic neuritis produces a mixture of red-green and blue-yellow deficits, although one axis is usually more affected than the other.

A wide variety of color vision tests are available to the clinician. Because most were designed to evaluate congenital red-green color vision deficiencies, many do not permit adequate testing of blue-yellow deficits

or optimum characterization of acquired color vision losses. As with any test of visual function, it is important that the testing conditions be standardized and performed in the proper manner. A particularly important factor for all clinical color vision test procedures is the use of proper lighting, both in terms of having an adequate amount of light for the test and having a light source with the proper spectral distribution.

Pseudoisochromatic Plates

Pseudoisochromatic plates are the most common color vision tests employed in clinical practice. A number of pseudoisochromatic plate tests are available, although the Ishihara and Hardy–Rand–Rittler are the most commonly used versions (Fig. 1.4). Each of these tests consists of a series of plates that contain colored dots of varying size and brightness. The tests are designed, so that persons with normal color vision see numbers, shapes, or letters as a consequence of grouping certain colored dots together to form a figure against the background of other dots. Depending on how the particular test is designed, persons with color deficiencies are either unable to see the figure because the figure dots are confused with the background dots, or they see a figure different from that seen by persons with normal color vision because figure dots and background dots are grouped together in an abnormal pattern. The variation in size and brightness of the dots is used to ensure that recognition of

Figure 1.4 Appearance of figures on the Hardy–Rand–Rittler and Ishihara pseudoisochromatic color plates.

figures is made on the basis of color discrimination and not other cues. Even children who are shy or do not know their colors may be able to trace the shapes. Other variations of pseudoisochromatic plates include winding paths of colored dots that the patient can trace. These are useful in young children, illiterates, and some neurologically ill patients who are unable to identify letters, numbers, or shapes.

Color vision testing using pseudoisochromatic plates is quick and easy to perform and therefore can be an excellent screening procedure for distinguishing normal color vision from congenital or acquired color vision deficits.

Farnsworth Panel D-15 Test

The Farnsworth Panel D-15 test is a color arrangement test consisting of 15 color caps that form a color circle covering the visual spectrum. A reference cap is permanently fixed in the arrangement tray; the other 15 caps are placed in a scrambled order in front of the patient. The patient's task is to select the cap that is closest in hue to the reference cap and place it next to the reference cap in the tray. The patient is then asked to continue to place the caps in the tray, one at a time, so that they are arranged in an orderly transition of hue. Patients with moderate to severe protan, deutan, or tritan color vision deficits will confuse colors across the color circle, so that the arrangement contains misplaced caps. On the back of each cap is a number to assist in scoring the test. On the D-15 scoring chart, the caps along the color circle are connected in a dot-to-dot fashion in the order represented in the tray, and the specific arrangement indicates the type of color deficiency. The Panel D-15 test does not indicate the degree of color deficiency, other than to separate color normals and mild anomalous trichromats from those with moderate to severe color vision deficiencies.

Farnsworth–Munsell 100 Hues Test

The Farnsworth–Munsell 100 Hues test permits both classification of the type of color vision deficiency and its severity. Despite its name, it consists of **85** colored caps that are arranged in roughly equal small steps around the color circle. The caps are divided into four boxes, and arrangements of caps are performed one box at a time. In each box, there are two reference caps, one at each end, that are permanently attached to the box. The other caps are taken out of the box, scrambled, and placed before the patient. The patient is then asked to arrange the caps, so that there is an orderly transition in hue from one reference cap to another. As with the panel D-15 test, the Farnsworth–Munsell 100 Hues test is designed, so that certain caps across the color circle will be confused by persons with both congenital and acquired color deficiencies. The caps are numbered on the back, and scoring is determined by the arrangement of the caps in the box. Depending on the type of color deficiency, specific caps across the color circle will be confused, resulting in greater arrangement errors in those locations. In this manner, the type of color vision deficit can be classified. In addition, the severity of the color deficiency can be quantified by determining an overall error score for arrangement errors. This test is rarely used in clinical practice.

Color comparison tests, although only qualitative in nature, can provide valuable information concerning subtle visual anomalies. In general, the best color to compare is red. Using pages from the pseudoisochromatic plates, red-colored bottle caps, or other brightly colored objects, comparisons of color appearance can be very effective in detecting subtle differences between the two eyes. The brightness or saturation of the colored objects may be less in one eye, making the object's color appear dim or washed out. Similarly, comparisons

Figure 1.5 Method of testing the visual field using a red test object. This method can be used to detect a subtle central or paracentral scotoma or hemianopia.

within the same eye across the vertical and horizontal midline or between central vision and the mid-periphery can detect subtle differences in color appearance that are indicative of damage to the visual pathways. For example, red may appear pink, orange or brown or the color may disappear completely (Fig. 1.5).

Visual Field Examination

Examination of the visual field is one of the fundamental portions of the afferent system evaluation. A variety of visual field test procedures can be employed, including confrontation, the Amsler grid, kinetic perimetry, and static perimetry. When evaluating a patient with an afferent system deficit, it is important to keep in mind the advantages and disadvantages of the various procedures.

General Principles

Perimetry and visual field testing have been clinical diagnostic test procedures for more than 150 years. Although instrumentation and testing strategies have changed dramatically over this time, the basic principle underlying conventional perimetry has remained the same. Detection sensitivity is determined for a number of locations throughout the visual field using a small target presented against a uniform background. The loss of sensitivity at various visual field locations serves as a noninvasive marker for identifying pathology or dysfunction of the visual pathways. The ability of perimetry to provide helpful clinical information has been responsible for its long-term use as a diagnostic procedure. Because perimetry can provide information about both the likely anatomic locus and disease process or processes for afferent system abnormalities, it remains a vital part of the neuro-ophthalmologic evaluation.

Perimetry and visual field testing fulfill several important diagnostic functions:

1 **Early detection of abnormalities.** Because many ocular and neurologic disorders initially are expressed as sensitivity loss in the peripheral visual field, perimetry is an important factor in identifying early signs of afferent system dysfunction. Perimetry is typically the only clinical procedure that evaluates the status of the afferent visual pathways for locations outside the macular region.
2 **Differential diagnosis.** The spatial pattern of visual field deficits and comparison of patterns of visual field loss between the two eyes also provide valuable differential diagnostic information. Not only can this information be helpful in defining the location of damage along the visual pathways, it also can assist in identifying the specific type of disease that has caused the damage.
3 **Monitoring progression and remission.** The ability to monitor a patient's visual field over time is important for verifying a working diagnosis, establishing if a condition is stable or progressive, and evaluating the effectiveness of therapeutic interventions.
4 **Revealing hidden visual loss.** Perhaps the most important role served by perimetry is the ability to detect afferent visual pathway loss that may not be apparent to the patient. Changes in central visual function typically are symptomatic. Peripheral vision loss, on the other hand, can often go unnoticed, especially if it is gradual and monocular. Paradoxically, even though a patient may be unaware of peripheral visual field loss, it can significantly affect the performance of daily activities such as driving, orientation, and mobility.

Some form of visual field testing should be performed on all patients, regardless of their presenting visual symptoms. It is not feasible nor is it necessary to perform a long quantitative visual field examination on all patients; however, a confrontation visual field should be performed as part of a standard neuro-ophthalmologic examination. When more sensitive measurements of the visual field are needed, automated static or manual kinetic perimetry can be performed.

Manual kinetic perimetry with the Goldmann perimeter has many advantages. As the perimetric stimulus presentation is done by a human, subjects can be cajoled into performing. When the perimetrist senses subject fatigue, he or she can provide a rest break. Unlike the fixed, 6-degree spaced grid of conventional automated perimetry, perimetry using the Goldmann or a similar apparatus allows for custom test point locations along with improvisation of strategies based on coexisting findings. Specific exploration strategies can be used for individual concerns. This allows for much more accurate mapping of defect shape and can be invaluable for the topographic localization of visual field defects. However, manual perimetry is less sensitive than conventional automated perimetry and it may be more time-consuming. Its most severe limitations, though, are that replacement parts for the perimeter are increasingly difficult to find and, even more importantly, many technicians are adequately trained (or not trained at all) in the performance of manual, kinetic perimetry.

Automated static perimetry has had a dramatic impact on improving the quality of care for patients with ocular disorders. Automatic calibration of instruments, standardized test procedures, high sensitivity and specificity, reliability checks ("catch trials"), and quantitative statistical analysis procedures are some of the many advantages of this method of perimetry. However, there are also disadvantages of automated perimetry, including prolonged test time, increased cognitive demands, fatigue, and lack of flexibility for evaluating difficult patient populations. We believe that there is no single method of visual field testing that is best for all circumstances and all patients. Automated perimetry is but one of many tools that the clinician can use to evaluate peripheral visual function, and the various forms of visual field testing should be regarded as **complementary** techniques, the utility and appropriateness of which are determined by the clinical circumstances and the question that is being addressed. There is no single method of data representation, analysis procedure, visual field index, or other method of evaluating visual field data that provides all of the essential clinical information. It is important to consider all of the information available, including reliability characteristics and the subjective clinical interpretation of the visual field. In addition, it should be kept in mind that although the test may be automated, the patient is not. It is inappropriate to begin an automated visual field test, leave a patient alone in a dark room, and expect the patient to remain alert, energetic, attentive, interested, and to maintain proper alignment and fixation throughout the test procedure. Some patients require periodic rest breaks, encouragement, and personal contact to perform visual field examinations in a reliable manner. It also is important to insure that proper test conditions, refractive characteristics, and other factors have been properly established before initiating the examination.

Specific Techniques for Testing Visual Fields

Confrontation Testing. Confrontation visual fields usually are performed with the patient seated in the examination chair and the examiner seated facing the patient at a distance of 2 to 3 ft. One of the patient's eyes is occluded using the palm of the patient's hand, an occluder paddle, or a patch, and the patient is asked to fixate with the uncovered eye on the examiner's nose

Figure 1.6 Method of testing the visual field by having the patient count fingers in the upper left, upper right, left, right, lower left, and lower right regions of each field.

or opposite eye. A variety of stimuli can be employed for confrontation visual fields (Fig. 1.6). The basic intent is to use a small, localized target, the presence or absence of which in the visual field can be readily determined by the patient. A confrontation visual field should include an examination of each of the four visual field quadrants, including the superior and inferior hemifields along the horizontal midline, the nasal and temporal hemifields along the vertical midline, and the central and peripheral visual field. Most examiners test patients using double simultaneous finger counting to survey the visual field for any dense quadrantic defect, although some authors recommend finger wiggling instead of counting. Finger counting or wiggling should be followed by a test of the central field. One such test, as noted above, is to use a red object and compare color perception between the two eyes or between parts of the visual field in each eye (Fig. 1.5). By combining several confrontation visual field tests, about 70% of neurologic field defects can be identified. Thus, formal perimetry usually is necessary when the patient has visual loss not explained by a general ophthalmologic examination.

Confrontation visual field techniques for infants and children can be quite challenging (Fig. 1.7). For infants and young children, simply holding up one hand and observing whether or not the child looks at it is the best one can do. Another option is to hold both hands up on either side of the child's fixation and then wave one or wiggle a finger and see if the child looks at the moving hand/finger. For older children, finger mimicking can be used to evaluate the peripheral visual field. The child mimics the examiner by holding up the same number of fingers he or she observes.

In many instances, simultaneous comparison of color saturation or brightness of stimuli between hemifields or between the two eyes is useful in distinguishing subtle anomalies. When the stimuli are presented in a

A

B

C

Figure 1.7 Examples of confrontation visual field testing in children. **A:** Startle response. **B:** Finger counting. **C:** Finger puppets.

double simultaneous fashion to the right and left of fixation, it is possible to detect homonymous defects. Subtle deficits across the vertical midline can be detected by asking the patient to indicate which of the two test objects is clearer or brighter. In addition, double simultaneous presentation can be used to detect the phenomenon of visual extinction—the lack of awareness of an object in a seeing area of the visual field when other seeing areas of the visual field are stimulated simultaneously.

The obvious advantages of confrontation visual field testing include its simplicity, flexibility, speed of administration, and ability to be performed in any setting, including at the bedside. The disadvantages of confrontation visual field testing include the

lack of standardization, the qualitative nature of the results, and the limited ability to detect subtle deficits and monitor progression or remission of visual loss. Because it is quick and easy to perform, confrontation visual field should be performed on all patients, regardless of their visual complaints.

Amsler Grid. Amsler grids are a series of charts, specifically designed to qualitatively analyze the disturbances of visual function which accompany the beginning and evolution of maculopathies. The charts are a series of lined and patterned grids that test the central visual field within 10 degrees of fixation when the plates are held at one-third of a meter from the eyes. Each square of the grid subtends 1 degree of visual angle, making the ability to define the location of small defects rather easy. The patient is asked to fixate a central spot on the grid, using one eye at a time, and is asked if he or she can see the spot. If not, the patient's finger can be placed on the center to help fixation. The patient is then asked to point out any regions in which the lines are missing, blurred, distorted, bent, or irregular.

This technique is well known to ophthalmologists who routinely examine patients with known or suspected macular disease because Amsler grids can be used to detect metamorphopsia or identify and plot small scotomas and other visual field defects that occur with macular scars, mild macular degeneration, central serous chorioretinopathy, and related disorders. It is perhaps less well recognized that small central or paracentral scotomas that occur with optic nerve disease also can be identified with the Amsler grid (Fig. 1.8). Indeed, the grid is particularly useful for identifying small central scotomas and other subtle central visual disturbances that are difficult to detect with more sophisticated automated and manual perimeters. Its main disadvantages are related to the qualitative, subjective nature of the information derived from the test.

The Amsler grid is quick and easy to administer. The patient is instructed to look at the central dot and asked if, in fact, he/she can see it. If not, the patient may have a central scotoma, and the examiner must query the patient regarding exactly what he/she DOES see. If the patient sees the dot, the examiner asks if the patient is aware that surrounding it are numerous squares. The examiner then asks the patient if any of the squares are distorted, missing, etc. The patient is then given a pen or pencil and asked to draw any areas of disturbance directly on the grid.

Static Perimetry. Static perimetry uses a stationary target, the luminance of which is adjusted to vary its visibility. It most often is performed with an automated perimeter such as the Humphrey Field Analyzer or the Octopus perimeter, with the former being by far the most widely used instrument. Measurements of

Figure 1.8 Amsler grid defects. **A:** Metamorphopsia and paracentral scotomas in a patient with a maculopathy. **B:** A small central scotoma in a patient with optic neuritis.

the increment threshold are obtained at a variety of visual field locations that usually are arranged in a grid pattern or along meridians (Fig. 1.9).

The amount of time required for static perimetry depends on several factors, including patient alertness and cooperation, the threshold strategy used, and the size of the field being tested. For example, using the Humphrey Field Analyzer, a full-threshold test usually takes about 10 to 12 minutes per eye, whereas use of the Swedish interactive threshold algorithm (SITA) that

Figure 1.9 Static perimetry using a Humphrey visual field analyzer. **A:** Full field using a 24-2 threshold test and SITA-Standard strategy. **B:** Tiny central scotoma in a different patient identified using a 10-2 threshold test and SITA-Standard strategy. This field defect would not have been identified using a 24-2 threshold test.

employs thresholds that are 1 to 2 dB higher than the full-threshold method results in a 50% (SITA-Standard strategy) to 70% (SITA-Fast) reduction in test time (about 4 to 6 minutes for SITA-Standard and 3 to 4 minutes for SITA-Fast). The shortening of test time is likely the result of a combination of less patient fatigue and interruption of the staircase procedure before threshold is reached. As far as the size of the field tested, most neuro-ophthalmologists use a 24-2 test, meaning that the central 24 degrees is tested superiorly, inferiorly, and temporally (the nasal field is tested out to 30 degrees because the developer of the program, Anders Heijl, wanted to be sure that the test captured early nasal steps!) (Fig. 1.9A), whereas others prefer a 30-2 test in which the entire field is tested out to 30 degrees. For patients whose history suggests one or more small central or paracentral defects, a 10-2 (i.e., 10 degree) field test is available (Fig. 1.9B).

Kinetic Perimetry. The Goldmann perimeter is a white hemispheric bowl of uniform luminance (31.5 asb) onto which a small bright stimulus is projected. It generally is used to perform kinetic perimetry, although static and suprathreshold static perimetry can also be tested with this perimeter. Unlike the Amsler grid and most automated perimeters, the Goldmann perimeter can be used to evaluate the entire visual field and is particularly useful when there is an extensive or a peripheral defect (Fig. 1.10). With one eye occluded, the patient fixates a small target in the center of the bowl with the uncovered eye, and the perimetrist monitors eye position by means of a telescope. A particular stimulus size and luminance is projected onto the bowl, the target is moved from the far periphery toward fixation at a constant rate of speed, typically 4 to 5 degrees per second, and the patient is instructed to press a response button when he/she first detects the stimulus. The location of target detection is noted on a chart, and the process is repeated for different meridians around the visual field. Isopters and scotomas are plotted in a manner similar to that described for the tangent screen examination, except that both the target size and luminance

Figure 1.10 Kinetic perimetry using a Goldmann perimeter. **A:** Full visual field. **B:** Large central scotoma associated with a full peripheral field. Static perimetry using a 10-2, 24-2, or 30-2 threshold would provide no useful information as the entire field would be absent. **C:** Far peripheral scotoma. Static perimetry using a 10-2, 24-2, or 30-2 threshold would not identify this scotoma as it is too far peripherally. **D:** Partial sparing of the temporal peripheral field (the temporal crescent) in a patient with a left inferior homonymous quadrantic defect (only the field of the left eye is shown). Static perimetry would not have shown the area of spared peripheral field.

Figure 1.11 Influences on visual field test results. **A:** An example of visual field results for ptosis before (**left**) and after (**right**) taping up the upper lid and brow. **B:** Example of trial lens rim artifact (**left**) and its disappearance (**right**) after realigning the patient. **C:** Refractive error introduced by improper lens correction (**left**) and results after proper lens was employed (**right**). **D:** Visual field results obtained in the same eye with a 1-mm (**left**) and a 3-mm (**right**) pupil diameter.

can be adjusted to vary stimulus detectability. This process produces a two-dimensional representation of the hill of vision that is basically a topographical contour map of the eye's sensitivity to light. Kinetic testing (at least 1 or 2 isopters) on the Goldmann perimeter can be performed in cooperative children as young as 5 or 6 years of age.

Interpretation of Automated Visual Field Information

A large amount of visual field information is derived from perimetric testing, especially from automated perimetry. Test conditions and stimulus parameters used, indicators of patient reliability and cooperation, physiologic factors (pupil size, refractive state, visual acuity, etc.), summary statistics and visual field indices, and other items are presented in conjunction with sensitivity values for various locations in the patient's visual field. Visual field sensitivity can also be represented in many different forms (numerical values, deviations from normal, gray scale representations, probability plots, etc.). The following discussion presents a brief overview of the various types of information provided on the final printed outputs. Because of its current popularity and widespread use, this discussion and most of the examples are derived from automated static perimetry using the Humphrey machine; however, some examples of kinetic testing using the Goldmann perimeter are presented for certain clinical cases, especially for situations in which kinetic testing provides more information about visual field status.

Several important pieces of information that should be checked on each visual field examination are the position of the eyelids, the refractive correction used for testing, pupil size, and visual acuity. Ptosis can produce a superior visual field defect that may be minimal or significant (Fig. 1.11A). High refractive corrections (greater than 6-diopter spherical equivalent) can sometimes produce trial lens rim artifacts (Fig. 1.11B). When a patient's spherical equivalent correction for perimetric testing exceeds 6 diopters, it is advisable to use a soft contact lens correction that is appropriate for the testing distance to avoid lens rim artifacts. Proper near refractive corrections that are appropriate for the near testing distance of the perimeter bowl and the patient's age must be used to minimize the likelihood of refraction scotomas and sensitivity reductions from blur (Fig. 1.11C). Small pupils (less than 2 mm diameter) can produce spurious test results, especially in older persons who may have early lenticular changes. If pupil size is small, the patient should be dilated to 3 mm or greater (Fig. 1.11D). Finally, the patient's visual acuity also can provide useful information when assessing generalized visual field sensitivity loss and the potential sources responsible for the loss.

Reliability Indices. The quality of information obtained from perimetry and visual field testing depends on a patient's cooperation, willingness, and ability to respond in a reliable fashion and maintain a consistent response criterion. It is important to have an assessment of patient reliability and consistency to properly evaluate the significance of visual field information. With manual perimetry, it is possible to monitor the patient's fixation behavior directly by means of a telescopic viewer. False-positive errors (responses when no stimulus is presented) and false-negative errors (failure to respond to a stimulus presented in a region previously determined to be able to detect equal or less detectable targets) can be monitored throughout the test procedure.

Automated test procedures not only have the capability of monitoring false-positive errors, false-negative errors, and fixation behavior in the same manner as described above but also can assess response fluctuation by retesting a sample of visual field locations. Also, indirect indicators of fixation accuracy (e.g., whether or not a patient responds to a target presented to the physiologic blind spot) can be monitored. An additional advantage of automated test procedures is that these **reliability indices** (false positives, false negatives, fixation losses, short-term fluctuations) can be immediately compared with those of age-adjusted normal control subjects, thereby providing an indication as to whether or not the patient's reliability parameters are within normal population characteristics (Fig. 1.12).

Some of the reliability indices for automated perimetry are not always accurate indicators of a patient's true performance. For example, false-negative rates are correlated with visual field deficits, that is, there is an increase in false-negative responses with increased field loss. Thus, high false-negative rates may be more indicative of disease severity than of unreliable patient responses. Excessive fixation losses can be caused by factors such as mislocalization of the blind spot during the initial phases of testing, misalignment or head tilt of the patient midway through testing, or inattention on the part of the technician administering the visual field examination. Also, one should be careful not to consider reliability indices as a replacement for technician interaction and monitoring of patients. Some patients are uncomfortable when left alone in a darkened room during automated perimetry testing. In addition, misalignment of the patient, drowsiness, and related factors can occur during testing and go undetected if the patient is not adequately monitored. As has been emphasized above, it is important to remember that it is the test procedure that is automated, not the patient.

Although reliability indices are helpful in determining if the visual field is accurate, they are not sufficient

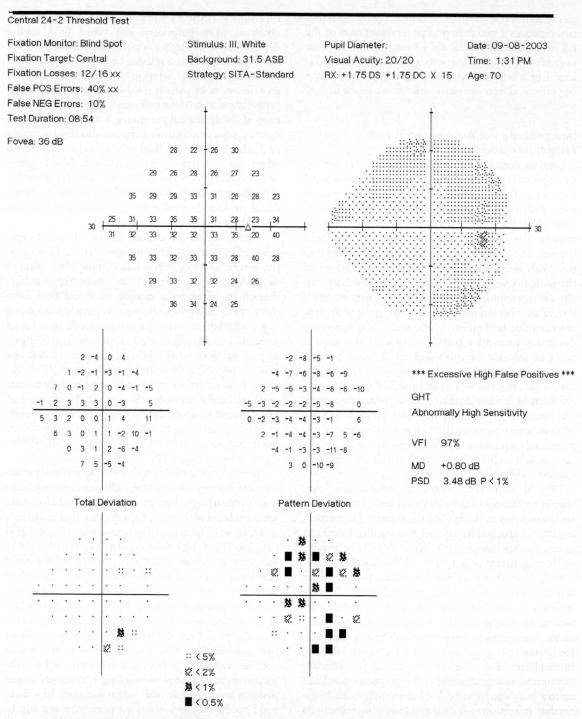

Central 24-2 Threshold Test

Fixation Monitor: Blind Spot

Fixation Target: Central

Fixation Losses: 12/16 xx

False POS Errors: 40% xx

False NEG Errors: 10%

Test Duration: 08:54

Fovea: 36 dB

Stimulus: III, White

Background: 31.5 ASB

Strategy: SITA-Standard

Pupil Diameter:

Visual Acuity: 20/20

RX: +1.75 DS +1.75 DC X 15

Date: 09-08-2003

Time: 1:31 PM

Age: 70

Total Deviation

Pattern Deviation

*** Excessive High False Positives ***

GHT

Abnormally High Sensitivity

VFI   97%

MD   +0.80 dB

PSD   3.48 dB P < 1%

:: < 5%

▨ < 2%

▨ < 1%

■ < 0.5%

Figure 1.12 Markedly abnormal reliability indices in a patient on whom static perimetry was attempted using a Humphrey Visual Field Analyzer. Note that the patient has multiple fixation losses, false-positive responses, and false-negative responses. When faced with this issue, the physician must decide whether to repeat the field at another time in the hope that the problems were because the patient had never undergone field testing before, use a different strategy that takes less time (e.g., SITA-Fast instead of SITA-Standard), or abandon this technique and use another, such as confrontation testing or kinetic perimetry.

to eliminate the possibility that a visual field defect is nonorganic in nature. It has been shown that both patients and otherwise normal subjects can "fool" the automated perimeter, producing a variety of abnormal fields despite maintaining reliability indices that are within normal limits.

Visual Field Indices. A distinct advantage afforded by automated perimeters is the ability to provide summary statistics, usually called **visual field indices.** The Mean Deviation (MD) on the Humphrey Field Analyzer refers to the average deviation of sensitivity at each test location from age-adjusted normal population values. They provide an indication of the degree of generalized or widespread loss in the visual field. The Pattern Standard Deviation (PSD) on the Humphrey Field Analyzer presents a summary measure of the average deviation of individual visual field sensitivity values from the normal slope after correcting for any overall sensitivity differences, that is, the MD. It represents the degree of irregularity of visual field sensitivity about the normal slope and therefore indicates the amount of localized visual field loss because scotomas produce significant departures from the normal slope of the visual field.

Probability Plots. Although automated perimeters provide a general assessment of the visual field by showing increasingly dark areas correlating with decreasing sensitivity (the gray scale) (Fig. 1.13), a major advantage of automated static perimetry is that a patient's test results are compared with age-adjusted normal population values. Thus, it is possible to determine the amount of deviation from normal population sensitivity values on a point-by-point basis for all visual field locations tested. A useful means of expressing this information is by means of **probability plots.** The Humphrey Field Analyzer has two methods of presenting this type of information. One is called the "Total Deviation Plot" and the other is called the "Pattern Deviation Plot." For the Total Deviation Plot, each visual field location has one of a group of different symbols indicating whether the sensitivity is within normal limits, or is below the 5%, 2%, 1%, or 0.5% of normal limits, respectively. In other words, visual field locations or indices that have a probability corresponding to *p* less than 1% means that this value is observed less than 1% of the time in a normal population of the same age. This provides an immediate graphic representation of the locations that are abnormal and the degree to which they vary from normal levels.

The Pattern Deviation Plot is similar to the Total Deviation Plot, except that the determinations are performed after the average or overall sensitivity loss has been subtracted, thereby revealing specific

locations with **localized** deviations from normal sensitivity values. The value of these representations is twofold. First, they provide an immediate indication of the locations with sensitivity loss. Second, the comparison of the Total and Pattern Deviation Plots provides a clear indication of the degree to which the loss is diffuse or localized. If the loss is predominantly diffuse, the abnormal locations will appear on the Total Deviation Plot, but all or most of these locations will be within normal limits on the Pattern Deviation Plot (Fig. 1.14A). If the deficit is predominantly localized, the Total and Pattern Deviation Plots will look almost identical (Fig. 1.14B). The degree of similarity between the Total and Pattern Deviation Plots thus gives an indication of the proportion of loss that is diffuse and localized. In some instances, the Total Deviation Plot may appear to be normal, but the Pattern Deviation Plot reveals a number of abnormal locations. This occurs when the patient's measured sensitivity is better than normal (Fig. 1.14C) or when the patient presses the response button too often ("trigger happy") (Fig. 1.14D). In general, the Pattern Deviation Plot is the most important diagram to view when assessing the results of automated field testing as it will often show subtle areas of abnormality that may not be apparent on the gray scale or may be hidden by general loss of sensitivity shown in the Total Deviation Plot.

Progression of Visual Field Loss. The determination of whether a patient's visual field improves, worsens, or remains stable over time is the most difficult aspect of visual field interpretation. Although there are several quantitative analysis procedures available for evaluating visual field progression, none of them enjoys complete acceptance by the clinical ophthalmic community. Nevertheless, the use of quantitative statistical analysis procedures may be helpful in monitoring a patient's visual field status.

There are several important factors to consider when evaluating a patient's visual field status over time. First, it is necessary to examine the test conditions that were present for each visual field examination. If different test strategies, target sizes, or other test conditions are different from one examination to another, it is difficult to compare the results because the type of test procedure and the stimulus size (and characteristics) can significantly alter the appearance of the visual field. Second, it is important to determine if there are any differences in patient conditions from one visual field to another. As noted above, if there are meaningful differences in pupil size, refractive corrections, visual acuity, time of day, or other factors (e.g., upper lid taped on one occasion and not on another occasion), this can have a dramatic effect

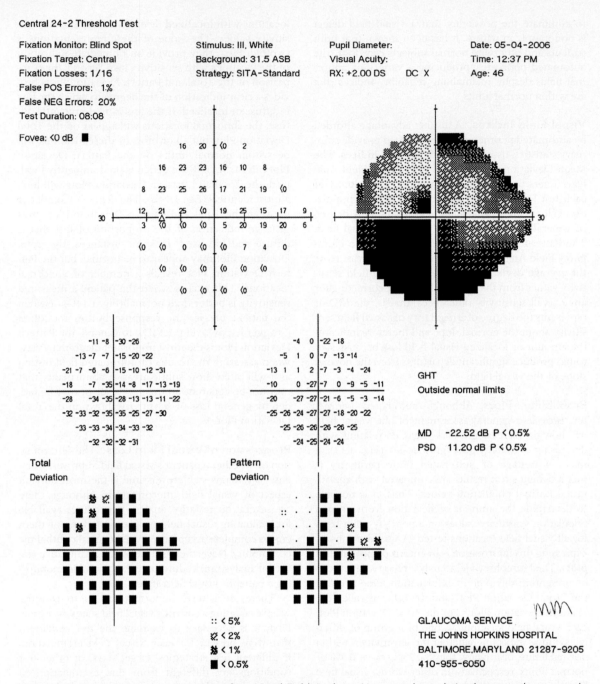

Central 24-2 Threshold Test

Fixation Monitor: Blind Spot	Stimulus: III, White
Fixation Target: Central	Background: 31.5 ASB
Fixation Losses: 1/16	Strategy: SITA-Standard
False POS Errors: 1%	
False NEG Errors: 20%	
Test Duration: 08:08	

Pupil Diameter:
Visual Acuity:
RX: +2.00 DS   DC X

Date: 05-04-2006
Time: 12:37 PM
Age: 46

Fovea: <0 dB ■

GHT
Outside normal limits

MD   -22.52 dB P < 0.5%
PSD   11.20 dB P < 0.5%

Total Deviation

Pattern Deviation

:: < 5%
✵ < 2%
✻ < 1%
■ < 0.5%

GLAUCOMA SERVICE
THE JOHNS HOPKINS HOSPITAL
BALTIMORE, MARYLAND 21287-9205
410-955-6050

Figure 1.13 Static perimetry using a Humphrey Visual Field Analyzer. Note good correlation between the gray scale (**above right**) and the Pattern Deviation Plot (**lower right**).

on the visual field results obtained on different visits (Fig. 1.11). Third, unless the visual field changes are dramatic, it is important to base judgments of visual field progression or stability on the basis of the entire series of visual fields that are available. It is not possible to distinguish subtle visual field changes from long-term variation on the basis of two visual fields

(e.g., comparing the current visual field to the previous visual field). In particular, patients with moderate to advanced visual field loss can sometimes exhibit considerable variations from one visual field to another. Also, factors such as fatigue and experience can produce significant differences in visual field characteristics. If it is suspected that a change in visual field

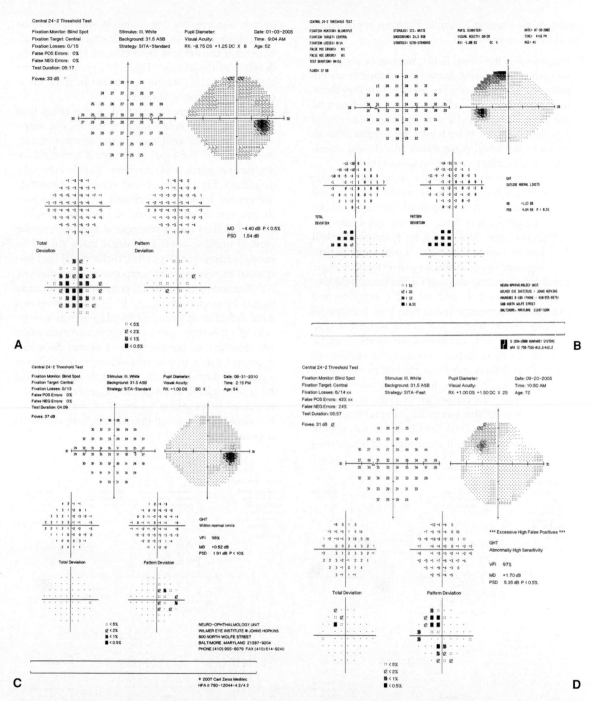

Figure 1.14 Pattern results as they are depicted on the gray scales, Total Deviation Plots, and Pattern Deviation Plots. **A:** Diffuse loss; **B:** Dense localized loss; **C:** Very mild localized loss; **D:** "Trigger happy" patient.

loss has occurred, it is best to repeat the examination on a separate visit to confirm the suspected change. Depending on which part of the sequence and which eye is examined, any two successive visual fields can reflect apparent improvement, progression, or stability of the visual field (Fig. 1.15).

Five-Step Approach to Visual Field Interpretation

One of the common errors that occur in visual field interpretation is the lack of attention to details and specific patterns of visual field loss before obtaining a global evaluation of the visual field. To avoid this tendency, we suggest a simple five-step approach to visual field interpretation:

1 Determine if the visual field is normal or abnormal for each eye separately. Automated perimetry results provide assistance with this task, because they show both point-by-point and summary comparisons of the patient's test results with age-matched normal population values. If both eyes are normal, both in terms of statistical comparison and clinical assessment, then further evaluation is unnecessary.

2 If one or both visual fields are abnormal, examine the ancillary information to determine if proper test conditions were employed, the appropriate near correction was used, and the pupil size was sufficiently large. Also, check for patterns of visual field loss that are indicative of a trial lens rim artifact, a droopy upper eyelid, or other nonpathologic conditions that may account for the visual field loss. Fatigue, drowsiness, and related conditions also can produce apparent visual field loss. It is crucial that the person who performs the perimetric testing, especially with automated perimetric tests, be attentive to these factors. A surprising number of visual field deficits can be attributed to nonpathologic influences. In some instances, it may be necessary to query the technician as to the state of the patient when he/she was undergoing testing.

3 Determine if the visual field is abnormal in both eyes or in only one eye. If the visual field is abnormal in only one eye, the defect almost always is caused by a disorder anterior to the optic chiasm (Fig. 1.16), whereas if the fields of both eyes are abnormal, the deficit is at the chiasm (Fig. 1.17), posterior to the chiasm (Fig. 1.18), **or** the patient has bilateral intraocular or optic nerve disease.

4 Determine the general location of the visual field loss for each eye independently. Specifically, determine if the visual field loss is in the superior or inferior hemifield, the nasal or temporal hemifield, or the central portion of the field. This is especially important for the nasal and temporal hemifield assessment. If the loss is extensive, determine where the greatest amount of visual field loss is present. If the visual field loss is bitemporal and respects the vertical midline, then a chiasmal locus should be strongly suspected (Fig. 1.17). If the visual field loss is nasal in one eye and temporal in the other eye (i.e., homonymous), then a retrochiasmal location should be suspected (Fig. 1.18). Binasal defects or a nasal deficit in only one eye should generate a suspicion of glaucoma, various nonglaucomatous optic neuropathies, or certain types of retinal disorders. A central defect in one or both eyes may indicate a macular disorder. With this simple step, a global view of visual field properties is generated, and a hierarchy of potential locations of damage along the visual pathway and probable disease entities is hypothesized.

Figure 1.15 Artifactitious field defect detected in a patient with a pituitary adenoma. **A:** On 7/23/02, the patient has only some nonspecific defects in both eyes. (*continued*)

Figure 1.15 (*continued*) **B:** On 10/17/02, 3 months later, the patient appears to have developed significant field defects in both eyes; however, note that the patient is 79 years old and the fields were obtained at about 4 PM. Before we recommended treatment of the adenoma, we brought the patient back 5 days later for repeat fields. **C:** Repeat fields performed earlier in the day (about 11:15 AM) on 10/22/02, show that the apparent worsening of the fields was spurious and probably related to fatigue.

5 Look at the specific shapes, patterns, and features of the visual field loss (Figs. 1.16 to 1.18). Does the defect respect either the horizontal or vertical meridians? What is the shape of the defect (arcuate, oval, circular, pie-shaped, irregular)? If there is visual field loss in both eyes, is it congruous (symmetric in the two eyes) or incongruous (more extensive visual field loss in one eye than in the other) (Fig. 1.19)? Do the edges of the defect have a steep or a gradual sloping profile? These and other

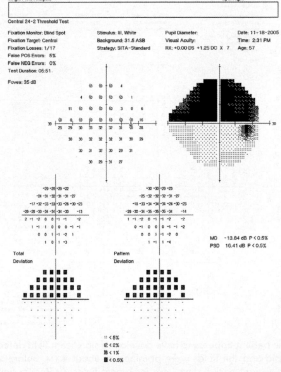

Figure 1.16 Examples of monocular field defects detected with a Humphrey Visual Field Analyzer. **A:** Central scotoma; **B:** Inferior arcuate defect; **C:** Superior altitudinal defect.

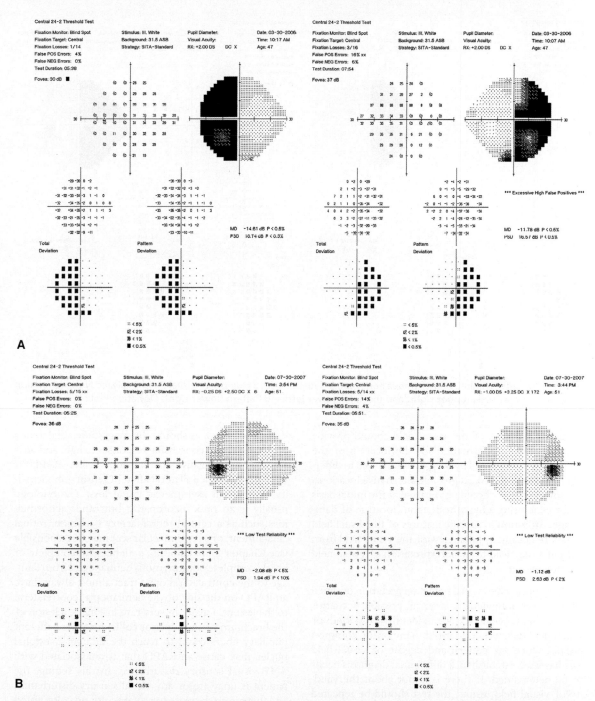

Figure 1.17 Examples of bitemporal field defects detected with a Humphrey Visual Field Analyzer. **A:** Severe bitemporal hemianopia. Note correlation between the gray scale (**above right**) and the Total (**lower left**) and Pattern (**lower right**) Deviation Plots. **B:** Very mild superior bitemporal quadrantic defect. Note that the gray scale does not clearly identify the defect, whereas it is obvious when looking at the Total Deviation and Pattern Deviation Plots.

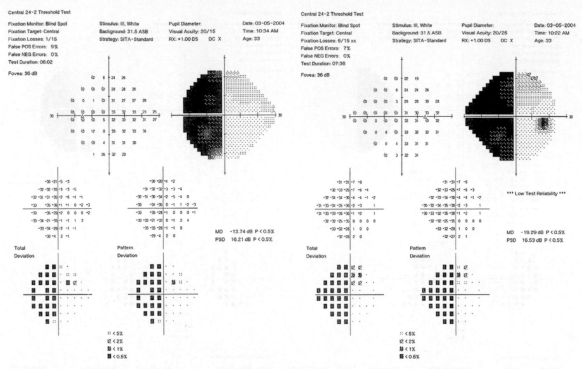

Figure 1.18 Left complete homonymous hemianopia detected with a Humphrey Visual Field Analyzer. Note correlation between the gray scale (**upper right**) and the Total (**lower left**) and Pattern (**lower right**) Deviation Plots.

specific features of the visual field should provide confirmatory information for the location of the damage determined by Step 4 or allow one to differentiate among several possible alternative locations. However, they should not be used as the initial basis for generating a hypothesis about location of damage. Attention to specific features of the visual field before getting a global view of the visual field from Step 4 may lead to misinterpretation of visual field information.

The approach to visual field interpretation outlined above is not intended to cover all possible scenarios but is rather meant as a guide to identify most kinds of visual field deficits and to avoid many of the common pitfalls. Once the pattern and degree of visual field loss has been established, a differential diagnosis needs to be determined. If there is doubt about the validity of visual field results, the test should be repeated when the patient is well rested (Fig. 1.15). Pathologic visual field changes usually are replicable, whereas nonpathologic visual field changes typically are not. If there is concern about fatigue affecting visual field results, a shorter test procedure should be employed.

Pupillary Examination

Examination of the pupils is an essential part of the afferent system evaluation. Pupil size for each eye

should be noted, as should the magnitude and latency of the direct and consensual responses to light and near stimulation. A relative afferent pupil defect (RAPD) is the hallmark of a unilateral afferent sensory abnormality or bilateral asymmetric visual loss. The etiology usually is an optic neuropathy, but other abnormalities such as a central retinal artery occlusion, retinal detachment, or a large macular scar may be responsible (see Chapter 2). In addition, patients with complete or nearly complete homonymous hemianopias from damage to the contralateral optic tract almost always have an RAPD on the side of the hemianopia (contralateral to the lesion). Finally, in very rare instances, a lesion of the brachium of the superior colliculus where afferent pupillary fibers travel to reach the Edinger–Westphal nuclei, may cause an RAPD that is unassociated with ANY visual sensory disturbance. In this setting, the patient is unaware of any visual sensory disturbance, and there is no decrease in visual acuity, no color vision deficit, and no visual field defect.

The presence or absence of an RAPD is one of the most crucial issues in dealing with a patient who has monocular or binocular but asymmetric visual loss as in such a setting, **an RAPD may be the only objective sign of organic and serious anterior visual pathway dysfunction.** Cataracts, refractive errors, and nonorganic visual loss NEVER cause a RAPD. Thus, an RAPD in a patient with a cataract, regardless of the cataract's

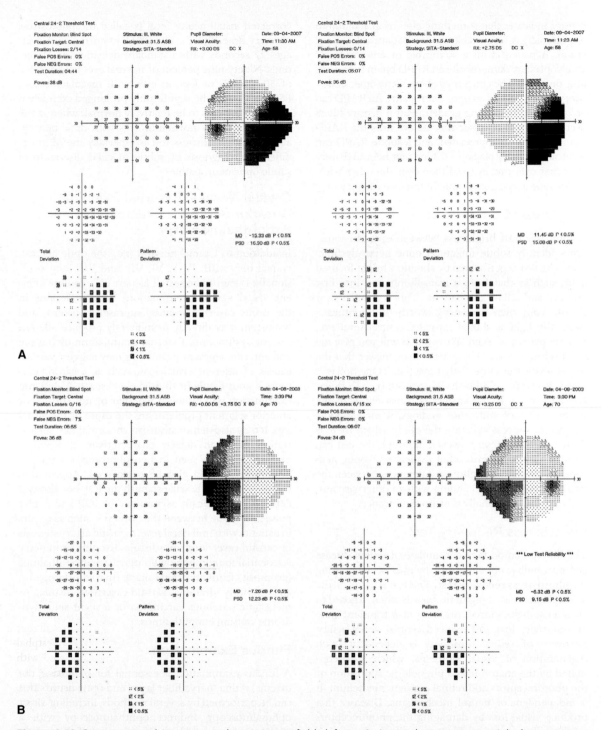

Figure 1.19 Congruous and incongruous homonymous field defects. **A:** Incomplete congruous right homonymous hemianopia from a left-sided occipital lobe infarct. **B:** Incomplete incongruous left homonymous hemianopia from a right-sided parietal lobe tumor.

density, indicates that something else (or in addition to the cataract) is responsible for the patient's decreased vision. A patient with a strabismic or anisometropic amblyopia may demonstrate an RAPD but in such a setting, one should be concerned about some other underlying process such as an optic neuropathy. An RAPD can be quantified by placing graded neutral density filters over the normal or lesser affected eye until the RAPD can no longer be appreciated, and a subtle RAPD can be brought out by placing a 0.3 log unit neutral density filter first over one eye and then over the other while performing a swinging flashlight test (see Chapter 14).

Brightness Comparison

A comparison of brightness between eyes can sometimes identify subtle unilateral optic nerve dysfunction. The test is performed by shining a bright focused light, such as that from a transilluminator, into first one eye and telling the patient "This is a dollar's (or choose your own currency!) worth of brightness." Next, the light is shined into the contralateral eye, and the patient is asked "How much will you give me for this brightness?" The patient may answer that the brightness is the same in that eye (i.e., "One dollar"); that it is less (i.e., "50 cents"); or more (i.e., "a dollar and 20 cents"). If the answer is consistent with the patient's history and other findings, it may support an organic process affecting the eye in which there is decreased brightness; however, although the test can be used to corroborate other evidence of optic neuropathy, subjective brightness differences between the two eyes as an isolated finding with an otherwise normal examination usually is of no significance.

Photostress Recovery Test

The differentiation between unilateral retinal disease and retrobulbar optic neuropathy may be aided using the **photostress recovery test.** This test is based on the principle that visual pigments bleach when exposed to an intense light source, resulting in a transient state of sensitivity loss and reduced central visual acuity. Recovery of retinal sensitivity is dependent upon regeneration of visual pigments, which are determined by the anatomic and physiologic apposition of the photoreceptors and retinal pigment epithelium. It is independent of neural mechanisms. Diseases that produce visual loss by damaging the photoreceptors or the adjacent retinal pigment epithelium cause a lag in regeneration of pigment, resulting in a delay in visual recovery following light stress.

The photostress test is performed by determining best-corrected visual acuity, shielding one eye, and then asking the patient to look directly at a bright focal light held 2 to 3 cm from the eye for about 10 seconds. The time needed to return to within one line of best-

corrected visual acuity level is called the photostress recovery time (PSRT). The PSRT in normal eyes averages 27 seconds with a standard deviation of 11 seconds. Ninety-nine percent of normal eyes have a PSRT of 50 seconds or less. In eyes with macular disease, PSRT is likely to be significantly prolonged even when the retina appears to be relatively normal, whereas the PSRT is relatively normal in eyes with optic neuropathies. The photostress test is especially useful in the differential diagnosis of subtle macular disease from subtle optic neuropathies.

Cranial Nerves, External Examination, Anterior Segment Examination, and Exophthalmometry

In addition to Cranial nerve II (i.e., the optic nerves), cranial nerves III, IV, V, VI, VII, and VIII (and occasionally I) should be tested as part of a routine afferent visual system examination, because lesions in the orbit, cavernous sinus, suprasellar cistern, and brainstem may directly or indirectly produce afferent system dysfunction. External examination of the eye and anterior segment evaluation may suggest various causes of afferent visual loss, such as a carotid-cavernous sinus fistula or thyroid eye disease. A slit lamp examination will establish whether or not corneal or anterior segment problems are the cause of the visual loss. It may also demonstrate iris abnormalities, such as transillumination defects characteristic of albinism or Lisch nodules seen in neurofibromatosis type 1. Tonometry should also be performed. Applanation tonometry not only will establish the IOP but also will detect any significant asymmetry of IOP and ocular pulse amplitude between the two eyes, such as occurs in patients with unilateral severe carotid artery stenosis or carotid-cavernous sinus fistula. Exophthalmometry is essential for someone who may have exophthalmos (proptosis) from an orbital mass, thyroid orbitopathy, an anteriorly draining carotid-cavernous fistula, or metastatic scirrhous carcinoma or a silent sinus syndrome causing enophthalmos.

Fundus Examination

A fundus examination is essential for evaluating the macula, retina, nerve fiber layer, and optic nerve. This can be performed by several methods, including direct ophthalmoscopy, indirect ophthalmoscopy with a 20-diopter hand-held lens. Examination of the macula with a 78- or 90-diopter hand-held lens or a corneal contact lens viewed through a slit lamp may identify the cause of visual loss as being from retinal dysfunction rather than neuro-ophthalmologic disease.

Performing a fundus examination on infants and young children can be a challenge. It is best to leave the room after performing the afferent system and motility evaluations, allowing a nurse or technician to administer dilating drops to preserve your rapport with the child. In the case of infants, it is best to ask the parents to withhold a feeding bottle until you return to the room. Most infants will readily accept a bottle at this point and will be cooperative during a cycloplegic refraction and dilated fundus examination. The soporific effect of the cycloplegic drops also may cause them to fall asleep.

After completing the cycloplegic refraction, the physician should perform a dilated fundus examination using both a hand-held direct ophthalmoscope and a 20-diopter lens in conjunction with an indirect ophthalmoscope, using a low level of illumination for both assessments. A lid speculum is not necessary for most pediatric neuro-ophthalmologic examinations because the macula and optic disc are the primary areas of interest. If a child becomes uncooperative, it may be necessary for the parents or an assistant to hold the child in a "lock-down" position (one person holding the arms outstretched over the ears with the other holding the feet) to complete the examination. This is a stressful and difficult situation for all concerned, and all rapport with the child is gone when this occurs. If it is not possible to perform an adequate dilated examination of the infant or child, it may be necessary to conduct an evaluation with the child under sedation.

Ancillary Testing

Despite taking a complete history and performing a complete examination, the physician may not be able to determine exactly what is responsible for a patient's visual symptoms. In such a setting, the two ancillary tests most likely to be helpful are ocular imaging and electrophysiologic studies.

Ocular Imaging

Optical coherence tomography (OCT) is a noninvasive and noncontact transpupillary imaging technique that can provide high-quality in vivo resolution (5 to 10 μm) of the retina and the optic nerve. The OCT creates a cross-sectional image using the principle of optical backscattering of light. It can be used to measure the average thickness of the peripapillary retinal nerve fiber layer (PRNFL) as well as its thickness in various sectors, macular volume, and thickness of the retinal ganglion cell layer. It is important to realize, however, that whereas OCT can be used to assess **structure,** it does not necessarily provide any information about **function.** For this, one may have to turn to electrophysiologic tests (see below). Nevertheless, in the appropriate setting, OCT can: (1) pro-

vide information that can help distinguish retinal from optic nerve disease, (2) allow objective monitoring of optic nerve axon damage in patients with neurologic disorders such as multiple sclerosis, (3) provide data that can guide treatment decisions for patients with compressive and other optic neuropathies, and (4) predict potential recovery or lack thereof after treatment (Figs. 1.20 and 1.21). A number of OCT instruments are available to the clinician, and improvements in imaging quality continue to be forthcoming.

Electrophysiologic Testing

Frequently, the physician is confronted with a patient who has unexplained loss of vision and an apparently normal fundus examination. Because electrophysiologic testing often provides diagnostic clues as to the etiology of the unexplained visual loss, it should be part of the neuro-ophthalmologic examination in selected patients. Electrophysiology provides a relatively objective method for evaluating the function of the visual system from the retina to the visual cortex. Several electrodiagnostic methods can be used to evaluate the status of individual components of the afferent visual pathways, including full-field (Ganzfeld), pattern, and multifocal electroretinography and both standard and multifocal VEPs.

The Full-field (Ganzfeld) Electroretinogram

Full-field ERGs are global retinal responses to a full-field flash stimulus and arise largely in the photoreceptor and inner nuclear layers of the retina. Modification of stimulus parameters and the adaptive state of the eye enable separation of the function of rod and cone systems and inner and outer retinal layers. Stimulation is provided by a Ganzfeld stimulator, an integrating sphere that provides uniform retinal illumination.

There are two main components of the ERG: an early cornea-negative a-wave and a cornea-positive b-wave (Fig. 1.22). The photoreceptors are responsible for the generation of the leading edge of the a-wave, whereas the cellular origin of the b-wave is a combination of cells in the Müller and bipolar cell layers (Fig. 1.22B).

The rod and cone components of the ERG may be separated on the basis of their respective spectral sensitivities by altering the retinal state of adaptation or by using different flicker rates for the stimulus. ERGs often are described as having photopic (light-adapted) and scotopic (dark-adapted) responses. The wavelength, intensity, and temporal properties of the stimulus, as well as the state of retinal adaptation, are all important in separating rod and cone system contributions.

The ERG is described by the temporal characteristics and amplitudes of the recorded waveform. The

Figure 1.20 Optical coherence tomography (OCT) in a 56-year-old man with a 1-year history of progressive visual loss in both eyes. Visual acuity was 20/50 OU. The fundi appeared normal. **A:** Visual field defects. **B:** OCT of the peripapillary retinal nerve fiber layer (PRNFL) shows no thinning in either eye, consistent with normal optic nerve function. (*continued*)

C

Figure 1.20 (*continued*) **C:** OCT of the maculae shows marked thinning bilaterally. A diagnosis of macular dystrophy was made after performance of a multifocal electroretinogram (see Figure 1.24).

temporal aspects of the waveform can be described by the latency and implicit times. Latency refers to the time between stimulus onset and response onset, whereas implicit time refers to the time needed for the response to reach maximum amplitude. Waveform amplitudes are measured from the baseline (which is usual for the a-wave) or as a peak-to-peak comparison (which is usual for the b-wave). The b/a-wave ratio can be used as an index of inner to outer retinal function.

The ERG can be affected by a number of factors. The implicit time of the waveform does not mature until 4 to 6 months of age, and the amplitude may be reduced until 1 year of age. The ERG may be greater in women than in men and may be reduced in myopes with more than 6 diopters of refractive error. There may be as much as a 13% reduction in ERG amplitude in the morning, which corresponds to the time of maximum photoreceptor disk shedding. Systemic drugs and anesthetics may also alter the ERG. In addition, the ERG can be altered if the subject blinks, moves the eye during stimulation, or is not concentrating on the stimulus.

A full-field ERG can provide important information about a number of retinal disorders that may simulate neuro-ophthalmologic problems. These include congenital stationary night blindness, congenital achromatopsia, retinitis pigmentosa (rod-cone dystrophy), retinitis pigmentosa sine pigmenta, cone-rod dystrophy, cone dystrophy, cancer-associated retinopathy (CAR), melanoma-associated retinopathy (MAR), and toxic retinopathies.

Pattern Electroretinography

The pattern electroretinogram (PERG) is the response of the retina to a centrally viewed isoluminant black

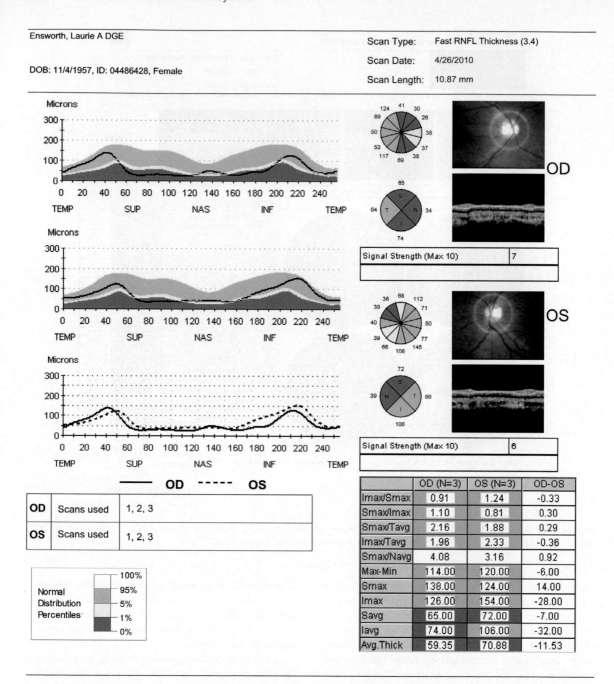

Ensworth, Laurie A DGE

DOB: 11/4/1957, ID: 04486428, Female

Figure 1.21 Optical coherence tomography (OCT) of the peripapillary retinal nerve fiber layer (PRNFL) in a 35-year-old woman with multiple sclerosis complaining of blurred vision in both eyes. She had 20/20 vision and normal color perception in both eyes. The visual fields showed mild reduction in sensitivity OU. The optic discs appeared normal. The OCT shows marked thinning of the PRNFL in both eyes, consistent with a significant bilateral optic neuropathy.

and white reversing checkerboard. The transient PERG has an initial negative wave at around 35 msec (N35), followed by a positive wave at approximately 50 msec (P50), and a late, large negative wave at around 95 msec (N95) (Fig. 1.23). The N95 component arises in the retinal ganglion cells, whereas the P50,

although mostly arising in the retinal ganglion cells, has significant contributions from structures anterior to the retinal ganglion cells, possibly the bipolar cells. A normal P50 component depends on the integrity of the macular cones and thus acts as an objective measure of macular function. Normal persons have

A Time (msec)

B Time (5 msec/div)

Figure 1.22 Full-field (Ganzfeld) electroretinogram (ERG). **A:** Normal ERG showing the cornea-negative a-wave and the cornea-positive b-wave. **B:** In a patient with visual loss in the right eye several years earlier associated now with optic disc pallor and some narrowing of the retinal arteries, the ERG of the left (L) eye has a normal a-wave *(arrow)* and a normal b-wave *(asterisk)*; however, although the ERG of the right (R) eye has a normal a-wave *(arrow)*, the b-wave amplitude is markedly diminished. This indicates that the photoreceptors are functioning, but there has been damage to the inner retinal Müller and bipolar cells. These findings are consistent with a previous central retinal artery occlusion. (Both figures courtesy of Dr. Mary A. Johnson.)

excellent symmetry in the waveforms between the two eyes, with amplitude ratios typically 0.8 to 0.9 in each eye. Because the N95 reflects RGC activity, the PERG can be used to determine RGC function in patients with primary RGC disease as well as optic nerve (i.e., axon) disease. This can be crucial in determining treatment windows and visual prognosis in patients with various optic neuropathies, including inflammatory (i.e., optic neuritis), ischemic, compressive, and toxic.

Multifocal Electroretinography

The human ERG recorded at the cornea in response to a full-field stimulus is a mass response generated by cells across the entire retina. Loss of half the retinal photoreceptors across the retina is associated with about a 50% reduction in ERG amplitude. Because the total cone population in the human retina is about 7 million, and the number of cones in the macula is at most 440,000, the macula contains only about 7% of the total retinal cone population. Thus, a full-field ERG is unable to detect abnormalities confined to small regions of the retina, including the fovea and macula. Fortunately, it is possible to assess macular function as well as retinal function in the posterior pole using multifocal ERG (mfERG).

mfERGs typically are generated using an array of 61 or 102 hexagonal elements that subtend a total angle of 55 degrees. Each stimulus element is illuminated according to a pseudorandom binary sequence; cross-correlation techniques enable the construction

of multiple responses from a single electrode. The mfERG, similar to the PERG, may be a useful complement to VEP testing (see below) but is highly dependent upon accurate fixation.

Nevertheless, it can be exceptionally helpful in patients with small field defects including central or paracentral scotomas and normal-appearing fundi in whom it is unclear if the cause is retinal, due to optic nerve dysfunction, or is nonorganic (Figs. 1.24 and 1.25).

Figure 1.23 Pattern-evoked electroretinogram (PERG) in a patient with a severe demyelinating right retrobulbar optic neuropathy. Visual acuity with the right was 20/200. The left eye had normal visual function. The PERG from the left eye (LE) shows normal P50 and N95 waveforms, whereas the PERG from the right eye (RE) shows a P50 waveform with slightly reduced amplitude and no N95 waveform. The findings in the right eye are consistent with normal overall retinal function but marked loss of retinal ganglion cells. (Courtesy of Dr. Graham Holder.)

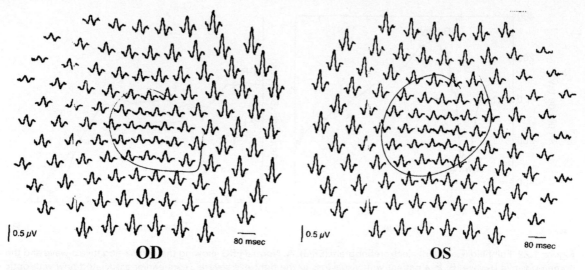

Figure 1.24 Multifocal electroretinogram (mfERG) in the patient whose optical coherence tomography is shown in Figure 1.20. The mfERG shows marked central reduction in both eyes consistent with a macular dystrophy.

Visual-evoked Potential

If the spontaneous occipital electroencephalogram (EEG) is recorded while brief flashes of light or an alternating black and white checkerboard pattern are presented to an eye, changes result in the occipital potential. These changes are called the **visual-evoked potential** (VEP), visual-evoked response (VER), or the visual-evoked cortical potential (VECP). The VEP thus is a gross electric potential of the visual cortex in response to visual stimulation. The VEP is limited mainly to the occipital region of the brain, with an amplitude between 1 and 20 µV. The VEP depends on the integrity of the entire visual pathway, although it remains to be determined if its components can truly be separated into anatomic correlates.

The VEP is measured by placing scalp electrodes over the occipital region (O$_z$) of both hemispheres, with reference electrodes attached to the ear. The patient then views the display, typically a xenon-arc photostimulator for flash VEPs and a television screen display with patterned stimuli for pattern VEPs. Recordings of the VEP may be made from either hemisphere with one or both eyes fixating. Typically, 100 to 150 stimulus presentations are generated, and time-locked signal averaging is used to extract the VEP waveform from the spontaneous EEG activity. The amplitude and latency of the waveform then are measured. A flash stimulus is used when no response is produced using a pattern stimulus. Thus, infants and patients with extremely poor acuity, dense media opacities, or poor fixation most commonly are tested with flash VEP. In most patients, however, a pattern stimulus is preferred for obtaining the VEP, because of the greater clinical utility and more reliable waveform generated with this stimulus. A repetitive pattern of light and dark areas (checkerboards, bar gratings) are phase reversed every 1 or 2 seconds. The pattern VEP is primarily generated from the central 5 degrees of the visual field, consistent with the anatomic correlates that the central 10 degrees of the visual field is represented by at least 50% to 60% of the posterior striate cortex and that the central 30 degrees is represented by about 80% of the cortex (see Chapter 12).

The amplitude of the pattern VEP is affected by a number of different factors. The size of the stimulus pattern can affect the amplitude of the VEP signal, as can the rate of alternation of the pattern. The VEP also varies with stimulus size and frequency, attention, mental activity, pupil size, fatigue, state of dark adaptation, color of the stimulus, background illumination, and even the emotional content of the stimulus. All of these factors emphasize the importance of using standardized and optimized test conditions (including the best refractive correction) for

Figure 1.25 Optical coherence tomography (OCT) of the peripapillary retinal nerve fiber layer (PRNFL) and multifocal electroretinogram (mfERG) in a 47-year-old woman complaining of blurred vision in the right eye. The patient's visual acuity was 20/40 OD and 20/15 OS. There was no relative afferent pupillary defect. Visual fields showed an enlarged blind spot on the right. The fundi appeared normal. **A:** OCT of the PRNFL shows no thinning. Thus, there is no evidence of optic nerve disease. **B:** mfERG shows marked central reduction in cone function in the right eye. A diagnosis of acute zonal occult outer retinopathy (AZOOR) was made.

Scan Type: Fast RNFL Thickness (3.4)
Scan Date: 8/9/2011
Scan Length: 10.87 mm

Microns (OD chart, axis 300/200/100/0; x-axis 0-240: TEMP SUP NAS INF TEMP)

OD: 105 132 104 / 63 92 / 49 48 / 53 67 / 122 155 119
114 / 55 T S N 69 / 132

Signal Strength (Max 10): 7

OS: 142 125 68 / 89 58 / 58 37 / 71 46 / 112 135 119
112 / 73 N S T 47 / 122

Signal Strength (Max 10): 6

	OD (N=3)	OS (N=3)	OD-OS
Imax/Smax	1.12	0.94	0.18
Smax/Imax	0.89	1.06	-0.17
Smax/Tavg	2.59	3.22	-0.63
Imax/Tavg	2.91	3.03	-0.12
Smax/Navg	2.08	2.07	0.01
Max-Min	122.00	121.00	1.00
Smax	143.00	151.00	-8.00
Imax	161.00	142.00	19.00
Savg	114.00	112.00	2.00
Iavg	132.00	122.00	10.00
Avg.Thick	92.43	88.34	4.09

—— OD ----- OS

OD	Scans used	1, 2, 3
OS	Scans used	1, 2, 3

Normal Distribution Percentiles
100%
95%
5%
1%
0%

A

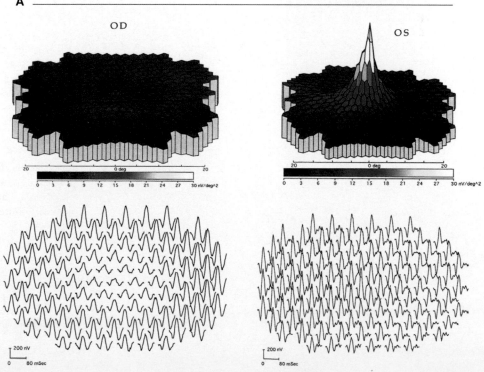

OD   OS

0 deg   0 3 6 9 12 15 18 21 24 27 30 nV/deg^2

200 nV
0   80 mSec

B

Figure 1.26 Visual-evoked potential (VEP) in a patient with a left retrobulbar optic neuritis. The VEP shows a marked reduction in amplitude and an increased latency of the P100 peak in the left eye. The P100 waveform on the right has both a normal amplitude and a normal latency. (Courtesy of Mary A. Johnson, PhD.)

clinical VEP testing, as well as establishing age-related normative standards for the procedures employed for each laboratory. In addition, it is crucial that the technician or physician performing the study be well trained.

Although VEP is characterized by several waveforms, the main one used in clinical practice is the positive wave that occurs at about 100 msec, called the P100 (Fig. 1.26). Both the latency and amplitude of the P100 are assessed. The latency increases in most optic neuropathies, particularly inflammatory (i.e., optic neuritis) and compressive. Patients with ischemic optic neuropathy may show P100s that have relatively normal latencies but reduced amplitudes.

A more recent development is the use of evoked potentials to map visual field function, the **multifocal VEP.** Electrical responses to pattern reversal stimuli presented pseudorandomly to the central visual field can be extracted from occipital scalp recordings. The clinical usefulness of this test in patients with optic nerve, cerebral and nonorganic visual loss remains under investigation, and it is used mainly as a research tool.

Anatomy and Physiology of the Retina and Optic Nerve

Distinguishing Retinal from Optic Nerve Disease

Anatomy and Physiology of the Retina
Cell Types and Layers of the Retina
Retinal Blood Vessels
Rod and Cone Through Pathways: Functional
    Considerations

Anatomy and Physiology of the Optic Nerve
Optic Nerve Head (Intraocular Optic Nerve)
Orbital Optic Nerve
Intracanalicular (Intraosseous) Optic Nerve
Intracranial Optic Nerve
Optic Nerve Physiology
Topographic Anatomy of the Optic Nerve

Topographic Diagnosis of Retinal Lesions
Distinguishing Retinal Disease from an Optic
    Neuropathy by Clinical Examination
Distinguishing Retinal Disease from an Optic
    Neuropathy by Visual Field
Appearance of the Optic Disc in Retinal Disease

Knowing the anatomy and physiology of the retina and optic nerve is crucial in understanding the similarities and differences in findings in patients with retinal versus optic nerve disease.

Anatomy and Physiology of the Retina

The retina is a unique part of the nervous system because it can be visualized, allowing the clinician to observe directly the effects of a wide range of diseases such as an infarction in evolution, deposition of metabolic storage products, or slowing of axoplasmic flow. The retina is also a favorite tissue for study by neuroscientists because it is thin and can be dissected easily from the eye because its cells are segregated into layers, and because there is at least a fundamental appreciation of its anatomic and physiologic organization.

The cellular structure of the retina is enormously complex. In humans, it contains over 100 million neurons, among which are about 30 different cell types that use at least 10 different neurotransmitters. Most architectural schemas underrepresent the intricacy of the retina because the degree to which information is shared among various cells depends on a variety of factors, including the region of the retina being illuminated, the characteristics of the light stimulus, and the state of adaptation of the retina to light. Given this complexity, one might imagine that a large number of symptoms would result from dysfunction of these many cell types. On the contrary, most clinically recognized diseases of the retina are caused by dysfunction of either photoreceptors or retinal ganglion cells (RGCs).

The human retina covers an area approximately 2500 mm^2 and extends from the ora serrata to the optic disc. The retina contains six classes of neurons (photoreceptors, horizontal cells, bipolar cells, amacrine cells, interplexiform cells, and RGCs) and two types of glial cells (astrocytes and Müller cells) that are arranged into three parallel layers, except in the perifoveal zone, where the retina thins to a single layer (Table 2.1; Figs. 2.1 and 2.2). The human retina is roughly 120 μm thick over most of its area, with a maximum thickness of 230 μm in the macula and a minimum thickness of 100 μm in the foveal pit.

Cell Types and Layers of the Retina

The **retinal pigment epithelium (RPE)** is a monolayer of cells derived from the outer wall of the optic vesicle. It is intimately associated with the outer segments of the photoreceptors (Fig. 2.1). The RPE is responsible for several essential functions. Most significantly, it (a) is integrally involved in the phototransduction cascade through regeneration of chromophore; (b) provides trophic support for photoreceptors; (c) is a transport barrier between the choriocapillaris and the sensory retina; (d) participates in ocular immune responses; (e) binds reactive oxygen species; and (f) absorbs excess radiation with their melanin granules.

T. Hengst © 1981
THE JOHNS HOPKINS UNIVERSITY

Figure 2.1 Cellular components of the fully developed primate retina, showing cellular relationships and major synaptic interactions. *OPL*, outer plexiform layer; *ONL*, outer nuclear layer; *ELM*, external limiting membrane; *OS*, outer segment; *As*, astrocyte; *G*, ganglion cell; *Am*, amacrine cell; *I*, interplexiform cell; *H*, horizontal cell; *B*, bipolar cell; *C*, cone; *R*, rod; *M*, Müller cell. The photoreceptor nuclei lie in the ONL, and a large stretch of the photoreceptors consists of their outer segments, which lie proximal (i.e., nearer to the retinal pigment epithelium) to their nuclei. The outer segments contain chromophore, which captures the energy from incoming light and initiates the ionic exchange that hyperpolarizes the photoreceptors. The inner segments of photoreceptors (not labeled) are the segments between the outer segments and the nucleus that contain a high concentration of mitochondria and endoplasmic reticulum.

Table 2.1	Cellular Organization of the Retina
Cell Layer	**Neuronal and Glial Nuclei**
Outer nuclear layer	Photoreceptors
Inner nuclear layer	Horizontal cells
	Bipolar cells
	Interplexiform cells
	Amacrine cells
	Müller cells
Ganglion cell layer	Ganglion cells
	Displaced amacrine cells
	Astrocytes

present in patients with various macular dystrophies, age-related macular degeneration, and central serous chorioretinopathy, but also in patients with severe stenosis of the ipsilateral internal carotid artery causing markedly reduced oxygen delivery to the photoreceptors. It can be detected clinically by performing a photostress test (see Chapter 1).

The second primary function of the RPE—membrane renewal—is just as important as RPE's role in phototransduction. Outer segments of rods and cones are shed on a daily basis. The outer segment of a human rod is entirely replaced over a period of 10 days and, although the timing of cone shedding is more variable, the involvement of the RPE in this process of shedding and renewal is integral. Disruption of the interaction between the RPE and the photoreceptors can lead to retinal degeneration, as occurs in hydroxychloroquine toxicity.

The **photoreceptor cells** of the retina are the sensory transducers for the visual system. They convert electromagnetic energy (i.e., light) into a neural signal. The photoreceptors contain visual pigments that, by absorbing photons of light, initiate the phototransduction process. These pigments absorb within the range of electromagnetic wavelengths that pass through the cornea and lens, generally between 400 and 700 nm. The two types of photoreceptors are the **rods** and the **cones**.

The visual cycle begins when the outer segment of a photoreceptor absorbs a photon, causing isomerization of 11-*cis*-retinol, the dark adapted form of rhodopsin, to all-*trans*-retinol. This reaction initiates the phototransduction cascade that ultimately influences propagation of nerve impulses through the retina (Fig. 2.3). The 11-*cis*-retinol must be continuously regenerated to maintain the ability of the photoreceptors to respond to light, and this regeneration is performed by the RPE. Patients in whom regeneration of photopigment is abnormally slow have a prolonged recovery of central vision following exposure of the retina to bright light. This phenomenon is

Figure 2.2 Section through center of fovea. Nuclei of rod receptor cells are indicated by *arrows*. Remaining receptor cells are foveal cone cells. *OS*, outer nuclear layer; *OF*, outer cone fiber; *OH*, outer fiber layer of Henle; *IN*, inner nuclear layer; *g*, ganglion cell; *CP*, capillary; *IM*, internal limiting membrane; *IS*, inner segment; *OM*, outer limiting membrane; *ON*, outer nuclear layer. (Reduced from ×400.) (Reprinted with permission from Yamada E. Some structural features of the fovea centralis in the human retina. *Arch Ophthalmol.* 1969;82:151–159.)

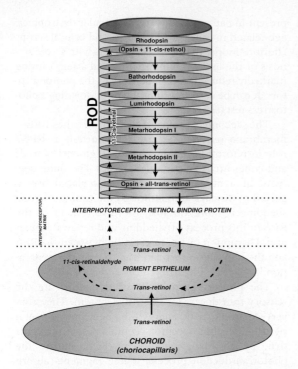

Figure 2.3 Phototransduction cascade. Schematic drawing of junction of rod, retinal pigment epithelium, and choroid to show the interrelationship among those structures required to regenerate photopigment. *trans*-Retinol is carried by the blood to the choriocapillaris where it can then enter the retinal pigment epithelium and contribute to the cycle.

Both rods and cones have inner and outer segments, both of which are located outside the boundary of the outer limiting membrane (Fig. 2.4). The inner segment contains the **ellipsoid**, a structure that is richly endowed with mitochondria. The ellipsoid is responsible for the high level of oxidative metabolism that occurs in photoreceptors. The **myoid** is the region between the ellipsoid and the nucleus of the photoreceptor. This region contains numerous cellular organelles. The outer segment is connected to the inner segment by a cilium, which contains nine pairs of microtubules arranged in a pattern that is characteristic of nonmotile cilia.

Rods contain rhodopsin, a molecule that is composed of the apoprotein, opsin, and 11-*cis*-retinol. Rhodopsin is present in very high concentrations within the membranes of the outer segment discs, which are oriented vertically to maximize capture of incident photons. Activation of the phototransduction cascade causes an intracellular decline in cyclic guanidine monophosphate (GMP) concentration within the rod outer segment, followed by closure of the cyclic GMP-gated cation channel and cessation of inflow of extracellular cations that normally generates the

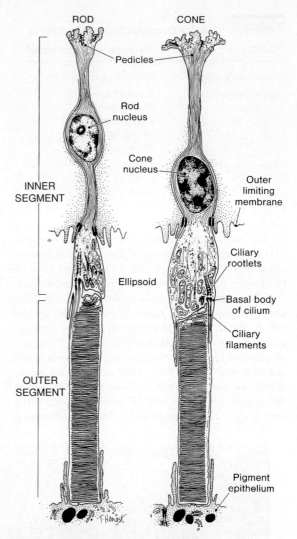

Figure 2.4 Ultrastructure of photoreceptors. Schematic drawing of photoreceptor cells showing the relationship of the inner and outer segments. The ellipsoid is located at the apex of the inner segment. (Reprinted with permission from Hogan MJ, Alvarado JA, Weddell JC. *Histology of the Human Eye: An Atlas and Textbook.* Philadelphia, PA: WB Saunders; 1971.)

dark current. The rod becomes hyperpolarized upon exposure to light, which decreases the amount of neurotransmitter released at the synaptic terminal.

Vitamin A is used in the process of phototransduction and regeneration of photopigment. Vitamin A must be replenished from the circulation, and failure to do so can result in a bilateral retinopathy that clinically may mimic a bilateral optic neuropathy; however, because rods are predominately affected in the retinopathy caused by deficiency of vitamin A, **nyctalopia** (night blindness) usually is the initial manifestation of this disorder. This symptom helps to distinguish the retinopathy from an optic neuropathy. Hypovita-minosis A is a highly significant problem in develop-ing countries, but also occurs in persons who live in developed countries but who have malabsorption syn-dromes or liver disease, who adhere to restrictive diets, or who have poor diets due to chronic alcohol abuse.

Cones also contain 11-*cis*-retinol but have differ-ent apoproteins than rods. The variation of the opsin moieties produces three different spectral response curves corresponding to the blue, green, and red cones, which are more appropriately called short- (S), medium- (M), and long- (L) wavelength cones to emphasize that their responsiveness is not limited to a single color but rather is spread across a portion of the visible spectrum. Congenital color blindness almost always results from defects in either the red or green photopigment gene, both of which are located on the X chromosome.

Humans have a cone:rod ratio of approximately 1:20, with each retina containing 140 million rods and 7 million cones. About 50% of the cones are located within the central 30 degrees of the visual field, an area that roughly corresponds to the size of the mac-ula. Rods are absent in the fovea and are in highest density in an elliptical ring, the center of which is the optic nerve head. There is an age-related decline in the number of rods in the human retina, with an annual loss of about 0.2% to 0.4%.

The density of foveal cones poses a problem in regard to their forward connections because their syn-aptic terminals (called cone pedicles) and the ganglion cells to which they connect have larger diameters than the cone inner segments themselves. Thus, each foveal ganglion cell soma is displaced away from the site of the cone that initiates its visual response. This realign-ment is accomplished by the nerve fiber layer (NFL) of Henle, an elongation of cones and rods between their nuclei and synaptic terminals.

The "midget" system refers to the anatomic pat-tern of cone outflow within the most central retina, although there is no specific boundary beyond which the midget pathway cannot be found. The midget sys-tem provides the most direct communication of spatial detail from outer to inner retina. In this system, out-put from one cone passes to one ON-center **and** one OFF-center bipolar cell with each bipolar cell connect-ing in turn to a single ON- **or** OFF-center ganglion cell. Thus, the divergence of signal from a foveal cone to a ganglion cell is 1:2. In the peripheral retina, by compar-ison, there is marked convergence of information from outer to inner retina, with perhaps up to 1500 rods influencing the function of one ganglion cell.

The **outer plexiform layer (OPL)** is the zone of synaptic connection between cells whose nuclei are in the outer and inner nuclear layers (Fig. 2.1). Cone pedicles and rod spherules, the synaptic specializations

of cones and rods, respectively, have several invagina-tions into which processes of horizontal and bipolar cells extend, creating "triads" of one bipolar cell and two horizontal cells.

The retina contains two types of **horizontal cells** (Fig. 2.1). The HII cell, the smaller of the two types, makes dendritic contact with cones and axon contact with rods, whereas both ends of the HII cell synapse only with cones. Horizontal cells seem to provide the anatomic substrate for the center-surround response characteristics observed in the physiologic recordings made from ganglion cells and some other inner ret-inal neurons. Specifically, the response of a ganglion cell to light that falls within the center of its receptive field is opposite to that, which occurs to light that falls in the surround (i.e., the portion of the receptive field beyond the center). The antagonistic center-surround organization emphasizes contrast within the visual scene, which enhances spatial resolution.

Bipolar cells receive input from photoreceptors and provide output to both amacrine cells and gan-glion cells (Fig. 2.1). Some bipolar cells receive input from rods, others from cones. Rod bipolar cells are the target of an apparent paraneoplastic immune attack in some patients with cutaneous malignant melanoma, so-called melanoma-associated retinopathy (MAR). The physiologic consequence of destruction of these cells is loss of the scotopic b-wave of the electroretino-gram (ERG).

The major excitatory neurotransmitter in the retina is glutamate, and this substance has a profound effect at the level of the bipolar cells. There are two physiologic types of bipolar cells: hyperpolarizing (OFF-center cells) and depolarizing (ON-center cells). These bipo-lar cells respond differently to changes in the ambient glutamate concentration within the OPL. Release of glutamate by photoreceptors initiates two opposing but parallel signals to the inner retina (Fig. 2.5).

Amacrine cells are so named because they lack axons. Their cell bodies are located primarily in the inner nuclear layer of the retina (Fig. 2.1). Some ama-crine cells are interneurons between bipolar and gan-glion cells. Others connect to fellow amacrine cells, forming a lateral pathway within the inner plexiform layer (IPL) similar to that formed by horizontal cells in the OPL. There are numerous subtypes of amacrine cells.

The cell bodies of the **interplexiform cells** reside in the IPL (Fig. 2.1). These cells are postsynaptic to amacrine and bipolar cells in the IPL and presynaptic to horizontal and bipolar cells. This cell thus appears to be unique in that it apparently conveys information from the inner to the OPL, against the standard direc-tion of neural transmission within the retina.

The retina contains several types of glial cells that have various functions. The most important are Müller

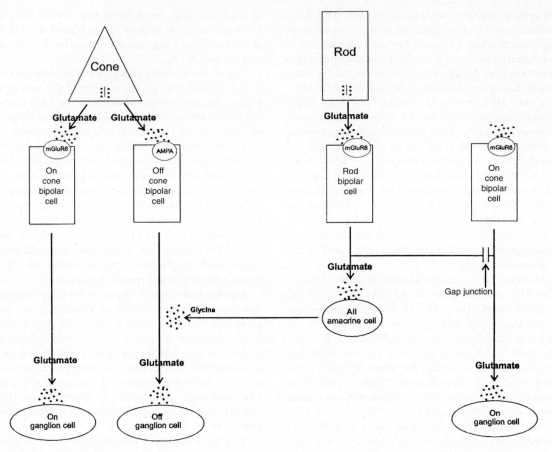

Figure 2.5 Schematic illustration of neurotransmitters used by cells of the rod and cone pathways. The neurotransmitters are released within the outer and inner plexiform layers. The mGluR6 and AMPA receptors of the bipolar cells are also depicted. The former uses a G protein to control the intracellular concentration of cGMP that, in turn, regulates the Na^+-Ca^{2+}-cGMP-gated ion channel.

cells and astrocytes. Müller cell somas are located in the inner nuclear layer, but processes from these cells extend throughout the entire retina (Fig. 2.1). The apical processes of **Müller cells** form the outer limiting membrane by making junctional complexes with one another and with photoreceptors. On the vitread side, apposed Müller cell end feet forms the inner limiting membrane. Lateral extensions from Müller cells contact neurons within cellular layers, synapses within plexiform layers, axons within the NFL, and blood vessels.

Despite all of their connections, Müller cells are not part of the direct pathway for transfer of neural signals. Instead, they exert substantial influence over signal transmission by (1) maintaining the local extracellular environment needed for proper neuronal function, particularly with respect to the extracellular concentration of potassium; (2) adjusting concentrations of extracellular neurotransmitters; and (3) possibly buffering pH levels.

Astrocytes are found only on the vitread side of the retina, within the nerve fiber and ganglion cell layers. Two morphologic types of astrocytes develop from stem cells in the optic nerve. Each cell type preferentially contacts either nerve fiber bundles or blood vessels. Oligodendrocytes are not present in the primate retina, which is consistent with the absence of myelin in these retinas. However, the observation of myelinated nerve fibers in the retinas of about 0.5% of normal persons suggests that such a migration can occur during, and even after, development (see Chapter 3).

The **inner plexiform layer** is the zone of synaptic connection of bipolar and amacrine cells to ganglion cells and is much thicker than the OPL (Fig. 2.1). The IPL can be divided into sublaminae a and b. Sublamina a is the more proximal layer. It is nearer the inner nuclear layer and is the zone within which bipolar, amacrine, and ganglion cells of the OFF-center pathway synapse. Sublamina b is the more distal layer. It is nearer the RGC layer and is the site of synaptic connections for the ON-center cell pathway.

The **retinal ganglion cell layer** is, in fact, composed not only of RGCs, but also of "displaced" amacrine cells, astrocytes, endothelial cells, and pericytes (Fig. 2.1). The human retina contains about 1.2 million RGCs, although there is a very wide interindividual variability. It has been calculated that 69% of the RGCs in the human retina subserve the central 30 degrees of the visual field and are located adjacent to the fovea.

Dendrites of RGCs branch in well-defined strata within the IPL, and the specific region of stratification varies with the particular cell type. ON-center and OFF-center cells have dendrites that terminate in sublamina b or a of the IPL, respectively. RGC axons terminate in either the magnocellular or parvocellular layers of the lateral geniculate nucleus (LGN), and this also depends on the cell type. In the primate retina, there may be as many as 10 or more subpopulations of RGCs.

RGCs can be subdivided into two main types based on cell size. About 80% of the cells are small cells that are called "beta" or "P" cells, for **parvocellular** cells. These cells, as their name implies, synapse in the parvocellular layers of the LGN. From 5% to 10% of primate RGCs are large cells that are called "alpha" or "M" cells, for **magnocellular** cells. The axons of these cells synapse in the magnocellular layers of the LGN. Together, the P and M RGCs comprise 85% to 90% of all primate RGCs. The remainder of the ganglion cells is present in small numbers, is less well studied, and has functions other than for visual perception, such as the pupillary light reflex (see below) and the retinohypothalamic pathway, the latter believed to be an integral part of the pathway that regulates circadian functions.

From a clinical standpoint, the P and M cells have great significance. The P cells are color opponent (i.e., the center of the receptive field is maximally responsive to either red or green light, whereas the inverse is true for the surround), have small receptive fields, and have low sensitivity to contrast in the visual scene. Color opponency is generated by connections at both the OPL and IPL. The receptive field center of P ganglion cells near the fovea approximately equals the diameter of a single cone. These cells have linear response characteristics, meaning that their firing rate is proportional to the degree to which the center of the receptive field is stimulated or inhibited. Cells with this response property are also called "X" cells. Given these characteristics, the P cells are probably the major neural input to the optic nerve for visual functions such as central (i.e., Snellen) acuity, color vision, and fine stereopsis.

The M cells are spectrally "broadband." Because of the combined input to these cells from all three cone types, their peak responsiveness at a given intensity of light is not determined by the wavelength. M cells have much larger receptive fields and are more responsive to luminance contrast than P cells. The majority of M cells have nonlinear responses to light. These cells typically show spikes of activity in response to changes in the visual scene, rather than showing activity that is proportional to the intensity of light and that matches the duration of light stimulation, as is the case with P cells. M cells with this physiologic profile are also called "Y" cells, to distinguish their responses from the X-like response profile of P cells. Lesions of the magnocellular pathway in monkeys impair high-temporal-frequency flicker and motion perception.

Most RGCs have several physiologic properties in common. First, their receptive fields have a concentric and antagonistic center-surround organization. This property probably derives at least in part from the effect of the lateral inhibition of horizontal and, possibly, amacrine, cells. Second, most respond either in an on or off manner to change in the luminance contrast or spectral distribution of light within their receptive field centers. This property is reflected in the location of dendritic ramification within the IPL. ON-center bipolar and ganglion cells ramify in sublamina b of the IPL, whereas OFF-center bipolar and ganglion cells ramify in sublamina a. Third, the responses to light of most RGCs are either sustained or transient, depending on the pattern of interconnections with amacrine cells within the IPL. Fourth, RGCs with sustained responses also show linearity of spatial summation; that is, the magnitude of their response is proportional to the degree of illumination within the center of the receptive field. In contrast, transiently responding RGCs briefly increase or decrease their firing rates in response to a change in illumination. Finally, RGCs maintain a continuous spontaneous discharge. This activity requires considerable energy but presumably has the advantage of allowing the cell to reflect more precisely the degree of illumination by either increasing or decreasing its firing rate.

As noted above, not all RGCs are P or M cells. Melanopsin (also called opsin 4, Opn4) is a photopigment that was first identified in frog skin and thereafter was detected in a small subpopulation of RGCs in vertebrates. These cells depolarize in response to light stimulation **without any synaptic input from rods and cones**; hence, their designation as intrinsically photosensitive RGCs (ipRGCs). The ipRGCs combine their direct, melanopsin-triggered photoresponses with signals derived from rods and cones and project to several targets in the diencephalon and midbrain involved in circadian rhythms and pupil responses to light (Fig. 2.6).

The ipRGCs constitute a small percentage of ganglion cells; in each human eye, about 3,000 of 1.5 million (0.2%) RGCs stain positively for melanopsin;

Figure 2.6 The melanopsin-containing intrinsically photosensitive retinal ganglion cells (ipRGCs) have a giant soma and long, sparsely branching dendritic processes that extend either into the outer (off) sublayer of the inner plexiform layer (M1 cells) or the inner (on) sublayer (M2 cells). These ipRGCs integrate their direct light responses with signals from rods and cones for non–imaging-forming functions. Rods provide excitatory inputs to ipRGCs sequentially via rod bipolar (RB), type II amacrine (AII), and cone bipolar (CB) cells. Red cones (RC, long wavelength, L-cones) and green cones (medium wavelength, M-cones) provide excitatory inputs to the proximal dendrites of ipRGC cells syn cone bipolar cells. In contrast, blue cones (BC, short wavelength, S-cones) trigger provide inputs presumably through cone bipolar cells and inhibitory amacrine (A) cells. The axons of ipRGCs exit the retina via the optic nerve and project to the suprachiasmatic nucleus (SCN), the subparaventricular zone (SPZ), the ventrolateral preoptic area (VLPO), and the intergeniculate leaflet (IGL) of the lateral geniculate nucleus (LGN), that are involved in circadian regulation, and to the olivary pretectal nucleus (OPN), which is a relay of the pupillary light reflex. Projections to the dorsal LGN provide an interface with the imaging-forming system; projections to dural-sensitive neurons in the posterior hypothalamus (Po) may contribute to light-induced exacerbation of migraine. *EW,* Edinger–Westphal nucleus; *GCL,* ganglion cell layer; *INL,* inner nuclear layer; *IPL,* inner plexiform layer; *NFL,* nerve fiber layer; *ONL,* outer nuclear layer; *OPL,* outer plexiform layer; *OS,* outer segment; *RPE,* retinal pigment epithelium. (Reprinted from Benarroch EE. The melanopsin system. Phototransduction, projections, functions, and clinical implications. *Neurology.* 2011;76:1422–1427, with permission.)

these cells are concentrated in the parafoveal region and at the far end of the nasal hemiretina. Like all RGCs, ipRGCs utilize the excitatory amino acid L-glutamate as their primary neurotransmitter; they also express pituitary adenylate cyclase-activating polypeptide (PACAP), which acts as a cotransmitter of glutamate in the retinohypothalamic pathway. There are several subtypes of ipRGCs that differ in their dendritic distribution in the IPL, melanopsin expression, physiologic responses to light, and connections. The melanopsin-containing ipRGCs are relatively spared in inherited mitochondrial optic neuropathies, may be selectively affected in glaucoma and may trigger photophobia in patients with migraine.

The **axon** of an RGC is relatively long, and the body of the cell is the sole site for production of the components needed to maintain the health of the axon. The axon is a dynamic structure that requires nearly constant repair of its membranes, a process that is partly achieved by transport of proteins, enzymes, and other subcellular components (including mitochondria) to, and detritus from, sites up to the synapse.

Axon transport is bidirectional and simultaneous, with velocities that can be divided broadly into fast (i.e., hundreds of mm/day) and slow (<10 mm/day). Slow anterograde transport, which largely carries components that remain within the cell such as cytoskeletal proteins, constitutes the bulk (about 85%) of all movement within the axon. At least five different classes of proteins are transported at different velocities within RGCs, and these relationships vary during development. Fast anterograde transport is used to carry neurotransmitter-containing vesicles. Retrograde transport, which is less well understood, proceeds at roughly half the maximum velocity of anterograde transport. It returns to the cell body substances that have been taken into the cell at its terminal synapse. Axon transport, whether anterograde or retrograde, is highly energy dependent, and the adenosine triphosphate (ATP) needed to sustain it is supplied by mitochondria that are distributed along the entire length of the axon.

The final common defect in pathologic swelling of the optic disc from almost any etiology is disruption of anterograde axonal transport of the RGC at the lamina cribrosa (see Chapter 4). The degree to which fast versus slow transport is disrupted probably varies according to the etiology.

Axons of RGCs synapse in the LGN, mesencephalon, pretectum, or one of several nuclei in the hypothalamus. The specific site of termination of the axon is related to the anatomy of the ganglion cell body. Generally, P- and M-cell axons synapse in the parvocellular and magnocellular layers, respectively. ON-center and OFF-center ganglion cells appear to remain functionally separated at the level of the LGN, although both channels converge at the visual cortex.

The **nerve fiber layer** of the retina is composed of axons of RGCs, astrocytes, components of Müller cells, and a very small number of efferent fibers to the retina, the functions of which are unknown (Fig. 2.1). The NFL is thinnest in the peripheral retina and thickest adjacent to the superior and inferior margins of the optic disc, where it measures about 200 μm in humans. The temporal and nasal NFL adjacent to the optic disc is about 1/10 as thick.

The gross organization of the NFL is characterized by three main features. The first is the papillomacular bundle, which contains nerve fibers originating from RGCs in the foveal area. Papillomacular fibers from RGCs on the nasal side of the fovea project directly to the optic disc, whereas those from RGCs on the temporal side of the fovea arch around the nasal fibers en route to the optic nerve (Fig. 2.7). The relatively early formation of the central retina relative to the peripheral retina gives rise to the second feature: the arching of axons from midperipheral and peripheral ganglion cells temporal to the fovea around the previously formed papillomacular bundle. A watershed line called the temporal raphe is present on the temporal side of the fovea, and this horizontal demarcation separates axons in the superior temporal retina from those in the inferior temporal retina. The raphe creates not only an anatomic separation, but also a physiologic separation between the superior and inferior regions of the temporal retina. The third anatomic feature of the NFL is the radial distribution of nerve fibers that enter the nasal aspect of the optic disc.

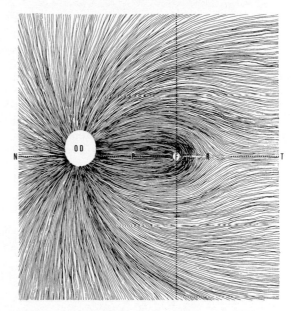

Figure 2.7 Drawing of the retinal nerve axons as they extend from the ganglion cells to the disc. The axons arising from ganglion cells in the nasal macula project directly toward the optic disc (OD) and comprise part of the papillomacular bundle (P). Axons from ganglion cells of the temporal macula have a slight arching pattern around the nasal macular axons. They form the remainder of the papillomacular bundle. Axons from nonmacular ganglion cells that are nasal to the fovea (F) have a straight or gently curved course to the optic disc, whereas axons from ganglion cells temporal to the fovea must arch around the papillomacular bundle and enter the disc at its superior and inferior poles. Note that the superior and inferior portions of the temporal retina are delineated by an anatomic landmark, the temporal raphe (R). The dotted lines delineate the nasal (N), temporal (T), superior, and inferior portions of the retina. Note that the temporal and nasal parts of the retina are defined by a vertical line through the fovea, not the optic disc. (Redrawn from Hogan MJ, Alvarado JA, Weddell JE. *Histology of the Human Eye. An Atlas and Textbook.* Philadelphia, PA: WB Saunders; 1971.)

The temporal–nasal demarcation of the retina (and, thus, the visual field) is a vertical line that passes through the **fovea**, not the optic disc. Fibers from RGCs located nasal to the fovea cross to the opposite side within the optic chiasm, whereas fibers from RGCs located temporal to the fovea remain uncrossed, passing through the chiasm into the ipsilateral optic tract. This vertical meridian, although reasonably precise from a clinical standpoint, is inexact at a cellular level. There is a small area of nasotemporal overlap on either side of the vertical meridian in which some axons from ganglion cells temporal to the fovea cross within the chiasm, and some axons from ganglion cells nasal to the fovea remain uncrossed. However, the mere presence of an overlap may have no significant visual consequences. A ganglion cell that is located on one side of the fovea does not necessarily receive input from a photoreceptor that is located on the same side. The much larger width of the cone pedicle compared with the foveal cone soma creates a packing problem that is only partly resolved by lateral displacement of cone pedicles and via the NFL of Henle. This lateral shift could theoretically connect photoreceptors on one side of the vertical meridian to seemingly displaced ganglion cells on the opposite side. Such an anatomic relationship would have no adverse visual consequences because it is the position of the photoreceptor and not the ganglion cell body that provides spatial cues to the brain.

There is, in addition to the specific arrangement of fibers in the NFL described above, an orderly arrangement of the fibers in the third dimension—that is, with respect to their vertical orientation as viewed in cross-section (Fig. 2.8). The nerve fibers are generally stratified such that axons from ganglion cells in the peripheral retina occupy a position adjacent to the ganglion cell layer, whereas axons from ganglion cells located more centrally lie more superficially in the NFL, adjacent to the vitreoretinal interface. To achieve this arrangement, fibers from increasingly central ganglion cells must cross fibers from more peripheral ganglion cells (Fig. 2.8A). This arrangement is maintained until the fibers are near the optic disc, at which point there is significant intermingling of more central axons with those that originated peripherally. Nevertheless, near the disc margin, most of the axons with a long course (i.e., from peripheral ganglion cells) are located deep within the NFL, whereas axons with a short course (i.e., from central ganglion cells) are located superficially. This arrangement results in the longest axons being positioned in the periphery of the anterior optic disc, and axons from more central ganglion cells being located more centrally in the anterior optic disc (Fig. 2.8B).

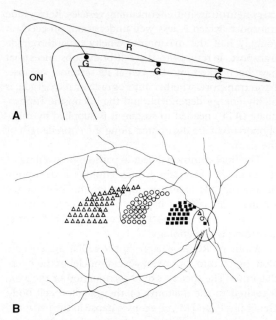

Figure 2.8 The three-dimensional organization of the nerve fiber layer in the primate retina and optic disc. **A:** Anterior–posterior organization of axons projecting from ganglion cells (G) located in peripheral, middle, and peripapillary retina (R) into the optic nerve (ON). Lamination of axons within retina is speculative. Only half of retina and optic nerve are represented, as if displayed in standard horizontal section. **B:** Horizontal topography of axon bundles from the arcuate fibers (i.e., those that course around the papillomacular bundle) as they project into the anterior portion of the optic nerve head. Peripherally located ganglion cells project to the peripheral aspect of the optic nerve (*triangles*), centrally located ganglion cells to the midperipheral aspect of the optic nerve (*circles*), and peripapillary ganglion cells to the center of the nerve (*squares*).

Table 2.2 provides a list of known neurotransmitters for the major classes of retinal cells, and Figure 2.5 shows some of the neurotransmitters used by the intraretinal cone and rod through pathways.

Table 2.2 Retinal Neurons and Some of Their Associated Neurotransmitters

Cell Type	Neurotransmitter
Photoreceptors	Glutamate
Horizontal cells	GABA

Bipolar cells:
    ON-center (depolarizing)
    OFF-center (hyperpolarizing)
	
	Glutamate
	Glutamate

Interplexiform cells	Dopamine, GABA
Amacrine cells	Acetylcholine, Glycine, GABA, Peptides, Dopamine

Retinal vasculature

Outer retina

Choroidal vasculature

Figure 2.9 Drawing showing the blood supply of the retina. Note that the choroidal circulation supplies the photoreceptors, whereas the inner retina is supplied by the retinal arteries.

Retinal Blood Vessels

The human retina receives its essential nutrients—oxygen and glucose—from both the retinal and the choroidal circulations. The border between these circulations is near the OPL. The choroidal circulation supplies the photoreceptors; the retinal arteries supply the inner retina (Fig. 2.9), although the latter do not enter a small area composed of the fovea and a varying degree of perifoveal retina. This avascular area is called the **foveal avascular zone** (Fig. 2.10). There is considerable interindividual variation in the size of the foveal avascular zone. In addition, the degree to which the inner retina is vascularized appears to correlate with the degree of oxidative metabolic demand, rather than with the thickness of the retina.

Figure 2.10 Fluorescein angiogram showing the foveal avascular zone.

The retinal vasculature is organized into specific laminae. Generally, four planes of capillaries can be recognized. The two more vitread layers bracket the inner nuclear layer, whereas the two other layers are located more superficially. Superficial retinal capillaries in humans can probably nourish ganglion cell bodies up to 45 μm away.

Retinal blood vessels are barrier vessels, analogous to the blood–brain barrier elsewhere within the central nervous system. These vessels are impermeable to particles larger than 2 nm. Astrocytes and pericytes almost certainly play a role in maintaining this nonspecific low permeability for capillaries within the NFL, whereas Müller cells probably play a similar role within deeper retina. The blood–retinal barrier is maintained not only by physical factors, such as the cells surrounding the retinal capillaries described above, but also by chemical factors. Specifically, autoregulation of retinal (and choroidal) blood vessels may be at least partially controlled chemically by hormonal products of the local vascular endothelium. These substances include vasodilators, such as nitric oxide and prostaglandins, and vasoconstrictors, particularly endothelin and the products of the renin-angiotensin system that are produced and released via angiotensin-converting enzyme, which is located on the endothelial cell membrane. In addition, adenosine and α_1-adrenergic receptors in retinal blood vessels have been shown to mediate vasodilation and vasoconstriction, respectively.

Rod and Cone Through Pathways: Functional Considerations

The complex anatomic and physiologic features of the retina combine to produce a well-defined reaction when the retina is stimulated with light. Light causes the photoreceptors to hyperpolarize, decreasing the release of glutamate from both rod and cone synaptic terminals. Horizontal cells then become hyperpolarized, suppressing the light response of the photoreceptors. Rod and cone outputs then diverge. Rod signals are transmitted to the rod bipolar cells via a sign-inverting signal. Thus, bipolar cells depolarize in response to light. The signal then is carried via the axons of the rod bipolar cells to sublamina b of the IPL, where there is a sign-conserving synapse on amacrine cells. (Rod bipolar cells do not make direct contact with ganglion cells.) The amacrine cells make gap junctions with cone-depolarizing bipolar cells, the axon terminals of which also ramify in sublamina b of the IPL, where the terminal of the amacrine cells contact ON-center ganglion cells via a conventional synapse. The amacrine cells also make conventional synapses on cone-hyperpolarizing bipolar cells through sign-reversing glycinergic synapses, and these bipolar cells terminate in sublamina a of the IPL and then make contact with OFF-center ganglion cells.

Cone output in the central retina uses the midget system of interconnections in which one foveal cone contacts two bipolar cells, each of which then contacts a single ganglion cell. A sign-conserving synapse is made on a cone-hyperpolarizing (OFF-center) bipolar cell, and a sign-conserving synapse is made with a cone-depolarizing (ON-center) bipolar cell. The two bipolar cells then terminate in the proximal (sublamina a) and distal (sublamina b) laminae of the IPL, respectively, wherein they make contact with an OFF-center (sublamina a) or an ON-center (sublamina b) ganglion cell. From this location, visual information is passed to the brain via the optic nerve. Visual information (i.e., spatial detail, color, contrast) is presented in parallel fashion to the brain, with major physiologic cell types in the retina, generally maintaining anatomic segregation at the LGN.

Anatomy and Physiology of the Optic Nerve

The **optic nerve** is not really a nerve. It is a part of the central nervous system. As such, it is a tract, and its axons are myelinated entirely by oligodendrocytes, not Schwann cells. The optic nerve carries about 1.2 million axons whose cell bodies are the RGCs and that synapse in one or more of at least eight primary visual nuclei.

Common nomenclature considers only the anterior portion of this retinofugal fiber projection to be the optic nerve. The optic chiasm is the site of a partial decussation of these fibers, and the optic tract is the posterior continuation of the same fiber tract to its termination in the LGN.

The optic nerve is about 50 mm long (Fig. 2.11), although there is some individual variation in length, especially with regard to its posterior half. It may be

Figure 2.11 Histologic section showing the four topographic sections of the normal optic nerve. *1*, intraocular; *2*, intraorbital; *3*, intracanalicular; *4*, intracranial; *OC*, optic chiasm. (Reprinted with permission from Hogan MJ, Zimmerman LE. *Ophthalmic Pathology. An Atlas and Textbook*. Philadelphia, PA: WB Saunders; 1962.)

Figure 2.12 Light photomicrograph showing architectural arrangement of the prelaminar (P), laminar (L), and retrolaminar (R) portions of the optic nerve. The retrolaminar segment of the optic nerve is darker because of the presence of myelin. Note the abrupt transition between myelinated and unmyelinated segments of the optic nerve, which occurs just posterior to the lamina cribrosa. (Courtesy of Dr. Harry A. Quigley.)

described as having four parts: (1) the intraocular portion (the optic nerve head or optic disc); (2) the intraorbital portion; (3) the intracanalicular (intraosseous) portion within the optic canal; and (4) the intracranial portion. The intraocular optic nerve can be further divided into three anatomically distinct zones: the prelaminar portion (anterior), the laminar portion (middle), and the retrolaminar portion (posterior) (Fig. 2.12). These zones have very different microanatomic arrangements.

Optic Nerve Head (Intraocular Optic Nerve)

Axons of the RGCs form bundles that constitute the NFL, which converges like spokes of a wheel at the optic nerve head. The optic nerve head is about 1 mm long (anterior–posterior); its diameter is 1.5 mm horizontally by 1.8 mm vertically at the level of the retina and a little wider in the retrolaminar space. It is a major zone of transition because nerve fibers pass from an area of high tissue pressure within the eye to a zone of low pressure that correlates with the intracranial pressure. At the same time, the nerve fibers leave an area in which their blood supply is from the central retinal artery alone to zones supplied by other branches of the ophthalmic artery. In addition, the axons become myelinated immediately at the posterior end of the optic nerve head (Fig. 2.12).

The optic nerve head is composed of four types of cells: ganglion cell axons, astrocytes, capillary-associated

Figure 2.13 Scanning electron micrograph of the lamina cribrosa, viewed from the vitreous cavity.

Figure 2.15 Appearance of a tilted optic disc. Note inferior conus.

cells, and fibroblasts. It also includes an oval grouping of 200 to 300 holes that perforate the choroid and sclera, forming a specialized structure called the **lamina cribrosa**, through which all retinal axons pass to exit the eye (Figs. 2.12 and 2.13).

The anterior surface of the optic nerve head is the clinically visible **optic disc**. The appearance of the disc depends on two important features: the size of the scleral canal and the angle of exit of the canal from the eye. The size of the canal varies somewhat among individuals; however, the volume of tissue passing through the hole appears to be more constant. The scleral canal may be thought of as a hole in the sclera. The larger the scleral canal, the more leftover space is present in the center of the disc,

leading to a larger physiologic cup size (Fig. 2.14A). The converse is also apt to be true. A small or absent physiologic cup often reflects a small scleral canal and a crowded optic nerve head (Fig. 2.14B). This "disc-at-risk" is a crucial factor in the pathogenesis of nonarteritic anterior ischemic optic neuropathy (see Chapter 7).

When the optic nerve head exits the sclera at less than a 90-degree angle, the RPE frequently ends before the edge of the canal proper, exposing a crescent-shaped halo of choroid and sclera (Fig. 2.15).

A

B

Figure 2.14 Appearance of a normal optic disc with a moderate central cup (**A**) and a "disc at risk" (for nonarteritic anterior ischemic optic neuropathy) (**B**). Note that the disc-at-risk is smaller than the normal disc and has no central cup.

Figure 2.16 Appearance of a tilted optic disc. The elevated superior portion of the disc simulates optic disc swelling. Note inferior conus.

In addition, with an oblique angle of exit at one side of the disc, nerve fibers must make a greater than 90 degree turn, giving a rolled edge to this rim of the disc that may simulate true swelling (Fig. 2.16) and, thus, be mistaken for papilledema (see Chapter 5). At

the opposite side of such a disc, fibers are exiting at less than a 90-degree angle, and the disc rim appears shallowly sloped.

The axons that comprise the NFL turn 90 degrees posteriorly as they enter the optic nerve head (Fig. 2.8). The axons then run in bundles surrounded by glial columns as they pass through the perforations of the lamina cribrosa. The fenestrated connective tissue and glia form a tight seal that helps keep the relatively high intraocular pressure from "leaking" into the retrolaminar tissues.

Within the optic nerve head, there are two types of blood vessels: capillary-sized vessels that directly supply the cells and the central retinal vessels (the central retinal artery and one or more central retinal veins) that pass through the nerve head. The ophthalmic artery originates from the ophthalmic segment of the internal carotid artery just as that vessel emerges from the distal dural ring of the cavernous sinus (Fig. 2.17). It then turns anteriorly and passes through the optic canal along with the optic nerve but separated from it by a covering of dura. Once within the orbit, the ophthalmic artery gives rise to several branches, one of which is the central retinal artery, which pierces the optic nerve sheath 10 to 12 mm behind the globe and runs anteriorly in the central aspect of the optic nerve to emerge in the center of the optic disc. This

Figure 2.17 The internal carotid artery blood supply to the orbit and eye, with emphasis on the ophthalmic artery and its major branches. Key for arteries: *16*, frontal branch; *17*, internal carotid; *18*, ophthalmic; *20*, posterior ethmoidal branch of the ophthalmic; *25*, superior peripheral arcade; *27*, lacrimal; *28*, recurrent meningeal; *35*, central retinal; *37*, muscular branches for the superior rectus, superior oblique, and levator palpebrae muscles; *38*, medial posterior ciliary; *39*, short ciliary; *40*, long ciliary; *41*, anterior ciliary; *42*, greater circle of the iris; *43*, lesser circle of the iris; *44*, episcleral; *45*, subconjunctival; *46*, conjunctival; *47*, marginal arcade; *49*, medial palpebral; *48*, vortex vein. (From BM Zide, GW Jelks. *Surgical Anatomy of the Orbit.* New York, NY: Raven Press; 1985.)

Figure 2.18 Blood supply to the intraocular optic nerve. Note three sources: choroidal feeder vessels, short posterior ciliary arteries, and the pial arterial network.

Figure 2.19 Retinochoroidal vessels (*arrows*) in a patient with chronic compression of the optic nerve by an optic nerve sheath meningioma.

artery does not contribute directly to the circulation of the optic nerve head. Instead, the blood supply to the optic nerve head derives from the circle of Zinn–Haller, which forms a ring about it. The circle of Zinn–Haller receives three major sources of blood. Much of its blood derives from the choroidal feeder vessels. A second source consists of about four short posterior arteries that feed into the circle directly. The third source of blood to this perineural arteriolar anastomosis is a small contribution from the pial arterial network. Feeding this capillary plexus are subdivisions of the ophthalmic artery via third- and fourth-order branches of posterior ciliary arteries, which enter the lateral aspect of the nerve head and vessels of the pial plexus and retrobulbar optic nerve posteriorly (Fig. 2.18).

The venous drainage of the optic nerve head is primarily via the central retinal venous system. Under certain conditions, however, such as chronic compression of the intraorbital optic nerve or after central retinal vein occlusion, preexisting connections between superficial disc veins and choroidal veins—retinochoroidal vessels—may enlarge and shunt venous blood from the retina to the choroid and then, via the vortex veins, to the superior and inferior ophthalmic veins (Fig. 2.19).

Orbital Optic Nerve

The orbital portion of the optic nerve is about 25 mm in length and thus exceeds the anterior–posterior distance from the back of the eye to the optic foramen by about 8 mm (Fig. 2.20). The redundancy of the sinuous optic nerve permits it to move freely during eye movements. There is also an allowance of up to 9 mm of proptosis before the optic nerve acts as a tether and distorts the globe or is stretched to the point of dysfunction.

The optic nerve increases in diameter from 3 mm just posterior to the globe to about 4.5 mm at the orbital apex. Throughout its orbital course, the nerve

is surrounded by dura, arachnoid, and pia mater (Figs. 2.20 and 2.21). The dura is the outermost sheath, a dense collagenous tunic that is continuous anteriorly with the sclera. At the apex of the orbit, the dura fuses with the periosteum and with the annulus of Zinn (Fig. 2.19). The arachnoid lies under the dura and is more cellular, less vascular, and less collagenous. Delicate trabeculae connect the arachnoid with

Figure 2.20 Sagittal section through a normal orbit showing the optic nerve (N). Note that the length of the nerve within the orbit appears to exceed the distance from the posterior aspect of the globe to the apex of the orbit. Also note that the intraorbital and intracanalicular portions of the nerve are covered by leptomeninges, the dural sheath of which is continuous with the periorbita lining the inner surface of the orbital walls and the dura lining the base of the skull. (Reprinted with permission from Unsöld R, DeGroot J, Newton TH. Images of the optic nerve: anatomic-CT correlation. *Am J Roentgenol.* 1980;135:767–773.)

Figure 2.21 Axial section of normal optic nerves (N), showing relationships to other orbital and intracranial structures. Note that the intraorbital and intracanalicular portions of the nerve are covered by a dural sheath that is continuous with the periorbita lining the inner surface of the orbital walls and the dura lining the base of the skull. *C*, optic chiasm. (Reprinted with permission from Unsöld R, DeGroot J, Newton TH. Images of the optic nerve: anatomic-CT correlation. *Am J Roentgenol.* 1980;135:767–773.)

the underlying pia (Fig. 2.22). The pia is the most vascular of the sheaths covering the optic nerve. It invests the capillaries as they enter the substance of the nerve. The subarachnoid space is continuous with the intracranial subarachnoid space and thus contains cerebrospinal fluid.

Figure 2.22 Cross-section electron micrograph of human optic nerve, showing relationships of the vaginal sheaths. Not the many trabeculae, some of which are extremely fine (T) connecting the Arachnoid (A) and the Pia mater (P). Dura (D). View of the intraorbital optic nerve from above showing relationships of the nerve to the ocular motor nerves and the posterior ciliary vessels.

The cellular organization of the myelinated orbital portion of the optic nerve is similar to that of the intraocular optic nerve head, although the retrobulbar nerve is twice as wide because of the addition of myelin. Bundles of nerve fibers are surrounded by connective tissue septa containing small arterioles, venules, and capillaries, forming a meshwork much like that in the lamina cribrosa. Astrocytes are here joined by oligodendrocytes, the specialized glial cells that provide membranes for myelination. All of the visual axons are myelinated from their exit from the eye to their synapse in the LGN. The axons from the largest RGCs are surrounded by the thickest myelin sheaths, thus providing them with faster nerve conduction velocities.

With the exception of the central retinal artery, there are few vessels larger than capillaries within the orbital portion of the optic nerve. The arterial input derives chiefly from the surrounding pial plexus. As the optic nerve leaves the eye, it is surrounded by about four posterior ciliary arteries that are branches of the ophthalmic artery. Within the midportion of the orbit, the ophthalmic artery initially runs inferolateral to the optic nerve until it crosses under (or occasionally over) it to proceed medially. At the optic foramen, the ophthalmic artery lies below and lateral to the nerve. The inferior division of the oculomotor nerve, the nasociliary artery, the abducens nerve, and the ciliary ganglion are all located lateral to the optic nerve in the posterior orbit (Figs. 2.17, 2.23, and 2.24). At the apex of the orbit, the optic nerve is surrounded by the four rectus muscles that originate from the fibrous circle of Zinn (Fig. 2.24).

Intracanalicular (Intraosseous) Optic Nerve

The optic nerve enters the optic canal through its anterior opening in the apex of the orbital roof about 5 cm posterior and 1.5 cm inferior to the supraorbital margin (Figs. 2.20 and 2.21). This anterior opening is called the **optic foramen**.

The optic canal itself is formed by the union of the two roots of the lesser wings of the sphenoid bone. The proximal (orbital) opening of the optic canal usually is elliptical in shape, with the vertical diameter being consistently greater than the horizontal. The distal (intracranial) opening is always elliptical, but its widest diameter is in the horizontal plane.

The thickness of the bony optic canal wall varies from medial (thinnest in mid-canal) to lateral (thickest in mid-canal), but also from anterior to posterior. The thin medial wall separates the optic nerve from the sphenoid and posterior ethmoid sinuses. The canal is about 10 mm in length, with the lateral wall being shorter (9 mm) than the medial wall (about 14 mm). Inferolaterally, the optic canal is separated from the

Levator palpebrae

Sup. rectus

Lacrimal gland

Sup. oblique and med. rectus retracted

Short ciliary ns.

Long ciliary ns.

Ophthalmic a.

Lat. rectus retracted

Nasociliary n.

Sup. div. of III

Ciliary ganglion

Sup. rectus

Abducens (VI)

Frontal n.

Inf. div. of III

Lacrimal n.

Nasociliary n.

Optic n. (II)

Ophthalmic a.

Carotid a.

Optic chiasm

Oculomotor n. (III)

Trochlear n. (IV)

Frontal n.

Trigeminal n. (V)

Figure 2.23 View of the posterior orbit showing the relationship of the optic nerve to the ocular motor nerves and extraocular muscles.

superior orbital fissure by a bony ridge that joins the lesser wing of the sphenoid to the body of the sphenoid bone—the **optic strut**.

The relationship between the paranasal sinuses and the optic canal is extremely important, particularly because in about 4% of patients, the nerves have areas covered only by the nerve sheaths and sinus mucosa but without any bone separating the intracanalicular portion of the optic nerve from the adjacent paranasal sinus. The paranasal sinuses may occasionally

Supraorbital n.
IV n.
Trochlea
Sup. oblique m.
Ant. ethmoidal n.
Inf. trochlear n.
Long ciliary n.
Med. rectus m.

Levator palpebrae m.
Sup. rectus m.
Lacrimal n.
Sup. div. III n.
Lat. rectus m.

Optic n. and a.
Inf. rectus m.
Ciliary ganglion
Inf. oblique m.

IV n.
Inf. div. III n.

Figure 2.24 Schematic drawing of the optic nerve sheaths showing their relationship to the optic nerve (ON) and to the surrounding sphenoid bone. The dura is tightly adherent to the bone within the optic canal. Within the orbit it divides into two layers, one of which remains as the outer sheath of the optic nerve, and the other becomes the orbital periosteum (periorbita). Intracranially, the dura leaves the optic nerve to become the periosteum of the sphenoid bone.

become ballooned out without erosion of bone. This condition, called "pneumosinus dilatans," may result in the optic canals appearing as tunnels surrounded by sphenoid and posterior ethmoid air cells. Pneumosinus dilatans in this region is usually associated with an adjacent optic nerve sheath meningioma.

Falc. lig.
Ant. root
CN II
Ant. clin.
Rec. a.
Car. a.
M1

Figure 2.25 Appearance of the intracranial optic nerve as it exits from the optic canal. Note that its exit, it is covered by the falciform ligament (Falc. Lig.). *Ant. clin.,* anterior clinoid process; *Ant. root,* superior aspect of the optic canal; *Car. a.,* internal carotid artery; *CN II,* optic nerve; *M1,* M1 segment of the middle cerebral artery; *Rec. a.,* recurrent artery of Heubner. (From Joo W, Funaki T, Yoshioka F, Rhoton AL Jr. Microsurgical anatomy of the carotid cave. *Neurosurgery.* 2012;70/ONS Suppl 2:300–312, with permission.)

The intraorbital optic nerve moves freely as the eye moves; however, the intracanalicular optic nerve is tightly fixed within the optic canal. The dura is adherent to the bone of the canal on one side and the optic nerve on the other. Thus, small lesions arising within the optic canal or at either of its openings may compress and significantly damage the optic nerve while they are still quite small.

Intracranial Optic Nerve

The intracranial portion of each optic nerve exits past a firm fold of dura, the falciform ligament, that covers it superiorly and to some extent on both sides (Fig. 2.25). The distance between the optic nerves as they exit from the optic canal averages 13 mm. The two nerves then extend posteriorly, superiorly, and medially to join at the optic chiasm.

The length of the intracranial segment of the normal optic nerve varies considerably. It is usually about 10 mm long, but it may be as short as 3 mm or as long as 16 mm. This portion of the nerve is about 4.5 to 5.0 mm in average diameter, but it is flattened and thus is wider in the horizontal plane than in the vertical plane. When the intracranial optic nerve is shorter than about 12 mm, the optic chiasm is positioned anteriorly, or "prefixed," and sits directly over the sella turcica. When the intracranial optic nerve is long (over

Prefixed chiasm   Normal chiasm   Postfixed chiasm

Figure 2.26 Schematic drawing of three sagittal sections of the optic chiasm and sellar region. **Left:** The position of a prefixed chiasm above the tuberculum sellae. **Center:** The position of a normal chiasm above the diaphragma sellae. **Right:** The position of a postfixed chiasm above the dorsum sellae.

18 mm), the chiasm is positioned posteriorly to the dorsum sellae, or "postfixed" (Fig. 2.26). The variation in the length of the optic nerve is extremely important with respect to the visual deficits caused by tumors in the suprasellar region (see Chapter 12).

The gyrus recti of the frontal lobes of the brain are above the optic nerves. On the ventral surface of each frontal lobe, the olfactory tract is separated from the optic nerve by the anterior cerebral and anterior com-

municating arteries. On the lateral side of the optic nerve, the internal carotid artery sometimes forms an immediate relationship as it emerges from the cavernous sinus. Because the intracranial optic nerve is in the region where the internal carotid artery bifurcates into the anterior cerebral and middle cerebral arteries, these vessels are often immediately adjacent to the optic nerve, as is the proximal portion of the posterior communicating artery (Fig. 2.27).

Figure 2.27 Blood supply to the dorsal aspect of the optic chiasm and intracranial optic nerves. ON, optic nerve; OT, optic tract.

Figure 2.28 Anatomy of the proximal portion of the oph-thalmic artery (Ophth. a.) as it enters the optic canal beneath the optic nerve (CN II). Note that there is a fine sheath sep-arating it from the nerve. *Car. a.,* internal carotid artery; *Clin. seg.,* clinoidal segment of the internal carotid artery; *Prox. ring,* proximal dural ring; *Dist. Ring,* distal dural ring. *Rec. br.,* A recurrent branch of the ophthalmic artery; *Sup. hyp. a.,* superior hypophyseal artery; *Clin. venous plex.,* clinoidal venous plexus. (From Joo W, Funaki T, Yoshioka F, Rhoton AL Jr. Microsurgical anatomy of the carotid cave. *Neurosurgery.* 2012;70/ONS Suppl 2:300–312, with permission.)

The internal carotid artery supplies the optic nerve via the ophthalmic artery, which enters the optic canal inferior and lateral to the optic nerve (Figs. 2.17 and 2.28). It is separated from the nerve, however, by a dural sheath that covers it throughout the length of the canal. The anatomic relationship of the optic nerve and the internal carotid artery and its branches account for the visual deficits that occur in some cases of dolichoectasia or aneurysms of the internal carotid, ophthalmic, and anterior cerebral arteries. Inferome-dially, the sphenoid sinus has an important relation-ship to the optic nerve.

Optic Nerve Physiology

As noted above, there are at least three classes of RGCs in humans. About 80% to 90% of these cells are of small-to-moderate size, are concentrated in the macula, have small-caliber axons, and project to the parvocellular layers of the dorsal LGN (the P-cell system). P cells have color-opponent physiology and are thought to subserve high-contrast, high-spatial fre-quency resolution. In contrast, large cells with large, fast-conducting axons comprise about 10% to 20% of the RGC population. These M cells project to the magnocellular layers of the LGN and are primarily involved with noncolor information of high-tempo-ral and low-spatial frequency. Conduction velocities in optic nerve fibers are much faster than those in the unmyelinated but similar caliber fibers in the retina, ranging from 1.3 to 20 m/s. The ipRGCs have a high threshold for activation, long response latency, and a prolonged duration of firing before return to baseline.

Topographic Anatomy of the Optic Nerve

Fibers from peripheral ganglion cells occupy a more peripheral position in the optic disc, whereas fibers from ganglion cells located closer to the optic disc occupy a more central position. The arrangement of fibers in the optic disc and distal optic nerve corresponds generally to the topographic distribution of fibers in the retina. Fibers from the superior portion of the retina are located in the superior part of the optic nerve head; fibers from the inferior retina are located inferiorly in this region; and nasal and temporal fibers are on their respective sides. The papillomacular bundle is a sector-shaped structure that occupies about one-third of the temporal optic disc, adjacent to the central vessels. This bundle of fibers gradually moves centrally in the more distal (pos-terior) portions of the orbital optic nerve. The gradual movement of the macular fibers to the center of the orbital optic nerve allows the uncrossed upper and lower retinal fibers to come together (Fig. 2.29). Dorsal (superior) and ventral (inferior) macular fibers retain their relative positions throughout the nerve, whereas crossed macular fibers lie nasal to the uncrossed fibers. Indeed, all the retinal fibers retain their relative posi-tions throughout the visual pathways; that is, upper fibers remain upper and lower remain lower, except in the optic tract and at the LGN, where there is a rotation of 90 degrees that becomes straightened out in the optic radiations (see Chapter 12).

Within the intracranial portion of the optic nerve, the axons lose their retinotopic order to some extent because some axons decussate within the optic chiasm and some do not. The macular fibers do not have a pre-cise localization in the posterior nerve and the gradual inclination inward of the macular fibers in the most posterior portions of the nerve allows for regrouping of the peripheral visual fibers.

Most of the visual axons, whether crossed or uncrossed, pass directly through the chiasm into the ipsi-lateral (uncrossed) or contralateral (crossed) optic tract. However, as they enter the chiasm, some ventral crossed fibers, primarily from the inferonasal retina of the con-tralateral eye and serving the superotemporal portion of the contralateral visual field, were historically believed to loop anteriorly 1 to 2 mm into the terminal portion of the opposite optic nerve before turning posteriorly to continue through the chiasm and into the optic tract (Fig. 2.30). This loop is called **Wilbrand's knee**. There is conflicting evidence as to whether Wilbrand's knee is a true anatomic structure or an artifact that develops in both humans and nonhuman primates with long-stand-ing unilateral optic atrophy. Regardless, Wilbrand's knee clearly exists from a clinical standpoint in that patients with a monocular optic neuropathy caused by a lesion that has damaged the distal optic nerve at its junction

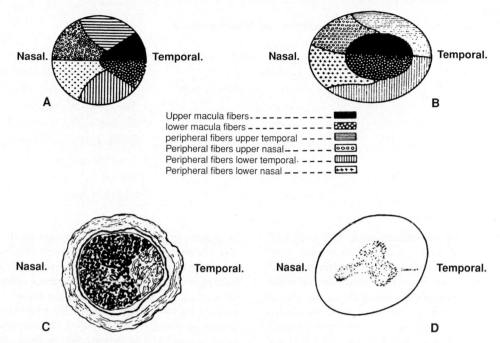

Upper macula fibers - - - - - - - - - -
lower macula fibers - - - - - - - - - - -
peripheral fibers upper temporal - - - -
Peripheral fibers upper nasal - - - - - -
Peripheral fibers lower temporal - - - -
Peripheral fibers lower nasal - - - - - -

Figure 2.29 Fiber arrangement in the optic nerve. **A:** In the distal portion of the optic nerve. **B:** In the proximal portion of the optic nerve. **C:** A transverse section of the optic nerve in its distal portion in a case of atrophy of the papillomacular bundle. **D:** Secondary degeneration in the proximal portion of the optic nerve after a macular lesion. (Reprinted with permission from Duke-Elder S. *Textbook of Ophthalmology*. Vol 1. St. Louis, MO: CV Mosby; 1932.)

Figure 2.30 Dark-field autoradiograph of a horizontal section through the optic chiasm of a macaque monkey. The right eye was enucleated 4 years earlier, at which time the left eye was injected with H3-proline. The radioactive label from the left eye appears bright. Note the extension of label representing Wilbrand's knee into the distal aspect of the atrophic right optic nerve. (Courtesy of Dr. Jonathan Horton.)

with the optic chiasm not infrequently have an asymptomatic superior temporal defect in the visual field of the contralateral eye (see Chapter 12).

Topographic Diagnosis of Retinal Lesions

Retinal diseases may be divided into two main groups: (1) those affecting the detecting apparatus—the receptor cells and their synapses; and (2) those affecting the conducting apparatus—the ganglion cells and their axons (i.e., the NFL). In many cases, the diagnosis is obvious from the appearance of the affected region of the retina. In other cases, however, it is possible to diagnose retinal dysfunction only from other aspects of the clinical examination. Indeed, patients with "unexplained visual loss" may, in fact, have a disorder of the retina that may not be obvious during a clinical examination. Features that help distinguish retinal disease from optic nerve disease are noted in Table 2.3.

Distinguishing Retinal Disease from an Optic Neuropathy by Clinical Examination

Central **visual acuity** may or may not be affected by disease that damages the retina. Disorders that cause

Table 2.3	Distinguishing Optic Neuropathies and Maculopathies	
Features	**Optic Nerve**	**Macula**
Presenting deficit	Dark/black area(s) in field	Distortions; floaters; cobwebs
Pain	Sometimes with eye movement	Rarely; not with eye movement
Refractive error	Unchanged	Sometimes hyperopia
Color vision	Very reduced	Normal or slightly reduced
Brightness sense	Very reduced	Variable; may have photophobia
Photostress test	Normal recovery	Prolonged recovery
Relative afferent pupillary defect	Present	Absent
Amsler grid	Scotoma	Metamorphopsia

dysfunction only of extramacular retina typically are unassociated with a reduction in central acuity, whereas macular disorders and disorders that damage the entire retina invariably reduce central vision. Most disorders that affect the macula are detected by a careful funduscopic examination, particularly when the macula is examined with a slit lamp biomicroscope using a corneal contact lens, a 78- or 90-diopter handheld lens, or a Hruby lens. Nevertheless, some disorders, such as central serous chorioretinopathy, cystoid macular edema, and epiretinal membrane formation (surface wrinkling retinopathy, cellophane maculopathy) can easily be overlooked (Fig. 2.31).

In other diseases that affect the macula, such as macular cone dystrophy, there often are no changes that can be observed in the macula even though the patient has decreased central vision and a visual field defect. In such cases, the diagnosis of retinal disease may be suspected if there is associated metamorphopsia (an irregularity or distortion in the appearance of viewed objects), photophobia, nyctalopia (night blindness), or hemeralopia (the inability to see as distinctly in a bright light as in a dim one). These symptoms occur much more often in patients with ocular disease than in patients with neurologic disease. Photophobia should be obvious during the examination. Metamorphopsia is usually caused by a distortion of the normal alignment of the photoreceptors. When there is increased separation among cones (and among rods to a lesser extent because of the central position of the lesion), there is an apparent decrease in the size of objects (micropsia). The foveal cones are already so close to each other that it is unlikely that an apparent increase in the size of objects (macropsia) can occur from further crowding together of these cells. Evidence of metamorphopsia may be detected in patients with and without the complaint of distortion of objects by using an Amsler grid. The results of a photostress test usually are abnormal

Figure 2.31 Subtle macular lesions causing visual loss. **A:** Subtle pigmentary change in the macula of a patient complaining of blurred vision in the left eye. **B:** Epiretinal membrane overlying the papillomacular bundle in a patient with distorted vision in the left eye.

Figure 2.32 Subtle macular lesions in two patients with unexplained visual loss thought to be due to malingering. **A and B:** A 13-year-old girl complained of loss of vision (20/80 OU) in both eyes. **A:** The left macula looks normal except for a blunted foveal reflex. **B:** Fluorescein angiography shows impressive pigment epithelial changes in the macula, consistent with her decreased vision. Identical changes were seen in the right fundus. A diagnosis of macular dystrophy was made. **C and D:** A 24-year-old man experienced recent painless blurred vision in his right eye (20/30). **C:** The foveal reflex is blunted. **D:** Fluorescein angiogram shows a pigment epithelial detachment with leakage superior to the fovea, consistent with a diagnosis of central serous chorioretinopathy.

in such patients, as are the results of fluorescein angiography, OCT, and/or multifocal electroretinography (Figs. 2.32 and 2.33) (see Chapter 1).

Color vision is often but not always abnormal in patients with retinal disease. For instance, patients with central serous chorioretinopathy and epiretinal membrane formation rarely have any significant dyschromatopsia, whereas patients with macular cone or cone–rod dystrophies usually do; such patients may even develop difficulties with color vision as the initial sign of the disease. In such cases, the correct diagnosis is not made until other studies such as electroretinography are performed. Retinal disorders are more likely to produce either generalized loss of color vision or a blue-yellow dyschromatopsia, but there are sufficient exceptions that make the pattern of color vision loss an unreliable diagnostic criterion.

A **relative afferent pupillary defect** can only be detected clinically in patients with unilateral or asymmetric retinal disease if the retinal disease is severe, affects most of the retina or the entire macula, and is obvious during a funduscopic examination (Fig. 2.34). If a relative afferent pupillary defect is observed in a patient with decreased visual acuity associated with some macular drusen, central serous chorioretinopathy, cystoid macular edema, an epiretinal membrane,

Figure 2.33 Unexplained visual loss from macular disease diagnosed by optical coherence tomography (OCT). The patient was a 54-year-old man with progressive visual loss in both eyes over several years. **A and B:** Right and left maculae show loss of the foveal reflex but appear otherwise normal. Fluorescein angiography showed no abnormalities. **C:** OCT of the peripapillary retinal nerve fiber layer shows no abnormalities in either eye. **D:** OCT of the maculae shows marked thinning bilaterally. The patient was diagnosed with a macular cone dystrophy.

or a normal-appearing fundus, a lesion affecting the optic nerve must be assumed.

Distinguishing Retinal Disease from an Optic Neuropathy by Visual Field

When the photoreceptors are affected, the defect in the visual field corresponds to the retinal defect in position, shape, extent, and intensity. When the ganglion cell or NFL is damaged, however, the field defect does not conform to the size and shape of the lesion but rather to the field represented by the RGCs whose fibers are damaged. Thus, a small lesion situated close to the optic disc that damages only photoreceptors

usually causes a small scotoma, whereas a lesion of the same size that damages the RGCs and nerve fibers in the same area may result in an extensive defect in the visual field. Conversely, a small lesion in the periphery that damages only a few fibers transmitting impulses from widely separated RGCs may produce such a small field defect that it may be difficult or even impossible to detect.

Any visual field defect that can be produced by an inner retinal lesion can also be produced by a lesion of the optic nerve. For example, damage to the papillomacular area of the retina results in a central scotoma that connects to the physiologic blind spot; this is a **cecocentral scotoma** (Fig. 2.35A). Cecocentral scotomas are

A   B

Figure 2.34 Macular lesions associated with an ipsilateral relative afferent pupillary defect. **A:** Extensive macular degeneration with hemorrhage. **B:** Scar from presumed ocular histoplasmosis. Note that both lesions are quite obvious and would not be overlooked during an ophthalmoscopic examination, even if the pupils were not dilated.

A   B

C

Figure 2.35 Optic nerve and retinal disease causing a cecocentral scotoma. **A:** Kinetic perimetry shows a dense cecocentral scotoma in the field of the right eye. This type of scotoma could be caused by optic nerve dysfunction such as that seen in a toxic optic neuropathy (**B**) or from retinal disease such as serous detachment of the retina involving the papillomacular bundle associated with an optic disc pit (**C**).

Figure 2.36 Optic nerve and retinal disease causing an arcuate field defect. **A:** Static perimetry reveals a dense inferior arcuate field defect. This type of defect could be caused by a superior branch retinal artery occlusion (**B**) or glaucoma with superior extension and an acquired pit (**C**).

typically present in patients with toxic and nutritional optic neuropathies and Leber hereditary optic neuropathy; however, retinal dysfunction such as a serous detachment of the retina extending from the optic disc to the macula also can cause such a scotoma (Fig. 2.35B and C). Similarly, an **arcuate visual field defect** can result from damage to retinal nerve fibers or ganglion cells in the superior or inferior arcuate nerve fiber bundles (Fig. 2.36A). This visual field defect may occur in patients with occlusion of the blood supply of the superior or inferior portion of the macula such as that, which occurs from a branch retinal artery occlusion or in patients with a glaucomatous or nonglaucoma optic neuropathy (Fig. 2.36B and C). In both settings, the scotoma is associated with normal visual acuity since it does not completely affect the macula. Indeed, virtually any lesion, whether ischemic, inflammatory, infiltrative, or compressive, can cause an arcuate field defect and may be located in either the retina or the optic nerve.

Annular or ring scotomas occur in a variety of conditions, most notably in patients with various pig-

mentary retinopathies. Ring scotomas may also occur in patients with open angle glaucoma, but in such cases, the ring is actually caused by the coalescence of upper and lower arcuate scotomas originating from the physiologic blind spot and extending across the vertical midline into the nasal visual field. Similar defects may be seen in various optic neuropathies, particularly those caused by ischemia, compression, and inflammation.

In general, a unilateral temporal or nasal hemianopia that respects the vertical midline is either nonorganic or caused by dysfunction of the optic nerve (see Chapter 4). Nevertheless, a unilateral hemianopia very rarely can be caused by sectoral retinitis pigmentosa.

The **blind spot** also plays a role in the interpretation of the visual field. It represents the negative scotoma that is the projection of the optic disc. The optic disc is located nasal to the fovea, and its center is slightly above it. Thus, the blind spot is temporal to the point of fixation, and its center is slightly below it.

A   B

Figure 2.37 Enlargement of the blind spot in a patient with papilledema. **A:** The blind spot of the left eye is enlarged. **B:** There is moderate (Frisén Grade 3) generalized swelling of the left optic disc. The patient had normal visual acuity in the eye and similar findings in the contralateral eye.

The blind spot becomes enlarged from peripapillary retinal dysfunction. This dysfunction can occur because the peripapillary retina is diseased, as occurs in patients with the so-called "big blind spot syndrome" and related disorders such as acute zonal occult outer retinopathy (AZOOR) and the multiple evanescent white dot syndrome (MEWDS), or because expansion of the optic disc tissue encroaches on the peripapillary retina, as occurs in optic disc swelling and in pseudopapilledema (Fig. 2.37).

Appearance of the Optic Disc in Retinal Disease

The optic nerve is composed primarily of axons whose cell bodies are the ganglion cells of the retina. Thus, any retinal disorder that directly or indirectly damages the ganglion cells or their axons in the retinal NFL will eventually produce optic atrophy. Indeed, damage to the ganglion cell body or the NFL is tantamount to damage to the optic nerve; that is, there will be visual

A   B

Figure 2.38 Optic atrophy in vitamin A deficiency. The patient was a woman who developed bilateral visual loss and cecocentral scotomas several years after a jejunoileal bypass for morbid obesity. An electroretinogram revealed evidence of a retinopathy affecting the photoreceptors, and laboratory studies revealed a reduced concentration of vitamin A in the patient's serum. The patient's visual function improved after vitamin A therapy. Both the right **(A)** and left **(B)** optic discs are pale. (Courtesy of Dr. Eric Eggenberger.)

loss, a relative afferent pupillary defect if the damage is unilateral or asymmetric, and ultimately optic atrophy. Because the central retinal arterial and venous circulations subserve the inner layers of the retina (including the ganglion cell and NFL s), retinal vascular occlusive events will result in inner retinal damage, visual loss, and eventual optic atrophy. Acute vascular events involving the retina—including central and branch retinal artery occlusions, ophthalmic artery occlusions, and central retinal vein occlusions—have a dramatic and distinct funduscopic appearance, permitting immediate correct diagnosis. However, over time, the retinal findings resolve, and the optic disc becomes pale. In such cases, subsequent narrowing and sheathing of

the retinal arteries or the presence of a visible embolus within the retinal circulation may provide clues as to the etiology of the original event.

Loss of the NFL and optic atrophy are not uncommon in patients with various photoreceptor dystrophies and degenerations, particularly those affecting the cones. Clues that suggest retinal cone dysfunction include profound dyschromatopsia, photophobia and hemeralopia, retinal arterial attenuation, and, eventually, changes in the appearance of the maculae, often resembling a bull's eye (bull's eye maculopathy). Bilateral secondary optic atrophy can be seen in patients with cone dystrophies, rod/cone dystrophies, paraneoplastic retinopathies, and the retinopathy of vitamin A deficiency (Fig. 2.38).

Congenital Anomalies of the Optic Disc

Anomalous Optic Disc Elevation (Pseudopapilledema)
Pseudopapilledema Associated with
Optic Disc Drusen
Anomalous Disc Elevation without Drusen

Optic Nerve Hypoplasia
Clinical Features
Associated Endocrinologic Deficiencies
Associated Central Nervous System Malformations
Systemic and Teratogenic Associations
Segmental Optic Nerve Hypoplasia
Pathogenesis

Excavated Optic Disc Anomalies
Morning Glory Disc Anomaly
Optic Disc Coloboma
Peripapillary Staphyloma
Megalopapilla
Optic Pit
Papillorenal Syndrome

Congenital Tilted Disc Syndrome

Optic Disc Dysplasia

Congenital Optic Disc Pigmentation

Aicardi Syndrome

Doubling of the Optic Disc

Optic Nerve Aplasia

Myelinated (Medullated) Nerve Fibers

Ophthalmologists and neurologists frequently are asked to evaluate patients with anomalous optic discs. A comprehensive evaluation requires an understanding of the ophthalmoscopic features, associated neuro-ophthalmologic findings, pathogenesis, and appropriate ancillary studies for each anomaly. Increased recognition of the ocular and systemic associations related to each anomaly has advanced our understanding of its pathogenesis. For instance, different forms of excavated optic disc anomalies that were previously lumped together as colobomatous defects are now subclassified. This has enhanced our ability to predict the likelihood of associated central nervous system (CNS) anomalies based solely on the appearance of the optic disc. In addition, the widespread clinical application of computed tomographic (CT) scans and magnetic resonance imaging (MRI) has enabled us to more accurately identify associated CNS anomalies and predict the likelihood of subsequent neurodevelopmental and endocrinologic problems.

Certain general principles are particularly useful in the evaluation and management of patients with anomalous optic discs.

1 Children with bilateral optic disc anomalies generally present in infancy with poor vision and nystagmus; those with unilateral optic disc anomalies generally present during their preschool years with sensory esotropia.
2 CNS malformations are common in patients with malformed optic discs. Small discs are associated with a variety of malformations of the cerebral hemispheres, pituitary infundibulum, and midline intracranial structures (septum pellucidum, corpus callosum). Large optic discs of the morning glory configuration are associated with the transsphenoidal form of basal encephalocele, whereas colobomatous optic discs may be associated with systemic anomalies and a variety of syndromes.
3 Any structural ocular abnormality that reduces visual acuity in infancy may lead to superimposed amblyopia. A trial of occlusion therapy may be warranted in young children with unilateral optic disc anomalies and decreased vision.

Anomalous Optic Disc Elevation (Pseudopapilledema)

Anomalous optic disc elevation (pseudopapilledema) may bear a striking resemblance to true optic disc swelling. As most patients with pseudopapilledema have no visual symptoms, this condition is often mistaken for papilledema. In most instances, a patient is noted to have elevated optic discs or blurred disc margins during the course of a routine examination. The diagnostic uncertainty and alarm created by this finding overshadows the fact that the patient has no other signs or symptoms of increased intracranial pressure. Many patients with pseudopapilledema thus are referred for neuro-ophthalmologic evaluation only after being subjected to neuroimaging, lumbar puncture, and extensive laboratory studies.

Pseudopapilledema may be caused by underlying optic disc drusen that may be superficial and obvious on funduscopic examination or deep ("buried") and identifiable only with ancillary studies such as optical coherence tomography, ultrasonography, or CT scanning. In other cases, no drusen are present. In such cases, the nerve may be smaller than normal (i.e., optic nerve hypoplasia) or tilted, resulting in general or focal elevation of the disc tissue.

Pseudopapilledema Associated with Optic Disc Drusen

The word drusen, of Germanic origin, originally meant tumor, swelling, or tumescence. The word was used in the mining industry approximately 500 years ago to indicate a crystal-filled space in a rock. Other terms for these lesions include **hyaline bodies** and **colloid bodies** of the optic disc. It is unfortunate that the term "drusen" is used both for these lesions and for the hypopigmented lesions of the retinal pigment epithelium that may precede the development of macular degeneration.

Drusen of the optic disc are homogeneous, globular concretions, often collected in larger, multilobulated agglomerations. They usually exhibit a concentrically laminated structure that is not encapsulated and contains no cells or cellular debris. Optic disc axons are atrophic adjacent to large accumulations of drusen, whereas axons not adjacent to the drusen are normal. Drusen take up calcium salts and must be decalcified before being cut into sections for histopathologic study. According to most investigators, drusen are composed predominantly of a mucoprotein matrix with significant quantities of acid mucopolysaccharides, small quantities of ribonucleic acid and, occasionally, iron. Drusen are insoluble in most of the common solvents.

The primary pathology of optic disc drusen appears to be an inherited dysplasia of the optic canal or of the optic disc and its vasculature, resulting in narrowing of the lamina cribrosa and, thus, of the exit space of optic nerve axons from the eye. The small optic disc size and absence of a central cup in eyes with disc drusen are consistent with the concept of axon crowding. The crowding, in turn, leads to abnormal axon metabolism, with deposition of calcium crystals in mitochondria of intact axons. The axons subsequently become disrupted, and the mitochondria are extruded into the extracellular space, where a higher concentration of calcium ions causes further calcium deposition into the mitochondria. Eventually, these calcified mitochondria coalesce to form drusen.

The prevalence of optic disc drusen depends on the method of analysis. For example, in a clinical series from Scandinavia, the prevalence of optic drusen was 0.3%, whereas the prevalence of drusen in autopsy series is, as might be expected, somewhat higher, varying between 0.4% and 2.0%. Men and women are equally affected, with bilateral drusen occurring in 67% to 85% of cases. The age at which visible drusen or pseudopapilledema caused by buried drusen is diagnosed varies widely, depending on the population studies. Familial drusen are transmitted as an autosomal-dominant trait. The prevalence of disc drusen in African Americans is low, possibly attributable to racial variation in optic disc size.

The evolution of disc drusen is a dynamic process that continues throughout life. It is rare to see visible drusen or significant optic disc elevation in an infant. During childhood, however, the affected optic disc begins to appear "full" and acquires a tan, yellow, or straw color (Fig. 3.1A). The buried drusen gradually impart a scalloped appearance to the margin of the disc and produce subtle excrescences on the disc surface that tend to predominate nasally (Fig. 3.1B). These later enlarge, calcify, and become more visible on the disc surface (Fig. 3.1C). As they enlarge, they sometimes deflect retinal vessels overlying the disc. In adulthood, the optic disc elevation diminishes, the disc gradually becomes pale, the nerve fiber layer thins, and discrete slits appear. This evolution reflects a slow attrition of optic axons over decades. Despite this progression, most patients remain asymptomatic and retain normal acuity.

Although all drusen are located anterior to the lamina cribrosa, drusen may be classified as superficial or buried. Superficial drusen can be identified easily by their ophthalmoscopic appearance. Buried drusen, however, can only be suspected by the general appearance of the optic disc and surrounding peripapillary retina but cannot be diagnosed with certainty without ancillary testing such as OCT or CT scanning.

Superficial drusen appear as round, slightly irregular excrescences that are present within and occasionally around the disc (Figs. 3.1B and C and 3.2). They may be scattered or form conglomerates that cover the disc, reflect whitish yellow light, are globular, and vary in size from minute dots to granules 2 or 3 times the diameter of a retinal vessel. In some cases, drusen located just below the disc surface may be illuminated when indirect lighting is used.

Drusen buried within the tissue of the disc produce moderate elevation of the surface of the disc, as well as blurring of its margins (Figs. 3.1A and B and 3.3). It is this appearance that mimics true disc swelling; however, the anomalously elevated disc is not hyperemic, and there are no dilated capillaries on its surface. In addition, despite obvious elevation of the disc, the surface vessels, even small ones, are not obscured, the physiologic cup is absent, and the peripapillary

Figure 3.1 Evolution from buried to visible optic disc drusen over 20 years. **A:** At initial diagnosis. **B:** 5 years later. **C:** 10 years later.

Figure 3.2 Visible optic disc drusen. Note globular glistening appearance with elevation of vessels overlying the optic disc.

retinal nerve fiber layer retains its normal linear pattern unless there are abnormalities indicative of nerve fiber layer atrophy. Anomalously elevated discs are smaller than normal and sometimes have an irregular border with pigment epithelial defects being present. The most elevated portion of the disc is usually the central area from which the vessels emerge. In a large percentage of cases, there are anomalous vascular patterns on the disc surface, including an increased number of otherwise normal vessels, abnormal arterial and venous branchings, increased tortuosity, vascular loops, and cilioretinal arteries.

The distinction between pseudopapilledema associated with buried drusen and papilledema (or other forms of optic disc swelling) can be difficult, but several clinical signs are particularly helpful (Table 3.1).

The differentiation between papilledema and pseudopapilledema caused by buried drusen is frequently aided by ancillary studies. Special photographic techniques may be useful in identifying superficial or buried optic disc drusen. Monochromatic (red-free) photography may highlight the glistening drusen against the intact or atrophic nerve fiber layer. Photographs taken with the filters normally used for fluorescein photography in place, but without injection of fluorescein, show that superficial disc drusen often demonstrate the phenomenon of autofluorescence (Fig. 3.4B). Fluorescein angiography also can facilitate the differentiation between true papilledema and pseudopapilledema. After intravenous fluorescein injection, drusen exhibit a true nodular hyperfluorescence corresponding to the location of the visible drusen (Fig. 3.4C). The late phases may be characterized by minimal blurring of the drusen that either fade or maintain fluorescence (i.e., stain). Unlike in papilledema, however, there is no visible leakage along the major vessels. Fluorescein angiography also may disclose venous anomalies (venous stasis, venous convolutions, and retinociliary venous communications) and staining of the peripapillary vein walls in eyes with optic disc drusen. In addition to the above photographic techniques, CT scanning (often obtained when papilledema is suspected), OCT (particularly using enhanced depth imaging), and ultrasonography will

A

B

Figure 3.3 Buried optic disc drusen. **A:** The right optic disc is elevated. Two druse are visible (*arrows*). **B:** The left optic disc is diffusely elevated, but it is not hyperemic and the vessels crossing its surface, even the smallest, are easily seen. A small subretinal peripapillary hemorrhage is present (*arrow*).

Table 3.1   Ophthalmoscopic Features Useful in Differentiating Acquired Optic Disc Swelling from Pseudopapilledema Associated with Buried Drusen

Optic Disc Swelling	Pseudopapilledema with Buried Drusen
Disc vasculature obscured at disc margins	Disc vasculature remains visible at disc margins
Elevation extends into peripapillary retina	Elevation confined to optic disc
Graying and muddying of peripapillary nerve fiber layer	Sharp peripapillary nerve fiber
Venous congestion	No venous congestion
± exudates	No exudates
Loss of optic cup only in moderate to severe disc swelling	Small cupless disc
Normal configuration of disc vasculature despite venous congestion	Increased major retinal vessels with early branching
No circumpapillary light reflex	Crescentic circumpapillary light reflex
Absence of spontaneous venous pulsations	Spontaneous venous pulsations may be present or absent

A

B

C

Figure 3.4 Fluorescent characteristics of optic disc drusen. **A:** Fundus photograph of optic disc drusen. **B:** Autofluorescence of drusen observed through a fluorescein filter but without injection of fluorescein dye. **C:** Late staining of drusen after fluorescein angiogram.

Figure 3.5 Methods of diagnosing buried optic disc drusen. **A:** Optical coherence tomography shows a circular appearance of a druse. **B:** B-scan ultrasonography in a patient with deep (buried) optic disc drusen. The area of disc elevation is clearly seen as is a focal area of brightness (*arrow*). **C:** Noncontrast axial computed tomographic scan (bone-window level) in a patient with bilateral buried drusen shows a focus of increased density at the site of each optic disc.

all demonstrate calcifications within the elevated optic disc associated with optic disc drusen (Fig. 3.5).

Although patients with pseudopapilledema are not immune to the neurologic and ophthalmologic disorders of the general population, there is no significant relationship between drusen and neurologic disorders.

Most patients with optic disc drusen are asymptomatic and remain so throughout life. Nevertheless, such patients occasionally experience visual loss.

Acute visual loss is rare in patients with optic disc drusen (see below); however, **peripheral visual field defects** eventually develop in up to 75% of eyes with disc drusen. In most cases, the field defects are asymptomatic (at least initially) because they develop over decades, reflecting the insidious atrophy of optic nerve fibers. Nevertheless, a minority of patients experience episodes of sudden, step-like visual field loss. Visual field defects are much more common in eyes with visible drusen than in those with pseudopapilledema. The defects are of many types, including nasal steps, arcuate defects, sector defects, enlargement of the blind spot; and concentric visual field constric-

tion (Fig. 3.6). A relative afferent pupillary defect may result from unilateral or asymmetric visual field loss in the absence of central acuity loss.

The pathogenesis of visual field loss in patients with optic disc drusen is unclear. In some cases, it is assumed that there is impaired axon transport in an eye with a small scleral canal, leading to gradual attrition of optic nerve fibers. In others, direct compression of prelaminar nerve fibers or of arterioles or capillaries supplying the anterior optic nerve are thought to be responsible.

At the heart of the controversy is whether or not drusen produce damage to nerve fibers through direct axon or vascular compression, or if they are merely an epiphenomenon of a chronic low-grade axon stasis that produces a slowly progressive diminution in optic axons. Several studies have been unable to correlate the location of visible disc drusen with the location of field defects.

Central visual loss is a rare but well-documented complication of disc drusen that should be considered only when no other causes can be identified. In these cases, the visual loss usually follows a series of

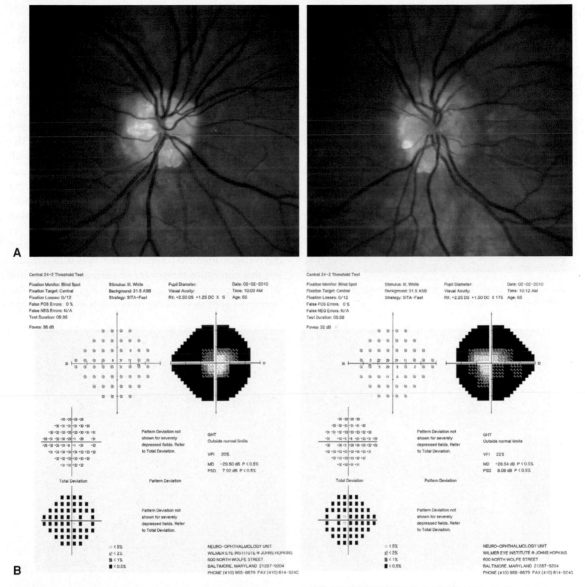

Figure 3.6 Visual fields in a patient with bilateral extensive optic disc drusen. **A:** Both optic discs are filled with drusen. **B:** There is marked constriction of the fields of both eyes.

episodic, step-like events that progressively diminish the peripheral visual field. In other cases, the decreased acuity is associated with a new field defect and true optic disc swelling associated with peripapillary retinal hemorrhages; that is, the picture of anterior ischemic optic neuropathy.

Prepapillary or peripapillary hemorrhages may develop in eyes with disc drusen. Such hemorrhages may be small, superficial, and located on the optic disc, in which case they tend to be single and prepapillary in location, in contrast to the multiple nerve fiber layer hemorrhages that characterize papilledema. In other cases, there may be a large, superficial hemorrhage

overlying the optic disc and, on occasion, extending into the vitreous. Most often, however, the hemorrhages associated with optic disc drusen are peripapillary, subretinal, or subepithelial, and circumferentially oriented around the disc (Figs. 3.3 and 3.7). Most patients with optic disc drusen and hemorrhages have a good visual prognosis.

Retinal vascular occlusions, both arterial and venous, can occur in patients with optic disc drusen. They tend to occur in young adults but rarely may be seen in children. Retinal vascular occlusions that occur in eyes with disc drusen could result from vascular crowding secondary to the small scleral canal size in eyes with drusen, anomalous

Figure 3.7 Peripapillary subretinal hemorrhage (*arrow*) in a patient with buried drusen.

optic disc vasculature that may make it more susceptible to the effects of disrupted hemodynamics, or mechanical displacement of the prelaminar vasculature by the calcified fixed drusen.

Transient visual loss occurred in 8.6% of the patients with disc drusen in one large study. This phenomenon may occur because of anomalous elevation of the optic disc. Like papilledema, optic disc drusen produce increased interstitial pressure and decreased perfusion pressure in the intraocular portion of the optic nerve. Thus, minor fluctuations in arterial, venous, or cerebrospinal fluid pressure may result in brief but critical decrements in perfusion, leading to transient obscurations of vision. Rarely, transient visual loss is a harbinger of retinal vascular occlusion in patients with disc drusen.

Peripapillary subretinal neovascularization is a rare but well-documented complication in eyes with disc drusen that can cause temporary or permanent visual loss when it occurs in the macular region (Fig. 3.8). This phenomenon appears to occur more often in children than

Figure 3.8 Subretinal neovascularization in a child with intrapapillary drusen. **A:** The right optic disc is moderately elevated and has blurred disc margins, but there is no hyperemia, there is no obscuration of the vessels crossing its surface, and the peripapillary retinal nerve fiber layer is not distorted. These features are consistent with anomalous elevation of the disc caused by buried drusen. **B:** The left optic disc also is elevated and several drusen can be seen within it. Temporal to the disc there is a large hyperpigmented area of subretinal neovascularization. **C:** In the arteriovenous phase of the fluorescein angiogram, there is diffuse staining of the left optic disc and there is both staining and leakage of dye from the area of subretinal neovascularization. (Courtesy of Drs. Sandra Brown and Monte del Monte.)

A   B

Figure 3.9 Optic disc drusen in a patient with retinitis pigmentosa. **A:** The optic disc is pale and there are drusen within the substance of the disc and at its margins. Note marked thinning of the retinal arteries. **B:** There is extensive pigment spicule formation in the mid-peripheral retina.

in adults. Optimum management of this complication remains unclear. Both observation and photocoagulation of the area of neovascularization have been used.

Optic nerve head drusen usually are unassociated with any systemic, ocular, or neurologic conditions. They were once thought to be more common in patients with brain tumors and in patients with migraine headaches; however, the concurrence of brain tumors or migraine and optic disc drusen probably reflects the frequent and often expedited referral of patients with headaches and optic disc elevation. On the other hand, drusen occasionally occur in patients with **retinitis pigmentosa**, in which cases the drusen often are located at the disc margin in the superficial retina and the disc is neither elevated nor anomalous but is flat and waxy yellow (Fig. 3.9).

There is an association between disc drusen and angioid streaks. Using ultrasonography or OCT, disc drusen can be detected in about 20% of patients with pseudoxanthoma elasticum and in 25% of patients with angioid streaks with no pseudoxanthoma elasticum.

Optic disc drusen also may occur as part of the **Riley–Smith syndrome** of macrocephaly, multiple hemangiomata, and pseudopapilledema.

Anomalous Disc Elevation without Drusen

Not all anomalously elevated optic discs are associated with superficial or buried drusen. For example, the morning glory syndrome is associated with disc elevation, the superotemporal portion of a tilted optic disc usually is elevated, dysplastic discs may show some degree of elevation, and hypoplastic discs often have generalized elevation that may seem out of proportion to the size of the disc (Fig. 3.10). Thus it is essential that patients with elevated optic discs but with no clinical or imaging evidence of drusen not be automatically assumed to have true optic disc swelling.

Optic Nerve Hypoplasia

Optic nerve hypoplasia is the most common optic disc anomaly encountered in ophthalmologic practice. According to one study, it occurs in 1 in 2,287 live births. In another study from Sweden, it was present in 17.3/100,000 children and adolescents younger than 18 years of age. It may be unilateral or bilateral.

Clinical Features

Ophthalmoscopically, the hypoplastic disc appears as an abnormally small optic nerve head (Fig. 3.11). It may appear gray or pale and is often surrounded by a yellowish mottled peripapillary halo, bordered by a ring of increased or decreased pigmentation ("double-ring" sign), which facilitates recognition of the anomaly (Fig. 3.12). Optic nerve hypoplasia often is associated with tortuosity of the retinal veins.

Optic nerve hypoplasia is characterized histopathologically by a subnormal number of optic nerve axons with normal mesodermal elements and glial supporting tissue. The double-ring sign correlates to a normal junction between the sclera and lamina cribrosa, which corresponds to the outer ring, and the termination of an abnormal extension of retina and pigment epithelium over the lamina cribrosa, which corresponds to the inner ring.

Figure 3.10 Anomalous optic disc elevation without drusen. The patient had no visual or systemic symptoms and a normal examination. **A:** The right optic disc is elevated, but it is not hyperemic nor is there any obscuration of the vessels crossing the disc surface. **B:** The left optic disc is also elevated. It also is smaller than normal. There were no drusen by either optical coherence tomography or B-scan ultrasonography.

Figure 3.11 Optic nerve hypoplasia. **A:** Bilateral hypoplasia. Note classic double-ring sign. **B:** Unilateral hypoplasia. The right optic disc (**left**) is about half normal size and there is a prominent double-ring sign. The left disc (**right**) is normal in size and configuration.

Figure 3.12 Optic nerve hypoplasia. The optic disc is small and surrounded by a rim of variably pigmented tissue.

Visual acuity in optic nerve hypoplasia ranges from 20/20 to no light perception, and affected eyes show localized visual field defects, often combined with generalized constriction. Because visual acuity is determined primarily by the integrity of the papillomacular nerve fiber bundle, it does not necessarily correlate with the overall size of the disc. The strong association of astigmatism with optic nerve hypoplasia warrants careful attention to correction of refractive errors. In addition, unilateral optic nerve hypoplasia may be associated with amblyopia, in which case occlusion therapy may result in visual improvement. Decreased vision associated with optic nerve hypoplasia should remain stable throughout the patient's life unless another process is superimposed such as cataract formation or retinal disease such as a traction retinal detachment or peripheral retinal nonperfusion as occur in some patients. Thus, any patient with progressive visual loss in the setting of optic nerve hypoplasia should be evaluated for some other underlying cause such as an intracranial mass compressing the anterior visual pathway.

It is often difficult to distinguish between a normal and a hypoplastic disc; indeed, large optic discs can be axonally deficient, and small optic discs do not preclude normal visual function. Other variables also must be considered, including the size of the central cup, the percentage of the nerve occupied by axons (as opposed to glial tissue and blood vessels), and the cross-sectional area and density of axons. Furthermore, segmental forms of optic nerve hypoplasia (see below) affect only one sector of the disc and, thus, not produce a diffuse diminution in the size of the disc. As such, it would seem prudent to reserve the diagnosis of optic nerve hypoplasia for patients with small optic discs who have reduced vision or visual field loss with corresponding nerve fiber bundle defects.

Associated Endocrinologic Deficiencies

Optic nerve hypoplasia frequently is associated with other CNS anomalies and these, in turn, may produce significant endocrinologic dysfunction. Septo-optic dysplasia (de Morsier syndrome) refers to the constellation of small anterior visual pathways, absence of the septum pellucidum, and thinning or agenesis of the corpus callosum. Growth hormone deficiency is the most common endocrinologic deficiency associated with optic nerve hypoplasia in this setting, but hypothyroidism, hypocortisolism, diabetes insipidus, and hyperprolactinemia also may occur. Estimates of the prevalence of pituitary hormone deficiency in children with septo-optic dysplasia are as high as 62%, but these clinical reports are strongly skewed toward cases with endocrinologic manifestations, and the true prevalence probably is closer to 15%. Children with septo-optic dysplasia and corticotropin deficiency are at risk for sudden death during febrile illness. This is explained by their impaired ability to increase corticotropin secretion to maintain blood pressure and blood sugar in response to the physical stress of infection. These children may have coexistent diabetes insipidus that contributes to dehydration during illness and hastens the development of shock. Some also have hypothalamic thermoregulatory disturbances signaled by episodes of hypothermia during well periods and high fevers during illnesses, which may predispose to life-threatening hyperthermia. Because corticotropin deficiency represents the preeminent threat to life in children with septo-optic dysplasia, a complete anterior pituitary hormone evaluation, including provocative serum cortisol testing and assessment for diabetes insipidus, should be performed in these children. In addition, children with an intact septum pellucidum and optic nerve hypoplasia still may have endocrinologic deficiency. In such children, anterior pituitary hormone deficiencies may evolve over time in some patients; thus, longitudinal reevaluation and periodic monitoring of anterior pituitary hormone function are indicated in children with posterior pituitary ectopia as well as in children who have clinical symptoms (history of hypoglycemia, dehydration, or hypothermia) or neuroimaging signs (absent pituitary infundibulum with or without posterior pituitary ectopia) of pituitary hormone deficiency.

Associated Central Nervous System Malformations

MRI is the optimum noninvasive neuroimaging modality for delineating CNS malformations in

Figure 3.13 Septo-optic dysplasia. **A:** "Bowtie" optic disc pallor and small-diameter optic disc in the right eye and normal optic disc in the left eye. **B:** Visual fields show temporal hemianopia in the right eye and a normal result in the left eye. **C:** Postcontrast T1 coronal MRI shows a thin right optic nerve just anterior to the optic chiasm, absent septum pellucidum, and normal-appearing pituitary gland (**left**); midorbital view shows a thin right optic nerve (**right**). (From Brooks DB, Subramanian PS. Monocular temporal hemianopia with septo-optic dysplasia. *J Neuroophthalmol.* 2006;26:195–196, with permission.)

patients with optic nerve hypoplasia. In optic nerve hypoplasia, coronal and sagittal T1-weighted MRI consistently demonstrates thinning and attenuation of hypoplastic prechiasmatic intracranial optic nerves (Fig. 3.13). In addition, there is diffuse thinning of the optic chiasm in patients with bilateral optic nerve hypoplasia, and focal thinning or absence of the side of the chiasm corresponding to the hypoplastic nerve in unilateral optic nerve hypoplasia. When MRI shows a decrease in intracranial optic nerve size accompanied by other features of septo-optic dysplasia, a presumptive diagnosis of optic nerve hypoplasia can be made.

In approximately 45% of cases with optic nerve hypoplasia, MRI demonstrates other intracranial structural abnormalities, including hemispheric migration anomalies (schizencephaly, cortical heterotopia, polymicrogyria), evidence of intrauterine or perinatal hemispheric injury (periventricular leukomalacia,

encephalomalacia, or porencephaly), midline fusion of the cerebral hemispheres (holoprosencephaly) and cerebellar hemispheres, and other intracranial anomalies including anencephaly, hydranencephaly, and transsphenoidal encephalocele. Abnormalities of the midbrain and hindbrain also have been described in children with septo-optic dysplasia.

Evidence of perinatal injury to the pituitary infundibulum (seen on MR imaging as posterior pituitary ectopia) is found in approximately 15% of patients with optic nerve hypoplasia. Normally, the posterior pituitary gland appears bright on T1-weighted images (Fig. 3.14A), probably because of the phospholipid membrane component of its hormone-containing vesicles. In posterior pituitary ectopia, MRI demonstrates absence of the normal posterior pituitary bright spot, absence or attenuation of the pituitary infundibulum, and an ectopic posterior pituitary bright spot where the upper infundibulum is normally located (Fig. 3.14B). It is unknown if posterior pituitary ectopia results from defective neuronal migration during embryogenesis or from a perinatal injury to the hypophyseal-portal system causing necrosis of the infundibulum.

In a child with optic nerve hypoplasia, posterior pituitary ectopia is almost pathognomonic of anterior pituitary hormone deficiency with normal posterior pituitary function while absence of a normal or ectopic posterior pituitary bright spot predicts coexistent antidiuretic hormone deficiency (i.e., diabetes insipidus). Cerebral hemispheric abnormalities are highly predictive of neurodevelopmental deficits. Absence of the septum pellucidum alone does not portend neurodevelopmental deficits or pituitary hormone deficiency. Thinning or agenesis of the corpus callosum is predictive of neurodevelopmental problems only because of its frequent association with cerebral hemispheric abnormalities. The finding of unilateral optic nerve hypoplasia does not preclude coexistent intracranial malformations. MRI thus provides critical prognostic information regarding the likelihood of neurodevelopmental deficits and pituitary hormone deficiency in the infant or young child with **unilateral** or **bilateral** optic nerve hypoplasia.

Systemic and Teratogenic Associations

Numerous environmental factors that are detrimental to the fetus are sporadically associated with optic nerve hypoplasia. These include maternal insulin-dependent diabetes mellitus, fetal alcohol syndrome, maternal ingestion of quinine, anticonvulsants, illicit drugs, and fetal or neonatal infection with cytomegalovirus or hepatitis B virus. Optic nerve hypoplasia occurs with increased frequency in firstborn children of young mothers. The majority of cases are sporadic,

A   B

Figure 3.14 Posterior pituitary ectopia in a patient with bilateral optic nerve hypoplasia. **A:** T1-weighted, mid-sagittal MRI in a normal person shows the posterior pituitary as a bright spot within the sella turcica (*arrow*). **B:** T1-weighted, mid-sagittal MRI in a patient with bilateral optic nerve hypoplasia shows an ectopic posterior pituitary (*arrow*).

although a handful of familial cases have been reported in siblings. The growing list of systemic and ocular disorders associated with optic nerve hypoplasia includes frontonasal dysplasia, aniridia, fetal alcohol syndrome, Dandy–Walker syndrome, Kallmann syndrome, Delleman syndrome, Duane syndrome, Klippel–Trenaunay–Weber syndrome, Goldenhar syndrome, linear nevus-sebaceous syndrome, Meckel syndrome, hemifacial atrophy, blepharophimosis, osteogenesis imperfecta, chondrodysplasia punctata, Aicardi syndrome, Apert syndrome, Potter syndrome, chromosome 13q-syndrome, trisomy 18, neonatal isoimmune thrombocytopenia, and bilateral microphthalmos.

Segmental Optic Nerve Hypoplasia

Some forms of optic nerve hypoplasia are segmental. An isolated superior segmental optic hypoplasia with an inferior visual field defect occurs in children of insulin-dependent diabetic mothers (Fig. 3.15).

A   B

Figure 3.15 Segmental optic nerve hypoplasia in a 21-year-old woman with juvenile diabetes mellitus. **A:** The right optic disc is normal in size and shape. **B:** The left optic disc is small and the vessels exit and enter superiorly. The patient had an inferior altitudinal field defect.

Congenital lesions of the retina, optic nerve, chiasm, tract, or retrogeniculate pathways are associated with segmental hypoplasia of the corresponding portions of each optic nerve. The term "homonymous hemioptic hypoplasia" describes the asymmetric form of segmental optic nerve hypoplasia seen in patients with unilateral congenital hemispheric lesions affecting the postchiasmal afferent visual pathways. In this setting, the nasal and temporal aspects of the optic disc contralateral to the hemispheric lesion show segmental hypoplasia and loss of the corresponding nerve fiber layers. This anomaly may be accompanied by a central band of horizontal pallor across the disc. The ipsilateral optic disc may range from normal in size to frankly hypoplastic. Homonymous hemioptic hypoplasia in retrogeniculate lesions results from transsynaptic degeneration of the optic tract.

Pathogenesis

The term "optic nerve hypoplasia" implies that the nerve is deficient in axons because of a primary failure of these axons to develop. A deficiency of axon guidance molecules (such as netrin-1) at the optic disc can lead to optic nerve hypoplasia. In addition to defects in optic nerve formation, the lack of netrin-1 function during development also results in abnormalities in other parts of the CNS, such as agenesis of the corpus callosum, and cell migration and axonal guidance defects in the hypothalamus. The timing of coexistent CNS injuries would suggest that some cases of optic nerve hypoplasia result from intrauterine destruction of a normally developed structure (i.e., an encephaloclastic event), whereas others represent a primary failure of axons to develop. In human fetuses, there is a peak of 3.7 million axons at 16 to 17 weeks of gestation, with a subsequent decline to 1.1 million axons by the 31st gestational week. This massive degeneration of supernumerary axons, termed "apoptosis," occurs as part of the normal development of the visual pathways and may serve to establish the correct topography of the visual pathways. Toxins or associated CNS malformations could augment the usual processes by which superfluous axons are eliminated from the developing visual pathways. Prenatal hemispheric injuries or malformations that injure the optic radiations can lead to retrograde transsynaptic degeneration and segmental hypoplasia of both optic nerves.

Reported cases of optic nerve hypoplasia in siblings are sufficiently rare that parents of a child with optic nerve hypoplasia can reasonably be assured that subsequent siblings are at little or no additional risk. Homozygous mutations in the *Hesx1* gene have been identified in two siblings with optic nerve hypoplasia, absence of the corpus callosum, and hypoplasia of the pituitary gland. Additional mutations in *Hesx1*

have been observed in children with sporadic pituitary disease and septo-optic dysplasia. Optic nerve hypoplasia may accompany other ocular malformations in patients with mutations in the *PAX6* gene.

Excavated Optic Disc Anomalies

Excavated optic disc anomalies (also called congenital cavitary optic disc anomalies [CODA]), include optic disc coloboma, morning glory disc anomaly, peripapillary staphyloma, megalopapilla, optic pit, and the "vacant optic disc" associated with papillorenal syndrome. In the morning glory disc anomaly and peripapillary staphyloma, an excavation of the posterior globe surrounds and incorporates the optic disc, while in the other conditions, the excavation is contained within the optic disc. The terms "morning glory disc," "optic disc coloboma," and "peripapillary staphyloma" are often transposed in the literature, causing tremendous confusion regarding their diagnostic criteria, associated systemic findings, and pathogenesis. It is important to emphasize that optic disc colobomas, morning glory optic discs, and peripapillary staphylomas are distinct anomalies, each with its own specific embryologic origin, and not simply clinical variants along a broad phenotypic spectrum.

Morning Glory Disc Anomaly

The morning glory disc anomaly is a congenital, funnel-shaped excavation of the posterior fundus that incorporates the optic disc, resembling the morning glory flower (Fig. 3.16A). Ophthalmoscopically, the disc is markedly enlarged, orange or pink in color, and may appear to be recessed or elevated centrally within the confines of a funnel-shaped peripapillary excavation (Fig. 3.16B and C). A wide annulus of chorioretinal pigmentary disturbance surrounds the disc within the excavation. A white tuft of glial tissue overlies the central portion of the disc. The blood vessels appear increased in number and often arise from the periphery of the disc. They often curve abruptly as they emanate from the disc, then run an abnormally straight course over the peripapillary retina. It is often difficult to distinguish arterioles from venules. Close inspection may reveal the presence of peripapillary or arteriovenous communications that can be confirmed by fluorescein angiography. The macula may be incorporated into the excavation. Neuroimaging shows a funnel-shaped enlargement of the distal optic nerve at its junction with the globe (Fig. 3.16D). Additional findings may include diffuse thickening with increased or decreased radiodensity of the orbital optic nerve, cavum vergae, and, most notably, transsphenoidal encephalocele.

The morning glory disc anomaly usually occurs as a unilateral condition, but bilateral cases have been

Figure 3.16 Morning glory syndrome. **A:** Appearance of the morning glory flower. **B and C:** The optic discs of two different patients show the classic features of the morning glory syndrome: An enlarged, funnel-shaped, excavated, and distorted optic disc that is surrounded by an elevated annulus of chorioretinal pigmentary disturbance. A tuft of white glial tissue overlies the center of both discs. **D:** MRI in a patient with morning glory syndrome shows a funnel-shaped enlargement of the distal optic nerve at its junction with the globe (*arrow*). (**D** courtesy of Dr. Gena Heidary).

reported. Visual acuity usually ranges from 20/200 to finger counting, but cases with 20/20 vision as well as no light perception have been reported. Unlike optic disc colobomas, which have no racial or gender predilection, morning glory discs are more common in females and rare in African Americans. The morning glory disc anomaly is usually not part of a multisystem genetic disorder. However, morning glory

disc anomaly has been described with ipsilateral orofacial hemangioma, suggesting an association with the PHACE syndrome (Posterior fossa malformations, large facial Hemangiomas, Arterial anomalies, Cardiac anomalies and aortic coarctation and Eye anomalies), which occurs only in girls. This is supported by findings of ipsilateral intracranial vascular dysgenesis in such patients. Atypical morning

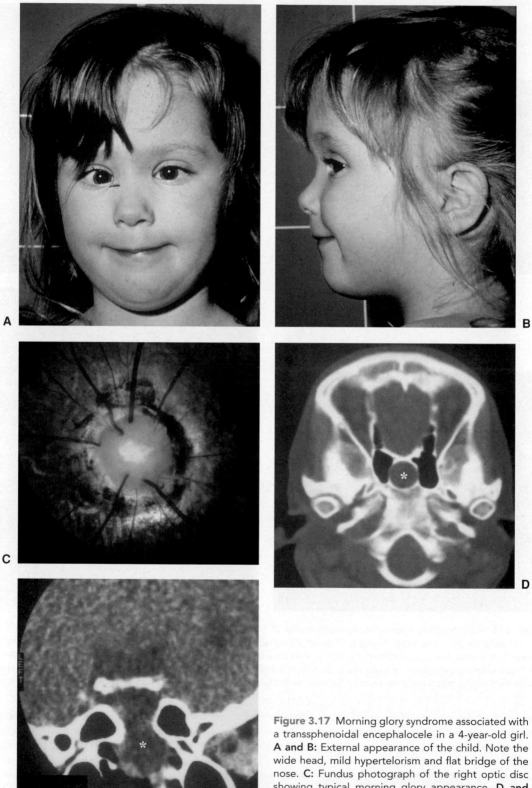

Figure 3.17 Morning glory syndrome associated with a transsphenoidal encephalocele in a 4-year-old girl. **A and B:** External appearance of the child. Note the wide head, mild hypertelorism and flat bridge of the nose. **C:** Fundus photograph of the right optic disc showing typical morning glory appearance. **D and E:** Axial (**D**) and coronal (**E**) computed tomographic scans showing the encephalocele (*asterisks*).

glory disc anomalies have also rarely been reported in patients with neurofibromatosis 2.

The association of morning glory disc anomaly with the transsphenoidal form of basal encephalocele is well established. The finding of V- or tongue-shaped infrapapillary depigmentation adjacent to a morning glory disc anomaly or other optic disc malformation is highly associated with transsphenoidal encephalocele. Transsphenoidal encephalocele is a rare midline congenital malformation in which a meningeal pouch, often containing the chiasm and adjacent hypothalamus, protrudes inferiorly through a large, round defect in the sphenoid bone. Patients with this occult basal meningocele have a wide head, flat nose, mild hypertelorism, a midline notch in the upper lip, and sometimes a midline cleft in the soft palate (Fig. 3.17). The meningocele protrudes into the nasopharynx, where it may obstruct the airway. Symptoms of transsphenoidal encephalocele in infancy include rhinorrhea, nasal obstruction, mouth-breathing, or snoring. These symptoms may be overlooked unless the associated morning glory disc anomaly or the characteristic facial configuration is recognized. A transsphenoidal encephalocele may appear clinically as a pulsatile posterior nasal mass or as a "nasal polyp" high in the nose, and surgical biopsy or excision of the lesion can have severe and even lethal consequences. Associated brain malformations include agenesis of the corpus callosum and posterior dilation of the lateral ventricles. Absence of the chiasm is seen in approximately one-third of patients at surgery or autopsy. Most of the affected children have no overt intellectual or neurologic deficits, but hypopituitarism is common.

In addition to transsphenoidal encephalocele, patients with the morning glory disc anomaly may have a Chiari I malformation or cerebellar tonsillar ectopia that may be overlooked on MRI. Morning glory disc anomaly also has been associated with hypoplasia of the ipsilateral intracranial vasculature, such ipsilateral intracranial vascular dysgenesis (hypoplasia of the carotid arteries and major cerebral arteries with or without Moyamoya syndrome). These reports underscore the need for MR angiography in the neurodiagnostic evaluation of patients with the morning glory disc anomaly.

Patients with a morning glory disc anomaly may experience both transient visual loss and permanent visual loss later in life. Serous retinal detachments occur in 26% to 38% of eyes with morning glory optic discs. These detachments typically originate in the peripapillary area and extend through the posterior pole, occasionally progressing to total detachments. In other cases with acquired visual loss, there is nonattachment and radial folding of the retina within the excavated zone.

Several authors have documented contractile movements in a morning glory optic disc, which may be related to fluctuations in subretinal fluid volume (Fig. 3.18 and **Video 3.1**). Subretinal neovascularization may occasionally develop within the circumferential zone of pigmentary disturbance adjacent to a morning glory disc.

The embryologic defect leading to the morning glory disc anomaly is debated. Some authors have suggested that the morning glory disc anomaly results from defective closure of the embryonic fissure and is but one phenotypic form of a colobomatous (i.e., embryonic fissure-related) defect. Others interpret the clinical findings of a central glial tuft, vascular anomalies, and a scleral defect, together with the histologic findings of adipose tissue and smooth muscle within the peripapillary sclera in presumed cases of the morning glory disc to signify a primary mesenchymal abnormality.

Optic Disc Coloboma

The term "coloboma," of Greek derivation, means curtailed or mutilated. It is used only with reference to the eye. Colobomas of the optic disc result from incomplete or abnormal coaptation of the proximal end of the embryonic fissure.

Optic disc coloboma is characterized by a sharply delimited, glistening white, bowl-shaped excavation

Figure 3.18 Morning glory syndrome with contractile movements. **A:** Disc appearance before contraction. **B:** Disc appearance during contraction. **See also Video 3.1.** (Photographs and video from Sawada Y, Fujiwara T, Yoshitomi T. Morning glory anomaly with contractile movements. *Graefes Arch Clin Exp Ophthalmol.* 2012;250:1693–1695, with permission.)

A
B

Figure 3.19 Coloboma of the optic disc in an eye with an old serous macular detachment. The disc is enlarged. A deep white excavation occupies most of the disc but spares its superior aspect. Note absence of inferior retinal nerve fiber layer and pigment epithelial disturbance in the macula. The patient had an extensive superior altitudinal visual field defect.

that occupies an enlarged optic disc (Fig. 3.19). The excavation is decentered inferiorly, reflecting the position of the embryonic fissure relative to the primitive epithelial papilla. The inferior neuroretinal rim is thin or absent, whereas the superior neuroretinal rim is relatively spared. Rarely, the entire disc appears excavated; however, the colobomatous nature of the defect still can be appreciated ophthalmoscopically because the excavation is deeper inferiorly. The defect may extend further inferiorly to include the adjacent choroid and retina, in which case microphthalmia frequently is present, as are iris and ciliary colobomas. CT scanning shows a crater-like excavation of the posterior globe at its junction with the optic nerve. Colobomatous malformations of the optic disc produce an inferior segmental hypoplasia of the optic nerve, with a C-shaped or quarter-moon–shaped neuroretinal rim confined to the superior aspect of the optic disc (Fig. 3.19).

Colobomas constitute the most common segmental form of optic nerve hypoplasia encountered in clinical practice. Indeed, MRI confirms that the intracranial portion of the optic nerve is reduced in size. The nosologic overlap between colobomatous derangement of the optic nerve and segmental hypoplasia reflects the early timing of colobomatous dysembryogenesis that results in primary failure of inferior retinal ganglion cells to develop.

Visual acuity, which depends primarily upon the integrity of the papillomacular bundle, may be mildly

to severely decreased in the eyes with an optic disc coloboma, with the level of vision being difficult if not impossible to predict from the appearance of the disc. Unlike the morning glory disc anomaly, which usually is unilateral, optic disc colobomas occur unilaterally or bilaterally with approximately equal frequency (Fig. 3.20) and may be sporadic or inherited in an autosomal-dominant manner.

Ocular colobomas may occur as part of a variety of genetic disorders such as the CHARGE syndrome (**C**ongenital **H**eart disease with choanal **A**tresia, **R**etardation of **G**rowth, urinary abnormalities, and **E**ar abnormalities with deafness), Walker-Warburg syndrome, Goltz focal dermal hypoplasia, Aicardi syndrome (see below), Goldenhar sequence, and linear sebaceous nevus syndrome. However, there is no association with basal encephalocele as is the case with the morning glory disc anomaly nor is there any association with the papillorenal syndrome even though the appearance of the colobomatous and papillorenal discs are somewhat similar (see below). The development of optic disc colobomas has been linked to a mutation of the *PAX6* gene.

Optic disc colobomas may be associated with a variety of ocular malformations, including retinal venous malformations, peripheral retinal nonperfusion with and without traction retinal detachment, macular holes, and orbital cysts that communicate with the anomalous disc.

Histopathologic examination of optic disc colobomas typically demonstrates intrascleral smooth muscle strands oriented concentrically around the distal optic nerve. Presumably, this pathologic finding accounts for the contractility of the optic disc seen in rare cases of optic disc coloboma. Heterotopic adipose tissue also is present within and adjacent to some optic disc colobomas. Eyes with an isolated optic disc coloboma can develop a serous macular detachment (Fig. 3.19A).

Unfortunately, many uncategorizable dysplastic optic discs (see below) are indiscriminately labeled as optic disc colobomas. This practice complicates the nosology of coloboma-associated genetic disorders. It therefore is crucial that the diagnosis of optic disc coloboma be reserved for discs that show an **inferiorly decentered**, white-colored excavation, with minimal peripapillary pigmentary changes. These ophthalmoscopic features are quite different from those of the morning glory disc anomaly (Table 3.2). The difference in appearance between these two anomalies as well as the profound differences in associated ocular and systemic findings between them (Table 3.3) lend further credence to the hypothesis that optic disc colobomas result from a primary structural dysgenesis of the **proximal** embryonic fissure, whereas the morning glory disc anomaly results from anomalous dilation

Figure 3.20 Optic disc colobomas. **A:** Bilateral colobomas. **B:** Unilateral coloboma. The right disc (**left**) is colobomatous. The left disc (**right**) is normal in both size and shape.

Table 3.2	Ophthalmoscopic Findings that Distinguish the Morning Glory Disc Anomaly from Optic Disc Coloboma	
Morning Glory Disc	**Optic Disc Coloboma**	
Optic disc lies within the excavation	Excavation lies within the optic disc	
Symmetrical defect (disc lies *centrally* within the excavation)	Asymmetrical defect (excavation lies *inferiorly* within the disc)	
Central glial tuft	No central glial tuft	
Severe peripapillary pigmentary disturbance	Minimal peripapillary pigmentary disturbance	
Anomalous retinal vasculature	Normal retinal vasculature	

Table 3.3 Associated Ocular and Systemic Findings that Distinguish the Morning Glory Disc from Isolated Optic Disc Coloboma	
Morning Glory Disc	**Optic Disc Coloboma**
More common in females; rare in blacks	No sex or racial predilection
Rarely familial	Often familial
Rarely bilateral	Often bilateral
No iris, ciliary, or retinal colobomas	Iris, ciliary, and retinal colobomas common
Rarely associated with multisystem genetic disorders	Often associated with multisystem genetic disorders
Basal encephalocele common	Basal encephalocele rare

Table 3.4 Ophthalmoscopic Findings that Distinguish Peripapillary Staphyloma from the Morning Glory Disc Anomaly	
Peripapillary Staphyloma	**Morning Glory Disc**
Deep, cup-shaped excavation	Less depth, funnel-shaped excavation
Relatively normal, well-defined optic disc	Grossly anomalous, poorly defined optic disc
Absence of glial and vascular anomalies	Central glial bouquet, anomalous vascular pattern

of the **distal** optic stalk. Nevertheless, anomalously excavated optic discs with overlapping features of the morning glory disc anomaly and optic disc coloboma occasionally are seen. These "hybrid" anomalies may represent instances of early embryonic injury affecting both the proximal embryonic fissure and the distal optic stalk.

Peripapillary Staphyloma

Peripapillary staphyloma is an extremely rare, usually unilateral anomaly, in which a deep fundus excavation surrounds the optic disc (Fig. 3.21). In this condition, the disc is seen at the bottom of the excavated defect

Figure 3.21 Peripapillary staphyloma in a patient with extremely high myopia. The optic disc is situated within a bowl-shaped excavation. Note extensive hypopigmentation surrounding a normal-appearing optic disc.

and may appear normal or show temporal pallor. The walls and margin of the defect may show atrophic changes in the retinal pigment epithelium and choroid. Unlike the morning glory disc anomaly, there is no central glial tuft overlying the disc, and the retinal vascular pattern remains normal, apart from reflecting the essential contour of the lesion (Table 3.4). Several cases of contractile peripapillary staphyloma have been documented.

Visual acuity usually is markedly reduced in eyes with a peripapillary staphyloma, but cases with nearly normal acuity have been reported. Affected eyes usually are emmetropic or slightly myopic, and eyes with decreased vision frequently have centrocecal scotomas. Although peripapillary staphyloma is clinically and embryologically distinct from the morning glory optic disc anomaly, these conditions frequently are transposed in the literature.

Although the peripapillary staphyloma usually occurs as an isolated phenomenon, it has been reported in association with transsphenoidal encephalocele, PHACE syndrome, linear nevus sebaceous syndrome, and 18q- (de Grouchy) syndrome.

The fairly normal appearance of the optic disc and retinal vessels in eyes with a peripapillary staphyloma suggests that the development of these structures is complete before the staphylomatous process begins. The clinical features of peripapillary staphyloma are most consistent with diminished peripapillary structural support, perhaps resulting from incomplete differentiation of sclera from posterior neural crest cells in the fifth month of gestation.

Megalopapilla

Megalopapilla is a generic term that connotes an abnormally large, excavated optic disc that lacks the numerous anomalous features of the morning glory disc anomaly, the inferior displacement of a coloboma, or the striking cilioretinal circulation of the papillorenal

Figure 3.22 Megalopapilla. Bilateral large optic discs with large central cups. The appearance is similar to that of glaucoma; however, unlike glaucomatous optic atrophy, the cups are horizontally oval and the peripapillary retinal nerve fiber layer appears intact despite the large cups. The patient had normal visual acuity, normal visual fields, and normal intraocular pressures.

syndrome (see below). Megalopapilla comprises two phenotypic variants. The first is a common variant in which an abnormally large optic disc (>2.1 mm in diameter) retains an otherwise normal configuration. This form of megalopapilla is usually bilateral and often associated with a large cup-to-disc ratio, which almost invariably raises the diagnostic consideration of normal-tension glaucoma (Fig. 3.22). However, the optic cup is usually round or horizontally oval with no vertical notching or encroachment, so that the quotient of horizontal to vertical cup-to-disc ratio remains normal, in contradistinction to the decreased quotient that characterizes glaucomatous optic atrophy. Because the axons are spread over a larger surface area, the neuroretinal rim may also appear pale, mimicking optic atrophy. Less commonly, the normal optic cup is replaced by a grossly anomalous noninferior excavation that obliterates the adjacent neuroretinal rim. The inclusion of this rare variant under the rubric of megalopapilla serves the nosologically useful function of distinguishing it from a colobomatous defect with the latter's important systemic and neurologic associative implications. Cilioretinal arteries are common in eyes with megalopapilla.

Visual acuity is usually normal in eyes with megalopapilla, but it may be mildly decreased. The visual field also is usually normal, although there may be an enlarged blind spot. Colobomatous discs are distinguished from megalopapilla by their predominant excavation of the **inferior** optic disc.

Pathogenetically, most cases of megalopapilla may simply represent a statistical variant of normal. However, it is likely that megalopapilla occasionally results from altered migration of optic axons early in embryogenesis, as evidenced by reports of megalopapilla in patients with anterior encephaloceles. Nevertheless, the rarity of an association between megalopapilla and CNS abnormalities suggests that neuroimaging is unwarranted in a patient with megalopapilla unless midline facial anomalies (e.g., hypertelorism, cleft palate, cleft lip, depressed nasal bridge) coexist.

Optic Pit

An optic pit is a round or oval, gray, white, or yellowish depression in the optic disc (Fig. 3.23). The estimated frequency of optic pits is about 1 in 11,000. Numerous reports of familial optic pits suggest an autosomal-dominant mode of transmission.

Optic pits commonly affect the temporal region of the optic disc but may be situated in any sector. Such temporally located pits often are accompanied by adjacent peripapillary pigment epithelial changes. One or two cilioretinal arteries emerge from the bottom or the margin of the pit in over 50% of cases. Although optic pits typically are unilateral, bilateral pits are present in 15% of cases. In unilateral cases, the affected disc is slightly larger than the normal disc. Visual acuity is typically normal unless there is fluid within or beneath the macula (see below). Although visual field defects are variable and often correlate poorly with the location of the pit, the most common defect appears to be a paracentral arcuate scotoma connected to an enlarged blind spot. Optic pits do not portend additional CNS malformations, although rare exceptions exist.

A

B

Figure 3.23 Optic pits. **A:** Oval white excavation occupies the temporal portion of the disc. **B:** Grayish temporal optic disc with extensive serous retinal macular detachment involving the entire papillomacular region.

A serous macular detachment develops in 25% to 75% of eyes with optic pits (Fig. 3.23B), usually in the third and fourth decades of life. Vitreous traction on the margins of the pit and tractional changes in the roof of the pit may be the inciting events that ultimately lead to this complication, which occurs most often in eyes with large optic pits and in eyes with temporally located pits. Spontaneous reattachment occurs in approximately 25% of cases. In others, vitrectomy with internal gas tamponade and laser photocoagulation can result in long-term improvement in acuity. Laser photocoagulation to block the flow of fluid from the pit to the macula is usually unsuccessful, perhaps because of the inability of laser photocoagulation to seal a retinoschisis cavity.

Histologically, optic pits consist of herniations of dysplastic retina into a collagen-lined pocket extending posteriorly, often into the subarachnoid space, through a defect in the lamina cribrosa. The source of intraretinal fluid in eyes with optic pits is controversial, but it appears to be cerebrospinal fluid from the subarachnoid space surrounding the optic nerve (Fig. 3.24).

The pathogenesis of optic pits remains controversial, Although some authors view them as a mild variant in the spectrum of optic disc colobomas, optic pits usually are unilateral, sporadic, and unassociated with systemic anomalies whereas colobomas are bilateral as often as unilateral, commonly hereditarily transmitted in an autosomal-dominant fashion, and often associated with a variety of multisystem disorders. In addition, it is rare for optic pits to coexist with iris or retinochoroidal colobomas, and optic pits usually occur in locations unrelated to the embryonic fissure.

Papillorenal Syndrome

The papillorenal syndrome (previously known as the renal-coloboma syndrome) is characterized by a distinct optic disc malformation that sometimes is mistaken for either a glaucomatous disc or an optic disc coloboma. In this syndrome, however, the excavated optic disc is normal in size unlike the enlarged colobomatous optic disc. In addition, the excavation in the papillorenal disc malformation is centrally positioned, not inferiorly positioned as occurs in the optic disc coloboma. The defining feature of the optic disc that is part of the papillorenal syndrome, however, is the multiple cilioretinal vessels that emanate from the periphery of the disc, associated with a variable attenuation of the retinal vessels (Fig. 3.25). Color Doppler imaging has confirmed the absence of central retinal circulation in patients with this syndrome.

Visual acuity usually is normal in patients with the papillorenal syndrome but occasionally is diminished secondary to choroidal and retinal hypoplasia and, in some cases, to late-onset serous retinal detachment. Binasal or arcuate visual field defects due to optic nerve dysfunction often are present, and these defects, coupled with the presence of central excavation in a normal-sized optic disc explains why the appearance of the papillorenal disc may be mistaken for that of normal-tension or open-angle glaucoma.

Families have been reported with an autosomal-dominant mode of transmission. In some patients, mutations have been found in the developmental gene *PAX2*. This malformation is attributed to a primary deficiency in angiogenesis involved in vascular development. In these patients, there is a failure of the hyaloid system to convert to normal central retinal vessels.

A

B

Figure 3.24 Optical coherence tomography (OCT) indicating the source of intraretinal fluid in a patient with an optic pit. **A:** Fundus photograph and swept-source optical coherence tomographic (SS-OCT) image of the left eye of a 66-year-old man with an optic disc pit. **Above**, Color fundus photograph. A gray, oval-shaped optic disc pit (*white arrow*) is present at the temporal margin of the disc along with some adjacent peripapillary pigmentary changes. The optic disc tissue other than the pit appears normal. *Black arrow* indicates the direction of the OCT scan. **Below**, Vertical SS-OCT image through the fovea shows retinoschisis, with tissue columns connecting the schisis cavities. **B:** Vertical **(upper left)** and horizontal **(upper right)** B-scan cross-sectional images near the optic disc pit. The retrobulbar subarachnoid space (*white arrows*) is clearly seen around the optic nerve. There is a direct communication between the retrobulbar subarachnoid space and the vitreous cavity (*red arrows*). *Blue arrow* indicates the optic nerve. *Red arrowhead* indicates a thin line of fluid that is presumably connecting with the retrobulbar subarachnoid space, but communication with this line and the schisis cavity (*white arrowhead*) is unclear. *Blue arrowhead* points to a part of a vitreous strand. *Yellow arrows* indicate the optic disc pit, and *green arrows* indicate the direction of the OCT scan. Lower, three-dimensional OCT reconstruction shows a break in the cup of the optic disc (*red arrow*). (From Katome T, Mitamura Y, Hotta F, et al. Swept-source optical coherence tomography identifies connection between vitreous cavity and retrobulbar subarachnoid space in patient with optic disc pit. *Eye.* 2013;27:1325–1326, with permission.)

Figure 3.25 Papillorenal syndrome in a 35-year-old man with chronic renal failure. Both optic discs show a central excavation with multiple cilioretinal arteries in place of the normal central retinal circulation. Visual acuity was 20/20 in each eye.

Figure 3.26 Tilted optic discs. Both optic discs are oval with the relative elevation of the superior-temporal portion compared to the inferior-nasal portion. This elevation is often mistaken for true disc swelling. Note situs inversus of the vessels and inferior retinochoroidal hypopigmentation.

Patients with the papillorenal syndrome have a variety of disorders in kidney function. In addition, some have other manifestations that may be related to their kidney disease, including gout and diabetes mellitus.

Congenital Tilted Optic Disc Syndrome

The tilted optic disc syndrome is a nonhereditary, usually bilateral condition in which the superotem-poral region of the optic disc is elevated and the inferonasal region is posteriorly displaced, resulting in an oval-appearing optic disc, with its long axis obliquely oriented (Figs. 3.26 and 3.27). This config-uration is accompanied by *situs inversus* of the retinal vessels, congenital inferonasal conus, thinning of the inferonasal RPE and choroid, a bitemporal (when the condition is bilateral) hemianopia that does not respect the vertical midline (Fig. 3.28), and an optic nerve that exits the globe at an extremely oblique angle that can be seen on MRI (Fig. 3.29).

Figure 3.27 Unilateral tilted optic disc. The right optic disc (**left**) is tilted with superior elevation and an inferior conus. The left optic disc (**right**) is normal in size and shape.

Figure 3.28 Kinetic perimetry showing a bitemporal field defect in the patient whose optic discs are shown in Figure 3.26. Note that the defects are scotomatous and do not "obey" the vertical midline as would be expected if the defects were caused by a lesion damaging the optic chiasm.

Figure 3.29 Magnetic resonance images (MRIs) in a patient with bilateral tilted optic discs. **A:** The right optic disc is slightly small and oval with mild blurring of its temporal margin. The left optic disc shows more obvious blurring of its nasal margin. **B:** Automated static perimetry (Humphrey, SITA standard 24–2) shows nonlocalizing visual field defects in both eyes. **C:** Precontrast T1 **(left)** and T2 **(right)** MRIs demonstrate oblique insertion of the optic nerve into the left globe (*arrows*) and posterior nasal flattening of the left globe (*arrowheads*). (From Tarver-Carr ME, Miller NR. Tilted optic discs visualized by magnetic resonance imaging. *J Neuroophthalmol.* 2006;26:282–283, with permission.)

Histopathologically, the superior or superotemporal portion of the disc is elevated, and there often is posterior ectasia of the inferior or inferonasal fundus and optic disc. The cause of the tilted disc syndrome is unknown, but the inferonasal or inferior location of the excavation suggests a pathogenetic relationship to retinochoroidal coloboma.

Patients with the tilted optic disc syndrome often have myopic astigmatism, with the plus-axis oriented parallel to the ectasia. The ocular imagery resulting from a tilted retina creates a type of curvature of field that subjectively may simulate astigmatic blur. The congenital tilted disc syndrome is bilateral in about 80% of cases. Familiarity with the tilted disc syndrome is crucial for the ophthalmologist, as affected patients may present with a bitemporal hemianopia, suggesting a chiasmal process, nasal disc elevation suggesting papilledema, or both. The bitemporal hemianopia in patients with tilted discs, however, typically is incomplete, does not respect the vertical midline, and is confined primarily to the superior quadrants (Fig. 3.28). It is, in fact, a refractive scotoma, usually secondary to regional myopia localized to the inferonasal retina. As far as the disc elevation is concerned, it is limited to the nasal or superior nasal disc, with the rest of the disc being flat, and there is no disc hyperemia, obscuration of disc vessels, or superficial disc or peripapillary hemorrhages as might be expected in true optic disc swelling.

It should be emphasized that patients with tilted optic discs can harbor a mass in the region of the optic chiasm, often a congenital tumor such as an optic glioma or craniopharyngioma. Thus, urgent neuroimaging should be performed in any patient with a tilted disc syndrome whose bitemporal hemianopia respects the vertical meridian. The tilted disc syndrome also has been documented in patients with craniofacial anomalies, including Crouzon disease and Apert disease as well as in patients with transsphenoidal encephalocele, congenital tumors of the anterior visual pathways, X-linked congenital stationary night blindness, Ehlers–Danlos syndrome (type III), and familial dextrocardia.

Optic Disc Dysplasia

Optic disc dysplasia is a term that connotes a markedly deformed optic disc that fails to conform to any recognizable diagnostic category (Fig. 3.30). The distinction between a nonspecifically "anomalous" disc and a "dysplastic" disc is somewhat arbitrary, however, and based primarily upon the severity of the lesion.

Dysplastic optic discs can occur in patients with a transsphenoidal encephalocele. In such a setting, there

Figure 3.30 Optic disc dysplasia. The optic disc is grossly malformed, and the retinal vessels emerge from the region of the disc in an anomalous pattern.

often is a discrete infrapapillary zone of V- or tongue-shaped retinochoroidal depigmentation such as that seen in patients with morning glory syndrome (see above). This finding should prompt neuroimaging. These juxtapapillary defects differ from typical retinochoroidal colobomas that widen inferiorly and are not associated with basal encephaloceles. Unlike the typical retinochoroidal coloboma, this distinct juxtapapillary defect is associated with minimal scleral excavation and no visible disruption in the integrity of the overlying retina.

Congenital Optic Disc Pigmentation

Congenital optic disc pigmentation is a condition in which melanin deposition anterior to or within the lamina cribrosa imparts a slate-gray appearance to the entire optic disc (Fig. 3.31). True congenital optic disc pigmentation is extremely rare, but it has been described in association with interstitial deletion of chromosome 17, Aicardi syndrome, and optic nerve hypoplasia. Congenital optic disc pigmentation is compatible with good visual acuity but may be associated with coexistent optic disc anomalies that decrease vision.

Aicardi Syndrome

Aicardi syndrome is a congenital cerebroretinal disorder of unknown etiology that occurs almost exclusively in females. The syndrome is characterized by infantile spasms, agenesis of the corpus callosum, an

Figure 3.31 Congenital optic disc pigmentation. Entire disc is gray, and the disc is hypoplastic with a surrounding zone of depigmentation, suggesting migration of peripapillary pigment onto the disc.

abnormal electroencephalographic pattern termed hypsarrhythmia, and a pathognomonic fundus appearance consisting of multiple depigmented "chorioretinal lacunae" clustered around an anomalous optic disc that may be colobomatous, hypoplastic, or have abnormal pigmentation (Fig. 3.32A). Histologically, the chorioretinal lacunae consist of well-circumscribed,

full-thickness defects limited to the retinal pigment epithelium and choroid. The overlying retina remains intact but is often histologically abnormal.

Other ocular abnormalities that may be present in the Aicardi syndrome include microphthalmos, retrobulbar cyst, pseudoglioma, retinal detachment, macular scar, cataract, pupillary membrane, iris synechiae, iris coloboma, and persistent hyperplastic primary vitreous. The most common systemic findings associated with Aicardi syndrome are vertebral malformations (fused vertebrae, scoliosis, spina bifida) and costal malformations (absent ribs, fused or bifurcated ribs). Other systemic findings include muscular hypotonia, microcephaly, dysmorphic facies, cleft lip and palate, auditory disturbances, and auricular anomalies. Aicardi syndrome also has been associated with choroid plexus papilloma.

CNS anomalies in Aicardi syndrome include agenesis of the corpus callosum, cortical migration anomalies (pachygyria, polymicrogyria, cortical heterotopias), and multiple structural CNS malformations (cerebral hemispheric asymmetry, Dandy–Walker variant, colpocephaly, midline arachnoid cysts) (Fig. 3.32B). Neuropathologic specimens show a characteristic profile, consisting of unlayered polymicrogyria, subcortical or periventricular heterotopias, and agenesis of the corpus callosum. This complex cerebral malformation suggests a problem in nerve cell proliferation and migration. An overlap between Aicardi syndrome and septo-optic dysplasia has been recognized in several patients.

Figure 3.32 Aicardi syndrome in a 2-month-old girl. **A:** An enlarged, malformed optic disc is surrounded by numerous, well-circumscribed, chorioretinal lacunae. **B:** Axial computed tomographic scan shows enlargement of the lateral and third ventricles as well as cystic dilation of the fourth ventricle, consistent with a Dandy-Walker malformation.

Severe mental retardation is present in almost all cases of Aicardi syndrome. The disorder is associated with decreased life expectancy, but some patients survive into their teenage years. It has been suggested that the size of the largest chorioretinal lacuna correlates with neurologic outcome, whereas age at presentation, type, and severity of seizures does not. Most children have medically intractable seizures, and 91% attain milestones no higher than 12 months.

Aicardi syndrome is thought to result from an X-linked mutational event that is lethal in males.

Doubling of the Optic Disc

Doubling of the optic discs is a rare anomaly in which two optic discs are seen ophthalmoscopically and presumed to be associated with a duplication or separation of the distal optic nerve into two fasciculi. Most cases have a "main" disc and a "satellite" disc, each with its own vascular system (Fig. 3.33). Most cases occur unilaterally and are associated with decreased acuity in the affected eye.

Optic Nerve Aplasia

Optic nerve aplasia is a rare nonhereditary malformation seen most often in a unilaterally malformed eye of an otherwise healthy person. The term implies complete absence of the optic nerve (including the optic disc), retinal ganglion and nerve fiber layers,

Figure 3.33 Doubling of the optic disc. Note "main" disc and "satellite" disc. (From Donoso LA, Magaragal LE, Eiferman RA. Ocular anomalies simulating double optic discs. *Can J Ophthalmol.* 1981;16:84–87. Photograph courtesy of Larry A. Donoso.)

and optic nerve vessels. Histopathologic examination usually demonstrates a vestigial dural sheath entering the sclera in its normal position (Fig. 3.34), as well as retinal dysplasia with rosette formation. Some early reports of optic nerve aplasia actually described patients with severe hypoplasia at a time when the latter entity was not clearly recognized.

Optic nerve aplasia usually is unilateral. When it occurs bilaterally, it is invariably associated with severe and widespread congenital CNS malformations.

Optic nerve aplasia may be diagnosed when there is no defined optic disc, there is only a whitish area where the disc should be, or when there is a deep avascular cavity surrounded by a whitish annulus in the site corresponding to the optic disc. In all of these settings, there also should be no central retinal blood vessels and no macular differentiation.

Children with true optic nerve aplasia are, as expected, blind in the affected eye. Neuroimaging may show both the eye and the bony orbit to be smaller than normal.

The cause of optic nerve aplasia is unknown; however, its frequent association with malformations such as microphthalmia, malformations in the anterior chamber angle, hypoplasia or segmental aplasia of the iris, cataracts, persistent hyperplastic primary vitreous, anterior colobomas, macular staphyloma, retinal dysplasia, or pigmentary disturbance suggests that the cause is fundamentally distinct from optic nerve hypoplasia.

Myelinated (Medullated) Nerve Fibers

Myelination of the anterior visual system begins centrally at the lateral geniculate body at 5 months of gestation. It proceeds distally, reaching the optic chiasm by 6 to 7 months, the retrobulbar optic nerve by 8 months, and the lamina cribrosa at term or shortly thereafter. Normally, myelin does not extend intraocularly; however, intraocular myelination of retinal nerve fibers occurs in 0.3% to 0.6% of the population by ophthalmoscopy and in 1% by postmortem examinations. In most eyes, the myelination is continuous with the optic disc, and the majority of patients have normal visual acuity.

The pathogenesis of myelinated nerve fibers remains largely speculative, but it has been suggested that a defect in the lamina cribrosa may allow oligodendrocytes to gain access to the retina and produce myelin there.

Ophthalmoscopically, myelinated nerve fibers usually appear as white striated patches at the upper and lower poles of the optic disc (Fig. 3.35). In these locations, they may impart a gray appearance to the optic

Figure 3.34 Myelinated nerve fibers. **A:** In one patient, the right optic disc is surrounded by myelinated, feathery nerve fibers. **B:** In another patient, myelinated nerve fibers extend superiorly and inferiorly from the left optic disc along the arcuate nerve fiber bundles. **C:** In a third patient, there is only a small region superior to the right optic disc where there are myelinated nerve fibers.

disc, and they also may simulate papilledema, both by elevating the adjacent portions of the disc and by obscuring the disc margin and underlying retinal vessels. Distally, they have an irregular fan-shaped appearance that facilitates their recognition. Small slits or patches of normal-appearing fundus color occasionally are visible within areas of myelination. Myelinated nerve fibers are bilateral in 17% to 20% of cases and, clinically, they are discontinuous with the optic disc in 19%. Isolated patches of myelinated nerve fibers occasionally are seen in the peripheral retina.

Retinal vascular abnormalities, such as telangiectasia or neovascularization, have been described within areas of myelinated nerve fibers. They sometimes are associated with vitreous hemorrhage, suggesting that the retinal vessels within patches of myelinated nerve fibers may harbor occult microvascular abnormalities.

Myelinated retinal nerve fibers do not usually reduce visual acuity; however, because myelinated fibers usually are adjacent to the optic disc, the blind spot often is enlarged in affected eyes. When the myelinated fibers surround the macula, there may be a ring scotoma, and isolated patches of myelination in the posterior pole or periphery may produce isolated scotomas that invariably are small than the size of the myelin patch would suggest. If the macula is affected, there may be a central scotoma, but this is an extremely rare occurrence.

Extensive unilateral (or rarely bilateral) myelination of nerve fibers can be associated with high myopia and severe amblyopia. However, unlike other forms of unilateral high myopia that characteristically respond well to occlusion therapy, the amblyopia that occurs in children with myelinated nerve fibers is notoriously refractory to this treatment. In such patients, myelination surrounds most of the disc. In addition, the macular region (although unmyelinated) usually appears abnormal, showing a dulled reflex or pigment dispersion.

Myelinated nerve fibers may occur in association with the Gorlin syndrome (multiple basal cell nevi). Myelinated nerve fibers may be familial, in which case the trait usually is inherited in an autosomal-dominant fashion. Isolated cases of myelinated nerve fibers also may occur in association with abnormal length of the optic nerve (oxycephaly), defects in the lamina cribrosa (tilted disc), anterior segment dysgenesis, and neurofibromatosis type 2. An autosomal-dominant vitreoretinopathy associated with myelination of the nerve fiber layer is characterized by congenitally poor vision, bilateral extensive myelination of the retinal nerve fiber layer, severe degeneration of the vitreous, high myopia, a retinal dystrophy with night blindness, reduction of the electroretinographic responses, and limb deformities.

Rarely, areas of myelinated nerve fibers may be acquired after infancy and even in adulthood, sometimes after a trauma to the eye. Progression of myelinated nerve fibers has been documented in children. Conversely, myelinated nerve fibers may disappear as a result of an acquired optic neuropathy, central retinal artery occlusion, and branch retinal artery occlusion.

Topical Diagnosis of Acquired Optic Nerve Disorders*

Appearance of the Disc
    Optic Disc Swelling
    Infiltration of the Optic Disc
    Optic Atrophy

Syndromes of Prechiasmal Optic Nerve Dysfunction
    Retino-Choroidal Vessels and the Syndrome of Chronic Optic Nerve Compression
    Distal Optic Nerve Syndrome
    Foster Kennedy Syndrome
    Bilateral Superior or Inferior (Altitudinal) Hemianopia
    Nasal Hemianopia

Damage to an optic nerve classically causes an abnormality in visual sensory function, a relative afferent pupillary defect, and, if the damage is irreversible, a change in the appearance of the optic disc. Acquired optic neuropathies can produce any type of visual field defect, including a central scotoma, cecocentral scotoma, arcuate field defect, altitudinal defect, or even a temporal or nasal hemianopic defect. Unless the optic neuropathy is bilateral or the lesion is located near the optic chiasm, the field defect produced by an optic nerve lesion is always monocular.

The visual field defects that occur with various optic neuropathies are not in themselves localizing. Rather, it is the demographics of the patient (age, gender), history of visual loss (rapid vs. slow onset, progressive vs. stable, painful vs. painless), the presence or absence of other neurologic or ocular signs (relative afferent pupillary defect, acquired color deficit, ocular motor paresis, proptosis, optociliary shunt veins, optic disc swelling, optic pallor), and the results of neuroimaging that most often allow the physician to diagnose an optic neuropathy, to localize the pathology along the course of the nerve, and to determine its etiology.

Appearance of the Disc

The optic disc has only two ways to respond to the many acquired pathologic processes that may affect the optic nerve. It can swell, or it can remain normal in appearance. If the pathologic process causes irreversible damage to the optic nerve, the disc will eventually become pale.

Optic Disc Swelling

True optic disc swelling of the optic disc occurs when there is obstruction of axonal transport at the lamina cribrosa (Fig. 4.1) and may result from compression, ischemia, inflammation, metabolic dysfunction, or toxic damage (Table 4.1). In some cases, infiltration of the proximal portion of the disc by inflammatory or malignant processes causes an appearance indistinguishable from true swelling. Mimics of true swelling such as congenital disc anomalies are discussed in Chapter 3.

Appearance

Useful funduscopic signs of early swelling of the optic disc include blurring of the nerve fiber layer around the disc, especially superiorly and inferiorly, and segmental obscuration of small vessels (typically arterioles) as they approach or cross the disc edge (Fig. 4.2A) (see Chapter 5). When disc swelling is fully developed (Fig. 4.2B), additional funduscopic changes can appear, including intraretinal hemorrhages and infarcts (cotton-wool spots) within the nerve fiber layer, hard exudates (sometimes in a star figure around or on the nasal half of the macula), and subhyaloid hemorrhage, occasionally breaking out into the vitreous cavity.

When disc swelling persists for several months or longer, the hemorrhages and exudates tend to resolve, and the initial hyperemia is replaced by a gray or yellow atrophic appearance. Other changes include development of "drusen-like" hard exudates in the superficial substance of the disc itself (Fig. 4.3). Neovascular membranes with subretinal hemorrhages and serous fluid can progressively develop. The peripapillary retinal vasculature may be narrowed with a sheathed quality. Optociliary shunt vessels may also appear on the optic disc, presumably secondary to chronic obstruction of normal retinal venous drainage through the central retinal vein by chronic disc swelling.

Optic disc swelling may not develop if significant optic atrophy is already present: "dead axons can't

*The authors acknowledge the past contributions of Alfredo A. Sadun and Madhu R. Agarwal to this chapter.

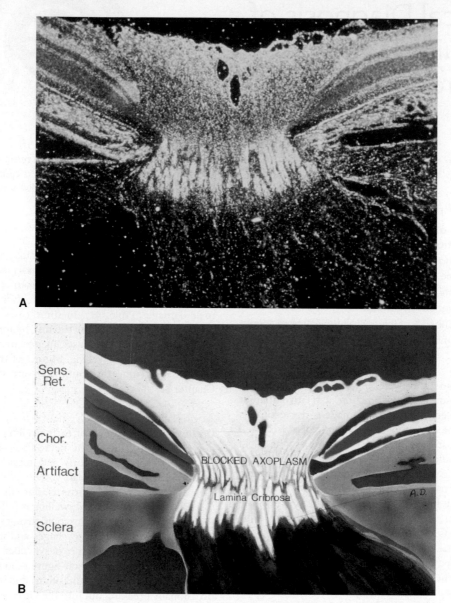

Figure 4.1 The final common denominator of optic disc swelling: obstruction of axon transport. **A:** Phase-contrast photomicrograph of a swollen optic disc in an animal with experimental papilledema shows accumulation of axon products (seen as *white material*) in the region of the lamina cribrosa. **B:** Artist's drawing of the photomicrograph. *Sens. Ret.*, sensory retina; *Chor.*, choroid. (Reprinted with permission from: Miller NR, Fine SL. *The Ocular Fundus in Neuro-Ophthalmologic Diagnosis: Sights and Sounds in Ophthalmology.* Vol 3. St. Louis, MO: CV Mosby; 1977.)

swell." This is particularly important to remember when the ophthalmoscopic appearance of an atrophic optic disc is being used to determine recurrence or exacerbation of a condition such as raised intracranial pressure (see Chapter 5).

Specific Etiologies

Patients with increased intracranial pressure may develop optic disc swelling. This condition is called **papilledema**. The symptoms and signs in patients with

papilledema generally are those typically associated with raised intracranial pressure, including headache, nausea, vomiting, and pulsatile tinnitus. Visual symptoms in such patients include transient obscurations of vision and diplopia. Loss of central vision, dyschromatopsia, a relative afferent pupillary defect, and visual field defects other than enlargement of the blind spot caused by the swollen disc are uncommon in patients with acute papilledema unless the lesion causing the increased intracranial pressure also directly damages

Table 4.1 The Differential Diagnosis of the "Swollen Disc"

Disc Elevation without True Swelling
Optic disc anomalies
  Drusen
  Tilted disc
  Crowded disc
Optic disc infiltration
True Disc Swelling
Elevated intracranial pressure
Inflammatory
  Infectious
  Demyelinating
  Sarcoidosis
Vascular
  Anterior ischemic optic neuropathy
    Arteritic
    Nonarteritic
  Central retinal vein occlusion
Compressive
  Neoplastic
    Meningioma
    Hemangioma
  Nonneoplastic
    Thyroid ophthalmopathy
Infiltrative
  Neoplastic
    Leukemia
    Lymphoma
    Glioma
  Nonneoplastic
    Sarcoidosis
Toxic/Metabolic/Nutritional deficiency
Hereditary
  Leber's hereditary optic neuropathy
Traumatic
Hypotony

the visual sensory system in some way, or there are hemorrhages or exudates in the macula. The optic disc swelling in papilledema is usually bilateral and symmetric, but it may be asymmetric or even unilateral. It may be very mild or extremely severe (see Fig. 4.2). Papilledema is discussed in Chapter 5.

Inflammation of the proximal portion of the optic nerve produces swelling of the optic disc. This condition, called **anterior optic neuritis** or **papillitis**, is characterized by relatively acute visual loss, usually in one eye; it is almost always associated with pain around or behind the eye. Eye movement often exacerbates the pain. The appearance of the optic disc ranges from very mild to severe swelling. Vitreous cells may be present, particularly overlying the swollen disc, but peripapillary hemorrhages are rarely seen. In most cases of anterior optic neuritis, vision continues to decline for several hours to several days. It then stabilizes and, after several days to several weeks, begins to improve.

Anterior optic neuritis typically occurs in young adults and is most often caused by demyelination, although it may also develop in patients with a variety of systemic disorders, such as catscratch disease, syphilis, Lyme disease, and sarcoidosis. Patients who develop optic neuritis that is unassociated with a systemic inflammatory or infectious disorder have an increased risk of developing clinical evidence of multiple sclerosis (MS) compared with the normal population.

A special form of anterior optic neuritis called **neuroretinitis** is characterized ophthalmoscopically by optic disc swelling associated with a macular star figure composed of lipid (Fig. 4.4). This form of optic neuritis is almost never caused by demyelination and

A   B

Figure 4.2 Variability in severity of papilledema. **A and B:** Mild papilledema in a 28-year-old woman with early obstructive hydrocephalus. The right disc (**A**) is somewhat more hyperemic and swollen than the left (**B**). (*continued*)

C

D

Figure 4.2 (*continued*) **C and D:** Severe papilledema in a 23-year-old woman with pseudotumor cerebri. Note numerous hemorrhages and cotton-wool spots surrounding the markedly swollen right (**C**) and left (**D**) optic discs. Also note hard exudates (lipid) in both maculae.

occurs most often in the setting of catscratch disease or in association with other systemic infectious diseases, as well as with sarcoidosis. Optic neuritis is discussed in Chapter 6.

Ischemia that affects the laminar or prelaminar portions of the optic nerve produces swelling of the optic disc. This condition, called **anterior ischemic optic neuropathy (AION)**, is characterized by monocular and usually painless visual loss associated with a relative afferent pupillary defect and a visual field defect

that is most often altitudinal or arcuate in nature. The loss of vision usually occurs over several hours to several days. It then stabilizes in most cases with only mild recovery if any. AION occurs most often in patients older than 50 years of age who have underlying systemic vasculopathies, particularly diabetes mellitus, systemic hypertension, and giant cell arteritis.

The optic disc swelling that occurs in AION may be hyperemic or pallid (Fig. 4.5) and is usually accompanied by one or more flame-shaped hemorrhages near

Figure 4.3 Drusen-like bodies (*arrows*) in chronic papilledema.

Figure 4.4 Neuroretinitis. The patient was a young woman who developed acute visual loss in the right eye. The right optic disc is swollen, and there is a *star figure* composed of lipid (hard exudate) in the macula. An evaluation revealed serologic evidence of Lyme disease. Neuroretinitis is not associated with the subsequent development of multiple sclerosis but is most often caused by an underlying systemic infection, such as catscratch disease, Lyme disease, or syphilis, or sarcoidosis.

Figure 4.5 Optic disc swelling in anterior ischemic optic neuropathy. **A:** Hyperemic swelling. **B:** Pallid swelling.

the margins of the disc (Fig. 4.6B). Most patients with nonarteritic AION have a congenitally small optic disc with an absent or small central cup (Fig. 4.6A), and this congenital abnormality is thought to be the major predisposing factor for the development of the disorder. Patients with arteritic AION, on the other hand, may have any sized optic disc. AION is discussed in Chapter 7.

Compression of the proximal portion of the optic nerve may produce optic disc swelling. The compression may be caused by a tumor, such as a cavernous hemangioma, meningioma, or schwannoma. In other cases, enlargement of structures normally in the orbit, such as the extraocular muscles in dysthyroid ophthalmopathy, causes optic nerve compression. Patients in whom such compression occurs initially may have no visual complaints and may have few, if any, signs of optic nerve dysfunction other than an enlarged blind spot on visual field testing. Alternatively, they may complain of insidious and slowly progressive visual loss. In such cases, there is invariably some degree of dyschromatopsia, a relative afferent pupillary defect, and a defect in the visual field of the affected eye. The optic disc is generally only mildly to moderately

Figure 4.6 The "disc at risk" in nonarteritic anterior ischemic optic neuropathy (NAION). **A:** Small left optic disc with no cup in a patient who had experienced an attack of NAION in the right eye several months earlier. **B:** NAION characterized by hyperemic disc swelling and peripapillary hemorrhages in the same eye several months later.

Figure 4.7 Optic disc swelling from compression of the anterior portion of the orbital optic nerve. **A:** Left optic disc of a 25-year-old man who noted mildly decreased vision in the left eye. Visual acuity was 20/25 and there was an ipsilateral relative afferent pupillary defect. The optic disc is moderately swollen. **B:** MRI orbit, T1-weighted axial view, shows that the mass compresses the lateral aspect of the optic nerve, displacing it medially. The patient's vision returned to normal, and the optic disc swelling resolved, after the mass was removed.

swollen and hyperemic (Fig. 4.7). Peripapillary hemorrhages are usually absent, but chorioretinal striae are present in some cases, particularly when the compressive lesion is adjacent to the globe. The diagnosis of anterior compressive optic neuropathy is made by neuroimaging of the orbit. Compressive optic neuropathy is discussed in Chapter 8.

Toxic and metabolic disorders may cause swelling of the optic disc. In such cases, the swelling is usually bilateral and mild. Central vision is often reduced, with visual loss progressing slowly over several weeks to months. Color vision is almost always markedly abnormal, regardless of the level of central vision. Bilateral central or cecocentral scotomas are the rule, in some cases being associated with mild to severe constriction of the peripheral visual field. In many but not all cases, eliminating the source of the toxicity or reversing the metabolic abnormality is associated with partial or complete recovery of visual function. Toxic and metabolic optic neuropathies are discussed in Chapter 10.

Infiltration of the Optic Disc

Infiltration of the proximal portion of the optic nerve by tumor or inflammatory cells can produce an appearance similar to true swelling of the optic disc (Fig. 4.8). The disc changes may be asymptomatic or associated with variable visual loss, dyschromatopsia, and a visual field defect. The infiltration may be unilateral or bilateral, and a relative afferent pupillary defect may be present if the infiltration is either unilateral or bilateral but asymmetric. Infiltration of the

optic nerve occurs most frequently in patients with malignant tumors, such as leukemia, lymphoma, and various carcinomas that spread to the central nervous system, but it may also occur in patients with systemic

Figure 4.8 Optic disc elevation from infiltration of the orbital portion of the optic nerve. The patient was an 11-year-old boy with acute lymphocytic leukemia that was thought to be in remission when he developed mild blurred vision in the right eye. Note moderate elevation of the right optic disc, associated with dilation of small disc vessels. Malignant cells were detected in the patient's cerebrospinal fluid. The disc elevation resolved and visual acuity improved after radiation therapy.

inflammatory disorders, including sarcoidosis. Infiltrative optic neuropathies are discussed in Chapter 8.

Optic Atrophy

Optic atrophy is not a disease. It is a morphologic sequela of disease—any disease—that causes irreversible damage to ganglion cells and axons of the optic nerve. The term "optic atrophy" is therefore a pathologic generalization applied to optic nerve shrinkage from any process that produces degeneration of axons in the anterior visual system (the retinogeniculate pathway), including ischemia, inflammation, compression, infiltration, and trauma. Although the pathologist can make the diagnosis of optic atrophy by direct observation of histopathologic changes in the optic nerve, the clinical diagnosis of atrophy is usually based on (1) ophthalmoscopic abnormalities of color and structure of the optic disc with associated changes in the retinal vessels and nerve fiber layer, and (2) defective visual function that can be localized to the optic nerve.

Nonpathologic Pallor of the Optic Disc
An absolute prerequisite to recognition of the abnormal disc is familiarity with normal disc color. The temporal side of the normal disc usually has less color than the nasal side. The degree of this temporal pallor is primarily related to the size of the physiologic cup, to the thin translucent character of the temporal nerve fiber layer, and possibly to the relative sparseness of capillaries on that side of the disc.

The normal physiologic cup may vary in size. When it extends almost to the temporal edge of the disc, the temporal side of the disc is pale. In addition, the temporal margins of some large physiologic cups are steep-walled. When the margins slope gradually downward from the margin of the disc, the crescent of sclera adjacent to the temporal, and occasionally to the inferior, margin of the disc is visible and appears a mottled grayish white. This crescent, known as a temporal (or sometimes inferior) conus, is exposed by retraction of the dark retinal pigment epithelium from the disc margin. It enhances the whitish appearance of such a disc.

Marked recession or excavation of a physiologic cup makes the center of a disc pale. The retinal vessels at the base of the cup are partially obscured as they pass through a thin rim of neural tissue that borders the excavation. It may be difficult to distinguish this type of cup from a glaucomatous cup. The pallor of the floor of a physiologic cup is directly related to the glistening whiteness of the lamina cribrosa or cribriform plate, a connective and elastic tissue structure with small sieve-like openings through which transparent nerve fiber bundles pass (see Chapter 2). Because the openings are irregular, direct light entering them is reflected in many directions, and the holes appear as grayish yellow ovals or dots. When this dotting is seen, it signifies that no abnormal opaque connective tissue is present over the surface of the cribriform plate.

Many infants have pale fundi; the optic discs in such cases also appear pale. A white-appearing disc is common in an eye with axial myopia. Because the optic nerve enters the globe obliquely, the contents of the disc, including the nerve fibers and the retinal vessels, are displaced nasally. The physiologic cup is shallow, and its extension to the temporal margin produces relative temporal pallor that is often exaggerated by a temporal conus.

Perceived optic disc color is affected by the chromatic spectrum of the illumination source (e.g., LED vs. halogen) and the presence or absence of cataract. Dense cataract may mask pallor; conversely, the examiner must be especially cautious in diagnosing apparent disc pallor in a patient with unilateral or bilateral pseudophakia.

Pathology and Pathophysiology of Optic Atrophy
Because the axons in the optic nerve arise from the ganglion cells located in the retina, damage to such axons may occur from numerous sources at several locations:

- From disease within the eye that damages the ganglion cells, the retinal nerve fiber layer, or the optic disc.
- From disease within or surrounding the intraorbital, intracanalicular, or intracranial portions of the optic nerve.
- From disorders that damage the optic chiasm, optic tracts, or lateral geniculate bodies.
- From disorders of the retrogeniculate pathways that produce transsynaptic (transneuronal) degeneration.

A disease may be focal, multifocal, or diffuse. It may destroy axons directly or by its effects on their investing glia or capillary blood supply. Focal disruption anywhere along an axon causes degeneration of the entire axon and its cell body, the retinal ganglion cell. When large numbers of axons undergo such degeneration, gross shrinkage or atrophy of the optic nerve becomes evident.

When an axon is irreversibly damaged, it undergoes two types of degeneration: **anterograde (wallerian)** and **retrograde**. Anterograde degeneration occurs in the distal portion of the axon that has been separated from its cell body, whereas retrograde degeneration occurs in the proximal segment of the nerve that remains in contact with the cell body. Programmed cell death, or apoptosis, results in a cascade of metabolic events that culminates in the loss of affected retinal ganglion cells by 6 to 8 weeks after the injury. The timing of this process does not vary regardless of the injury location, and thus damage to the retrobulbar portion of the optic nerve, the optic chiasm, and the optic tract all cause pathologic and visible degeneration of the ganglion cell bodies at about the same time.

Regeneration of axons in the optic nerve in human and nonhuman primates is quite limited and abortive. However, some degree of remyelination does occur after the injury. This remyelination results from the activity of uninjured, injured but surviving, and newly generated oligodendroglia.

Transsynaptic (transneuronal) **degeneration** is a secondary degenerative reaction of neurons that occurs in a number of areas of the brain. For example, transneuronal degeneration is a well-established phenomenon in the cells of the lateral geniculate body following destruction of parts of the retina. Recent MRI data show a similar phenomenon may occur with acquired optic neuropathies such as glaucoma. However, the most profound transsynaptic changes occur following lesions in the immature brain. This type of transsynaptic degeneration occurs most often in patients with occipital lobe damage in utero or during early infancy.

Loss of function within the central nervous system is consistently associated with a reduction of blood supply to the affected tissue, regardless of the primary pathogenetic process. When the optic nerve degenerates, its blood supply is reduced, and small vessels that were once visible in the normal nerve can no longer be seen with an ophthalmoscope. In addition to reduction of blood supply, formation of glial tissue is said to occur with optic atrophy.

Other factors that may account for the normal pink appearance of the optic disc are its thickness and the cytoarchitecture of nerve fiber bundles passing between glial columns containing capillaries. Light entering the disc is normally conducted along the transparent nerve fiber bundles, much like fiberoptic pathways. The light diffuses among adjacent columns of glial cells and capillaries and acquires the pink color of the capillaries. Thus, light rays that exit through the tissue via the nerve fiber bundles are pink and give the disc its characteristic color. The axon bundles of an atrophic optic disc have been destroyed, and the remaining astrocytes are arranged at right angles to the entering light. Thus, little light passes into the disc substance to traverse the capillaries that, although still present, are surrounded by layers of astrocytes. Because the light is reflected from opaque glial cells and does not pass through capillaries, it remains white, and the optic disc thus appears pale. In some areas, loss of tissue also allows light to pass directly to the opaque scleral lamina, and this adds to the pale color of the disc.

Ophthalmoscopic Features of Optic Atrophy

The evaluation of optic disc color is a routine but often challenging problem. The lack of color in an optic disc is difficult to assess, record, compare, and describe. The normal color of the optic disc depends on its composition and the relationship of the components to each other and to the light that is reflected or refracted from the disc surface. Because the neural elements are gray, the pink color of the disc is also related to its blood vessels.

Pallor of the optic disc is often graded as mild, moderate, or severe; however, such distinctions are subjective and unreliable. More objective evaluation of the pale optic disc can be obtained by detailed observation of its configuration and neural tissue; its veins, arteries, and capillaries; and the peripapillary retinal nerve fiber layer (PRNFL) that surrounds it. Pallor of the optic disc may be diffuse or confined to one sector (Fig. 4.9).

In the early stages of atrophy, the optic disc loses its reddish hue, and the substance of the disc slowly disappears (Fig. 4.10). In the end stages of the atrophic process, retinal vessels of normal caliber still emerge centrally through the otherwise avascular-appearing disc. In many cases, the changes that develop during the progression to atrophy do not result in a significant change in the central cup of the optic disc. Despite the occasional confusion between glaucomatous and nonglaucomatous optic neuropathy that occurs in patients with pathologic cupping and pallor of the optic disc, a careful clinical examination almost always results in the correct diagnosis. Glaucomatous visual field defects occur only after extensive cupping is present, and acuity loss occurs even later. In such cases, there is usually absence of at least a portion of the neuroretinal rim, and any remaining rim tissue has a normal color (see Fig. 4.11B). In nonglaucomatous optic neuropathies, significant loss of visual acuity, color vision, and field may occur in combination with only mild cupping. In addition, the optic discs in such cases rarely have any areas in which the neuroretinal rim is completely absent, and the remaining rim is often pale (see Fig. 4.11A). Optical coherence tomography (OCT) of the PRNFL also may assist in differentiating the two entities. Deep, pathologic cupping is more likely to occur with severe ischemic processes such as arteritic AION (Fig. 4.11).

Focal destruction of nerve fiber bundles is one of the common pathologic denominators of disease that affects the inner retinal layers, optic disc, retrobulbar optic nerve, or a combination of these structures. The normal appearance of the PRNFL consists of fine curvilinear striations that overlie the retinal vessels, causing them to be seen slightly out of focus. Slit-like or small wedge defects in the PRNFL (Fig. 4.12A and B) may evolve into larger areas of PRNFL loss or become more numerous and impart a "raked" fundus

A   **B**

Figure 4.9 Sectoral and diffuse pallor of the optic disc. **A:** Temporal pallor in a myopic, tilted optic disc of a patient with multiple sclerosis and a history of right optic neuritis. **B:** Diffuse pallor after ischemic optic neuropathy. Visual acuity was counting fingers only with severe visual field loss. Note that the remaining neuroretinal rim is pale but intact, without the formation of an expanded optic cup as would be expected with advanced glaucoma damage.

appearance (Fig. 4.12C to E). Within the wedge, the entire retina takes on a flat granular appearance with no striations being appreciated (Fig. 4.12E and F). In addition, vessels in this area, having lost their surrounding nerve fiber covering, appear darker than normal and stand out sharply in relief. A prominent light reflex usually emanates from alongside the vessels, presumably as a result of draping of the inner lim-

iting membrane directly over the vessels (Fig. 4.12G). OCT of the PRNFL may detect early PRNFL changes in optic neuropathy before ophthalmoscopic sigs are visible. Clinical detection of nerve fiber layer atrophy is possible in nonhuman primates only after a loss of 50% of the neural tissue (approximately 25μ) in a given area. In contrast, OCT may detect PRNFL thinning of 7 to 9μ.

A   **B**

Figure 4.10 Early pallor of the optic disc. **A:** A 23-year-old patient developed intermittent left eye blurred vision and was found to have an optic nerve sheath meningioma. There is mild swelling and hyperemia at presentation. **B:** The patient declined treatment, and during serial examinations, early pallor is seen, especially temporally, with some loss of fine vascularity.

A

B

Figure 4.11 Optic disc cupping in glaucomatous and nonglaucomatous optic atrophy. **A:** Nonglaucomatous cupping. Note pallor and thinning of the neuroretinal rim. **B:** Glaucomatous cupping. Note normal appearance of the remaining neuroretinal rim.

In most cases of optic atrophy, the retinal arteries are narrowed or attenuated. In some instances, the narrowing is minor in nature; in others, such as severe nonarteritic AION, the vessels appear thread-like or are completely obliterated, especially around the edges of the disc (Fig. 4.13). Not all cases of optic atrophy are associated with retinal vascular changes, however. Indeed, in eyes with optic atrophy from damage to the retrolaminar optic nerve, the retinal vessels are often unaffected. Thus, eyes in which significant retinal vascular narrowing is associated with optic atrophy presumably have suffered an additional insult directly affecting the retinal vasculature.

Differential Diagnosis of Optic Atrophy

When optic atrophy is complete, it is often impossible to determine its etiology solely from the appearance of the optic disc. However, the atrophy caused by central retinal artery occlusion and ischemic optic neuropathy can often be differentiated from other entities because of the associated retinal arteriolar attenuation and sheathing. Macular OCT will demonstrate thinning of all inner retinal layers, not just the RNFL, in retinal artery occlusion.

Acquired temporal pallor is the most common expression of segmental optic atrophy and may be confirmed by OCT of the PRNFL. Its presence in combination with clinical findings of preserved peripheral visual fields and central acuity loss suggests a toxic, nutritional, or hereditary optic neuropathy (see Chapter 10). When superior or inferior disc pallor is present, an ischemic etiology is more likely.

The specific organization of the retinal nerve fiber layer results in specific patterns of nerve fiber layer and optic atrophy in patients with visual loss from optic chiasmal and retrochiasmal-pregeniculate lesions. In patients with chiasmal lesions, for example, temporal field defects are mirrored by loss of fibers from ganglion cells nasal to the fovea. The atrophy is most impressive directly nasal and temporal to the disc because the superior and inferior arcuate nerve fiber bundles are composed of fibers from ganglion cells both temporal and nasal to the fovea and are relatively spared. "Band" or "bow-tie" atrophy may result (Fig. 4.14).

In patients with congenital or neonatal homonymous hemianopia, or in patients with pregeniculate homonymous hemianopias, the eye contralateral to the lesion has temporal field loss and shows the pattern of nerve fiber and optic nerve atrophy described above—band atrophy of the optic disc. The eye ipsilateral to the lesion has a complete nasal field loss with loss of ganglion cells temporal to the fovea. Because the nerve fibers from these ganglion cells primarily comprise the superior and inferior arcuate bundles, these regions show extensive loss of nerve fibers, and the disc atrophy is more diffuse. The characteristic features of the fundi of such individuals are thus a bow-tie or band atrophy in the contralateral eye and reduced visibility of the superior and inferior arcuate nerve fiber bundles in the ipsilateral eye.

Although the presence or absence of pathologic pallor of the optic disc cannot be directly equated with visual function, it should be obvious that no judgment of pallor is meaningful until and unless the pallor is correlated with optic nerve function. The data should be obtained from careful testing of visual

Figure 4.12 Appearance of atrophy of the peripapillary retinal nerve fiber layer. **A:** Monochromatic red-free photograph shows mild nerve fiber bundle defects (seen as *dark streaks*) in the inferior arcuate fiber bundle. **B:** Artist's drawing of similar small defects. **C:** Monochromatic red-free photograph shows two large defects in the peripapillary retinal nerve fiber layer in the inferior arcuate region of the left eye in a patient with radiation-induced optic neuropathy. Note that compared with **A**, the defects in this photograph are darker, wider, and more distinct from the surrounding nerve fiber layer. **D:** Artist's drawing of moderate defects in the peripapillary retinal nerve fiber layer; the darker appearance results from both widening and deepening of the defects. **E:** Monochromatic red-free photograph shows a single broad defect in the peripapillary retinal nerve fiber layer in the inferior arcuate region of the right eye in a patient with early glaucoma and inferior extension of the optic cup. The defect is dark and quite distinct from the otherwise normal peripapillary nerve fiber layer, with a granular appearance of the fundus within the defect caused by loss of the axons. **F:** Complete loss of the peripapillary retinal nerve fiber layer in a patient with severe glaucoma. No linear striations can be seen, the peripapillary region has a distinct granular appearance, and the retinal vessels are seen clearly because of the absence of overlying nerve fibers.

Figure 4.13 Atrophic peripapillary vasculature in severe arteritic AION. The vessels are narrowed and attenuated adjacent to the diffusely pale optic disc and become more normal in appearance closer to the macula.

acuity and color vision, as well as quantitative perimetry, examination of the pupils, and electrophysiologic studies when appropriate (see Chapter 1). An optic disc may appear to be pale, yet meticulous clinical and electrophysiologic testing of visual function may fail to disclose any abnormality. OCT also may demonstrate a normal PRNFL thickness. In such cases, it is most likely that the pallor is physiologic rather than pathologic. Conversely, an optic disc occasionally appears normal despite severe and even long-standing

Figure 4.14 "Band" or "bow-tie" atrophy of the right optic disc in a patient with a temporal hemianopia caused by a pituitary adenoma. Note horizontal band of atrophy across the right disc, with preservation of the superior and inferior portions of the disc.

visual acuity or field loss caused by optic nerve dysfunction. In most of these cases, careful examination of the optic disc and PRNFL, both by ophthalmoscopy and OCT, will provide evidence of retinal nerve fiber atrophy.

Syndromes of Prechiasmal Optic Nerve Dysfunction

Retino-Choroidal Vessels and the Syndrome of Chronic Optic Nerve Compression

Chronic optic nerve compression may cause a specific syndrome characterized by progressive loss of vision, optic disc swelling that is followed or accompanied by optic atrophy, and the appearance of dilated venous channels called **retino-choroidal vessels**. These shunt veins are congenital connections between the retinal and choroidal venous circulations. When there is chronic compression of the optic nerve, particularly when the lesion is within the orbit, these veins enlarge and shunt blood from the retinal to the choroidal venous circulation, thus allowing the retinal venous blood to bypass the obstructed central retinal vein and exit the orbit via the choroidal circulation, vortex veins, and ophthalmic veins (Fig. 4.15). Sphenorbital meningiomas most commonly cause this syndrome, although it may also be caused by chronic papilledema, optic gliomas, or arachnoid cysts of the optic nerve. Retino-choroidal vessels also can appear in patients after chronic central retinal vein occlusion, often without evidence of optic nerve dysfunction.

Distal Optic Nerve Syndrome

Where the optic nerve joins the chiasm, at the anterior angle of the chiasm, its particular fiber anatomy provides another opportunity for anatomic diagnosis. The crossed and uncrossed fibers are separated at this level but are quite compact, and a small lesion affecting either the crossed or the uncrossed fibers may produce a unilateral hemianopic defect. Such a defect is called a "junctional scotoma." In such cases, it is not uncommon to find an asymptomatic scotoma in the upper temporal field of the **opposite** eye (Fig. 4.16). This scotoma results from damage to ventrally located fibers originating from ganglion cells located inferior and nasal to the fovea that, upon reaching the distal end of the optic nerve, loop anteriorly about 1 to 2 mm into the contralateral optic nerve (**Wilbrand's knee**, see Chapter 2).

Foster Kennedy Syndrome

Intracranial lesions that exert direct pressure on one optic nerve usually produce optic atrophy. As

Figure 4.15 Acquired retino-choroidal vessels. **A to C:** Three fundus photographs showing optociliary shunt veins in patients with optic atrophy from chronic compression of the optic nerves. Note varying size of the vessels, which are shunting venous blood from the retinal to the choroidal circulation so that it can exit the eye via the vortex veins to the superior and inferior ophthalmic veins rather than via the central retinal vein. **D and E:** Axial MRI (D, T1 with gadolinium contrast and fat suppression) and axial CT (**E**, with contrast) of orbits in two different patients showing optic nerve sheath meningiomas associated with optociliary shunt vessels. **F:** Artist's drawing depicting retinal venous compression at the lamina cribrosa from tumor-induced pressure exerted at the optic nerve head.

Figure 4.16 Two examples of the syndrome of the distal optic nerve (anterior chiasmal syndrome). **A:** Kinetic perimetry in a patient with decreased vision in the right eye from a pituitary adenoma shows a dense temporal defect with a central scotoma in that eye. In addition, however, there is a superior temporal defect in the visual field of the contralateral eye. **B:** Static perimetry in another patient with loss of vision in the left eye from a pituitary adenoma shows almost complete loss of the central field in that eye as well as a small superior temporal defect in the visual field of the right eye.

these lesions enlarge, they may eventually produce increased intracranial pressure. When the compressed optic nerve is significantly atrophic by the time intracranial pressure becomes increased, the increased intracranial pressure produces papilledema only in the contralateral eye. Unilateral optic atrophy and contralateral papilledema, when associated with anosmia, are the hallmarks of the so-called **Foster Kennedy syndrome** (Fig. 4.17). This syndrome occurs most often with frontal lobe tumors and olfactory groove meningiomas.

In some cases, this syndrome of optic atrophy in one eye and papilledema in the other eye is falsely localizing; that is, the optic atrophy is not on the ipsilateral side to the tumor but on the contralateral side. In addition, a "Foster Kennedy syndrome" consisting of optic atrophy on one side and optic disc swelling on the other side may result from asymmetric optic nerve compression from an intracranial mass in the absence

of increased intracranial pressure. Most importantly, a true Foster Kennedy syndrome is extremely rare. It is much more common to see optic atrophy on one side with optic disc swelling on the opposite side in cases of bilateral sequential optic neuritis or ischemic optic neuropathy. In such cases, the symptoms and signs are profoundly different and should cause no difficulty in diagnosis.

Bilateral Superior or Inferior (Altitudinal) Hemianopia

The question often arises in a patient with bilateral visual field defects if a single lesion accounts for the field defects or if there are bilateral optic nerve lesions. Bilateral central, cecocentral, and arcuate defects all suggest dysfunction of both optic nerves. Unilateral visual field loss in all or most of the upper or lower portion of the field results from a lesion of the retina

Figure 4.17 Foster Kennedy syndrome of unilateral optic atrophy, contralateral papilledema, and anosmia. The patient was a 34-year-old woman with severe headaches and progressive loss of vision in the right eye. A neurologic examination revealed anosmia and some degree of confusion. Visual acuity was 20/400 OD and 20/25 OS. There was a right relative afferent pupillary defect. **A:** The right optic disc is diffusely pale. **B:** The left optic disc shows chronic swelling. **C:** Axial CT scan with contrast reveals a large enhancing mass along the right sphenoid wing, consistent with a meningioma. **D:** Coronal CT scan with contrast shows the upward extension of the mass as well as enlargement of the lateral ventricles.

or optic nerve. Similarly, bilateral visual field defects of this type usually represent bilateral lesions damaging the retinas or optic nerves. In many of these cases, one eye is affected before the other. In such cases, the cause is typically bilateral nonarteritic AION. In rare cases, a simultaneous bilateral ischemic optic neuropathy can occur (Fig. 4.18).

Rarely, a large prechiasmal lesion compresses both optic nerves, producing bilateral altitudinal field defects. The more insidious onset of the visual field

loss, combined with a failure of the defect to respect the horizontal meridian strictly, helps in differentiating compression from the common causes of altitudinal defects (ischemia, optic neuritis).

Some patients with bilateral optic neuropathies—particularly those who develop bilateral simultaneous or sequential AION—develop a superior altitudinal defect in one eye and an inferior altitudinal defect in the other. Such patients may experience binocular diplopia or difficulty reading caused by decompensation

Figure 4.18 Bilateral inferior altitudinal visual field defects in a patient with simultaneous bilateral posterior ischemic optic neuropathy. The patient was a 62-year-old man who awoke from robotic prostatectomy with visual field loss in both eyes. Visual acuity was 20/25 OU. **A:** Static perimetry in both eyes shows incomplete inferior altitudinal scotomas. **B:** Optic disc appearance 2 months later, with superotemporal pallor in both eyes. (From Weber, Colyer MH, Lesser RL, et al. Posterior ischemic optic neuropathy after minimally invasive prostatectomy. *J Neuroophthalmol.* 2007;27:285–287.)

of a pre-existing vertical or horizontal phoria. Normally, partial overlap of the superior or inferior fields of the two eyes permits fusion of images and helps stabilize ocular alignment. However, in a patient with a complete superior altitudinal defect in one eye and an inferior altitudinal defect in the fellow eye, no overlap exists, and a pre-existing asymptomatic phoria becomes a tropia with either vertical or horizontal separation or overlap of the two remaining hemifields. Patients thus complain of diplopia and may have

difficulty reading because of doubling or inability to see printed letters or words (Fig. 4.19). This condition, called the **hemifield slide phenomenon**, was initially described in patients with bitemporal hemianopic field defects (see Chapter 12).

Nasal Hemianopia

Most organic nasal visual field defects are actually arcuate in nature, and the most common causes are

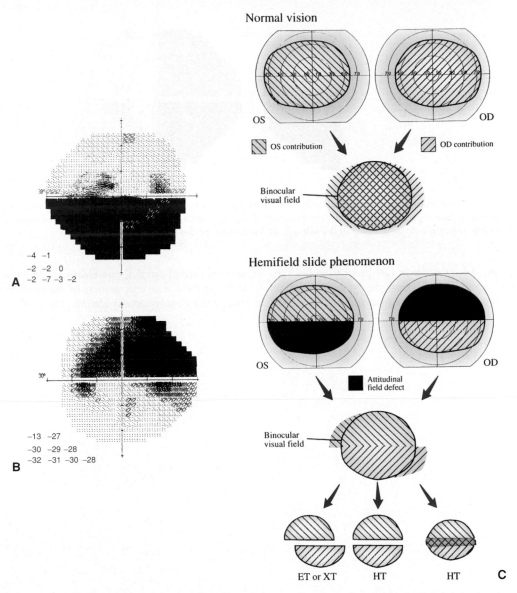

Figure 4.19 Hemifield slide phenomenon from bilateral optic neuropathy. Inferior altitudinal defect in the visual field of the right eye (**A**) and superior altitudinal defect in the visual field of the left eye (**B**) from bilateral ischemic optic neuropathy. **C:** Artist's drawing shows that such defects can produce a vertical or horizontal hemifield slide phenomenon from loss of overlapping portions of the visual fields. Affected patients may complain of vertical, horizontal, or diagonal diplopia.

chronic pathology of the optic disc, such as chronic papilledema and optic nerve head drusen. In some cases, however, a true unilateral hemianopia or bilateral nasal hemianopias occurs, with the defects having no connection to the blind spot and respecting the vertical meridian. Such field defects result from damage to the temporal aspects of one or both optic nerves.

Binasal hemianopia is an exceedingly infrequent visual field defect. Although a "binasal hemianopia" is sometimes said to occur in patients with intracranial tumors that grow between the intracranial optic nerves, pushing them laterally against the anterior cerebral or internal carotid arteries, the field defects in such cases are usually arcuate, not hemianopic, and do not respect the vertical midline. True binasal quadrantic or

Figure 4.20 Bilateral complete nasal hemianopia in a 34-year-old woman with a suprasellar aneurysm that displaced both optic nerves laterally against the supraclinoid portion of the internal carotid arteries. The field defect resolved after clipping of the aneurysm. **A:** Visual field of the left eye. **B:** Visual field of the right eye.

hemianopic defects occur in rare patients with a variety of intracranial lesions, including pituitary tumors, meningiomas, suprasellar aneurysm, dolichoectatic internal carotid arteries, optochiasmatic arachnoiditis, hydrocephalus with enlargement of the third ventricle, and primary empty sella syndrome (Fig. 4.20).

Papilledema*

Measurements of Intracranial Pressure

Ophthalmoscopic Appearance of Papilledema
    Stages of Papilledema
    Other Signs of Papilledema
    Chronic Papilledema
    Postpapilledema Atrophy
    Unilateral or Asymmetric Papilledema

Diagnosis of Papilledema

Course

Pathogenesis of Papilledema

Symptoms and Signs of Papilledema
    Nonvisual Manifestations
    Visual Manifestations

Etiology of Papilledema
    Intracranial Masses
    Disorders of CSF Flow
    Syndromes of Elevated Venous Pressure
    Trauma
    Craniosynostoses
    Extracranial Lesions
    General Considerations
    Conditions Associated with Papilledema

Idiopathic Intracranial Hypertension
(Pseudotumor Cerebri)
    Diagnosis of IIH
    Etiology of IIH
    Pathophysiology of IIH Not Associated with Other
        Factors
    Complications
    Treatment
    Special Circumstances

The term **papilledema** is often mistakenly applied to any type of swelling of the optic disc regardless of the etiology. Although it is true that swelling of the optic papilla can theoretically be denoted as "papilledema,"

---

*The authors acknowledge the past contributions of Deborah L. Friedman to this chapter.

the term has a particular, ingrained meaning to most clinicians. It should be used **only** for optic disc swelling that results from increased intracranial pressure (ICP). Other forms of disc swelling caused by local or systemic processes should be designated with respect to the presumed etiology—for example, "anterior ischemic optic neuropathy" or "anterior optic neuritis"—or in general terms, such as "optic disc swelling" or "optic nerve head edema."

Measurements of Intracranial Pressure

Normal cerebrospinal fluid (CSF) pressure in adults, measured by lumbar puncture (LP) with the patient in the left lateral decubitus position, varies between 80 and 250 mm of water; in children, pressures as high as 280 mm of water can be normal. Contrary to popular belief, CSF pressure is not dependent on weight or height, although pressure readings may be spuriously elevated when the patient coughs, strains, or holds his or her breath during the procedure. Prone positioning may falsely elevate the measured pressure, particularly in obese patients. In addition, ICP both in normal persons and in patients with increased ICP can fluctuate widely. Continuous monitoring of ICP of patients with idiopathic intracranial hypertension (IIH) has shown irregular variations ranging from 50 to 500 mm of water over a 24-hour period. Lumbar CSF pressure is often lower than the true ICP in patients with infratentorial tumors that block communication between the ventricular system and the spinal subarachnoid space.

LP is generally a safe procedure, but in certain situations it carries significant risk. Except under extraordinary circumstances, a neuroimaging study (computed tomography or magnetic resonance imaging (MRI)) should always be performed prior to the LP to make sure there is no mass effect in the brain. Removal of fluid from the spinal canal may allow the compressed brain to shift downward and to impact at the tentorial incisura or the foramen magnum, often with fatal results. LP occasionally induces an acquired Chiari malformation that may be reversible. Post-LP headaches may occur in up to 40% of patients after a lumbar tap. These headaches typically worsen when the patient is in the upright position and resolve when in supine position. Other symptoms of having low CSF pressure mimic those of increased ICP with visual disturbances and diplopia from sixth nerve paresis.

Ophthalmoscopic Appearance of Papilledema

There are several classification systems for papilledema. The disc appearance can be described according to the duration of papilledema (early; fully developed; chronic; and atrophic). However, the Frisén grading system (Table 5.1) is most useful as it classifies the papilledema grade by severity.

Stages of Papilledema

Stereoscopic viewing of a **normal optic disc (Frisén stage 0)** often reveals mild nasal elevation of the nerve fiber layer. With the direct ophthalmoscope the nasal disc margin may appear indistinct compared to the temporal disc rim. The vessels are generally seen coursing across the optic nerve head, although, rarely, a portion of a major vessel may be obscured in the upper pole (Fig. 5.1A).

In very early papilledema (Frisén stage 1), there is hyperemia of the optic disc, blurring of the peripapillary retinal nerve fiber layer, swelling of the optic disc, blurring of the disc margins, peripapillary flame-shaped hemorrhages, and absent spontaneous venous pulsations (SVPs) (Fig. 5.1B). There may be disruption of the normal radial nerve fiber layer arrangement with grayish opacity accentuating nerve fiber bundles. The absence of SVP is thought by some investigators to be an early sign of papilledema. Indeed, pulsations usually cease when ICP exceeds about 200 mm of water. However, reports of absent SVP with normal ICP and preserved SVP with ICP elevation inform us that SVP is not a reliable indicator of ICP status.

Early papilledema (Frisén stage 2) is characterized by obscuration of the optic disc borders, elevation of the nasal border, and a complete peripapillary halo (Fig. 5.1C).

As the severity of papilledema increases to **moderate papilledema (Frisén stage 3)**, the margins of the optic disc become obscured and elevated. The

Table 5.1   Papilledema Grading System (Frisén Scale)
Stage 0—Normal Optic Disc Blurring of nasal, superior, and inferior poles in inverse proportion to disc diameter Radial nerve fiber layer (NFL) without NFL tortuosity Rare obscuration of a major blood vessel, usually on the upper pole
Stage 1—Very Early Papilledema Obscuration of the nasal border of the disc No elevation of the disc borders Disruption of the normal radial NFL arrangement with grayish opacity accentuating nerve fiber layer bundles Normal temporal disc margin Subtle grayish halo with temporal gap (best seen with indirect ophthalmoscopy) Concentric or radial retrochoroidal folds
Stage 2—Early Papilledema Obscuration of all borders Elevation of the nasal border Complete peripapillary halo
Stage 3—Moderate Papilledema Obscurations of all borders Increased diameter of optic nerve head Obscuration of one or more segments of major blood vessels leaving the disc Peripapillary halo—irregular outer fringe with finger-like extensions
Stage 4—Marked Papilledema Elevation of the entire nerve head Obscuration of all borders Peripapillary halo Total obscuration on the disc of a segment of a major blood vessel
Stage 5—Severe Papilledema Dome-shaped protrusions representing anterior expansion of the optic nerve head Peripapillary halo is narrow and smoothly demarcated Total obscuration of a segment of a major blood vessel may or may not be present Obliteration of the optic cup

diameter of the optic nerve head increases, often resulting in enlargement of the physiologic blind spot. The optic cup may still be preserved at this stage. An important finding is that the edematous, opaque nerve fiber layer obscures one or more segments of major

---

Figure 5.1 A: Frisén grade 0 swelling with very mild disc elevation and no loss of disc margin clarity. **B:** Frisén grade 1 (very early papilledema) with a "C"-shaped halo of edema sparing the temporal disc. **C:** Early (Frisén grade 2) papilledema with 360 degrees of peripapillary retinal nerve fiber layer swelling and margin obscuration. **D:** Moderate (Frisén grade 3) papilledema with obscuration of major blood vessels as they leave the disc inferiorly. **E:** Marked (Frisén grade 4) papilledema with numerous peripapillary hemorrhages. Hemorrhage is not part of the Frisén classification system. **F:** Severe papilledema (Frisén grade 5) with loss of all normal anatomic landmarks of the optic disc. Lipid in the papillomacular bundle is also seen.

blood vessels leaving the disc. The gray peripapillary halo becomes more apparent and may have an irregular outer fringe with finger-like extensions conforming to the nerve fiber layer (Fig. 5.1D).

Marked papilledema (Frisén stage 4) is characterized by elevation of the entire optic nerve head. The optic cup is often obliterated. There is obscuration of all the borders of the nerve with a prominent peripapillary halo. Edema and infarction of the nerve fiber layer cause total obscuration on the disc of a segment of a major blood vessel. The retinal veins are often engorged and tortuous (Fig. 5.1E).

Severe papilledema (Frisén stage 5) is present when the optic nerve protrudes anteriorly with a dome-shaped configuration. The optic cup is obliterated and the peripapillary halo is narrow and smoothly demarcated. Often, there are no appreciable landmarks to distinguish the optic nerve head from the surrounding retina. Obscuration of segments of major blood vessels may or may not be present (Fig. 5.1F).

Other Signs of Papilledema

Other signs of papilledema may contribute to visual impairment but are often not helpful in determining the severity of papilledema. Flame-shaped, nerve fiber layer hemorrhages, cotton wool spots (focal retinal infarcts), and tortuous vessels on or surrounding the disc are common. In chronic cases, circumferential retinal folds (Paton lines) often develop; linear or curvilinear choroidal folds also may be observed (Fig. 5.2). Choroidal folds from increased ICP often result in acquired, progressive hyperopia. Hard exudates and

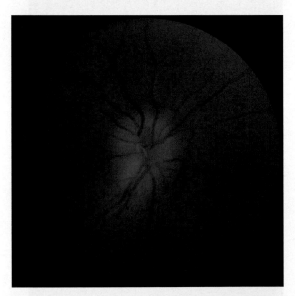

Figure 5.2 Circumferential chorioretina folds temporal to the optic disc (Paton lines) in a patient with papilledema from obstructive hydrocephalus.

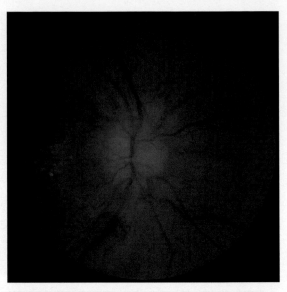

Figure 5.3 Macular star figure in a patient with papilledema requiring optic nerve sheath fenestration. The incomplete star in the papillomacular bundle is characteristic and may persist for months after papilledema resolves. Occasionally a complete star figure is seen.

hemorrhages may occur in the peripapillary region and in the macula, producing decreased central vision (Fig 5.3). Because nerve fibers in the macula have a radial orientation, hemorrhages and exudates in this region can assume a fan or star shape. Since vascular compromise on and around the optic disc is responsible for these macular changes, the star figure in such cases is usually asymmetric, being more prominent on the nasal side of the fovea toward the disc.

Hemorrhages are frequently present with papilledema, although they are not incorporated into the Frisén staging system. Nerve fiber layer hemorrhages are the most common and indicate that the edema is acute to subacute (Figs. 5.1E and F). A small nerve fiber layer hemorrhage in the peripapillary region may be an extremely important sign of early papilledema. Such a hemorrhage appears as a thin, radial streak on the disc or near its margins and is presumably caused by rupture of a distended capillary within or surrounding the disc.

When the increase in ICP is rapid, subhyaloid hemorrhages may be present in addition to the more common intraretinal hemorrhages (Fig. 5.4). These hemorrhages may break into the vitreous in some cases. Rarely patients with papilledema develop macular and peripapillary subretinal neovascularization, especially when the papilledema is chronic. The presence of peripheral retinal hemorrhages in addition to hemorrhages in the posterior pole suggests extensive retinal venous congestion produced by significantly elevated ICP.

Figure 5.4 Subhyaloid hemorrhage with papilledema in a patient with rapid intracranial pressure rise from cerebral venous sinus thrombosis.

Chronic Papilledema

When papilledema persists, hemorrhages and exudates slowly resolve, and the disc develops a rounded appearance (Fig. 5.5). The central cup, which may be retained in the acute phase of papilledema, ultimately becomes obliterated. Over a period of months, the initial disc hyperemia changes to a milky gray appearance, with hard exudates becoming apparent in the superficial disc substance. These exudates resemble optic disc drusen and may result in a misdiagnosis of pseudopapilledema (see Chapter 4, Fig. 4.3).

Most patients with chronic papilledema have evidence of nerve fiber layer atrophy. The appearance of the atrophy ranges from slit-like defects to diffuse loss. Nerve fiber layer atrophy can be appreciated by viewing through the red-free filter of a direct ophthalmoscope or slit lamp biomicroscope.

Occasionally, papilledema persists for a long period of time without significant visual symptoms. This situation occurs primarily in patients with IIH.

Postpapilledema Atrophy

With time, untreated papilledema subsides, the disc becomes atrophic, and the retinal vessels become narrow and sheathed. Some patients have persistent pigmentary changes or choroidal folds in the maculae (Fig. 5.6). The time required for papilledema to evolve into optic atrophy depends upon many factors, including the severity and constancy of the increased ICP. Atrophic changes can appear within weeks or days following the initial observation of acute papilledema in some cases, particularly if the rise in ICP is rapid, severe, and sustained. In such cases, the disc appearance may rapidly progress to fully developed papilledema and then to postpapilledema optic atrophy without ever having gone through a stage of chronic papilledema. Still in other cases, many months or even years may elapse before atrophy develops. In such

Figure 5.5 Chronic, severe papilledema. Note round compact appearance of the optic disc and lack of hemorrhages despite capillary dilation.

Figure 5.6 Postpapilledema optic atrophy and pigmentary changes in the retina in a patient who previously had severe papilledema. Note pallor of the optic disc, narrowed sheathed retinal vessels, and pigmentary changes superotemporal to the disc.

cases, the appearance of the fundus is typically that of chronic papilledema that gradually melts away into atrophy. In some cases of chronic papilledema, optociliary shunt veins develop. These vessels, which are pre-existing veins that connect the retinal and choroidal venous circulations, enlarge because the increased ICP either directly compresses the central retinal vein or indirectly compresses it by compressing the optic nerve (Fig. 5.7). In either case, the vessels shunt venous blood from the retinal to the choroidal venous circulation. Optociliary shunt veins may disappear after the ICP is surgically lowered or following optic nerve sheath decompression (ONSD) surgery.

Optic atrophy that results from chronic papilledema has a specific pattern of axonal loss. Loss of peripheral axons with sparing of central axons has been demonstrated in several postmortem studies. Good central visual acuity despite severe papilledema and optic atrophy is found in most patients with chronic papilledema (Fig. 5.8).

Unilateral or Asymmetric Papilledema

Papilledema is usually bilateral and relatively symmetric in the two eyes. In some instances, it is strictly unilateral or at least much more pronounced in one eye than in the other (Fig. 5.9). Some patients may have had pre-existing atrophy before the development of increased ICP (the pseudo-Foster Kennedy syndrome; see below and in Chapter 4). If there are not enough viable nerve fibers, papilledema cannot occur ("dead axons don't swell"). However, if sufficient nerve fibers remain, papilledema may develop even though the optic disc is pale. In the Foster Kennedy syndrome, patients with frontal lobe or olfactory groove tumors develop the triad of optic atrophy in one eye; papilledema in the other eye; and anosmia. The optic nerve ipsilateral to the tumor is generally atrophic because of compression. A rise in CSF pressure in the optic nerve sheath is a prerequisite condition for development of papilledema. Optic nerve

Figure 5.7 Development of optociliary shunt veins in a patient with chronic papilledema from pseudotumor cerebri. **A:** Marked (Frisén stage 4) papilledema. Note the small vessel located on the surface of the disc at 8 o'clock (*arrow*). **B:** As disc swelling resolves, the previously noted vessel becomes more apparent (*arrow*). **C:** Disc swelling has almost completely resolved. The vessel at 8 o'clock appears larger than previously, and clearly represents a retinal–choroidal shunt (*arrow*).

Figure 5.8 Preserved central acuity after severe papilledema. **A:** Marked (Frisén grade 4) papilledema; visual acuity was 20/50 with almost complete visual field loss. **B:** Postpapilledema atrophy with severe pallor. **C:** Visual field improvement with spared central island of vision; visual acuity was 20/20.

compression prevents elevated intrasheath pressure and produces ipsilateral atrophy of optic nerve fibers. Similarly, patients with unilateral optic disc dysplasia may develop papilledema only on the side of the previously normal disc.

When unilateral papilledema occurs in a patient with an apparently normal optic disc on the opposite side, it often results from some congenital anomaly of the optic nerve sheath or lamina cribrosa that prevents transmission of pressure to the optic nerve head on the side where the papilledema is absent. Both animal and human studies show that circulation of CSF may not occur between the optic nerve sheath space and the basal cisterns, thus preventing transmission of elevated ICP to the nerve. Conversely, elevated intrasheath pressure may persist despite medical or surgical lowering of ICP. In most patients with apparent unilateral papilledema, careful observation of the

"normal" optic disc often discloses minimal hyperemia, a blurred nerve fiber layer, or disc swelling that is easily overlooked in the face of significant papilledema on the opposite side.

Careful stereoscopic ophthalmoscopy, fluorescein angiography, and/or OCT imaging may be necessary to detect subtle papilledema. Nevertheless, purely unilateral papilledema has been described with IIH, cerebral tumors, abscesses, and intracranial hemorrhage caused by aneurysm, aqueductal stenosis, and traumatic brain injury.

Diagnosis of Papilledema

The most important method of diagnosing disc edema is careful ophthalmoscopic examination, assessing the features described above. An examination that includes

A   B

Figure 5.9 Asymmetric papilledema in an 18-year-old woman with pseudotumor cerebri. **A:** The right optic disc has Frisén stage 3 papilledema. **B:** Left eye with Frisén stage 1 papilledema. Transient visual loss and visual field changes were seen in the right eye only.

red-free ophthalmoscopy and slit lamp biomicroscopy with a hand-held lens is usually sufficient to determine whether disc edema is present. Once the diagnosis of disc edema is established, the associated clinical features suggest papilledema (i.e., disc edema from increased ICP) versus primary optic neuropathy with disc edema (such as anterior ischemic optic neuropathy, anterior optic neuritis, etc.). Classically, visual acuity is normal until late in papilledema while visual acuity is abnormal in other optic neuropathies. Other symptoms and signs such as headaches, pulsatile tinnitus, and diplopia also may suggest raised ICP.

On occasion, the diagnosis of true disc edema remains uncertain and the possibility of pseudo–disc edema is raised (see Chapter 3). In such cases, fluorescein angiography may be used to confirm early papilledema with both early and late peripapillary dye leakage observed. Orbital echography also may be useful in cases of questionable papilledema. This test can reliably determine if the diameter of the optic nerve is increased and, if so, whether or not the increase is caused by CSF surrounding the nerve. It can also easily detect buried optic disc drusen. Spectral domain OCT, using protocols to evaluate peripapillary retinal thickness and volume, also can reliably differentiate subtle papilledema from pseudoswelling.

The differential diagnosis of papilledema includes anomalous elevation of one or both optic discs and true optic disc swelling from a cause other than increased ICP (see Chapter 4). In most cases, such patients have no neurologic or systemic symptoms or signs referable to increased ICP, and this lack of man-

ifestations should help the physician focus on other possibilities.

Anomalous elevation of the optic discs is probably caused most often by buried optic disc drusen; however, hypoplastic discs may be anomalously elevated, and tilted optic discs often show elevation of their superior and nasal portions. In addition, some optic discs are anomalously elevated but do not contain drusen, nor are they small or tilted (see Chapter 3). In all cases, a careful ophthalmoscopic examination combined with ultrasonography, fluorescein angiography, and/or OCT should differentiate anomalously elevated optic discs from true optic disc swelling.

True optic disc swelling that mimics papilledema may be caused by local ocular disease, such as intraocular inflammation. Eyes in which optic disc swelling occurs in the setting of inflammation invariably show other evidence of inflammation, particularly aqueous or vitreous cells and, in some cases, sheathing of retinal vessels. Retinal vascular disturbances such as retinal vein occlusion can also produce optic disc swelling. In such cases, there may be no way to determine the cause of the disc swelling without performing appropriate neuroimaging studies and a LP. Patients with optic perineuritis (perioptic neuritis) have optic disc swelling that is also indistinguishable from papilledema unless there is associated intraocular inflammation. Nonarteritic anterior ischemic optic neuropathy can mimic papilledema, particularly when it is asymptomatic. Rare patients with anterior optic neuritis have normal central visual acuity; however, such patients invariably complain that they have decreased vision, and other tests of visual function in such patients (e.g., contrast sensitivity, visual fields) usually reveal an abnormality inconsistent with papilledema. Finally, optic discs infiltrated by inflammatory or neoplastic cells may appear similar to papilledema. The diagnosis in such cases can usually be made by neuroimaging, with or without a LP.

Course

The rapidity with which papilledema can develop depends to a large extent on the etiology of the increased ICP. Papilledema may develop within 2 to 8 hours when there is sudden intracranial or epidural hemorrhage. In addition, minimal papilledema may exist and suddenly become fully developed over several hours in certain settings, such as encephalitis associated with a cerebral abscess. Occasionally, there is an apparently paradoxical development, or increase in the severity, of papilledema several days to a week after normalization of increased ICP.

Fully developed papilledema may disappear completely within hours, days, or weeks, depending on the way in which ICP is lowered. For instance, papilledema can resolve 6 to 8 weeks after a successful craniotomy to remove a brain tumor, within 2 to 3 weeks after lumboperitoneal shunting in patients with IIH, and within days after optic nerve sheath fenestration.

In most cases, retinal venous and disc capillary dilations begin to regress as soon as ICP is lowered to a normal level. During the next few days to weeks, presumably because of the change in hemodynamics at the disc, new hemorrhages may appear; but these are of no significance and disappear within a short time. Gradually, disc hyperemia and elevation resolve. The last abnormalities to disappear are blurring of the disc margins and abnormalities of the peripapillary retinal nerve fiber layer. In some cases, optic atrophy appears as papilledema resolves. There may be extensive sheathing of vessels and gliosis indicating the nature of the etiology in such cases; however, in many cases, the atrophy is indistinguishable from that caused by inflammation, vascular disease, or trauma.

It is difficult to predict the visual prognosis in a patient with papilledema, although both rapid development of papilledema and severe papilledema herald a poorer outcome. Ominous signs include narrowing of the retinal arteries, often with sheathing, and loss of the peripapillary retinal nerve fiber layer. When these changes are seen, irreversible damage to optic nerve tissue has already occurred. Similarly, the onset of disc pallor while papilledema is still present is also an indication that the visual prognosis is poor, even if ICP is lowered immediately because the pallor is caused by loss of axons. Most patients with these changes have clinical evidence of visual dysfunction, including visual field defects and abnormal contrast sensitivity. Loss of visual acuity is the last visual parameter to be affected, much as is the case in patients with chronic open-angle glaucoma. Once a patient with papilledema begins to experience, or is found to have, deficits in these parameters, the visual prognosis is extremely tenuous. Severe venous engorgement, retinal hemorrhages, and hard and soft exudates have no prognostic significance.

Papilledema may be observed at any age, including in infants and children who still have open cranial sutures or fontanelles. Although papilledema is uncommon in infants and children with congenital hydrocephalus, studies have found papilledema or postpapilledema optic atrophy in 56% to 90% of children with brain tumors.

Symptoms and Signs of Papilledema

Both nonvisual and visual symptoms occur in patients with papilledema. As a general rule, the nonvisual symptoms are more severe and bothersome to the patient, although visual symptoms can be both distressing and indicative of impending permanent visual dysfunction.

Nonvisual Manifestations

Headache is one of the earliest symptoms of increased ICP, although there may be a considerable increase in ICP without headache. Neither the severity of the headache nor its location has any value in determining whether an intracranial mass is present, and if so, its location. An exception to this rule is the meningioma that infiltrates the dura over the convexity of the cerebral hemispheres and produces a palpable swelling and local pain at the site of the lesion. In some patients, headache associated with increased ICP is increased by coughing, straining, and Valsalva maneuvers. This is an inconstant phenomenon, but its presence may suggest a ball-valve action of a lesion within the ventricular system. It is believed that headache associated with increased ICP is caused by stretching of the meninges, whereas sharply localized pains in such cases may be explained on the basis of damage to sensory nerves at the base of the skull or localized dysfunction of meningeal nerves.

Nausea and vomiting are frequently associated with significantly increased ICP, although so-called projectile vomiting is rare. Vomiting, bradycardia, difficulty swallowing, and eventual respiratory failure may all be explained by herniation of the medulla into the foramen magnum.

Loss of consciousness, generalized motor rigidity, and pupillary dilation are terminal effects of increased ICP. Loss of consciousness presumably occurs from compression of the cerebral cortex and the reduction of its blood supply. Herniation of the hippocampal gyrus through the tentorium from increased ICP results in crowding of the temporal lobe into the incisura of each side. Tentorial herniation thus places pressure on the crura cerebri, resulting in generalized motor rigidity. Finally, direct pressure on the oculomotor nerves or dorsal midbrain produces bilaterally dilated pupils that do not respond to light stimulation.

Patients with increased ICP may, on occasion, develop spontaneous **CSF rhinorrhea**. In some cases, there is a history of previous trauma; in others, there is a congenital anomaly at the base of the skull. When spontaneous, CSF fistulas are usually located in the region of the cribriform plate. Up to 50% of patients with spontaneous CSF leakage have increased ICP.

Visual Manifestations

Patients with early, and even fully developed, papilledema are usually visually asymptomatic, with neither visual acuity nor color vision being affected. In some of these patients, the only abnormality found on careful testing is mild to moderate enlargement of the physiologic blind spot. Other patients may be aware of the physiologic blind spot, and such patients may complain of a negative scotoma in the field of vision of one or both eyes. Other patients have variable loss of visual acuity, color vision, visual field, or a combination of these visual parameters. Patients may have retinal or vitreous hemorrhages or exudates that reduce central acuity (Fig. 5.3, 5.10). In others, the intracranial mass causing high ICP also produces a visual sensory deficit in one or both eyes by a separate mechanism, such as direct compression of a portion of the visual sensory pathway (e.g., compression of the occipital lobe by a meningioma, producing a homonymous field defect), indirect compression of part of the pathway via a secondary effect on surrounding brain (e.g., gyrus rectus compression of the optic nerves producing a bilateral optic neuropathy in a patient with a frontal lobe tumor), or infiltration of a part of the pathway (e.g., infiltration of the optic chiasm by a germinoma, producing a bitemporal hemianopia).

Patients with papilledema may experience **brief, transient obscurations of vision.** During these episodes, vision may vary from mildly blurred to complete blindness. Some patients describe a rapid grayout of vision, whereas others experience positive visual phenomena—such as photopsias, phosphenes, and even scintillating scotomas—that obscure their vision. In all cases, recovery of vision is invariably rapid and complete. The obscurations may affect only one eye, alternate eyes, or both eyes simultaneously. They usually last only a few seconds, although attacks lasting several hours sometimes occur. Some patients experience up to 20 to 30 such episodes a day, with the obscurations often precipitated by changes in posture, particularly from sitting to standing or from lying down to sitting or standing; rare patients experience gaze-evoked amaurosis, a phenomenon much more commonly observed in patients with orbital lesions that compress and deform the optic nerve.

Transient visual obscurations have little prognostic value. Indeed, in many patients with transient obscurations, papilledema resolves completely without any detectable visual deficit. Conversely, patients with papilledema may develop permanent visual damage without ever having experienced transient visual obscurations. The cause of these obscurations is most likely related to transient compression or ischemia of the optic nerve.

Concentric enlargement of the blind spot is the most common—and frequently the only—**visual field defect** in patients with papilledema. Compression, detachment, and lateral displacement of the peripapillary retina appear to be the major reasons that the blind spot increases in size in patients with papilledema; however, the blind spot may be enlarged even when there is no obvious retinal displacement or detachment. In this setting, the enlarged blind spot represents a refractive scotoma caused by acquired peripapillary hyperopia, which, in turn, results from elevation of the retina by peripapillary subretinal fluid.

Early visual field defects, generally arcuate scotomas or nasal steps, in eyes with papilledema are not uncommon on automated static perimetry. Constriction of the visual fields is an ominous and often late sign that portends a poor outcome. The field defects are usually worse nasally than temporally and may persist after papilledema resolves (Fig. 5.11). Thus, an eye may have only a temporal island of vision before becoming completely blind.

Loss of visual field in the setting of papilledema is usually slow and progressive. Sudden loss of visual field in this setting suggests a local cause, such as ischemia. Superimposed ischemic optic neuropathy presumably occurs from occlusion of prelaminar disc arterioles caused by increased tissue pressure in the optic disc. These vessels may be more sensitive to increased intraocular pressure than are other vessels in the ocular fundus.

Patients with papilledema caused by intracranial mass lesions or meningitis (septic, aseptic, carcinomatous, lymphomatous) can **lose central vision** acutely or progressively from the effects of the underlying process on the optic nerves. In other cases, permanent loss of central vision results from the nonspecific effects of increased ICP on the optic nerve and begins with slowly progressive visual field constriction. In such cases, loss of central acuity is usually a

A

B

C

D

Figure 5.10 Papilledema associated with bilateral visual loss related to macular hard exudate. The patient was a 9-year-old girl with headaches, decreased vision, and constricted visual fields in both eyes. **A and B:** There is marked papilledema and macular exudate (**C and D**) in both eyes. After optic nerve sheath fenestration, papilledema improved (**E and F**) but central acuity remained abnormal because of persistent macular lipid (**G and H**). (*continued*)

late phenomenon, although it may occur over several weeks in cases with markedly increased ICP.

Acute loss of vision occurs in some patients with papilledema, usually from local causes. Some patients lose central vision because they develop hemorrhages or exudates in the maculae. Others develop ischemic optic neuropathy or retinal vascular occlusions that may be related to the underlying process (e.g., a coagulopathy) or to the rapid rate at which the ICP has risen. Finally, rare patients, many of them children, seem to have a fulminant course characterized by a rapid progression from normal vision to profound and permanent visual loss.

Even in the setting of normal visual acuity and a full visual field, patients with papilledema may have abnormal visual function evidenced by decreased contrast sensitivity and/or delayed latency of the P100 when visual-evoked potentials are measured.

Increased ICP may result in **diplopia** via compression or stretching of the abducens nerve at the base of the skull. The damage may be unilateral or bilateral; some patients have a comitant esotropia worse for distance than for near, which is often called "divergence insufficiency." Trochlear nerve palsies may occur rarely in patients with increased ICP, presumably from compression of either the dorsal midbrain or the

E

F

G

H

Figure 5.10 (continued)

nerves themselves by a ballooned suprapineal recess. Such palsies are often misdiagnosed as skew deviation if quantitative testing of eye movements or a Biel-schowsky head tilt test is not performed, although true skew deviation can exceptionally occur in patients with increased ICP.

Etiology of Papilledema

The craniospinal cavity is an almost rigid bony enclosure completely filled by tissue, CSF, and circulating blood. Within this enclosure, CSF is constantly produced at the rate of 500 mL/d, or 0.35 mL/min. Almost all of the production is by the choroid plexus within the lateral ventricles. The secretion of CSF is dependent on sodium-potassium–activated ATPase as well as the enzyme carbonic anhydrase. CSF flows from the lateral ventricles through the interventricular foramina into the third ventricle and mixes with the CSF produced in that ventricle. The CSF then flows through the cerebral aqueduct (of Sylvius) into the fourth ventricle, and out into the subarachnoid space through the foramina of Luschka and Magendie. In the subarachnoid space, CSF flows rostrally from the posterior fossa through the lower ventral basal cisterns and tentorial notch to reach the interpeduncular and chiasmatic cisterns. The CSF then flows dorsally through the communicating cisterns to reach the dorsal cisterns, and lateral and superiorly from the chiasmatic cistern into the cisterns of the Sylvian fissure. From the cisterns and Sylvian fissures, CSF moves

Figure 5.11 Visual field defects in papilledema. **A and B:** This patient has resolved papilledema with mild optic disc pallor and a gliotic appearance to both discs. **C and D:** An inferior nasal step visual field defect is seen in both eyes, left eye worse than right, corresponding to the severity of prior papilledema.

outward and superiorly over the cerebral convexities where it is absorbed.

The main route of absorption of CSF is passively through the arachnoid granulations that protrude into the venous sinuses and diploic veins. These vessels drain to the internal jugular vein and other extracranial veins. CSF is also absorbed in the spinal sac. Many factors influence CSF formation, including toxins, medications, and neurotransmitters while CSF absorption is affected by venous pressure and meningeal processes that may affect the arachnoid granulations.

The volume of blood, brain, and CSF within the cranial cavity must be in equilibrium, suggesting that a change in the volume of one component must be offset by a reciprocal change in another. As little as 80 cc of rapidly added volume (CSF, blood, edema, tissue, etc.) may raise ICP to a fatal level. Table 5.2 details the mechanisms involved in intracranial hypertension.

Table 5.2 Causes of Increased Intracranial Pressure

Space-occupying lesions
 Neoplasm
 Abscess
 Inflammatory mass
 Hemorrhage
 Infarction
 Arteriovenous malformation

Focal or diffuse cerebral edema
 Trauma
 Toxic
 Anoxia

Reduction in the size of the cranial vault
 Craniosynostosis
 Thickening of the skull

Blockage of CSF flow
 Noncommunicating hydrocephalus

Reduction in CSF resorption
 Communicating hydrocephalus
 Meningeal processes
  Infectious meningitis (bacterial, viral, fungus, parasitic)
  Inflammatory (aseptic) meningitis
  Carcinomatous meningitis
  Elevated CSF protein
   Spinal canal tumors
   Guillain–Barré syndrome
   Chronic inflammatory demyelinating polyneuropathy (CIDP)
 Elevated venous pressure

Increased CSF production
Idiopathic intracranial hypertension (pseudotumor cerebri)

Intracranial Masses

Intracranial masses such as tumors produce increased ICP through most of the mechanisms mentioned above. They may act solely as space-occupying lesions; they may produce focal or diffuse cerebral edema, and they may block the outflow of CSF by direct compression of CSF drainage pathways or by infiltration of the arachnoid villi or the cerebral venous sinuses. Other potential mechanisms are the production of increased protein or blood products that secondarily block the arachnoid villi, and by directly producing CSF.

Papilledema is not a common finding in brain tumor patients in the MR imaging era; in the past, 60% to 80% of patients with cerebral tumors had papilledema. Tumors that are situated below the tentorium (infratentorial), which may obstruct the aqueduct, are more likely to produce papilledema than those situated above it (supratentorial). Associated symptoms and signs usually allow a proper diagnosis; however, tumors in certain locations may produce

papilledema without lateralizing or localizing signs, particularly if they are supratentorial and situated within the nondominant hemisphere or within one of the lateral ventricles. This emphasizes the importance of examining the fundus of all patients with chronic or new-onset headaches.

Papilledema may occur with any type of intracranial mass. Neither the type of intracranial tumor nor its rate of growth correlates well with the development of papilledema.

Disorders of CSF Flow

Aqueductal stenosis often presents in childhood. It may be congenital, in which case it may or may not be associated with a Chiari malformation, or it may be acquired from intracranial infections. Presentation in infancy is accompanied by macrocephaly. Adults may have headaches, dorsal midbrain syndrome, meningitis, hemorrhage, endocrine disturbances from compression of the pituitary gland, seizures, gait disturbances, and CSF rhinorrhea.

Subarachnoid hemorrhage usually produces papilledema either by blocking CSF flow within the ventricular system (obstructive hydrocephalus) or by blocking CSF absorption at the arachnoid granulations. Papilledema occurs in 10% to 24% of patients with aneurysmal subarachnoid hemorrhage. Papilledema can develop several hours after the hemorrhage, or it may develop only after several weeks of increased ICP.

Meningitis and encephalitis produce severe cerebral edema, and resultant raised ICP, although obstructive hydrocephalus and impaired CSF absorption by arachnoid granulations may also occur. However, the reported frequency of papilledema with meningitis is fairly small, and the papilledema tends to be mild and transient. Papilledema is more likely to occur in patients with tuberculous meningitis (25% of cases) and cryptococcal meningitis than in any other type of infectious meningitis. These patients may have fulminant papilledema, and severe visual loss from secondary optic atrophy is common. Any type of meningeal process may be associated with papilledema. It is found in about 20% of patients with viral encephalitis. It is also common in noninfectious processes such as sarcoidosis or carcinomatous meningitis. This is why CSF analysis is an essential step in the diagnosis of papilledema. It must be emphasized that in almost all CNS infections and inflammations as well as neoplasms, swelling of the optic nerve may occur without increased ICP, presumably from inflammation or infiltration of the optic nerve or optic nerve sheath. In such cases, differentiating between papilledema and perineuritis is impossible, because in both cases, there is normal visual function. Only when a LP is performed in a patient with a meningeal process and disc swelling, and the CSF is found to be under normal pressure with an increased protein and pleocytosis, can the true inflammatory or infiltrative etiology of the disc swelling be ascertained.

Syndromes of Elevated Venous Pressure

Obstruction or impairment of cerebral venous drainage may result in increased ICP and papilledema. Indeed, most of the CSF drainage occurs passively into the cerebral venous sinuses at the level of the arachnoid granulations. When one (or more) cerebral venous sinus is occluded, the venous pressure rises and the CSF is not resorbed properly into the venous sinuses, thereby producing increased ICP.

Although cerebral venous thrombosis often produces neurologic symptoms and signs, it can also present with an isolated syndrome of raised ICP indistinguishable from IIH. The venous sinus obstruction is most often caused by compression or thrombosis, with the sinuses most often affected being the superior sagittal and transverse (lateral) sinuses. There are numerous local and systemic causes of cerebral venous sinus obstruction (Table 5.3).

Occlusion of one jugular vein (if it is the principal vein draining the intracranial space) or both jugular veins may also produce increased ICP and papilledema by producing increased venous pressure (Table 5.3).

It is very important to rule out venous hypertension from cerebral venous thrombosis or internal jugular vein thrombosis when evaluating a patient with isolated raised ICP. Indeed, the prognosis of these disorders is often poor unless a thorough workup is obtained, and appropriate treatment is rapidly initiated.

Trauma

Papilledema occurs in 20% to 30% of persons who have suffered severe cranial injuries, both with and without an associated skull fracture. In most of these cases, the increased ICP is caused by a severe subarachnoid hemorrhage or a significant intracerebral, subdural, or epidural hematoma. In other cases, the increased ICP is caused by cerebral venous thrombosis or by diffuse or localized cerebral edema.

Papilledema that develops in patients after head trauma is usually mild and may develop immediately, several days after the injury, or up to 2 weeks later. A sudden, severe, but transient increase in ICP is usually responsible for the immediate development of papilledema, whereas sustained but mild to moderately elevated ICP accounts for papilledema that appears during the first week after injury. Papilledema in the second week or later results from impaired CSF absorption and consequent communicating hydrocephalus or delayed focal or diffuse cerebral swelling.

Table 5.3 Etiologies of Obstruction/Impairment of Cerebral Venous Drainage

Cerebral venous thrombosis
  Primary hematologic
    Antiphospholipid antibody syndrome
    Thrombophilia (antithrombin III deficiency, protein S deficiency, resistance to activated protein C, prothrombin gene mutation)
    Thrombocythemia
    Polycythemia
    Disseminated intravascular coagulation
    Hyperviscosity syndrome
  Systemic conditions associated with coagulopathy
    Behçet disease
    Systemic lupus erythematosus
    Neurosarcoidosis
    Cancer
    Pregnancy/postpartum
    Renal disease (nephrotic syndrome)
    Infections
    Post surgery
Local infections
    Mastoiditis
    Facial/orbital cellulitis
    Meningitis
  Traumatic
  Tumors (compression of a sinus)
  Dural arteriovenous fistula
Transverse sinus stenosis
Occlusion of internal jugular vein
    Iatrogenic
    Indwelling catheter
    Surgery
    Traumatic
    Tumors (extravascular)
Increased venous pressure
    Right cardiac insufficiency
    Superior vena cava syndrome
    Morbid obesity
    Hyperviscosity syndrome

Craniosynostoses

The intracranial vault may become smaller in certain types of craniosynostoses. Among patients with premature synostosis of the cranial sutures, 12% to 15% eventually develop papilledema. However, simple cranial synostosis (oxycephaly, scaphocephaly, trigonocephaly, or plagiocephaly) is almost never associated with papilledema, whereas about 40% of patients with craniofacial dysostosis (Crouzon syndrome) or acrocephalosyndactyly (Apert syndrome) develop papilledema.

If papilledema is going to develop in a patient with a craniosynostosis, it usually does so before the age of 10 years. It is often chronic by the time it is detected, possibly because such patients may not undergo a careful examination of the ocular fundi unless they complain of visual disturbances. However, papilledema may develop at any age.

Extracranial Lesions

The association of increased ICP and papilledema with **tumors in the spinal canal** is an unusual but well-documented phenomenon. Most of these tumors are intradural; however, extradural spinal tumors can also cause increased ICP associated with papilledema. In some cases, the tumors are located in the high cervical region, and the explanation for the increased ICP in such cases is thought to be upward swelling of the tumor with compression of the cerebellum and obstruction of CSF flow through the foramen magnum. This mechanism seems unlikely to be the explanation in the majority of cases, however, because over 50% of spinal cord lesions associated with papilledema are ependymomas or neurofibromas that are usually located in the thoracic and lumbar regions. These tumors can produce extremely high concentrations of protein in the CSF, and it is therefore likely that increased ICP and papilledema in such cases is caused by the decreased CSF absorption that results from blockage of the arachnoid granulations by protein. In other cases, recurrent subarachnoid hemorrhage, which occurs commonly from bleeding from the surface of ependymomas, may also cause reduced CSF absorption from blockage of the arachnoid villi by blood or blood products.

Papilledema is an uncommon complication of **Guillain–Barré syndrome (GBS)**. Its pathogenesis remains uncertain, although it is postulated that protein in the arachnoid villi and granulations alters cerebral venous dynamics or causes partial venous thrombosis, leading to increased ICP. Increased ICP, often associated with papilledema, occurs more often in patients with **chronic inflammatory demyelinating polyneuropathy (CIDP)** than in patients with acute GBS. It seems to be caused in most cases by the markedly increased protein concentration that is one of the laboratory hallmarks of the disease; however, patients with CIDP can develop papilledema even with only a mildly increased concentration of protein in the CSF.

The **POEMS syndrome** is an unusual multisystem disorder that is characterized by polyneuropathy (*P*), organomegaly (*O*), endocrinopathy (*E*), monoclonal gammopathy (*M*), and skin changes (*S*). Patients with POEMS syndrome not infrequently develop ICP associated with papilledema. In addition, optic disc swelling may occasionally occur in patients without evidence of increased ICP. The POEMS syndrome may be a variant of multiple myeloma, and the associated monoclonal immunoglobulin may mediate multiple systemic manifestations. Patients with multiple myeloma can also develop increased ICP and papilledema, but the mechanism is unknown.

Idiopathic Intracranial Hypertension (Pseudotumor Cerebri)

IIH describes a syndrome defined by four criteria: (1) increased ICP, (2) no hydrocephalus on neuroimaging, (3) no evidence of an intracranial mass lesion or cerebral venous thrombosis, and (4) normal CSF composition. Most, but not all patients have papilledema. The term IIH was intended to replace "pseudotumor cerebri" in most cases of this syndrome, in recognition of the fact that the underlying cause was not known in most patients. Nonetheless, "pseudotumor cerebri" is once again being used more commonly in recognition of our identification of a putative cause of high ICP in an increasing percentage of IIH patients (see below).

The pseudotumor cerebri (PTC) syndrome was first described by Quincke in 1897. The terminology used historically in the literature gives a sense of the various conditions previously described under the term "pseudotumor cerebri": toxic hydrocephalus, otitic hydrocephalus, hypertensive meningeal hydrops, pseudoabscess, ICP without brain tumor, brain swelling of unknown cause, and papilledema of indeterminate etiology. The most popular and enduring term "pseudotumor cerebri" was first used in 1914. Noting that the condition was not caused by a tumor or malignancy, Foley introduced the term "benign intracranial hypertension" in 1955. However, the term "benign" also implies a favorable process or the absence of harm. As significant visual morbidity may result from PTC, the use of the prefix "benign" was challenged and is no longer considered an acceptable terminology.

The overall incidence of IIH is unknown and varies throughout the world. It approaches zero in countries in which the incidence of obesity is low, and it is common in countries or regions within countries with an increased incidence of obesity. As the obesity rate in developing nations has risen, so has the incidence of IIH. Historical incidences of 0.9 to 2.2 per 100,000 in the general population have been reported, with a 5 to 10 times greater incidence in obese women between ages 15 and 44. The age range in patients with PTC in general and IIH in particular is broad. Children and even infants are not infrequently affected, and such patients may have a higher incidence of permanent visual loss. The peak incidence of the disease, however, seems to occur in the third decade of life, with a female preponderance as high as 97% in a prospective study, causing some researchers to question whether true IIH occurs in males.

The occurrence of IIH in family members is uncommon but well recognized. No common metabolic or endocrinologic abnormalities have been found in such patients.

Diagnosis of IIH

The diagnostic criteria for IIH are (a) symptoms and signs solely attributable to increased ICP; (b) elevated CSF pressure; (c) normal CSF composition; (d) normal neuroimaging studies; and (e) no other etiology of intracranial hypertension identified. Each of these criteria is discussed below.

Clinical Manifestations

The most common presenting symptom in patients with IIH is headache, occurring in about 85% of cases. The headache is usually generalized, worse in the morning, and aggravated by cerebral venous pressure increased through some type of Valsalva maneuver (coughing, sneezing, etc.). Headaches may improve dramatically or resolve after LP, confirming their relationship to intracranial hypertension. Other common nonvisual manifestations of IIH include nausea, vomiting, dizziness, and pulsatile tinnitus. Pulsatile tinnitus is often described as a "whooshing sound," which may be uni- or bilateral and is usually relieved after LP. Focal neurologic deficits in patients with IIH are extremely uncommon, and their occurrence should make one consider alternative diagnoses. Patients with chronic IIH may occasionally develop cognitive disturbances and depression.

Visual manifestations of IIH are usually preceded by headache and occur in 35% to 70% of patients. These symptoms are identical with those described by patients with increased ICP from other causes, including transient visual obscurations, loss of vision from macular hemorrhages, exudates, pigment epithelial changes, retinal striae, choroidal folds, subretinal neovascularization, or optic atrophy, and/or horizontal diplopia from unilateral or bilateral abducens nerve paresis. Other ocular motor deficits have been rarely reported and should suggest cerebral thrombosis or a meningeal process rather than IIH. The papilledema that occurs in over 90% of patients with IIH is identical with that which occurs in patients with other causes of increased ICP. There is no correlation between severity of optic disc swelling and age, race, or body weight in patients with IIH, although men may have worse swelling than women. On occasion, IIH is asymptomatic and papilledema is discovered during a routine eye examination.

Ancillary Testing

To satisfy the criteria required to diagnose IIH, a patient must undergo neuroimaging studies followed by a LP. It is inappropriate to diagnose IIH without a LP or in the setting of abnormal CSF.

Neuroimaging Studies. Head CT is often the first test performed in patients with papilledema and is sufficient to detect most intracranial lesions that could produce raised ICP and to exclude obstructive hydrocephalus. However, this study is insufficient to exclude Chiari malformations, posterior fossa abnormalities, isodense lesions not associated with ventriculomegaly, gliomatosis cerebri, meningeal abnormalities, or cerebral venous thrombosis. Thus, MRI with contrast is required to diagnose IIH. In many cases, MR venography or CT venography should also be considered (see below). Rarely, a patient's body habitus exceeds the capacity of the MR gantry, and a head CT with contrast with CT venogram should be obtained.

Brain MRI may show typical signs of increased ICP. An asymptomatic empty sella, resulting from chronically increased ICP, is present in over half of cases. Other radiographic signs include dilation of the perineuronal subarachnoid space surrounding the optic nerves, protrusion of the optic papilla into the posterior aspect of the globe, and flattening of the posterior sclerae.

Cerebrospinal Fluid Examination. CSF examination is required for the diagnosis of IIH to confirm an elevated opening pressure and exclude a meningeal process producing high ICP. LP should be performed in the lateral decubitus position, relaxed with the legs partially extended. The pressure may be artifactually elevated if the patient is crying, performing a Valsalva maneuver, or is in severe pain. The opening pressure should be measured with a manometer, and adequate CSF should be obtained for assessment of cellular content, concentrations of protein and glucose, and any other tests deemed appropriate by the treating physician. In obese patients, LP is more easily performed with fluoroscopic guidance; prone positioning may elevate the opening pressure by up to 50 mm of water. For the diagnosis of IIH, the CSF opening pressure should be 250 mm (25 cm) of water or greater. In children, a value over 280 mm water is considered abnormal. Because CSF pressure normally fluctuates, multiple CSF pressure measurements or prolonged CSF pressure monitoring is sometimes required for diagnosis. The CSF contents by definition are normal in IIH.

A secondary cause for the elevated ICP should be considered in all patients but particularly in nonobese women and men, regardless of age or body habitus because such patients are much less likely to have IIH. A particularly careful history is necessary in such patients, with special attention given to any underlying systemic inflammatory or infectious disease, associated disorders such as anemia or sleep apnea, or ingestion or exposure to an inciting agent. Cerebral venous disease also should be carefully ruled out.

Table 5.4	Exogenous Substances Most Classically Associated with Idiopathic Intracranial Hypertension

Antibiotics
   Tetracycline
   Minocycline
   Doxycycline
   Nalidixic acid
Beta-human chorionic gonadotropin hormone
   withdrawal
Chlordecone (Kepone)
Corticosteroids withdrawal
Cyclosporine
Danazol administration or withdrawal
Growth hormone
Leuprolide acetate (Lupron)
Levonorgestrel implants (Norplant)
Lithium carbonate
Retinoids
   Vitamin A
   Isotretinoin
   All-*trans*-retinoic acid

Figure 5.12 CT angiogram of head in a patient with pseudotumor cerebri, with the venous phase shown in a 3D reconstruction. The right transverse sinus is dominant and has a focal stenosis at its distal aspect (*arrow*).

Etiology of IIH

IIH occurs primarily in young obese women, and occasionally men, with no evidence of any underlying disease. However, as noted above, a pseudotumor syndrome may develop in a number of different settings, including obstruction or impairment of cerebral venous drainage, endocrine and metabolic dysfunction, exposure to exogenous drugs and other substances, withdrawal of certain drugs, and systemic illnesses. Tables 5.4 and 5.5 list some of these purported associations. Except for those cases in which venous occlusive disease can be demonstrated, the exact mechanisms of increased ICP in these settings remain undetermined and a definite causal association unproven.

As noted above, uncompensated **obstruction of cerebral venous drainage** may cause increased ICP

Table 5.5	Systemic Illnesses Associated with Idiopathic Intracranial Hypertension

Obesity
Hyperthyroidism
Anemia
Chronic respiratory insufficiency
Pickwickian syndrome
Polycystic ovarian syndrome
Obstructive sleep apnea
Renal disease (nephrotic syndrome)
Sarcoidosis
Systemic lupus erythematosus
Systemic hypertension

and may mimic IIH. Such patients may be thought to have IIH unless the cerebral veins and venous sinuses are imaged using standard MRI, MR angiography, or CT angiography. Distal transverse sinus stenosis (uni- or bilateral) may be seen in over 90% of IIH patients versus fewer than 10% of obese controls, and they may obstruct venous outflow and thus CSF drainage (Fig. 5.12). In some cases, the stenosis is a consequence of high ICP, but in many instances the obstruction persists despite ICP lowering (i.e., by LP). In some cases, endovascular stenting of such stenotic venous sinuses may relieve symptoms of ICP.

Patients with **endocrine and metabolic dysfunction** can also develop IIH (Table 5.5). Obesity is the most common finding in patients with IIH, and recent weight gain has been associated with worsening of vision in such patients. In many of these patients, there is also a history of menstrual irregularity. However, attempts to uncover specific underlying endocrinologic disturbances in patients with this form of IIH have been unsuccessful. IIH not infrequently occurs during **pregnancy**.

Patients who are exposed to, or ingest, a variety of **exogenous substances** can develop PTC (Table 5.4). For some of these substances, a causative relationship is supported by only a single case report and is tenuous at best. For other drugs, such as tetracyclines, vitamin A, growth hormone, and cyclosporine, the association between exposure or ingestion and the development of increased ICP is well documented in numerous reports and investigations.

Increased ICP and papilledema in patients with meningitis and encephalitis is not IIH by definition.

In many of these cases, the ventricular system is obstructed physically and ventricular dilation develops. In other cases, such as meningeal carcinomatosis and lymphomatosis, Whipple disease, neuroborreliosis, and neurosarcoidosis, the ventricular system appears normal, but the CSF contains white blood cells, malignant cells, increased protein content, or a combination of these. Some **systemic diseases** can produce increased ICP, papilledema, normal-sized ventricles, and normal CSF content—a clinical picture consistent with IIH (Table 5.5). Anemia and sleep apnea need to be looked for as they may be associated with increased ICP and papilledema.

Optic disc swelling occurs in some patients with severe systemic hypertension, and is not always associated with other funduscopic signs of hypertensive retinopathy. This emphasizes that blood pressure should be carefully checked in patients with apparent papilledema and headaches.

Rarely, a syndrome resembling IIH has been reported with systemic inflammatory disorders such as **sarcoidosis** or **systemic lupus erythematosus**. Such a diagnosis should be made with caution as most patients have an inflammatory meningeal process or cerebral venous thrombosis.

Pathophysiology of IIH Not Associated with Other Factors

The pathogenesis of IIH remains unknown. A number of hypotheses have been suggested but none explain all IIH syndromes. It is logical to think that diminished absorption of CSF and cerebral edema may produce IIH. Indeed, patients with IIH may have both a defect in CSF resorption and an increased cerebral volume associated with a noncompliant ventricular system that resists dilation. Venous hypertension has long been proposed as one of the main mechanisms of IIH. Indeed, venous hypertension is common in obese patients with IIH, especially those with sleep apnea. In addition, cerebral transverse venous sinus stenoses often found in these patients may also produce venous hypertension. Because this disorder is more common in young obese women, it has been suggested that hormonal changes (excess of estrone) may increase the secretion of CSF by the choroid plexus. Vitamin A and retinol are also thought to play a role in IIH.

Complications

The natural history of IIH is variable. While it can be a self-limited condition, the feared complication of IIH is permanent visual loss, which is severe in up to 25% of patients. IIH may recur years after successful treatment, with weight gain as the major risk factor for recurrence. Depression is common in IIH patients who often develop chronic headaches.

Treatment

The primary goals of treatment are to preserve vision and alleviate headache symptoms. The treatment of IIH in adults and children is similar. Both medical and surgical treatments are used, often in combination. Prospective randomized clinical trial data now exist for treatment of mild IIH; the treatment of more severe disease remains based on case series data and anecdotal experience. IIH is considered an "off label" usage for all medications currently prescribed to treat the disorder.

Most patients with IIH require careful follow-up by a neurologist (who will manage the headaches) and an ophthalmologist (who will monitor the visual function and perform repeated formal visual field testing). Follow-up is decided on a case-by-case basis based on the severity of visual symptoms. Some patients need to be evaluated weekly until vision stabilizes or improves, while others who have good visual function may only need to be seen every few months. Therapeutic decisions are made individually based on each patient's characteristics. Particularly important to consider are (1) the presence and severity of headaches; (2) the degree of visual loss at presentation; (3) the rate of progression of visual loss; (4) the presence of an identifiable underlying etiology or aggravating factor (e.g., medication-induced IIH, anemia, sleep apnea, etc.).

Medical Treatment
Medical therapy is usually the first-line treatment in patients with IIH. It follows the LP performed as part of the diagnostic workup (which is the most efficient way to reduce ICP rapidly and improve symptoms and signs). When the primary problem is headache in the setting of good vision, medical treatment is usually sufficient and surgery not necessary. In asymptomatic patients with papilledema, close observation of visual function without specific therapy may be employed once an underlying etiology is excluded. If a secondary cause is identified, it should be treated appropriately. For example, implicated exogenous agents should be discontinued.

Weight loss is advised for obese patients based on both prospective and retrospective analyses. Even modest weight loss of 3% to 6% may result in symptomatic improvement. Severe caloric restriction to 400 kcal/d in a prospective study did lead to IIH resolution in almost all patients. When weight loss efforts fail, bariatric surgery may be considered. Such surgery is generally successful in producing weight reduction.

Obese patients with intracranial hypertension secondary to hypoxia and hypercapnia (i.e., the Pickwickian syndrome, obstructive sleep apnea) may respond not only to weight loss, but also to treatment of obstructive sleep apnea.

Carbonic anhydrase inhibitors decrease production of CSF and have a mild diuretic effect. The most commonly used agent is acetazolamide (between 1 and 4 g/d in adults). A prospective clinical trial of the treatment of mild IIH (defined as ≤7 dB of visual field loss on automated perimetry) demonstrated that acetazolamide use may lead to more rapid resolution of papilledema and visual dysfunction than weight loss alone. High doses are often limited by side effects, which include paresthesias of the extremities, lethargy, and altered taste sensation. Alternatively, methazolamide (Neptazane) may be used and is sometimes better tolerated than acetazolamide. Other diuretics may be used, such as furosemide and chlorthalidone. Spironolactone and triamterene may be considered in patients who are allergic to carbonic anhydrase inhibitors and other sulfonamide-containing diuretics. Combining diuretics, or using them with carbonic anhydrase inhibitors, may produce hypokalemia and should be done with extreme caution.

Although systemic corticosteroids may be beneficial in the treatment of isolated raised ICP associated with various systemic inflammatory disorders, such as sarcoidosis and systemic lupus erythematosus, they are not generally recommended for routine use in IIH. Indeed, rebound increase in ICP is common, and weight gain is an undesirable side effect in the obese population most affected by IIH. Corticosteroids should be reserved for the urgent treatment of patients with severe visual loss while arranging a definitive surgical procedure.

Headaches from IIH often improve dramatically after a LP. They most often can be managed medically as for chronic migraine or tension headaches. The majority of IIH patients also have headache that is unrelated to ICP, and appropriate treatment must be prescribed to discourage medical noncompliance with IIH therapy and analgesic abuse.

LPs have a very limited therapeutic role, and patient management by serial LP should be avoided, as the symptomatic relief is temporary in most cases. Patients with severe headache and/or vision loss may be managed with continuous lumbar drainage via spinal catheter until definitive surgical treatment can be performed.

Surgical Procedures

Surgery is performed in patients with severe optic neuropathy at initial presentation or when other forms of treatment fail to prevent progressive visual loss. It is rarely performed for the treatment of headaches alone. The decision of whether to proceed with a CSF shunting procedure or an ONSD depends largely on the local resources available. Retrospective analysis shows that both procedures protect vision; headache relief is much less predictable. ONSD may be preferred in patients with severe visual loss associated with disc edema but mild headaches, and a CSF shunting procedure in patients with visual loss, disc edema, and severe headaches. More than one type of surgical procedure may be necessary.

CSF diversion, either by **ventriculoperitoneal** or **lumboperitoneal shunting**, is quite effective in lowering ICP in patients with IIH. Most patients treated with a shunt experience rapid normalization of ICP and resolution of papilledema, often with improvement in visual function after shunting. Acute visual loss can occur, albeit very rarely, in patients with severe papilledema when the ICP is normalized rapidly. Both types of shunt tend to obstruct over time, and over half of patients ultimately require one or more shunt revisions, frequently within months after their initial insertion. Complications of the shunt procedure include spontaneous shunt obstruction, usually at the peritoneal end, excessively low pressure, infection, radiculopathy, and migration of the tube, resulting in abdominal pain. Some patients also develop a Chiari malformation after lumboperitoneal shunting that may or may not be symptomatic. Although the risks of shunting are generally minor, fatal tonsillar herniation after shunting in IIH has been reported. Use of a programmable valve may help prevent complications that arise from CSF overdrainage.

Optic nerve sheath fenestration (ONSF) is an efficient way to treat papilledema. In this procedure, a window or multiple slits are made in the dural sheath of the optic nerve immediately behind the globe. The procedure immediately reduces pressure on the operated nerve, with resultant improvement in visual function. While some studies report improvement of the fellow eye with unilateral surgery, the surgeon should not hesitate to operate on the fellow eye if continued visual decline occurs. Although some patients relate that ONSF improves their headaches, there is probably little effect on ICP in most cases, and the decrease in papilledema and visual improvement are related to the local decrease in optic nerve sheath pressure rather than from a generalized decrease in ICP. The mechanism of long-term effectiveness from ONSF may be fibrous scar formation between the dura and optic nerve creating a barrier to protect the anterior optic nerve from the intracranial CSF pressure.

The risks of optic nerve sheath fenestration, although low, are nevertheless significant. They include transient or permanent loss of vision from retinal vascular occlusion or optic nerve ischemia, diplopia, and infection. Some patients require a repeat procedure as vision may worsen months to years later. Nevertheless, most adults and children have stabilization or improvement of vision following optic nerve sheath fenestration.

Venous sinus stenting may be performed in select patients with cerebral venous sinus stenosis causing reduced cerebral venous outflow. Rapid resolution of both papilledema and headache has been reported with venous sinus stenting. Although bilateral stenosis often is found, unilateral stenting (often on the dominant side) usually proves adequate to relieve symptoms. We recommend that candidates for this procedure (i.e., patients with medically refractory disease and severe vision loss and/or headache) undergo CT venography immediately after LP to confirm the stenosis persists despite temporary ICP lowering. Catheter venography is then used to record a pressure gradient, and a stent is placed across the stenotic segment. Prolonged antiplatelet therapy is required after treatment to avoid intrastent thrombosis.

Special Circumstances

Pregnancy

Women who develop IIH during pregnancy are diagnosed and treated similarly to nonpregnant women. Most women do well, with little or no permanent visual loss. There is no contraindication to pregnancy in women with a history of IIH and no special provisions are required for delivery unless other medical complications are present. The majority of patients may be managed with careful neuro-ophthalmic follow-up. Acetazolamide may be used after 20 weeks gestation. If vision deteriorates, corticosteroids may be used. ONSF or lumboperitoneal shunting may be performed if needed, although there is a theoretical risk of shunt malfunction from peritoneal catheter obstruction as the uterus enlarges. Isolated raised ICP arising in the postpartum period or following fetal loss should raise the suspicion of cerebral venous sinus thrombosis.

Fulminant IIH

There is a small subgroup of patients with IIH who experience a rapid onset of symptoms and precipitous visual decline. They often have significant visual field loss, central visual acuity loss, and marked papilledema at presentation. Macular edema or ophthalmoparesis may also be present. A progressive or "malignant" course requires rapid and aggressive treatment that often includes a surgical procedure. Intravenous corticosteroids and insertion of a lumbar drain are often used while waiting for a more definite treatment. Cerebral venous sinus thrombosis and a meningeal process are important diagnostic considerations in these patients.

Optic Neuritis*

6

Idiopathic Demyelinating Optic Neuritis
   Acute Idiopathic Demyelinating Optic Neuritis
   Chronic Demyelinating Optic Neuritis
   Asymptomatic (Subclinical) Optic Neuritis

Optic Neuritis in Other Primary Demyelinating Diseases
   Neuromyelitis Optica (Devic Disease)
   Myelinoclastic Diffuse Sclerosis (Encephalitis
      Periaxialis Diffusa, Schilder Disease)
   Encephalitis Periaxialis Concentrica (Concentric
      Sclerosis of Baló)

Causes of Optic Neuritis Other than Primary Demyelination
   Infectious and Parainfectious Optic Neuritis
   Postvaccination Optic Neuritis
   Inflammatory Optic Neuritis
   Miscellaneous Causes of Optic Neuritis

Optic Neuritis in Children

Neuroretinitis

Optic Perineuritis

Optic neuritis is a term used to refer to inflammation of the optic nerve. When it is associated with a swollen optic disc, it is called **papillitis** or **anterior optic neuritis.** When the optic disc appears normal, the terms **retrobulbar optic neuritis** or **retrobulbar neuritis** are used. In the absence of signs of multiple sclerosis (MS) or other systemic disease, the optic neuritis is referred to as isolated, monosymptomatic, or idiopathic. The pathogenesis of isolated optic neuritis is presumed to be demyelination of the optic nerve, similar to that seen in MS. It is likely that most cases of isolated acute optic neuritis are a forme fruste of MS.

Optic neuritis can be caused by disorders other than MS and related demyelinating diseases. In addition, two variants of optic neuritis occasionally occur. **Neuroretinitis** is a term used to describe inflammatory involvement of both the intraocular optic nerve and

the peripapillary retina. **Optic perineuritis,** also called "perioptic neuritis," describes inflammatory involvement of the optic nerve sheath, without inflammation of the nerve itself.

Idiopathic Demyelinating Optic Neuritis

Optic neuritis usually is a primary demyelinating process. It almost always occurs as an isolated phenomenon or in patients with MS. Patients in whom optic neuritis occurs as an isolated phenomenon have a higher risk of the subsequent development of MS than the normal population. There are three forms of primary demyelinating optic neuritis: acute, chronic, and subclinical.

Acute Idiopathic Demyelinating Optic Neuritis

Acute demyelinating optic neuritis is by far the most common type of optic neuritis that occurs throughout the world and is the most frequent cause of optic nerve dysfunction in the young adult population. Much of our knowledge regarding this form of optic neuritis was obtained from the Optic Neuritis Treatment Trial (ONTT), a prospective study in which patients with a first episode of unilateral optic neuritis were randomized to corticosteroid treatment (either intravenous or oral) or placebo. The investigators in this trial enrolled 455 patients with acute unilateral optic neuritis. Although the primary objective of the trial was the assessment of the efficacy of corticosteroids in the treatment of optic neuritis, the trial also provided information about the clinical profile of optic neuritis, its natural history, and its relationship to MS.

Demographics
The annual incidence of acute optic neuritis is estimated in population-based studies to be between 1 and 5 per 100,000. In Olmstead County, Minnesota, where the Mayo Clinic is located, the incidence rate is estimated to be 5.1 per 100,000 person-years and the prevalence rate 115 per 100,000.

The majority of patients with acute optic neuritis are between the ages of 20 and 50 years, with a mean

*The authors acknowledge the past contributions of Craig H. Smith to this chapter.

age of 30 to 35 years; however, optic neuritis can occur at any age. Females are affected more commonly than males by a ratio of approximately 3:1.

Clinical Presentation

The two major symptoms in patients with acute optic neuritis are loss of central vision and pain in and around the affected eye.

Loss of central visual acuity is reported by over 90% of patients. Vision loss is typically abrupt, occurring over several hours to several days. Progression over a longer period of time can occur but should make the clinician suspicious of an alternative disorder. The majority of patients describe diffuse blurred vision, although some recognize that the blurring is predominantly central. Occasionally, patients complain of a loss of a portion of peripheral field, such as the inferior or superior region, often to one side. The visual loss is monocular in most cases, but in a small percentage, particularly in children, both eyes are simultaneously affected.

Pain in or around the eye is present in more than 90% of patients with acute optic neuritis. It is usually mild, but it may be severe and even more debilitating to the patient than the loss of vision. It may precede or occur concurrently with visual loss, usually is exacerbated by eye movement, and generally lasts no more than a few days. The presence of pain helps differentiate this condition from other causes of optic neuropathies such as anterior ischemic optic neuropathy, which typically produces painless visual loss (see Chapter 7).

Up to 30% of patients with optic neuritis experience positive visual phenomena, called **photopsias,** both at the onset of their visual symptoms and during the course of the disorder. These phenomena are spontaneous flashing black squares, flashes of light, or showers of sparks, sometimes precipitated by eye movement or certain sounds.

Examination of a patient with acute optic neuritis reveals evidence of optic nerve dysfunction. Visual acuity is reduced in most cases but varies from a mild reduction to no light perception. Contrast sensitivity and color vision are impaired in almost all cases. The reduction in contrast sensitivity is typically worse than the visual acuity loss, as is the reduction in color plate recognition (Ishihara or Hardy–Rand–Rittler). Even when the patient can detect all the pseudoisochromatic figures correctly, careful comparison of the appearance of a single plate by each eye may reveal a striking difference in color and brightness between the two eyes.

Visual field loss can vary from mild to severe, may be diffuse or focal, and can involve the central or peripheral field. Indeed, almost any type of field defect can occur in an eye with optic neuritis. Among 415 patients in the ONTT with baseline visual acuity of hand motions or

better, automated perimetry of the central 30 degrees of visual field revealed diffuse visual field loss in 48% of patients and focal loss in 52%. Focal nerve fiber bundle type defects (altitudinal, arcuate, and nasal step) were present in 20% of patients; pure central or centrocecal defects in 8%; and hemianopic defects in 5%.

A relative afferent pupillary defect is demonstrable in almost all unilateral cases of optic neuritis. When such a defect is not present, either there is a coexisting optic neuropathy in the fellow eye (e.g., from previous or concurrent asymptomatic optic neuritis), or the visual loss cannot be attributed to optic neuritis or another optic neuropathy.

Patients with optic neuritis also can be shown to have a reduced sensation of brightness in the affected eye, either by simply asking them to compare the brightness of a light shined in one eye and then the other, or by more complex tests using polarized lenses or flickering lights of varying frequencies.

About one-third of Caucasian patients with acute optic neuritis have some degree of disc swelling (Fig. 6.1); disc swelling is more prevalent in optic neuritis patients of Asian, African, and Caribbean origin. Although the swelling is usually mild, it may be so severe that it mimics the choked disc seen in patients with papilledema (Fig. 6.2). The degree of disc swelling does not correlate with the severity of either visual acuity or visual field loss. Disc or peripapillary hemorrhages and segmental disc swelling are less common in eyes with acute optic neuritis than in eyes with anterior ischemic optic neuropathy. Over approximately 4 to 6 weeks, the optic disc may become pale, even as the

Figure 6.1 Anterior optic neuritis. There is significant swelling and hyperemia of the disc with dilated surface capillaries.

Figure 6.2 Severe anterior optic neuritis mimicking papilledema. Note hyperemia and elevation of the disc and several peripapillary retinal hemorrhages.

visual acuity and other parameters of vision improve (Fig. 6.3). The pallor may be diffuse or sectoral, most often in the temporal region.

Slit lamp examination in eyes with demyelinating optic neuritis is almost always normal, but a very mild anterior or posterior uveitis may be observed. Sheathing of retinal veins may also occur, especially in patients with MS. When the cellular reaction is extensive, etiologies other than demyelination should be considered, including sarcoidosis, syphilis, catscratch disease, and Lyme disease (see p. 140, Infectious and Parainfectious Optic Neuritis).

Bilateral simultaneous acute optic neuritis is uncommon in adults, although the relative frequency increases when evaluating populations of patients with established MS. The ONTT showed a relatively high percentage of presumably asymptomatic fellow eye deficits at baseline: 14% with visual acuity abnormalities, 22% with color vision abnormalities, and 48% with visual field defects. The majority of the fellow eye deficits resolved over several months, suggesting that such abnormalities may be caused by subclinical but concurrent acute demyelination in the fellow optic nerve. In contrast to adults, acute optic neuritis is often symptomatically bilateral and simultaneous in children and is presumed related to infection (see p. 142, Optic Neuritis in Children).

Diagnostic Studies

Studies in patients with presumed acute optic neuritis are performed for one of three reasons: (1) to exclude another cause of optic neuropathy, particularly a compressive lesion; (2) to determine if a process other than demyelination is responsible for optic nerve inflammation; and (3) to determine the visual and neurologic prognosis.

With the widespread availability of magnetic resonance imaging (MRI), computed tomographic (CT) scanning has little or no role in the evaluation of patients with presumed optic neuritis. MRI will show optic nerve enlargement, T2 hyperintensity, and/or enhancement with gadolinium contrast in most cases of optic neuritis (Fig. 6.4). However, these findings are nonspecific, as a similar appearance can be observed in patients with infectious, and other inflammatory optic neuropathies. The most important application of MRI

A   B

Figure 6.3 Optic atrophy after acute, retrobulbar optic neuritis. **A:** In acute phase, visual acuity in the left eye is 20/300 with a central scotoma, but the optic disc is normal. **B:** Three months later, visual acuity has returned to 20/30, but the optic disc is pale, particularly temporally, and there is mild nerve fiber layer atrophy.

A   B

Figure 6.4 Magnetic resonance imaging (MRI), T1 weighted with gadolinium contrast and fat saturation, of the optic nerve in acute demyelinating optic neuritis. **A:** Axial image shows enhancement of the right optic nerve *(arrow)* with "spillover" to the optic nerve sheath leading to enhancement of this structure as well *(arrowheads)*. **B:** Coronal image shows enlargement and enhancement of the right optic nerve.

in patients with optic neuritis is in the identification of signal abnormalities in the white matter of the brain, usually in the periventricular region, consistent with demyelination (Fig. 6.5).

Other tests are similarly nonspecific in differentiating acute demyelinating optic neuritis from the less

Figure 6.5 Magnetic resonance imaging (MRI) of the brain of a patient with isolated optic neuritis and no previous history of neurologic dysfunction. T2/FLAIR-weighted sagittal MRI shows multiple ovoid periventricular white-matter lesions.

common systemic and local infectious and inflammatory optic neuropathies, and obtaining a thorough medical history is required to identify patients who may need additional testing. Therefore, diagnostic testing should be performed on a case-by-case basis to rule out common disorders such as syphilis, sarcoidosis, catscratch disease, Lyme disease, or systemic lupus erythematosus (SLE).

The role of CSF analysis in the evaluation of patients with acute optic neuritis is not clear. Although the presence of oligoclonal banding in the CSF is associated with the development of MS, the powerful predictive value of brain MRI for MS has reduced the role of lumbar puncture in the evaluation of patients with optic neuritis. Lumbar puncture can help define a very low risk population for MS if both CSF and MRI are normal. CSF studies in patients with optic neuritis are mostly useful to rule out another inflammatory or infectious disorder.

Visual Prognosis

The natural history of acute demyelinating optic neuritis is to worsen over several days to 2 weeks, and then to improve. Initial recovery is usually rapid and then slows, but further improvement may occur for 1 year after the onset of visual symptoms. Among patients in the ONTT who received placebo, visual acuity began to improve within 3 weeks of onset in 79% and within 5 weeks in 93%. For most patients in this study, recovery of visual acuity was nearly complete by 5 weeks after onset. Two-thirds of patients recover central acuity of 20/20 or better, and less than 15% of patients have worse acuity than 20/40. Other parameters of visual function, including contrast sensitivity, color perception, and visual field, improve in conjunction with improvement in visual acuity.

Although the overall prognosis for visual acuity after an attack of acute optic neuritis is extremely good, some patients have persistent severe visual loss after a single episode. Furthermore, even patients with improvement in visual function to "normal" may complain of movement-induced photopsias or transient loss of vision with overheating or exercise (Uhthoff symptom). Uhthoff symptom is most common in patients with other evidence of MS, but it is also experienced after isolated optic neuritis, by patients with chronic or subclinical optic neuritis, and occasionally by patients with optic neuropathies from other causes. Two major hypotheses regarding Uhthoff symptom are that (1) elevation of body temperature interferes directly with axon conduction, and (2) exercise or a rise in body temperature changes the metabolic environment of the axon, which, in turn, interferes with conduction.

Subjectively, patients with recovered optic neuritis frequently complain that their vision in the affected eye is "not right," or that colors are "washed out." One cause of these symptoms is probably related to subtle abnormalities in the visual field in which patients experience abnormally rapid disappearance of focal visual stimuli and abnormally rapid fatigue in sensitivity. These patients typically complain that when they look at something, it appears as if they have "holes" in their vision.

Recurrent attacks of optic neuritis may occur in either eye. The 10-year ONTT recurrence rate was 35%. The risk of recurrence was increased (41%) in the ONTT group treated with oral steroids compared with those receiving intravenous steroids or placebo (25%).

Neurologic Prognosis

Optic neuritis occurs in about 50% of patients with MS and is the presenting manifestation in about 20%. Both retrospective and prospective studies have been performed to determine the prognosis for the development of MS in patients who experience an attack of acute optic neuritis. Although retrospective studies provide figures ranging from 11.5% to 85%, most prospective studies support the higher figures. Among 95 incident cases of optic neuritis in Olmstead County, Minnesota, the estimated risk of MS was 39% by 10 years, 49% by 20 years, 54% by 30 years, and 60% by 40 years. The average time interval from an initial attack of optic neuritis until other symptoms and signs of MS develop varies considerably; most studies found that the majority of persons who develop MS after optic neuritis do so within 7 years of the onset of visual symptoms.

Without question, the most highly predictive baseline factor for progression to MS is the presence of one or more lesions in the periventricular white matter on MRI, a phenomenon noted in 50% to 70% of patients

with isolated optic neuritis. This was demonstrated by several studies, including the ONTT. Among patients with isolated optic neuritis in the ONTT, the cumulative percentage developing MS within 5 years was 16% in patients with normal MRI and 51% in patients with more than two lesions on the brain MRI. At 15 years from onset of optic neuritis, 72% of patients with even one typical MRI lesion at baseline (regardless of the number of lesions) had developed MS, while only 25% of those who had a normal MRI at baseline had developed MS (Fig. 6.6). Other risk factors for the development of MS among ONTT patients were Caucasian race, a family history of MS, history of previous ill-defined neurologic complaints, and a previous episode of optic neuritis. However, none of these factors affected the risk of developing MS as much as the results of MRI. Among patients with normal MRI, negative risk factors included male gender, absence of pain, mild visual acuity loss, and optic disc swelling. Although the ONTT did not support any correlation between age of onset and the development of MS, other studies suggest that the younger the age of onset of optic neuritis, the greater the subsequent risk for MS. Winter onset of optic neuritis also may be a risk factor.

The ONTT and the Longitudinal Optic Neuritis Study (LONS) have revealed a particularly low MS-risk group. Among the patients who had a normal brain MRI, none of the patients with severe disc edema, macular star, or disc hemorrhages developed MS at 15 years. These findings emphasize the role of the ophthalmologist in defining the prognosis of optic neuritis.

Treatment

Corticosteroids are the main treatment option for patients with acute idiopathic optic neuritis. The ONTT had three treatment groups: (1) oral prednisone (1 mg/kg/d) for 14 days; (2) intravenous methylprednisolone sodium succinate (250 mg four times a day for 3 days) followed by oral prednisone (1 mg/kg/d) for 11 days; and (3) oral placebo for 14 days. Each regimen was followed by a short oral taper (20 mg on day 15, 10 mg on days 16 and 18). Most patients in all three treatment groups had a good recovery of vision with only 10% of patients in each group having a visual acuity of 20/50 or worse in the affected eye at 6 months of follow-up. Among the three groups 1 year after the onset of visual symptoms, there was no significant difference in mean visual acuity, contrast sensitivity, color vision, or visual field. However, patients treated with the regimen of intravenous methylprednisolone followed by oral prednisone recovered vision faster than patients in the other two groups. The benefit of this treatment regimen was greatest in the first 15 days of follow-up and decreased subsequently. Patients treated with oral prednisone alone did not recover vision any faster and had no better visual outcome. A metaanalysis of 12

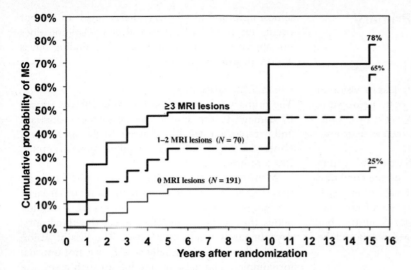

Figure 6.6 Progression to multiple sclerosis during 15 years of follow-up in the Optic Neuritis Treatment Trial (ONTT)/Longitudinal Optic Neuritis Study (LONS). The cumulative probability of multiple sclerosis was 50% in the entire ONTT cohort, but subjects with no MRI lesions had a 25% probability compared with a 72% probability for subjects with one or more lesions. (Adapted from: Optic Neuritis Study Group. Multiple sclerosis risk after optic neuritis: final optic neuritis treatment trial follow-up. *Arch Neurol.* 2008;65:727–732.)

randomized controlled clinical trials of steroid treatment in MS and optic neuritis confirmed these results. Initial data analysis at 2 years identified a reduced risk for progression to MS in patients with an abnormal brain MRI who were treated with intravenous corticosteroid; however, this apparent effect was not evident at subsequent time points.

Importantly, ONTT patients treated with oral prednisone alone had an increased rate of recurrent attacks of optic neuritis in the previously affected eye and an increased rate of new attacks of optic neuritis in the fellow eye compared with patients in the other two groups.

Management Recommendations

The question of whether long-term treatment of patients with optic neuritis and abnormal brain MRI should be initiated to decrease the subsequent risk of MS remains debated. By definition, such patients have clinically isolated syndrome (CIS), and numerous studies have been performed to evaluate the ability of prophylactic therapy to prevent progression to definite MS. Strong prospective data regarding the efficacy of interferon beta-1a, interferon beta-1b, and glatiramer acetate (CHAMPS, ETOMS, and PreCISe Study, respectively) in preventing progression have been collected and support the use of these agents in patients with CIS. The benefits and risks of such treatment versus observation should be reviewed with all CIS patients (by referral to an appropriate specialist if needed).

Chronic Demyelinating Optic Neuritis

Chronic optic neuritis is less common than acute optic neuritis. However, numerous patients with MS have no history of acute visual loss (painful or otherwise), but nevertheless complain that their vision is not normal and have evidence of unilateral or bilateral optic nerve dysfunction. Such patients may complain of a static disturbance of vision, a slowly progressive loss of vision in one or both eyes, or, occasionally, a stepwise loss of vision unassociated with periods of recovery.

Most patients with chronic unilateral or bilateral demyelinating optic neuropathies develop visual symptoms after other signs and symptoms of MS have developed, and it is for this reason that the percentage of patients with MS and evidence of chronic progressive optic neuritis increases the longer patients are followed. Nevertheless, slowly progressive visual loss or complaints of blurred or distorted vision in one or both eyes are the first symptoms underlying neurologic disease in some patients.

Asymptomatic (Subclinical) Optic Neuritis

A substantial percentage of patients with MS have clinical or laboratory evidence of optic nerve dysfunction even though they have no visual complaints and believe their vision to be normal. Evidence for optic neuritis in a patient who is visually asymptomatic may be clinical, electrophysiologic, psychophysical, or a combination of these. While high-contrast (Snellen) visual acuity is typically normal, low-contrast acuity is often reduced. Optical coherence tomography of the peripapillary retinal nerve fiber layer (RNFL) and macular ganglion cell complex (GCC) has proven particularly useful in the evaluation of patients with MS. Data from a large cohort of MS patients both with and without a history of acute optic neuritis show a statistically significant reduction in both RNFL and GCC thickness in MS patients compared with normal controls, regardless of optic neuritis history. Visual-evoked potentials often showed delayed P100 latency as well, confirming chronic demyelination.

Optic Neuritis in Other Primary Demyelinating Diseases

Neuromyelitis Optica (Devic Disease)

The association of acute or subacute loss of vision in one or both eyes caused by acute optic neuropathy preceded or followed within days to weeks by a transverse or ascending myelopathy is known as neuromyelitis optica (NMO) or Devic disease.

NMO occurs primarily in children and young adults, but all ages may be affected, and the condition has been described in patients over the age of 60 years. Both sexes are equally affected. It represents less than 1% of demyelinating disease in Western countries but may be more prevalent than typical MS in Asia and the Caribbean.

Pathology

In contrast to the demyelinating lesions of MS, destructive lesions of both white and gray matter are the hallmark of NMO. The optic nerves and spinal cord are invariably damaged while lesions of certain posterior fossa structures including the area postrema are frequently seen as well. Cerebral and cerebellar lesions are less common but may be present and do not exclude the diagnosis of NMO.

The majority of NMO patients have serum and/or CSF antibodies to aquaporin-4, a water channel protein that is found in high concentration in the cell membranes of astrocyte foot processes. This antibody, named NMO-IgG, has been shown to be pathologic in animal models of NMO and induces complement activation and tissue destruction. For example, aquaporin-4 is expressed throughout the brain and is not increased in optic nerve and spinal cord. Thus, specific involvement of certain areas of the central nervous system and not others may occur because of differences in permeability of the blood–brain barrier. Antibodies against myelin-oligodendrocyte glycoprotein (MOG) may be associated with a milder form of NMO, and overlap in clinical spectrum between patients who have one or the other antibody is being studied.

There are additional histopathologic features of NMO that may help differentiate it from MS. Cavitary tissue excavation is seen frequently in NMO but almost never in MS. Gliosis is characteristic of MS but occurs rarely in NMO. Cortical demyelination does not appear to occur in NMO as a late finding but is almost always seen in MS.

Clinical Manifestations

The primary features of NMO are visual loss caused by damage to the anterior visual sensory pathways and paraplegia caused by damage to the spinal cord. Other visual and neurologic manifestations are much less common.

Many patients with NMO develop a mild febrile illness several days or weeks before the onset of visual or neurologic manifestations. If vision loss is not simultaneous, the second eye usually is affected within hours, days, or rarely weeks after onset. The loss of vision is typically rapid and usually severe. It is not unusual for complete blindness to develop. In such cases, the pupils become dilated and nonreactive to light. When some vision remains, the size of the pupils and their reactivity to light stimulation are related to the severity of visual acuity and visual field loss. The rapid, bilateral loss of vision that occurs in patients with NMO is in sharp contrast to the loss of vision in optic neuritis, which tends to be unilateral and not as severe. Pain in or around the eyes precedes the loss of vision in a minority of cases, again distinguishing the condition from typical idiopathic optic neuritis in which pain is an almost universal feature.

As in demyelinating optic neuritis, visual field defects that develop in patients with NMO are variable. In many instances, vision is so poor when the patient is first examined that it is impossible to plot the field defect. Nevertheless, central scotomas seem to be the most common defect observed, with some patients developing concentric contraction of one or both fields. The ophthalmoscopic appearance of the optic discs varies considerably. A majority of patients have mild swelling of both optic discs. Some patients, however, have substantial disc swelling that may be associated with dilation of retinal veins and extensive peripapillary exudates, and others have normal appearing optic discs. With time, most patients develop pallor of the discs regardless of their initial appearance (Fig. 6.7). In some of these cases, there is slight narrowing of retinal vessels.

Figure 6.7 Ophthalmoscopic appearance in neuromyelitis optic spectrum disorder (NMOSD). This 37-year-old Caucasian woman developed severe left eye vision loss and 1 week later lost vision in the right eye as well. At its nadir, visual acuity was hand motions OD and no light perception OS. She received intravenous corticosteroid treatment and was subsequently maintained on immunosuppression with intravenous rituximab infusions. She recovered visual acuity of 20/30 OD and 20/150 OS and was left with cecocentral scotoma. **A and B:** Ophthalmoscopic appearance of the right and left ocular fundi, respectively, shows pallor of the optic discs associated with atrophy of the retinal nerve fiber layer, especially in the papillomacular bundles. **C:** Spectral domain OCT of the peripapillary retinal nerve fiber layer also demonstrates the extensive loss within the papillomacular bundles extending into the adjacent superior and inferior quadrants.

A

B

ZEISS

	OD	OS	
Exam Date:	3/7/2013	3/7/2013	CZMI
Exam Time:	11:02 AM	11:02 AM	
Serial Number:	4000-4553	4000-4553	
Signal Strength:	9/10	9/10	

Gender: Female
Doctor: Unknown

ONH and RNFL OU Analysis:Optic Disc Cube 200x200   OD ● | ● OS

RNFL Thickness Map

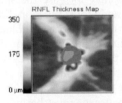

	OD	OS
Average RNFL Thickness	70 μm	51 μm
RNFL Symmetry	68%	
Rim Area	1.39 mm²	0.82 mm²
Disc Area	1.90 mm²	0.82 mm²
Average C/D Ratio	0.51	0.10
Vertical C/D Ratio	0.47	0.07
Cup Volume	0.072 mm³	0.000 mm³

RNFL Thickness Map

RNFL Deviation Map

Disc Center (-0.15,-0.06) mm
Extracted Horizontal Tomogram

Extracted Vertical Tomogram

RNFL Circular Tomogram

Neuro-retinal Rim Thickness
— OD - - - OS

RNFL Thickness
— OD - - - OS

Diversified:
Distribution of Normals
NA 95% 5% 1%

RNFL Quadrants

RNFL Clock Hours

RNFL Deviation Map

Disc Center (-0.78,-0.03) mm
Extracted Horizontal Tomogram

Extracted Vertical Tomogram

RNFL Circular Tomogram

C

Some recovery of vision usually occurs in patients with NMO. Visual acuity usually begins to improve within 1 to 2 weeks after visual symptoms begin, with maximum improvement occurring within several weeks to months. The peripheral fields usually begin to recover before there is noticeable improvement in the central field defects. Nevertheless, some patients have severe and permanent visual loss in both eyes.

Although optic neuritis usually precedes transverse myelitis, the sequence may be reversed. Regardless of which manifestation develops first, the interval between manifestations may be days, weeks, or months. In some cases, the blindness and paraplegia occur simultaneously. The onset of the paraplegia, like that of visual loss, usually is sudden and severe, and it may be associated with a mild fever. There may be severe radicular pain, and urinary retention may be present or develop shortly after the onset of motor weakness. Ascending paralysis may paralyze respiration and cause death at an early stage of the disease. Rarely, there is peripheral nerve involvement. Most patients recover motor function to some extent but have residual paraparesis, some have persistent and complete paralysis, and rare patients have complete recovery.

The mortality rate in patients with NMO was reported in the past to be as high as 50%, but improvement in supportive care has greatly reduced this rate, and we would estimate that death occurs in less than 10% of cases now. The disease tends to occur as a single episode without recurrences, unlike MS. Nevertheless, occasional recurrences of both visual loss and paraplegia, both separate and simultaneous, can occur.

Diagnosis

During the active stage of NMO, the CSF usually shows evidence of an inflammatory process. There often is a mild lymphocytic pleocytosis; the concentration of protein in the CSF may be increased, but intrathecal synthesis of IgG is usually not increased and oligoclonal bands are rarely detected. Neuroimaging rarely shows intracranial lesions, aside from the anterior visual pathways. However, MRI may show abnormal T2-weighted signals and enhancement with gadolinium in the optic nerves, chiasm, and spinal cord.

About 70% of patients with NMO have detectable NMO-IgG in serum or CSF; specificity of NMO-IgG is about 95%. A subset of patients with some symptoms of NMO (i.e., bilateral optic neuritis or transverse myelitis, but not both) has been identified with NMO-IgG positivity.

Not only there are important pathologic differences and differences in CSF findings between MS and NMO (see p. 132, Diagnostic Studies), but also there are important clinical differences: (1) NMO is not uncommon in the first decade of life, whereas MS rarely occurs in patients under 10 years of age; (2) the occurrence of bilateral optic neuritis associated with myelitis is rarely recorded in cases of pathologically proven MS; (3) bilateral blindness is extremely unusual in MS but is the rule in NMO; and (4) some serologic and neuroimaging findings seem specific to NMO.

Patients with severe vision loss from optic neuritis who do not recover good visual function, as well as patients with optic neuritis and spinal cord but not brain lesions on MRI, should be screened for the presence of NMO-IgG. The constellation of severe vision loss and atypical MRI findings for MS falls into an **NMO spectrum disorder**. A positive NMO-IgG test carries a high risk of recurrent optic neuritis and further vision loss as well as risk of progression to transverse myelitis with accompanying morbidity. A frank discussion of the risks and benefits of prophylactic treatment with immunosuppression must be held with patients, and careful surveillance regardless of treatment choice must be maintained.

Treatment

Acute treatment of NMO with corticosteroids and plasmapheresis may increase the speed of recovery of both visual and motor function. Long-term immunosuppressive therapy with azathioprine, mycophenolate mofetil, and rituximab should be considered, particularly if the patient is NMO-IgG positive. Azathioprine may be less effective in preventing relapse than the other two agents but is less expensive. The duration of treatment must be individualized but is usually not less than 24 months.

Myelinoclastic Diffuse Sclerosis (Encephalitis Periaxialis Diffusa, Schilder Disease)

Although original descriptions of **Schilder disease** may have inadvertently included examples of adrenoleukodystrophy and subacute sclerosing panencephalitis, there remains a characteristic group of patients with a noninherited demyelinating disease related to MS that is most commonly referred to now as **myelinoclastic diffuse sclerosis**. The characteristic lesion in these patients is a large, sharply outlined, asymmetric focus of demyelination with severe, selective myelinoclasia that often affects an entire lobe or cerebral hemisphere. There is typically extension across the corpus callosum and damage to the opposite hemisphere. Both hemispheres are symmetrically affected in some cases. Careful examination of the optic nerves, brainstem, cerebellum, and spinal cord often discloses typical discrete lesions consistent with MS, and histopathologic examination of both large and small foci reveals the characteristic features reminiscent of MS, including fibrillary gliosis with formation of giant multinucleated or swollen astrocytes and perivascular cuffing with inflammatory infiltrates containing plasma cells. The axons themselves may show little damage. Indeed, both the clinical and histopathologic features of myelinoclastic diffuse sclerosis disease suggest that it is closely related to MS and probably is a variant of it.

Myelinoclastic diffuse sclerosis occurs most often in children and young adults. Untreated, it is characterized by a progressive course that may be steady and unremitting or punctuated by a series of rapid worsening. A change in personality may be the first evidence of the disease. Cerebral blindness may be an early feature of the disease, particularly in adults. Central deafness may also occur. Other manifestations include dementia, homonymous visual field defect, varying degrees of hemiparesis and quadriparesis often culminating in plegia, and pseudobulbar palsy. The brainstem and cerebellum are affected in some cases, resulting in nystagmus, intention tremor, scanning speech, and spastic paraplegia.

Visual loss occurs in approximately 60% of cases, most often as a result of damage to the postchiasmal visual pathways, producing homonymous hemianopic or quadrantic visual field defects or cerebral blindness. Involvement of the visual association areas may also cause visual difficulties. Occasionally patients develop demyelination in the optic chiasm, producing bitemporal field defects. Optic neuritis occurs less frequently than in patients with MS, although the true incidence is not known. Rarely, papilledema occurs.

The CSF may show changes similar to those seen in typical MS. The intracranial pressure is usually normal, but in some patients the pressure is elevated. The protein concentration of the CSF is usually slightly increased, and there may be a mild lymphocytic pleocytosis. The IgG content is often increased, as is the CSF IgG index. Oligoclonal bands may be present and myelin basic protein may be extremely elevated. Neuroimaging studies show large, multifocal areas of extensive demyelination. In some cases, these lesions are similar in appearance to tumors or abscesses.

The diagnosis of myelinoclastic diffuse sclerosis may be suspected when a child or young adult develops evidence of a subacute or chronic progressive neurologic disease with neuroimaging and laboratory evidence of focal hemispheric demyelinating disease but without adrenal dysfunction or abnormal long-chain fatty acids.

Most patients with myelinoclastic diffuse sclerosis improve after being treated with corticosteroids or immunosuppressants, although recurrence within 4 years may occur in up to 70% of patients. A more fulminant initial course may be associated with better outcome and less long-term disability. Patients who improve clinically generally show disappearance or shrinkage of the lesions seen on neuroimaging studies.

Encephalitis Periaxialis Concentrica (Concentric Sclerosis of Baló)

Encephalitis periaxialis concentrica clinically resembles myelinoclastic diffuse sclerosis but differs from it pathologically. Patients rapidly develop a variety of neurologic symptoms and signs separated in time and space, including visual loss and diplopia. The visual loss is usually caused by damage to postgeniculate visual pathways and is characterized by homonymous field defects or cerebral blindness, although optic nerve involvement can occur.

The pathologic changes consist of alternating bands of demyelination and preserved myelin in a series of concentric rings in the cerebral white matter. The predominant feature of the bands of myelin is remyelination. The lesion likely originates as a small focus of acute demyelination around a perivascular inflammatory cuff, and the concentric bands are actually alternating areas of demyelination and remyelination. Some patients not only have pathologic changes consistent with encephalitis periaxialis concentrica but also have lesions typical of acute MS, suggesting that the former disease may actually be a variant of the latter.

Neuroimaging studies initially may be normal in patients with encephalitis periaxialis concentrica; however, eventually both CT scanning and MRI show multiple lesions consistent with demyelination. Similarly, analysis of the CSF at an early stage of the disease may reveal normal findings, but later analysis may show mild to moderate pleocytosis, increased protein, an increased IgG index, and multiple oligoclonal bands. The diagnosis can only be made conclusively by pathologic examination, either by biopsy or on postmortem studies.

Without treatment, encephalitis periaxialis concentrica usually progresses inexorably and is invariably fatal within a few weeks to a year. Treatment with systemic corticosteroids, however, may result in both immediate and long-term improvement in neurologic symptoms and signs. Early diagnosis thus is extremely important.

Causes of Optic Neuritis Other than Primary Demyelination

In a small percentage of cases, a primary demyelinating process in the optic nerve or the central nervous system is not the cause of unilateral or bilateral anterior or retrobulbar optic neuritis. Instead, the condition develops in the setting of, or as the presenting manifestation of, an underlying or recent systemic infection, vaccination, or systemic inflammatory disease.

Infectious and Parainfectious Optic Neuritis

Inflammation of the optic nerve can result from direct infection of the nerve by a variety of infectious agents such as viruses and bacteria. In addition, systemic or central nervous system infections can trigger an immune response that results in inflammation of the optic nerve.

Parainfectious optic neuritis typically follows the onset of a viral, or less often a bacterial, infection by 1 to 3 weeks. It is more common in children than in adults and is thought to occur most often on an immunologic basis, producing demyelination of the optic nerve. The optic neuritis may be unilateral, but it is often bilateral (Fig. 6.8). The optic discs may appear normal or swollen. Swelling of the peripapillary retina may be observed in patients with anterior optic neuritis. If a star figure composed of lipid and exudate develops in the macula of the affected eye, the condition is called **neuroretinitis** (see p. 142, Neuroretinitis). If there is evidence of optic nerve dysfunction and the intracranial pressure is normal, the inflammation is assumed to be affecting the periphery of the nerve and is called **perioptic neuritis** or **optic perineuritis** (see p. 144, Optic Perineuritis). Parainfectious optic neuritis, whether viral or bacterial, may occur in patients with no evidence of neurologic dysfunction or in association with a meningitis, meningoencephalitis, or encephalomyelitis—so-called acute disseminated encephalo-

myelitis (ADEM). When neurologic manifestations are present, patients have typical abnormalities in the CSF, such as a lymphocytic pleocytosis and an elevated protein concentration. Patients with encephalitis usually have disturbances on electroencephalography, and they may also have lesions on brain imaging, whereas patients with encephalomyelitis may show lesions in both the brain and spinal cord. Both enlargement and enhancement of the optic nerves may be demonstrated on MRI.

Visual recovery following parainfectious optic neuritis is usually excellent without treatment. Whether corticosteroids hasten recovery in patients with postviral optic neuritis is unknown, this treatment is reasonable to consider, particularly in cases in which visual loss is bilateral and severe.

Optic neuritis may occur in association with **infections** by a large number of both DNA and RNA viruses including adenovirus, coxsackievirus, cytomegalovirus, hepatitis A virus, human herpes virus 4 (Epstein–Barr virus), human immunodeficiency virus (HIV) type 1, and the measles, mumps, rubeola, rubella, and varicella zoster viruses. Bacterial infections can also produce optic neuritis and include syphilis, Lyme disease, catscratch disease, anthrax, β-hemolytic streptococcal infection, brucellosis, meningococcal infection, tuberculosis, typhoid fever, and Whipple disease.

Optic neuritis in **syphilis** is not rare, and it is particularly common in patients also infected with HIV. The optic neuritis of syphilis can be unilateral or bilateral and anterior or retrobulbar. When the condition is anterior, there is usually some cellular reaction in the vitreous, which serves to distinguish it (and other

A   B

Figure 6.8 Bilateral anterior optic neuritis. The patient is a 14-year-old girl who suffered bilateral visual loss 2 weeks following a flu-like illness. **A and B:** Both optic discs show severe swelling with peripapillary hemorrhages, as well as preretinal hemorrhage OS. Visual acuity was 20/400 in the right eye and counting fingers in the left eye acutely, but returned to normal within 6 weeks, and disc swelling completely resolved.

systemic inflammatory diseases that cause anterior optic neuritis) from demyelinating optic neuritis, in which the vitreous is usually clear. The diagnosis of syphilis is established using a variety of serologic and CSF assays. Treatment with intravenous penicillin produces visual recovery in many cases; however, the disease may be difficult to cure, particularly in patients who are HIV positive. Syphilis can also cause both neuroretinitis and optic perineuritis (see p. 142, Neuroretinitis, and p. 144, Optic Perineuritis).

Anterior, and rarely retrobulbar, optic neuritis can occur in patients with Lyme borreliosis (**Lyme disease**). This disorder is a spirochetal infection that is transmitted through the bite of a tick infected with the etiologic agent, **Borrelia burgdorferi**. The diagnosis of Lyme disease is made by serologic detection of infection or by finding the organism or its nucleic acid in the serum, CSF, or both. Treatment with antibiotics is usually effective, particularly in the early stages of the disease. As is the case with other systemic infectious processes that can cause optic neuritis, Lyme disease can also cause neuroretinitis or optic perineuritis (see p. 142, Neuroretinitis, and p. 144, Optic Perineuritis).

Many infectious agents that do not normally cause optic neuritis can do so in patients who are immunocompromised from drugs or disease. Such optic neuritis is particularly common in patients who are infected with **HIV** and in patients with AIDS. Optic neuritis, both anterior and retrobulbar, can develop in HIV-infected patients with cryptococcal meningitis, cytomegalovirus infection, herpesvirus infections, syphilis, tuberculous meningitis, and a variety of fungal infections. Rare patients with toxoplasmosis also develop optic neuritis. In some cases, such infections cause neuroretinitis, whereas in others, optic perineuritis occurs. Some patients with AIDS develop optic neuritis that is related to HIV alone, although it is not clear if the pathogenesis is direct infection or an immune-mediated parainfectious process.

In the preantibiotic era, spread of infection from the paranasal sinuses to the optic nerve was not unusual. However, this is now a rare occurrence, and most cases of **sinusitis** in patients with optic neuritis are fortuitous. Nevertheless, some patients with acute severe sinusitis develop a secondary optic neuritis from spread of infection. Spread of infection from the sphenoid sinus to the posterior optic nerve in the apex of the orbit or within the optic canal can produce isolated loss of vision. Aspergillosis and other fungal infections such as mucormycosis (especially in diabetic patients) should be considered in this clinical setting.

Postvaccination Optic Neuritis

Optic neuritis occurs rarely after vaccinations against both bacterial and virus infections. Most cases are bilateral, and both anterior and retrobulbar forms of optic neuritis may occur. Optic neuritis may develop after vaccinations with bacille Calmette-Guérin (BCG), hepatitis B virus, rabies virus, tetanus toxoid, and variola virus; combined smallpox, tetanus, and diphtheria vaccine; and combined measles, mumps, and rubella vaccine. Influenza vaccine is commonly associated with the development of optic neuritis. Most cases of postvaccination optic neuritis appear to be of the anterior variety and typically occur within 1 to 3 weeks of the vaccination. Visual recovery is common but may occur over several months.

Inflammatory Optic Neuritis

Granulomatous inflammation of the optic nerve may occur in **sarcoidosis**, producing a typical anterior or retrobulbar optic neuritis. In some cases, the optic neuritis occurs during the course of the disease, whereas in others it is the presenting manifestation. Clinical findings may be indistinguishable from those of demyelinating optic neuritis. However, the optic disc may have a characteristic lumpy, white appearance that suggests a granulomatous etiology, and there may be an inflammatory reaction in the vitreous or even the anterior chamber. The optic neuritis associated with sarcoidosis is usually extremely sensitive to steroids. In most cases, recovery of vision is rapid after treatment is instituted, although vision may decline again once steroids are tapered or stopped. It must be emphasized that rapid recovery of vision with corticosteroid treatment and subsequent worsening when the steroids are tapered is atypical for demyelinating optic neuritis and suggests an infiltrative or nondemyelinating inflammatory process, such as sarcoidosis.

Patients with **SLE, polyarteritis nodosa, and other vasculitides** can experience an attack of what seems clinically to be typical acute optic neuritis. This phenomenon occurs in about 1% of patients with SLE. In rare cases, the optic neuropathy is the presenting sign of the disease. The pathogenesis is most likely related to ischemia from vasculitis. The clinical profile of optic neuropathy in SLE and other vasculitides can be an acute anterior or retrobulbar optic neuropathy associated with pain or a slowly progressive loss of vision that mimics a compressive lesion.

Autoimmune optic neuropathy is a distinct variety of optic nerve inflammation. It is usually isolated, without any neurologic or systemic symptom or sign suggesting an underlying inflammatory disorder. Patients experience recurrent episodes of visual loss that are usually very sensitive to steroids. Despite prolonged therapy with corticosteroid or steroid-sparing immunosuppressant agents, visual function tends to deteriorate over time. Although workup for evidence of a connective tissue disease remains negative, some

A

B

Figure 6.9 Optic disc swelling in a patient with pars planitis (chronic cyclitis). The patient was initially believed to have papilledema. **A:** The left optic disc is hyperemic and slightly swollen. The hazy appearance is due to the presence of vitreous cells. **B:** Fluorescein angiogram of the left macula shows cystoid macular edema, characteristic of this disorder. The opposite eye had a similar ophthalmoscopic appearance.

patients have abnormal skin biopsies, with perivascular infiltrate and immune complex deposition within the dermis. Antibodies against optic nerve antigens may be detected in patient sera but do not guide therapy.

Miscellaneous Causes of Optic Neuritis

Optic neuritis can rarely occur in a large variety of conditions including almost all infections and systemic inflammatory disorders. In most cases, associated symptoms and signs suggest the diagnosis and isolated optic neuritis is only rarely the first sign of a systemic disease. Workup is usually obtained to rule out the most common causes of optic neuritis; subsequent tests are decided on a case-by-case basis.

Intraocular inflammation alone may cause optic disc swelling; however, in such cases, visual acuity is usually not significantly affected from damage to the optic nerve (Fig. 6.9). In such patients, visual acuity is limited only by the degree of vitreous inflammation or by secondary changes that occur in the macula (e.g., cystoid edema).

Optic Neuritis in Children

Optic neuritis in children has several unique characteristics that distinguish it from optic neuritis in adults: (1) it is more often anterior, with disc swelling in more than 70% of cases; (2) it is more often a bilateral simultaneous condition (up to 60% of cases); (3) it often seems to occur within 1 to 2 weeks after a known or presumed viral infection or vaccination; (4) it is less often associated with the development of MS (15% to 44% of cases); and (5) it is often steroid sensitive and steroid dependent. The visual prognosis in children

with optic neuritis appears to be quite good but not all children achieve a good visual result. All children with optic neuritis should be evaluated with MRI and a lumbar puncture. An infectious and inflammatory workup should also be obtained.

Neuroretinitis

Neuroretinitis is characterized by acute unilateral visual loss in the setting of optic disc swelling and hard exudate arranged in a star figure around the fovea (Fig. 6.10). Some cases of neuroretinitis are associated with particular infectious diseases, whereas others occur as apparently isolated phenomena.

Neuroretinitis affects persons of all ages, although it occurs most often in the third and fourth decades of life, with no gender predilection. The condition is usually painless, but some patients complain of an eye ache that may worsen with eye movements. Visual acuity at the time of initial examination can range from 20/20 to light perception. The degree of color deficit is usually worse than the degree of visual loss would suggest. The most common field defect is a cecocentral scotoma, but central scotomas, arcuate defects, and even altitudinal defects may be present, and the peripheral field may be nonspecifically constricted. A relative afferent pupillary defect is present in most patients unless the condition is bilateral. The degree of optic disc swelling is variable; in severe cases, splinter hemorrhages may be present. A macular star figure composed of lipid (hard exudates) may not be present when the patient is examined soon after visual symptoms begin, but it becomes apparent within days to weeks and tends to become more prominent even

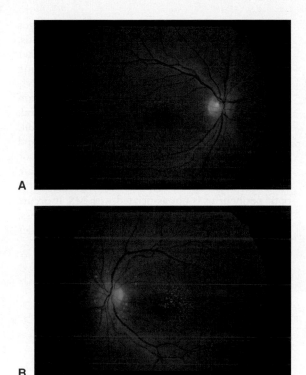

A

B

Figure 6.10 Neuroretinitis in 28-year-old woman who presented with subacute left eye vision loss. She also had accompanying facial weakness, and she was treated for presumed Lyme disease. **A:** Normal right optic disc and macula. **B:** Left optic nerve and macula about 6 weeks after onset of vision loss, showing resolving left optic disc swelling with peripapillary exudate as well as an extensive, nearly complete macular star figure. Extensive involvement of the temporal fovea confirms this is neuroretinitis and not macular exudate simply from optic disc edema, which occurs on the nasal side of the fovea in the papillomacular bundle.

as the optic disc swelling resolves (Fig. 6.10). Small, discrete, usually white, chorioretinal lesions may occur in both the symptomatic and asymptomatic eyes. Posterior inflammatory signs consisting of vitreous cells and venous sheathing as well as occasional anterior chamber cell and flare may occur. Fluorescein angiography in patients with acute neuroretinitis demonstrates diffuse disc swelling and leakage of dye from vessels on the surface of the discs. The retinal vessels may show slight staining in the peripapillary region; however, the macular vasculature is entirely normal.

Neuroretinitis is usually a self-limited disorder with a good visual prognosis. Typically over 6 to 8 weeks, the optic disc swelling resolves, and the appearance of the disc becomes normal or mildly pale. The macular exudate progresses over about 7 to 10 days, then remains stable for several weeks before gradual resolution occurs over 6 to 12 months. Most patients

ultimately recover good visual acuity, although some complain of persistent metamorphopsia or nonspecific blurred vision from mild disruption of the macular architecture. Most patients do not experience a subsequent attack in the same eye, and only a small percentage of patients develop a similar attack in the fellow eye.

In many cases, neuroretinitis is related to an infectious or parainfectious (i.e., immune-mediated) process that may be precipitated by a number of different agents. Catscratch disease, a systemic infection caused by the pleomorphic gram-negative bacillus **Bartonella henselae**, is the most common infectious process associated with neuroretinitis. Patients with catscratch fever usually have a history of contact with a cat, especially a kitten. They complain of malaise, fever, muscle aches, and headache. Examination typically reveals local lymphadenopathy. Some patients also have symptoms of arthritis, hepatitis, meningitis, or encephalitis; others are systemically and neurologically asymptomatic.

Other common infections that cause neuroretinitis are the spirochetoses, especially syphilis, Lyme disease, and leptospirosis. Neuroretinitis frequently occurs in patients with secondary and tertiary (late) syphilis. There is usually a history of previous sexual contact, a chancre, or prior treatment for syphilis or other sexually transmitted diseases. Neuroretinitis may develop in patients with secondary syphilis as part of the syndrome of syphilitic meningitis. In such cases, it is usually bilateral and associated with evidence of meningeal irritation and multiple cranial neuropathies. It may also occur as an isolated phenomenon in patients with secondary syphilis, in which case it is often associated with uveitis and may be either unilateral or bilateral. Neuroretinitis occasionally occurs in patients with late syphilis, usually in patients with meningovascular neurosyphilis. Neuroretinitis is commonly associated with an antecedent viral syndrome, suggesting a possible viral etiology for up to 50% of cases; however, viruses are rarely cultured from the CSF of such patients, and serologic evidence of a concomitant viral infection is usually lacking. Proposed causative viral agents include herpes simplex, hepatitis B, mumps, and the herpes viruses associated with the acute retinal necrosis (ARN) syndrome. Other presumed etiologies for neuroretinitis include toxoplasmosis, toxocariasis, and histoplasmosis.

Noninfectious systemic inflammatory disorders may also produce neuroretinitis such as sarcoidosis. One condition that is **not** associated with neuroretinitis is MS. Although the rate of development of MS after an attack of typical optic neuritis is substantial (Fig. 6.6), there is no increased tendency for patients who experience an attack of neuroretinitis to develop MS. Thus, the designation of an attack of acute optic neuropathy as an episode of neuroretinitis rather than anterior optic neuritis substantially alters the neurologic prognosis in the patient being evaluated.

Treatment of neuroretinitis depends on whether there is an underlying infectious or inflammatory condition that requires therapy. The prognosis for most cases of idiopathic neuroretinitis is excellent. Recurrent cases may benefit from long-term immunosuppression.

Optic Perineuritis

Optic perineuritis, also called periopic neuritis, is a condition in which only the periphery of the optic nerve is inflamed. Optic perineuritis is a form of orbital inflammatory pseudotumor; it may develop in isolation or it may be associated with other signs of orbital pseudotumor such as scleritis and myositis. In many cases of optic perineuritis, there are neither ocular symptoms nor signs other than disc swelling that is usually bilateral. The absence of visual dysfunction is explained by the absence of inflammation of the optic nerve itself. When perineuritis is bilateral, the differentiation from papilledema is often difficult, and it may be necessary to perform neuroimaging and lumbar puncture for diagnosis. Finally, enlargement of the optic nerve sheath on neuroimaging may simulate optic nerve sheath meningioma. As in neuroretinitis, optic perineuritis is **not** associated with MS. It occurs most often in association with an infectious process, such as syphilis, or a systemic inflammatory disorder such as sarcoidosis or Wegener granulomatosis.

Ischemic Optic Neuropathies*

7

Anterior Ischemic Optic Neuropathy
  Arteritic Anterior Ischemic Optic Neuropathy
  Nonarteritic Anterior Ischemic Optic Neuropathy
Posterior Ischemic Optic Neuropathy
Ischemic Optic Neuropathy in Settings of
  Hemodynamic Compromise
Radiation Optic Neuropathy
Ischemic Optic Disc Edema with Minimal
  Dysfunction

Ischemic syndromes of the optic nerve (ischemic optic neuropathy [ION]) are classified according to (a) the location of the ischemic damage of the nerve and (b) the etiologic factor, if known, for the ischemia. **Anterior** ischemic optic neuropathy (AION) includes syndromes involving the optic nerve head, with visible optic disc edema. **Posterior** ischemic optic neuropathy (PION) incorporates those conditions involving the intraorbital, intracanalicular, or intracranial portions of the optic nerve, with no visible edema of the optic disc. While several specific etiologic factors have been identified in ION, the most critical for initial management is giant cell, or temporal arteritis (GCA); therefore, ION is typically classified as either **arteritic** (usually due to GCA) or **nonarteritic** (Table 7.1). Nonarteritic ION is most often idiopathic, but specific risk factors and etiologies such as systemic hypotension and radiation injury have been identified. Finally, several syndromes of optic disc edema with relatively mild dysfunction, including preinfarct optic disc edema and diabetic papillopathy, are presumed to represent optic nerve ischemic edema along a spectrum of severity.

Anterior Ischemic Optic Neuropathy

AION typically presents with the rapid onset of painless unilateral visual loss developing over hours to days. An altitudinal visual field defect (typically inferior)

is the most common pattern of loss (Fig. 7.1) but arcuate scotomas, cecocentral defects, and generalized depression are also frequently seen. Visual acuity and color vision are decreased if the field defect involves fixation but may be normal if an arcuate pattern spares the central region. The pupil in the affected eye has a relative afferent pupillary defect present unless pre-existing or concurrent optic neuropathy in the fellow eye makes its pupillary response equally sluggish. The optic disc is edematous at onset; the edema may be pallid, but it is not uncommon to see disc hyperemia, particularly in the nonarteritic form (Fig. 7.2). The disc most often is diffusely swollen, but a segment of more prominent edema is frequently present (Fig. 7.3). Flame hemorrhages are commonly located adjacent to the disc, and peripapillary retinal arteriolar narrowing may occur (Fig. 7.4).

Arteritic Anterior Ischemic Optic Neuropathy

Although it often produces a severe and devastating optic neuropathy, GCA is the cause for AION in a relatively small minority (5.7%) of cases, with an estimated annual incidence in the United States of 0.57 per 100,000 over age 60. AION is, however, the most common cause of visual loss in GCA, accounting for 71% to 83% of cases, with retinal artery occlusion, choroidal ischemia, PION, and retrochiasmal ischemia less common. The mean age of onset for AAION is 70 years, with only rare occurrence under age 60. GCA occurs more frequently in women and with increasing age. It is most common in Caucasians and is unusual in African-American and Hispanic patients.

Clinical Manifestations
Arteritic anterior ischemic optic neuropathy (AAION) usually occurs in association with other systemic symptoms of the disease. Headache is the most common symptom while jaw claudication and temporal artery or scalp tenderness are the most specific for the disorder. The syndrome of polymyalgia rheumatica (PMR), including malaise, anorexia, weight loss, fever, proximal joint arthralgia, and myalgia, is frequently reported. So-called occult GCA, without overt systemic symptoms or sometimes without abnormal blood testing, occurs in up to 20% of patients with GCA and visual loss.

*The authors acknowledge the past contributions of Anthony C. Arnold to this chapter.

Table 7.1 Disorders and Drugs Associated with the Occurrence of Anterior Ischemic Optic Neuropathies

Arteritic anterior ischemic optic neuropathy
  Giant cell arteritis +++
  Periarteritis nodosa
  Churg–Strauss syndrome
  Wegener granulomatosis
  Connective tissue diseases such as systemic lupus
    erythematosus
  Rheumatoid arthritis
  Relapsing polychondritis

Nonarteritic anterior ischemic optic neuropathy
  Anomalous optic nerve:
    "Disc-at-risk": Small crowded optic nerve
    Papilledema
    Optic nerve head drusen
  Elevated intraocular pressure (acute glaucoma,
    ocular surgery)
  Radiation-induced optic neuropathy
  Diabetes mellitus
  Other vascular risk factors (atherosclerosis)
  Hypercoagulable states[a]
  Acute systemic hypotension/anemia:
    Bleeding
    Cardiac arrest
    Perioperative (especially cardiac and spine
      surgeries)
    Dialysis (CRF)
  Sleep apnea
  Drugs:
    Amiodarone
    Interferon alpha
    Vasoconstrictor agents (such as nasal
      decongestant)
    Erectile dysfunction drugs

[a]Hypercoagulable states are rarely responsible for AION and should only be tested in younger patients without other risk factors for AION.

In addition to systemic symptoms, certain associated local signs may aid in the diagnosis of AAION. Induration of the temporal region, decreased or absent temporal artery pulse, and cordlike firmness or nodularity of the temporal artery all may be seen. Ischemic scalp necrosis has been documented in GCA, and it may masquerade as herpes zoster dermatitis, with facial pain and even a vesicular reaction of the affected skin. Rarely, vasculitic ischemia of the central nervous system occurs, including mental status alterations, brain stem and cerebellar syndromes, and damage to the retrochiasmal afferent visual pathways. In cases of CNS involvement, there is a marked predilection (7:1) for the vertebrobasilar circulation.

AAION typically presents with severe visual loss (visual acuity less than 20/200 in 57.8% to 76.5% of cases, frequently hand motion or worse) developing rapidly over hours to days. While the initial presentation is often unilateral, bilateral simultaneous AION is more commonly arteritic than nonarteritic, and its occurrence raises suspicion for GCA. The persistent visual loss of AAION is preceded in 7% to 18% of cases by transient visual loss similar to that of carotid artery disease (but not seen in nonarteritic anterior ischemic optic neuropathy [NAION]), although the episodes may be of shorter duration. The pallid type of optic disc edema (Fig. 7.5) is seen more frequently in the arteritic than in the nonarteritic form. Cotton-wool patches (Fig. 7.6) indicative of concurrent retinal ischemia may be seen, but not expected in NAION. Retinal arterial occlusion may occur simultaneously with the optic neuropathy, especially cilioretinal artery occlusion (Fig. 7.7). Peripapillary choroidal ischemia may be associated with the optic neuropathy, exacerbating the visual loss. The optic disc of the fellow eye in AAION most frequently is of normal diameter, with a normal physiologic cup, as opposed to that in NAION, which tends to be small in diameter, with little or no physiologic cup (see below).

If untreated, AAION results in severe damage of the affected optic nerve. Recovery of useful vision after initial involvement is unusual, even with prompt therapy. In cases with unilateral presentation, estimates for development of AAION in the fellow eye without therapy range from 54% to 95%. Time to second eye involvement varies greatly, but it may occur within hours to days. The optic disc edema typically resolves over 4 to 8 weeks, with resultant optic atrophy and generalized attenuation of retinal arterioles. Excavation of the optic disc (see Fig. 7.6) occurs frequently after AAION but is unusual in NAION (see Fig. 7.8).

Diagnostic Confirmation

The most important initial step in the management of AION is the assessment for evidence of GCA. A tentative diagnosis may be made on the basis of advanced age and typical clinical symptoms in conjunction with elevation of the erythrocyte sedimentation rate (ESR) or C-reactive protein (CRP). Most cases of active GCA show markedly elevated ESRs (mean 70 mm/hr, often above 100 mm/hr). When the level is not extremely high, however, interpretation of the value becomes more difficult, as normative data are imprecise. As a rule, we recommend the clinically useful guideline that the upper level of normal, in mm/hr, is calculated by dividing patient age by 2 in males and patient age plus 10 by 2 in females. However, by these criteria, the level may be normal in up to 22% of patients with GCA. Conversely, the ESR rises with age, and levels above the listed upper limit of normal for the laboratory are common (up to 40% over 60 mm/hr) in patients over 70 without arteritis. Moreover, the test is nonspecific, elevation confirming only the presence of any active inflammatory process or other disorder affecting red

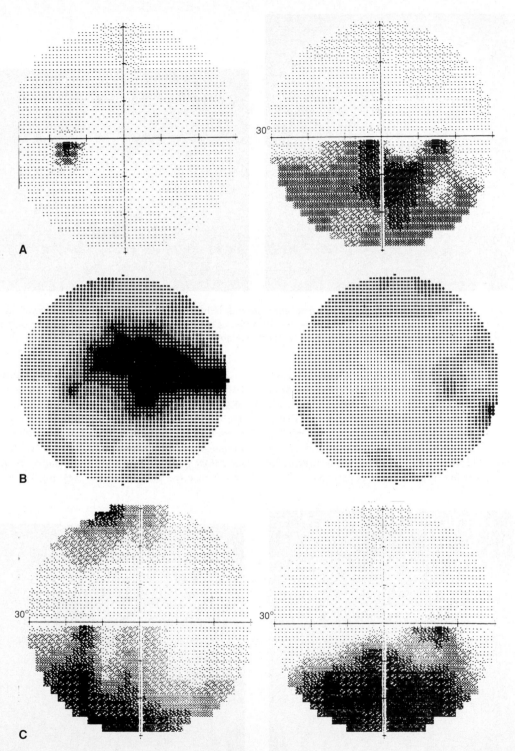

Figure 7.1 Automated quantitative perimetry in AION. Broad arcuate (altitudinal) defect **(A)** is most common, with central **(B)** and less severe arcuate **(C)** defects also frequently noted.

A

B

Figure 7.2 Ophthalmoscopic appearance of nonarteritic anterior ischemic optic neuropathy. **A:** Pallid swelling of the optic disc associated with a few small flame-shaped hemorrhages at the disc margin. **B:** Hyperemic swelling of the optic disc associated with numerous hemorrhages and a few soft exudates.

cell aggregation. In studies of temporal artery biopsy–negative cases with such elevation, the most common associated diseases have been occult malignancy (most frequently lymphoma) in 18% to 22%, other inflammatory disease in 17% to 21%, and diabetes in 15% to 20%. Patients with chronic renal disease commonly have elevated ESR as well, confounding the interpretation of this test in this group of ION patients.

Additional blood abnormalities are common in GCA and may have prognostic value. Measurement of C-reactive protein, levels of which do not rise with age or anemia, increases diagnostic accuracy and is currently recommended in conjunction with the ESR. In one study, specificity of 97% for GCA was attained for AION patients with ESR levels above 47 mm/hr and C-reactive protein above 2.45 mg/dL (normal

Figure 7.3 Segmental optic disc edema in NAION. The optic disc is edematous, with more prominent involvement inferiorly.

Figure 7.4 Peripapillary retinal arteriolar narrowing in AION. The vessels are focally attenuated overlying the disc, widening as they course toward the retinal periphery.

Figure 7.5 Bilateral simultaneous anterior ischemic optic neuropathy in a patient with GCA and no light perception in either eye. The right and left optic discs show markedly pale swelling.

Figure 7.6 Progressive optic atrophy and pseudoglaucomatous cupping after an attack of AAION. **A:** Right optic disc at the time of initial visual loss. Note pale optic disc swelling, peripapillary hemorrhage, and cotton-wool spot. **B:** Eight weeks after visual loss, the optic disc swelling has resolved, and both the hemorrhage and the cotton-wool spot are resolving. Note narrowing of retinal vessels. **C:** Four months after visual loss, the optic disc is pale and now has a large cup. The retinal vessels, especially the arteries, are markedly narrowed.

Figure 7.7 AAION with associated cilioretinal artery occlusion. In addition to the optic disc edema, there is a focus of retinal edema in the distribution of the cilioretinal artery.

less than 0.5). Fibrinogen is commonly elevated and may supplement C-reactive protein levels in increasing accuracy over the use of ESR alone. Thrombocytosis is seen in up to 50% of patients with GCA; its presence has been shown to be a marker for positive temporal artery biopsy and may be a predictor of visual loss, but not necessarily CNS involvement.

Histopathologic studies in AAION demonstrate vasculitis of the short posterior ciliary vessels supplying the optic nerve head, in addition to variable involvement of the superficial temporal, ophthalmic, choroidal, and central retinal arteries. Fluorescein angiographic data support involvement of the short posterior ciliary arteries in AAION. Delayed filling of the optic disc and adjacent choroid (Fig. 7.9) is consistently noted, and has been suggested as one useful factor in distinguishing arteritic from nonarteritic AION.

GCA is confirmed by a positive temporal artery biopsy, which is strongly recommended in any case of suspected arteritic AION. The certainty of biopsy-proven GCA provides support for long-term systemic corticosteroid therapy, which is often required for up to a year and may be associated with severe systemic complications. A negative biopsy, however, does not rule out GCA. A false-negative biopsy may result from (a) discontinuous arterial involvement ("skip lesions"), undetected in 4% to 5% due to insufficient length (minimum 3 to 6 cm recommended) of specimen or insufficiently detailed step sectioning; (b) unilateral involvement with biopsy of the uninvolved temporal artery; (c) improper handling of specimens; or (d) review by a pathologist inexperienced in the diagnosis of acute and healed arteritis.

The false-negative error rate for unilateral temporal artery biopsy has been estimated at 5% to 11%. Although the overall discordance rate for bilateral biopsies is low (1% to 3% in the largest series), there is substantial variation, even in major academic institutions with experienced pathologists, with rates as high as 13.4%. A recent paper reported discordance between the localization of symptoms and the side of positive biopsy in three patients out of 62 with positive biopsies. Considering the severe consequences of

A   B

Figure 7.8 A 66-year-old woman presenting with 2-day history of vision loss due to NAION. **A:** Right optic disc at presentation showing diffuse hyperemic swelling with RNFL. **B:** Six months later, complete resolution of edema, temporal pallor, and preservation of relatively small cup.

Figure 7.9 Fluorescein angiography in AAION. The optic disc and adjacent choroid show marked filling delay.

missed diagnosis, the relatively low risk of procedural complications, and the benefit of biopsy proof in the long-term management of these patients, we consider bilateral biopsy in all clinically suspicious cases.

Therapy

If GCA is suspected, therapy should be instituted immediately, as patients are at high risk for further visual loss in the affected eye, involvement of the fellow eye, and systemic complications of vasculitis, including stroke and myocardial infarction. Initial treatment should not await diagnostic confirmation by temporal artery biopsy. A delay of 7 to 10 days has no significant effect on the results. High-dose intravenous methylprednisolone at 1 g/d for the first 3 to 5 days is most often recommended, particularly when the patient is seen in the acute phase since this mode of therapy produces higher blood levels of medication more rapidly than oral therapy. As these patients are often elderly with multiple and complex medical problems, careful systemic monitoring is required. Daily infusions as an outpatient can also be organized with less expense than admission; however, requires very close surveillance. Oral prednisone at doses of at least 1 mg/kg/d is recommended after intravenous therapy (or initially if the intravenous route is not used) and is tapered slowly, monitoring for control of systemic symptoms and ESR and CRP levels; therapy is usually maintained for at least 6 to 9 months, often up to a year and longer. Patients can demonstrate recurrence of disease at any point, hence need to be monitored carefully throughout their course, preferably in conjunction with an internist or rheumatologist.

Systemic symptoms typically subside within a week, a response so characteristic that if it is absent, an alternate disease process should be strongly considered. Alternate-day corticosteroid therapy is inadequate for GCA. Some degree of visual recovery in the affected eye may be obtained on therapy but is not generally anticipated. However, the major goal of therapy, other than prevention of systemic vascular complications, is to prevent contralateral visual loss. Thrombocytosis in GCA and its possible predisposition to visual loss suggests the possibility that antiplatelet therapy may be of benefit in conjunction with corticosteroids, in particular for patients with luminal obliteration observed on biopsy; however, this has not been systematically studied. In severe cases, a few reports have shown benefit in the acute phase of admission for concomitant IV steroids and heparin infusion.

Nonarteritic Anterior Ischemic Optic Neuropathy

Most (95%) cases of AION are nonarteritic. NAION is the most common acute optic neuropathy in patients over 50 years of age, with an estimated annual incidence in the United States of 2.3 to 10.2 per 100,000 population, accounting for at least 6,000 new cases annually. The disease occurs with significantly higher frequency in the Caucasian population than in black or Hispanic individuals. There is no gender predisposition. The mean age at onset in most studies ranges from 57 to 65 years. In the Ischemic Optic Neuropathy Decompression Trial (IONDT), a multicenter prospective study of newly diagnosed patients with NAION begun in 1992, mean age was 66 years, probably somewhat biased by the exclusion criterion for patients under 50.

Clinical Presentation

NAION presents with loss of vision occurring over hours to days. Although some authors have proposed that visual loss from NAION is most frequently reported upon awakening, this was not confirmed in the IONDT. NAION typically presents without pain, although some form of periocular discomfort has been reported in 8% to 12%; in the IONDT, 10% reported minor ocular discomfort. In contrast to patients with optic neuritis, those with NAION usually do not report pain with eye movement. Headache and other symptoms associated with GCA are absent. Episodes of transient visual loss as seen in GCA are rare, but vague intermittent symptoms of blurring, shadows, or spots were reported in 5% of patients in the IONDT. The initial course may be static, with little or no fluctuation of visual level after initial loss, or progressive, with either episodic, stepwise decrements or steady decline of vision over weeks prior to eventual stabilization. The progressive form has been reported in 22% to 37% of nonarteritic cases.

Table 7.2	Ischemic Optic Neuropathies			
	Arteritic	**Nonarteritic**	**Diabetic Papillopathy**	**Posterior**
Age	Mean 70 yr	Mean 60 yr	Variable (<50)	Variable
Gender	F > M	F = M	F = M	F = M
Associated symptoms	Headache, jaw claudication, transient visual loss	Usually none	Usually none	None unless arteritic or postoperative
Visual acuity	<20/200 in >60%	>20/60 in >50%	>20/40 in >75%	Usually poor
Disc	Pale swelling common	Pale or hyperemic	Hyperemia, telangiectasia	Normal
	Cup normal + choroid ischemia	Cup small	Cup small	Variable
ESR	Mean 70 mm/hr	Usually normal	Usually normal	Elevated if arteritic
FA	Disc delay Choroid delay	Disc delay	Disc delay	Not studied
Natural history	Rarely improve Fellow eye 54–95%	16–42.7% improve Fellow eye 12–19%	Resolves 2–10 mo Bilateral 40%	Rarely improves Bilateral >60%
Treatment	Systemic steroids	None proven	None proven	Steroids if arteritic

NAION usually presents with less severe visual loss than AAION, with visual acuity better than 20/200 in 58% to 66% of patients (Table 7.2). In the IONDT, 49% had initial visual acuity of at least 20/64, 66% better than 20/200. Color vision loss in NAION tends to parallel visual acuity loss, as opposed to that in optic neuritis, in which color loss is often disproportionately greater than visual acuity loss. Visual field defects in NAION may follow any pattern related to optic nerve damage, but altitudinal loss, usually inferior, occurs in the majority, ranging from 55% to 80% of reported cases.

The optic disc edema in NAION may be diffuse or segmental, hyperemic or pale, but pallor occurs less frequently than in the arteritic form. A focal region of more severe swelling is often seen and may display an altitudinal distribution, but it does not consistently correlate with the sector of visual field loss. In the IONDT, 25% of patients demonstrated sectoral disc edema, but higher incidence of this finding has been reported in other retrospective series. Focal hyperemic telangiectatic vessels may appear on the optic disc of an eye with NAION within days to weeks after the onset of symptoms. This phenomenon has been interpreted as luxury perfusion, a vascular autoregulatory response to ischemia characterized by dilation of blood vessels and increased perfusion of tissues in a region surrounding an infarct. It is associated with focal early disc hyperfluorescence and corresponds to a spared region of the visual field. In some instances, this vascular response is so impressive that it is misin-

terpreted as a capillary hemangioma or neovascularization of the disc. Peripapillary retinal hemorrhages are common (Fig. 7.10), seen in 72% in the IONDT. Retinal exudates are unusual, but both soft and hard exudates may occur (7% in the IONDT). The retinal arterioles are focally narrowed in the peripapillary region (Fig. 7.4) in up to 68% of cases. The optic disc in the contralateral eye is typically small in diameter and demonstrates a small or absent physiologic cup (Fig. 7.10A). The disc appearance in such eyes has been described as the "disc at risk," referring to structural crowding of the axons at the level of the lamina cribrosa, associated mild disc elevation, and disc margin blurring without overt edema.

Histopathology and Pathophysiology

NAION is presumed to result from circulatory insufficiency within the optic nerve head, but the specific location of the vasculopathy and its pathogenetic mechanism remain unproven. Indeed, there has been no definite histopathologic documentation of the vasculopathy resulting in NAION. Implication of both the posterior ciliary arteries and the choroid has been based on indirect evidence. Recent data suggest that vasculopathy within the paraoptic branches of the short posterior ciliary arteries may play a major role, with resultant infarctions predominantly located in the retrolaminar region of the optic nerve head. Although carotid occlusive disease occasionally results in optic nerve ischemia, most often in the setting of more general ocular ischemia and occasionally with associated

Figure 7.10 Development of optic atrophy after AION. **A:** Appearance of the left optic disc before visual symptoms in the left eye. The patient subsequently developed decreased vision in the left eye associated with an inferior altitudinal field defect. **B:** The left optic disc is swollen and hyperemic. There are numerous flame-shaped, peripapillary, intraretinal hemorrhages. **C:** Two months later, the left optic disc is diffusely pale, the retinal arteries are narrowed, and the nerve fiber layer edema is no longer visible.

cerebral ischemia, the vast majority of cases of NAION are unrelated to carotid disease.

Similarly, the mechanisms involved in the development of optic disc ischemia in NAION remain unclear. Whether ischemia results from local arteriosclerosis with or without thrombosis, venous congestion, generalized hypoperfusion, vasospasm, failure of autoregulation, or some combination of these processes is not known. While structurally small, "crowded" optic discs are associated with NAION, the mechanism by which this contributes to ischemia (perhaps via a compartment syndrome) has not been fully elucidated. The role of nocturnal hypotension is debatable but generally avoided as much as possible by taking antihypertensive medications in the morning rather than at night. Multiple risk factors for vasculopathy and coagulopathy have been associated with NAION, but conclusive large-scale epidemiologic studies have not been performed (Table 7.1). Whatever the cause for impaired blood flow in the optic nerve vasculature, persistent hypoperfusion may require impairment in the normal autoregulatory mechanisms of the optic nerve head.

NAION has been reported in association with many conditions that may predispose to decreased optic nerve head perfusion via microvascular occlusion. Several cross-sectional case series have estimated the prevalence of systemic diseases that might predispose to vasculopathy in patients with NAION. Systemic hypertension was documented in 34% to 50% of patients (47% in the IONDT). Diabetes was reported in 5% to 25% (24% in the IONDT), with statistically significant increased prevalence in all ages in all but one study. Diabetes was associated with the development of NAION at a younger age in most series as well. Several studies have provided support for a robust and reproducible association between NAION and obstructive sleep apnea. The association of NAION with other vascular events such as stroke and myocardial infarction, and with other vascular risk factors, such as smoking, hypercholesterolemia, hypertriglyceridemia, hyperhomocysteinemia, and prothrombotic factors, is inconsistent.

NAION has been associated infrequently with a multitude of additional factors and disorders that may

Figure 7.11 A 65-year-old man presenting with bilateral sudden visual dysfunction consistent with optic neuropathy, characterized by altitudinal and peripheral constriction on VF, dyschromatopsia, 20/100 OD and 20/80 OS. He had been taking amiodarone 800 mg daily for 4 months. Upon cessation of amiodarone, acuity, fields, and optic nerve edema improved markedly over weeks.

be causative, either due to optic disc structure or other features that might affect optic disc perfusion pressure, including hyperopia, optic disc drusen, elevated intraocular pressure, cataract surgery, and migraine. A growing number of reports showing a convincing temporal association between the use of phosphodiesterase-5 inhibitors and the development of NAION, have provided greater acceptance of the likelihood of an association, if not causality in susceptible individuals. Amiodarone may produce a toxic optic neuropathy that is similar yet distinct from typical NAION (see Fig. 7.11). In contrast to typical NAION, most reported cases thought to be associated with amiodarone present with bilateral simultaneous involvement, an element of peripheral field constriction, and some reversibility upon cessation of the medication.

Clinical Course

Untreated, NAION generally remains stable, most cases showing no significant improvement or deterioration over time. Some spontaneous improvement of visual acuity is not uncommon; however, degree of visual field loss tends to be more permanent. In the IONDT, recovery of at least three Snellen acuity lines was found in 42.7% of patients who had initial visual acuity worse than 20/64. Visual acuity at 6 months was 20/200 or worse in 52% of the randomized (initial visual acuity 20/64 or worse) patients in the IONDT. After stabilization of vision, usually within 2 months, recurrent or progressive visual loss in an affected eye is extremely unusual and should prompt evaluation for another cause of optic neuropathy.

The optic disc becomes visibly atrophic, either in a sectoral (Fig. 7.12) or diffuse pattern (see Fig. 7.10C), usually within 4 to 6 weeks. Eventual involvement of the contralateral eye was reported in 14.7% of patients in the IONDT after a median follow-up of 5 years. A history of diabetes and baseline visual acuity of 20/200 or worse in the study eye, but not age, sex, aspirin use, or smoking were significantly associated with new NAION in the fellow eye. The IONDT found second eye visual acuity within three lines of the first in approximately half of the patients.

Occurrence in the second eye produces the clinical appearance of the "pseudo-Foster Kennedy

Figure 7.12 Sectoral optic atrophy after NAION.

syndrome," in which the previously affected disc is atrophic and the currently involved nerve head is edematous. Significantly impaired visual function in the eye with disc edema distinguishes this condition from the true Foster Kennedy syndrome, in which disc edema is due to elevated intracranial pressure and therefore does not produce visual loss acutely in the edematous eye.

Diagnosis

NAION must be differentiated from idiopathic, syphilitic, tuberculous, sarcoid-related, and Lyme disease-related anterior optic neuritis, particularly in patients under 50 years of age. Other important entities on the differential include infiltrative optic neuropathies, anterior orbital lesions producing optic nerve compression, idiopathic forms of optic disc edema, and diabetic papillopathy.

In patients with a typical presentation of NAION, without symptoms or signs to suggest GCA, and with normal ESR and C-reactive protein levels, we do not routinely perform additional testing. Evaluation by a primary care physician for evidence and control of risk factors such as hypertension, diabetes, and hyperlipidemia is essential. Neuroimaging is not performed unless the patient presents with substantial pain or follows an atypical course, such as prolonged optic disc edema or continued progressive or recurrent visual loss more than 2 months after initial presentation. The value of additional testing for vasculopathic and prothrombotic risk factors remains unclear. Carotid studies are not routinely performed unless prominent pain or other signs of orbital or ocular ischemia are present. For NAION in the typical age group, we do not routinely assess homocysteine levels, but in patients under 50, we proceed with this testing since elevated levels are amenable to therapy. We do not test for prothrombotic risk factors unless there is other evidence of personal or familial thrombosis, and we do not screen for vasculitides other than GCA unless there is clinical evidence for them.

Therapy

There is no proven effective therapy for NAION. No medications have been proven useful in the acute phase, and in the IONDT, optic nerve sheath decompression surgery for NAION was not beneficial and was potentially harmful. Over the years, investigators have studied the use of levodopa, brimonidine, corticosteroids, and pentoxifylline to name a few; however, the lack of reproducibility of results has precluded development of a consensus opinion or global practice guideline. Numerous case reports and small case series have purported a potential benefit from intravitreal injection of anti-VEGF medications; however, with a control group such findings must be interpreted with

caution. An experimental monkey model of NAION has provided a much needed mechanism to study such hypotheses—IVFAs in monkeys with induced AION showed no difference between those eyes injected with anti-VEGF or sham injection.

Similarly, there is no proven prophylactic measure for NAION. Although aspirin has a proven effect in reducing stroke and myocardial infarction in patients at risk, published data regarding its role in decreasing the severity of optic neuropathy and the incidence of fellow-eye involvement after the initial episode show no consistent positive effect. However, many experts recommend the use of aspirin after an initial episode of NAION, even if only for its role in decreasing risk for stroke and myocardial infarction in this vasculopathic population group. In the appropriate clinical scenario, it is certainly reasonable to suggest avoidance of any potentially associated medications such as phosphodiesterase-5 inhibitors or (controversially) amiodarone for individuals already having experienced NAION in one eye. Discussion with the patient's cardiologist is most appropriate in such a setting.

Posterior Ischemic Optic Neuropathy

Although the anterior form of ION is far more common than the posterior variety, ischemia of the retrobulbar portions of the optic nerve occurs in many settings, both arteritic and nonarteritic. Ischemia can independently affect the posterior portion of the optic nerve because of the distinct and separate arterial supplies of the anterior and posterior portions of the optic nerve. The anterior optic nerve is supplied by the short posterior ciliary artery and choroidal circulations while the retrobulbar optic nerve is supplied intraorbitally by a pial plexus arising from the ophthalmic artery, and intracranially by branches of the ipsilateral internal carotid, anterior cerebral, and anterior communicating arteries.

PION is a syndrome of acute visual loss with characteristics of optic neuropathy without initial disc edema but inevitably develop optic atrophy over time. Occasionally, a small amount of disc edema appears within the first week or so after acute visual loss, presumably as a result of propagation of swelling forward along the course of the optic nerve from the point of original ischemia.

In a multicenter, retrospective review covering 22 years, 72 patients with PION were classified into the three groups: perioperative PION, arteritic PION, and nonarteritic PION. The nonarteritic group accounted for 38 of the 72 patients, exhibited similar risk factors, and followed a clinical course precisely like that of NAION. In contrast to perioperative and arteritic PION, which were characterized by severe visual loss with little or no recovery, nonarteritic PION was less severe and showed improvement in 34% of patients. It is important to recognize this nonarteritic form in patients with acute optic neuropathy but no optic disc edema, a scenario that may be mistaken for optic neuritis. Such patients, as in some patients with AION and disc edema, particularly those with ischemic white matter lesions on MR imaging, might be incorrectly started on immunomodulatory therapy to reduce the risk of multiple sclerosis. PION differs from optic neuritis by its occurrence in older age groups, lack of pain on eye movements, and lack of enhancement of the affected optic nerve(s) on MRI.

The differential diagnosis includes compressive and infiltrative optic neuropathies, although the onset in PION is typically more abrupt. In all cases, neuroimaging is indicated to help differentiate between these possibilities. NAION typically shows no enhancement of the optic nerves on MR, presumably due to limitation to the optic nerve head. GCA PION may occasionally show enhancement of the optic nerve(s) on MRI. Although enhancement is not seen in nonarteritic or postsurgical PION, diffusion-weighted imaging can show features characteristic of acute cytotoxic edema (see Fig. 7.13).

Ischemic Optic Neuropathy in Settings of Hemodynamic Compromise

Systemic hypotension, blood loss, and anemia may produce optic nerve ischemia. The most commonly reported causes of blood loss associated with ION are (a) spontaneous gastrointestinal or uterine bleeding and (b) surgically induced hemorrhage, related most frequently to lumbar spine or cardiac bypass procedures, although a number of other surgeries have also been reported (see below). Less often, hypotensive episodes in the setting of chronic anemia without blood loss (as in chronic hemodialysis) may result in ION.

The optic neuropathy that occurs in these settings is typically bilateral, although unilateral cases occur. Visual loss is often severe. AION (with optic disc edema) accounts for the majority of cases, although PION is not infrequent. Visual loss may occur immediately after the episode or may be delayed as much as 2 to 3 weeks in cases of AION. It has been postulated that delayed visual loss is caused by vasoconstriction in the ciliary artery system secondary to activation of the renin–angiotensin pathway as a late response to blood loss.

Patients in whom visual loss occurs after **spontaneous hemorrhage** are usually 40 to 60 years old and debilitated. Most of these patients have experienced repeated episodes of bleeding, but cases following a single episode of massive hemorrhage with secondary hypotension have been reported. The visual loss is usually bilateral, but it may affect both eyes asymmetrically or be unilateral, and any degree of visual loss is possible. Both AION and PION have been reported in this setting, although AION is more common. The most frequent sites are the gastrointestinal tract in men and the uterus in women. A combination of both anemia and hypotension is frequently present when visual loss occurs in this setting.

ION occurs in the setting of various surgical interventions, most commonly cardiopulmonary bypass, and lumbar spine surgery. Indeed, lumbar spine surgery may carry an increased risk for postoperative ION, usually PION, compared with other surgeries. The American Society of Anesthesiologists (ASA) established the international ASA Postoperative Visual Loss (POVL) Registry in 1999 with the goal of acquiring a large database with detailed information on patient characteristics and perioperative conditions. Preliminary results confirm that at least two-thirds of cases are associated with spine surgery and that ION can occur even with the head suspended in Mayfield tongs with no external compression of the eyes and face. Indeed, perioperative ION can occur in young patients, with relatively short prone durations, with little blood loss, a normal hematocrit, and without hypotension. Nonetheless, this review has identified a number of potential risk factors for **perioperative ION**. These include prolonged surgeries (>6 hours) in the prone position with orbitofacial vascular congestion, anemia, blood loss (>1 L), hypotension, hemodilution, hypovolemia, hypoxia, and use of vasoconstricting agents. The purposeful maintenance of relative systemic hypotension to control intraoperative hemorrhage and the prolonged prone position may contribute to the development of some cases of perioperative ION, although it remains a rare but devastating, likely multifactorial complication. While aggressive fluid replacement and transfusion of blood products seem appropriate in cases where deficiencies are detected, there are no controlled studies of these interventions, and no therapy has been proven to significantly improve visual outcome in perioperative ION. It is suggested that colloids should be used in addition to crystalloids to maintain fluid volume in such patients. In addition, if possible, surgeons may plan to stage procedures anticipated to be prolonged in individuals with the proposed risk factors.

It is important to distinguish visual loss from postoperative ION with associated facial edema from the

Figure 7.13 DWI in posterior ischemic optic neuropathy. **A:** A 48-year-old man with chronic renal failure presenting with acute onset of light perception-only vision in his left eye, and no optic disc swelling. He had admitted to concomitant use of cocaine and heroin within the previous 24 hours, creating significant lability in blood pressure. **B:** DWI image on left showing hyperintensity along right optic nerve, with corresponding hypointensity on ADC (right image) consistent with cytotoxic edema.

prolonged prone position from those cases of visual loss secondary to direct compression of the eye from malpositioning. In the latter cases, which have been termed the "headrest syndrome," direct compression results in ocular ischemia, with severe orbital congestion, ecchymoses, and most often central retinal artery occlusion.

ION related to **hypotension** most often presents in patients with chronic renal failure and dialysis. The hypotension may be acute, temporally associated with the dialysis procedure, or it may be chronic.

Most patients are also chronically anemic. The accelerated diffuse vasculopathy that occurs in this disease may predispose to the development of ION, as may previous chronic hypertension, with possible arteriosclerosis and impaired autoregulation of the optic disc vascular supply. Visual loss from hypotension-induced ischemia in this setting may respond to rapid volume replacement and restoration of normotension. Maintenance of an SBP >100 and hemoglobin above 10 has been suggested for such patients undergoing chronic hemodialysis.

Radiation Optic Neuropathy

Radiation optic neuropathy (RON) is thought to be an ischemic disorder of the optic nerve that usually results in irreversible severe visual loss months to years after radiation therapy to the brain and orbit. It is most often a retrobulbar process. RON occurs most frequently after irradiation of the paranasal sinus and other skull base malignancies, but it may develop after radiation treatment for pituitary adenomas, parasellar meningiomas, craniopharyngiomas, frontal and temporal gliomas, optic nerve sheath meningiomas, and intraocular tumors. It has also been reported after low-dose radiation therapy for dysthyroid orbitopathy, although only in patients with diabetes mellitus. Pathologic specimens of optic nerves with RON show ischemic demyelination, reactive astrocytosis, endothelial hyperplasia, obliterative endarteritis, and fibrinoid necrosis, reflecting the presumed pathogenesis of both direct effects to replicating glial tissue and secondary effects from damage to vascular endothelial cells. The risk of RON appears to increase significantly at doses over 50 Gy, but both the total dose of radiation given and the daily fractionation size are important factors in determining the risk of delayed radiation necrosis in the central nervous system. However, RON should be considered even in situations where "safe" doses of radiation therapy have supposedly been administered, especially in optic nerves already compromised by tumor compression or chemotherapy, which may lower the threshold for radiation-related injury.

The syndrome typically presents with acute, painless visual loss in one or both eyes. Visual loss in one eye may be rapidly followed by visual loss in the fellow eye. Episodes of transient visual loss may precede the onset of RON by several weeks. The onset of visual symptoms associated with RON may be as short as 3 months or as long as 8 years after radiation therapy, but most cases occur within 3 years after radiation, with a peak at 1.5 years. Visual acuity loss ranges widely, and progression of visual loss over weeks to months is common. Spontaneous visual recovery is unusual. Final vision is no light perception in 45%, with a total of 85% of reported eyes with RON having final visual acuity of 20/200 or worse.

The affected optic disc is often pale initially, related to prior damage from tumor with possible superimposed radiation injury; less frequently it is edematous. Cases with disc edema at onset often have associated radiation retinopathy, with cotton-wool patches, hard exudates, and retinal hemorrhages, secondary to irradiation of intraocular or orbital structures. The visual field may show altitudinal loss or a central scotoma. A junctional syndrome with an optic neuropathy and contralateral temporal hemianopia may occur in patients with damage to the distal optic nerve. Patients with radionecrosis of the optic chiasm typically develop a bitemporal hemianopia that initially may suggest recurrence of the tumor for which the patient was initially irradiated, but superimposed optic neuropathy may involve the nasal visual fields as well.

The differential diagnosis of RON includes recurrence of the primary tumor, secondary empty sella syndrome with optic nerve and chiasmal prolapse, arachnoiditis, and radiation-induced secondary parasellar tumor. These conditions typically present with slowly progressive visual loss in contrast to the rapid evolution of RON. MR imaging is the diagnostic procedure of choice to distinguish tumor recurrence from RON. In RON, the unenhanced T1- and T2-weighted images may show no abnormality, but on T1-weighted enhanced images (Fig.7.14), there is marked enhancement of the optic nerves, optic chiasm, and even the optic tracts in some cases. The enhancement usually resolves in several months, at which time visual function usually stabilizes. Occasionally, enhancement may even precede visual loss.

Treatment for RON is controversial. Although delayed radionecrosis in the central nervous system can be treated with some success with systemic corticosteroids, which are effective in reducing tissue edema and may have some beneficial effect on demyelination, their use in RON, in oral or intravenous form, has produced disappointing results. Similarly, the use of anticoagulation to reverse or stabilize central nervous system radionecrosis does not appear to provide significant benefit in patients with RON. To the extent that RON is an ischemic process, hyperbaric oxygen therapy has a theoretical basis for effectiveness, but clinical results are not uniform and overall disappointing for nervous system–based radionecrosis. Visual improvement has been documented with therapy only in those treated within 72 hours; after 2 weeks, therapy is most likely ineffective. There are anecdotal case reports of benefit derived from intravitreal injection of anti-VEGF medications, but further study is needed.

Ischemic Optic Disc Edema with Minimal Dysfunction

Patients may develop **disc swelling from NAION before** they have **any visual symptoms**. In such cases, the patient may be thought to have papilledema or a compressive optic neuropathy from an orbital mass. Often, however, the asymptomatic disc swelling is noted in the fellow eye of a patient with a history of a previous attack of NAION, and the diagnosis

Figure 7.14 Radiation optic neuropathy in a 65-year-old woman who had undergone transsphenoidal resection of a non-secreting pituitary macroadenoma followed by radiation therapy totaling 5,500 cGy 18 months earlier. **A:** T1-weighted MR image, coronal view, shows enlargement of the left side of the optic chiasm. **B:** T1-weighted MR image, coronal view, after intravenous injection of paramagnetic contrast material, shows enhancement of the enlarged region. **C:** T1-weighted MR image, axial view, after intravenous injection of paramagnetic contrast material, shows enhancement and enlargement of the distal portion of the left optic nerve and the left side of the optic chiasm. **D:** T1-weighted gadolinium enhanced coronal section of 67-year-old woman presenting with bilateral severe visual loss to level of LP OU (progressed over 2 months) 14 months after XRT for left sphenoid wing meningioma.

is less confusing. On the basis of vasculopathic risk factors, lack of evidence for other causes of disc edema, evidence of NAION in the fellow eye, and the later development in some patients of NAION in the asymptomatically edematous eye, the disc edema has been presumed ischemic in origin.

An atypical form of NAION called **diabetic papillopathy** occurs most commonly in young diabetic patients. In most instances, transient unilateral or bilateral disc swelling develops in a diabetic (most often type 1 but not exclusively) who has minimal if any visual symptoms, and the swelling resolves spon-

taneously within several weeks. In some cases, there is a transient arcuate field defect; in others, the field defect persists. In most cases, however, there is only enlargement of the blind spot. When visual acuity is initially affected, it usually recovers as the disc swelling resolves. Eyes with diabetic papillopathy usually show prominent, dilated, telangiectatic vessels over the disc that mimic optic disc neovascularization (Fig. 7.15) but do not share the same fluorescein angiographic features. This phenomenon is akin to the luxury perfusion phenomenon described after typical NAION. As disc swelling resolves, these vessels usually disappear,

Figure 7.15 Appearance of diabetic papillopathy. The patient was an 18-year-old man with juvenile diabetes mellitus who was noted to have optic disc swelling during a routine eye examination. He had no visual complaints. Note dilated telangiectatic vessels mimicking neovascularization on the surface of both the right **(A)** and left **(B)** optic discs.

although they may occasionally persist. Diabetic papillopathy may develop in eyes with evidence of both preproliferative and proliferative diabetic retinopathy as well as in eyes with no evidence of retinopathy. Patients with diabetic papillopathy, like patients with typical NAION, often have a disc at risk. Thus, although the clinical features of diabetic papillopathy are different from those of typical NAION, this condition probably exists on a spectrum with NAION with a similar pathogenesis.

Compressive and Infiltrative Optic Neuropathies*

Compressive Optic Neuropathies
  Compressive Optic Neuropathies With Optic
    Disc Swelling (Anterior Compressive Optic
    Neuropathies)
  Compressive Optic Neuropathies Without Optic
    Disc Swelling (Retrobulbar Compressive Optic
    Neuropathies)
  Visual Recovery Following Decompression
Infiltrative Optic Neuropathies
  Tumors
  Inflammatory and Infectious Infiltrative Optic
    Neuropathies

Compressive Optic Neuropathies

Compressive Optic Neuropathies With Optic Disc Swelling (Anterior Compressive Optic Neuropathies)

Lesions within the orbit, occasionally within the optic canal, and extremely rarely intracranially, may compress the optic nerve, resulting in optic disc swelling (Fig. 8.1). Such lesions include tumors, infections, inflammations, and even adnexal structures that have become swollen or enlarged by disease. Specific orbital disorders include optic gliomas, meningiomas, hamartomas (e.g., hemangiomas, lymphangiomas), choristomas (e.g., dermoid cysts), and other malignancies (e.g., carcinoma, lymphoma, sarcoma, multiple myeloma), as well as inflammatory orbital pseudotumor and thyroid ophthalmopathy.

In most cases of anterior compressive optic neuropathy, there is progressive visual loss associated with proptosis; however, in many patients, visual acuity remains normal or near normal, and there is almost no external evidence of orbital disease despite obvious disc swelling. This clinical picture occurs particularly in patients with orbital hemangiomas adjacent to the optic nerve and in patients with primary optic nerve sheath meningiomas. In such patients, careful testing of color vision

may reveal subtle defects, and there may occasionally be a relative afferent pupillary defect despite retention of normal acuity. The visual field of the affected eye generally shows only enlargement of the blind spot or mild paracentral changes on automated perimetry. When other signs of orbital disease are not present (e.g., proptosis, limitation of ocular motility, orbital congestion), these patients may be thought to have unilateral papilledema from increased intracranial pressure. In such cases the workup may include MRI and MRV and potentially a lumbar puncture with opening pressure measurement. However, it should be noted that orbital disease is the most common cause of unilateral disc swelling without visual loss; hence, in such cases, in particular if there is an absence of signs or symptoms of raised ICP, orbital imaging is essential.

In addition to classical orbital signs, patients with orbital disease may develop various folds or striae that occur at the posterior pole, adjacent to the optic disc (Fig. 8.2). These folds may be horizontal, vertical, or oblique and tend to be coarser than those observed with intracranial pressure syndromes. Transient monocular visual loss can occur in patients with orbital lesions. The visual loss usually occurs only in certain positions of gaze, and vision immediately clears when the direction of gaze is changed. It is assumed that either direct pressure on the optic nerve or interruption of blood supply is responsible for this phenomenon.

Computed tomographic (CT) scanning and magnetic resonance imaging (MRI) offer superb topographic depiction (size, shape, and location) of lesions, and standardized echography provides supplementary information that often helps in refinement of the differential diagnosis. CT scanning is particularly useful for imaging bone, calcium, and metallic foreign bodies (suspicion of the latter being a contraindication for the use of MRI), whereas MRI excels at defining inflammatory and intrinsic disease of the visual pathway and parasellar area. MRI is particularly suited to imaging the intracanalicular optic nerve. With the use of fat-saturation techniques and gadolinium, demarcation of optic nerve sheath meningiomas can be optimized, and better differentiated from infiltrative disorders of the optic nerve.

When inflammatory conditions involve the orbit, such as **"idiopathic orbital inflammation (orbital**

---

*The authors acknowledge the past contributions of Nicholas J. Volpe to this chapter.

Figure 8.1 Optic disc swelling in a patient with a large left orbital cavernous angioma. **A:** The right optic disc is normal in appearance. **B:** The left optic disc is moderately swollen. **C** and **D:** Axial **(C)** and coronal **(D)** T1-weighted enhanced MR images show the large mass that is compressing the orbital portion of the left optic nerve.

pseudotumor)" the optic nerve may be compressed with secondary disc swelling. Affected patients usually experience visual loss, pain, proptosis, and congestion, and the presence of an orbital process is rarely in question. Infrequently, meningiomas of the orbital apex produce a similar clinical picture.

Patients with **thyroid eye disease** may develop evidence of a compressive optic neuropathy associated with optic disc swelling (Fig. 8.2). In such patients, congestive symptoms almost always precede visual loss resulting from the compression of the optic nerve at the orbital apex (see Fig. 8.2). Presenting visual acuities are typically 20/60 or worse, with central scotomas often combined with arcuate defects. Treatment options for thyroid-associated compressive optic neuropathy include intravenous or oral steroids and orbital decompression. Radiation therapy may also be effective, but its effects are often delayed and therefore more acutely effective treatments with steroids or surgery should be given in conjunction with radiation.

Anterior compressive optic neuropathy may result from primary **optic nerve sheath meningioma** (ONSM). Optic nerve sheath meningiomas surround the optic nerve and result in impaired axonal transport (leading to disc swelling) and also interfere with the pial blood supply to the optic nerve. The tumor occurs most commonly in middle-aged women and is usually unilateral. Patients present with slowly progressive vision loss, mild proptosis, double vision, transient visual obscurations, and gaze-evoked amaurosis. Examination reveals a color vision defect, afferent pupillary defect, and visual field defects including central scotomas, enlarged blind spots, and generalized constriction. The optic disc may be pale or swollen, and retinochoroidal shunt vessels may be present (Fig. 8.3; see Chapter 4). These tumors may expand rapidly during pregnancy producing a much more dramatic clinical picture in this setting.

Neuroimaging demonstrates focal or diffuse, tubular or fusiform, optic nerve enlargement (Fig. 8.3).

Figure 8.2 Optic disc swelling and choroidal folds in a patient with thyroid eye disease. **A:** External appearance of the patient showing lid retraction, proptosis, and orbital congestion. **B:** The patient's left optic disc shows hyperemia, swelling, and blurring of the peripapillary retinal nerve fiber layer. Horizontal chorioretinal folds extend across the posterior pole toward the macula. **C** and **D:** Axial **(C)** and coronal **(D)** CT images show greatly enlarged extraocular muscles surrounding and compressing the optic nerves within the orbit. The right fundus also showed optic disc swelling but no folds were seen.

MRI is often diagnostic, showing the tumor to be separated from the optic nerve proper, allowing distinction from gliomas (Fig. 8.4). MRI is particularly good at imaging the intracanalicular optic nerve, and delineating the extent of intracranial extension of the ONSM. On CT, calcification can be seen in one-third of patients as linear bright lines extending over the length of the optic nerve (tram-track sign) (Fig. 8.3). Clinical findings and neuroimaging generally establish the diagnosis and biopsy is almost never needed. In the rare equivocal case, biopsy is only recommended in an eye with very poor vision, after a thorough systemic workup including LP (often serial), empiric treatment including steroids with failure to improve vision, and threat to the contralateral optic nerve via the chiasm.

Natural history data suggest that ONSMs can remain stable or improve over several years. If progression is documented, radiation therapy is the best treatment available. Newer partially fractionated stereotactic delivery protocols may slowly replace conventional fractionated conformal external beam radiotherapy. Surgical excision of these lesions to improve vision is usually not possible because of the tumor involvement of the pial blood supply to the optic nerve. Portions of the tumor are occasionally removed to treat blind or uncomfortable eyes (proptosis), to decompress associated mass effect, or reduce the risk of intracranial extension.

Patients with meningiomas confined entirely to the optic canal may occasionally present with blurred vision and optic disc swelling. The mechanism by which disc swelling occurs in such cases is not clear, but it presumably results from direct compression of the optic nerve with blockage of axonal transport. It is very rare to see optic disc swelling from compression of the **intracranial portion** of the optic nerve.

Intracranial lesions, particularly sphenoid wing meningiomas, not infrequently extend through the

Figure 8.3 Optic disc swelling in a patient with a primary optic nerve sheath meningioma. **A:** The left optic disc is moderately swollen and there are several retinochoroidal vessels on its surface (*arrows*). Note also horizontal retinal striae in the papillomacular bundle. **B:** Non-contrast orbital CT scan, axial view, demonstrates the characteristic "tram-track" sign along the left optic nerve. Note the linear hyperdensities along the nerve due to extensive calcification within the optic nerve sheath meningioma.

Figure 8.4 Magnetic resonance imaging of a primary optic nerve sheath meningioma in a 42-year-old woman with slowly progressive visual loss in her right eye. **A** and **B:** Contrast-enhanced T1-weighted axial **(A)** and coronal **(B)** images show an enhancing mass surrounding the right optic nerve, which appears as a normal-sized, hypo-intense structure within the mass. The appearance is completely different from that of an optic nerve glioma in which the nerve itself is seen to be enlarged.

optic canal, compressing the intracranial, intracanalicular, and intraorbital optic nerve in the process. Optic disc changes, from swelling to pallor, may be minimal in such cases even when the lesion is quite large.

Compressive Optic Neuropathies Without Optic Disc Swelling (Retrobulbar Compressive Optic Neuropathies)

The importance of early diagnosis of compressive lesions that affect the retrobulbar portions of the optic nerve and do not cause optic disc swelling cannot be overemphasized. Early decompression of the optic nerves or chiasm may result in significant return of visual function, whereas delayed diagnosis may result in progressive visual failure and irreversible visual loss, neurologic dysfunction, or death. Intracranial, intracanalicular, and occasionally posterior orbital compressive lesions usually do not produce disc swelling or significant neurologic or systemic manifestations. Thus, by the time such lesions cause visible optic pallor, significant damage to the optic nerve has often already occurred, preventing return of visual function even with otherwise successful decompression. The physician managing a patient with unexplained unilateral visual loss must be aware of the characteristic history and early findings in patients with a retrobulbar compressive optic neuropathy.

In cases of prechiasmal optic nerve compression, progressive, painless dimming of vision is noted at an early stage. Although these patients may read the 20/25 or even 20/20 Snellen letters with the affected eye, they do so slowly and with great difficulty compared with the ease with which they read the 20/15 line with the opposite eye. There is usually some type of visual field defect, particularly when tested with automated perimetry, but the nature of the defect does not in isolation suggest the etiology of the visual loss. Compression of the optic nerve may produce **any** type of field defect, including an altitudinal, arcuate, hemianopic, central, or cecocentral scotoma. Although a hemianopic field defect or a "junctional" scotoma in the superior temporal field of the opposite eye strongly suggests a compressive lesion, it is the insidious, progressive nature of the symptoms that is most often the critical feature of the compressive process.

Two important abnormalities that are nearly always present in a patient with retrobulbar compressive optic neuropathy are unilateral dyschromatopsia and an ipsilateral relative afferent pupillary defect. The afferent defect is usually obvious even when visual acuity is minimally reduced and provides the observer with absolute evidence that the visual difficulty is caused by

something other than a simple refractive error, incipient cataract, or focal macular disease. Once a relative afferent pupillary defect is detected in a patient with an apparently normal fundus who is complaining of progressive dimming of vision, compression must be ruled out by neuroimaging, preferably gadolinium-enhanced MRI. The evaluating physician should have a low threshold for imaging in such cases, alerting the radiologist as precisely as possible about the region of interest.

The optic disc of a patient with a compressive optic neuropathy may appear normal or show a variable degree of pallor. Asymmetric cupping of the optic disc is not usually a prominent feature, but it may occur and be quite prominent in some patients (Fig. 8.5). In such cases, the visual loss may be thought to have resulted from glaucoma, particularly when there is an arcuate defect, but pallor of the neuroretinal rim indicates the nonglaucomatous nature of the lesion. Optic atrophy in one eye and disc swelling in the other may

A

B

C

Figure 8.5 Optic disc cupping in a patient with compression of the right optic nerve by a carotid-ophthalmic aneurysm. The patient was a 32-year-old woman with slowly progressive visual loss in the right eye. **A:** Cupped and pale right optic disc. **B:** Normal left optic disc. **C:** CT angiography shows a large aneurysm at the junction of the right internal and ophthalmic arteries.

result from asymmetric optic nerve compression or from tumor-induced direct optic nerve compression in one eye and papilledema from increased intracranial pressure in the other (Foster Kennedy syndrome) (see Chapter 4).

Causes of retrobulbar optic nerve compression include intraorbital and intracranial benign and malignant tumors (most commonly pituitary tumors, meningiomas, and craniopharyngiomas); aneurysms (Fig. 8.5); inflammatory lesions (particularly of the paranasal sinuses); primary bone disease (e.g., osteopetrosis, fibrous dysplasia, craniometaphyseal dysplasia, Paget disease); orbital fractures; dolichoectatic intracranial vessels; congenital and acquired hydrocephalus; thyroid eye disease; and orbital hemorrhage. Meningiomas arising from the planum sphenoidale or olfactory groove, pituitary tumors, and aneurysms are the most commonly identified lesions causing retrobulbar compressive optic neuropathy without disc swelling.

The **sudden onset of unilateral visual loss**, combined with signs of retrobulbar optic nerve dysfunction, usually suggests a diagnosis of optic neuritis or ischemic optic neuropathy. In rare instances, however, compressive lesions produce acute monocular visual loss, presumably from hemorrhage or from sudden interruption of the vascular supply to the optic nerve. This phenomenon probably occurs most frequently in patients with pituitary apoplexy, but it has also been reported in patients with pituitary tumors and meningiomas during pregnancy and in otherwise healthy patients upon awakening. Sudden onset of monocular visual loss can also occur from a ruptured ophthalmic artery aneurysm, fibrous dysplasia, orbital hemorrhage, subperiosteal abscess, orbital cellulites, and mucocele (particularly of the sphenoid sinus).

Visual Recovery Following Decompression

Restoration of visual function is not only possible following surgical decompression, but it can begin within hours to days after surgery, sometimes with full recovery. "Medical decompression" of the optic nerve with bromocriptine in patients with prolactin-secreting pituitary tumors has yielded similar improvements in visual function. Although it is not surprising that prompt decompression may restore visual function in patients rendered suddenly blind by pituitary apoplexy, it is not intuitively obvious that patients who have lost all light perception for days or weeks can occasionally experience dramatic visual recovery following decompression surgery. There is no correlation between the rapidity of visual loss and the rapidity of visual return. Recent studies using optical coherence tomography have demonstrated utility in the use of this technology in terms of visual prognosis following

decompression; preoperative RNFL measurements of over 80 microns portend a better prognosis and may be more helpful than features such as degree of optic atrophy, depth of visual field defect, or color vision or acuity measurements.

It has been theorized that there are three stages of visual recovery after decompression of the anterior visual pathway:

1 Relief of visual pathway compression is initially followed by **rapid recovery** of some vision within minutes to hours. This recovery can be likened to the relief of conduction block after an arm or leg "goes to sleep."
2 This initial recovery is followed by **delayed recovery** of additional function over weeks to months. This improvement may be related to progressive remyelination of previously compressed demyelinated axons.
3 Finally, there is an even longer period of improvement, taking many months to years. The mechanism by which this **late recovery** occurs is unknown.

Infiltrative Optic Neuropathies

The optic nerve can become infiltrated by a variety of different processes, primarily tumors and inflammatory processes (Table 8.1). The most common lesions that infiltrate the optic nerve are tumors and inflammatory or infectious processes. Tumors may be primary or secondary. The most common inflammatory disorder is sarcoidosis; the most common infectious agents are opportunistic fungi. Such processes typically produce one of three clinical pictures: (1) optic disc elevation with evidence of an optic neuropathy, (2) optic disc elevation with no evidence of optic nerve dysfunction, and (3) a normal-appearing optic disc associated with evidence of an optic neuropathy.

Infiltration of the proximal portion of the optic nerve, either anterior or just posterior to the lamina cribrosa, produces elevation of the optic disc. When the prelaminar portion of the nerve is infiltrated, the elevation of the disc is caused by the infiltrative process and is not true disc swelling. When the retrolaminar portion of the nerve is infiltrated, the disc elevation is caused by true swelling of the disc, and the appearance is indistinguishable from the disc swelling caused by such diverse entities as increased intracranial pressure, ischemia, and inflammation.

Tumors

Primary Tumors

Primary tumors that infiltrate the optic nerve are far more common than secondary ones. The most

Table 8.1   Lesions That Infiltrate the Optic Nerve

Primary Tumors
  Optic glioma
  Benign/malignant ganglioglioma
  Malignant teratoid medulloepithelioma
  Capillary hemangioma
  Cavernous hemangioblastoma
  Other

Secondary Tumors
  Metastatic carcinoma
  Nasopharyngeal carcinoma and other contiguous
    tumors
  Lymphoreticular tumors
    Lymphoma
    Leukemia
  Other

Infections and Inflammation
  Sarcoidosis
  Idiopathic perioptic neuritis
  Bacteria
  Virus
  Fungi

A

B

Figure 8.6 Optic nerve glioma in an 8-year-old child. **A:** External appearance of the child, showing moderate left proptosis and hypotropia. **B:** Axial, T1-weighted, contrast-enhanced MRI shows marked enlargement and enhancement of the left optic nerve as well as thickening of the subdural/subarachnoid space surrounding the nerve.

common primary tumor is the **optic nerve glioma** (Fig. 8.6). Optic pathway gliomas represent 1% of all intracranial tumors and 1.5% to 3.5% of all orbital tumors. Gliomas confined to the optic nerve constitute about 25% of all optic pathway gliomas, with the remainder infiltrating the optic chiasm and optic tracts in addition to one or both optic nerves. Seventy percent of patients with optic pathway gliomas develop visual symptoms or signs in the first decade of life, and 90% of the lesions are detected by the second decade.

Patients with gliomas confined to the optic nerve have three clinical presentations that are determined in part by the location, size, and extent of the tumor. When the glioma is confined to the orbital portion of the nerve or the bulk of the lesion is within the orbit, the patient typically develops proptosis associated with evidence of an anterior optic neuropathy with a swollen optic disc. Patients with optic nerve gliomas can develop retinochoroidal shunt vessels, although not as commonly as seen with optic nerve sheath meningiomas. Hyperopia may be induced by the increased volume of the optic nerve pressing on the globe, often also causing retinal striae.

When the tumor is located posteriorly in the orbit, and especially when the process begins in, or is limited to, the intracanalicular or intracranial portions of the nerve, the presentation is that of a slowly progressive or relatively stable retrobulbar optic neuropathy. In most of these cases, the optic disc on the affected side is pale and these patients do not typically have proptosis. Sometimes gliomas in these locations are discovered incidentally, often on routine screening MRI in

patients with neurofibromatosis type 1 (NF-1). Such patients have no visual complaints and may or may not have evidence of visual dysfunction.

On neuroimaging, optic nerve gliomas typically appear as fusiform enlargement of the orbital portion of the optic nerve, with or without concomitant enlargement of the optic canal (Fig. 8.6). Although gliomas may enhance, the enhancement usually is not nearly as pronounced as is typically seen with a meningioma. Two important signs help differentiate optic nerve gliomas from other lesions. One is an unusual "kinking" of the optic nerve within the orbit (Fig. 8.7). The other is a double-intensity tubular thickening of the nerve, best seen on MRI. This sign is called the "pseudo-CSF" signal because the increase in T2 signal surrounding the nerve may be misinterpreted as a CSF signal (Fig. 8.8). The genesis of this signal is perineural arachnoidal gliomatosis that occurs in optic nerve gliomas in patients with NF-1.

Figure 8.7 Kinking of the right optic nerve in a patient with neurofibromatosis type 1.

Approximately 29% of optic pathway gliomas occur in the setting of NF-1. Therefore, any patient found to harbor an optic pathway glioma should be assessed for evidence of NF-1, and patients with cutaneous lesions consistent with NF-1 should be screened for optic pathway gliomas and other intracranial lesions that occur in patients with neurofibromatosis. Among visually asymptomatic children with NF-1, neuroimaging reveals optic pathway gliomas in about 15% of cases.

The optimal treatment of optic nerve gliomas is highly variable. The natural history of these benign lesions is generally good, with long-term useful visual function and few, if any, neurologic complications. Most optic nerve gliomas do not change substantially in size over many years, especially those presenting in childhood. Some, however, rapidly enlarge and extend along the nerve to the chiasm and even into the third

Figure 8.8 Pseudo-CSF sign in a patient with a right optic nerve glioma. Note that the enlarged right optic nerve is surrounded by what appears to be CSF but that, in fact, is tumor in the subarachnoid/subdural space.

ventricle. Others suddenly expand from intraneural hemorrhage. Conversely, rare lesions exhibit spontaneous regression. Patients with optic nerve glioma with unequivocal sparing of the chiasm at presentation who later develop chiasmal involvement are exceedingly unusual. However, the possibility of intracranial extension exists in any given patient and for this reason patients are followed with serial neuro-ophthalmic examinations and MRI scanning. The natural history and prognosis may be better in patients with NF-1–associated tumors.

Patients with optic nerve gliomas are generally not treated with either chemotherapy or radiation therapy unless there is clear evidence of progression with the lesion extending into the optic chiasm, fellow optic nerve, or hypothalamus. Radiation therapy is probably effective in improving vision and disease-specific survival probability in gliomas of the anterior visual pathway that are clearly progressing clinically. Because of the risk of radiation to the developing brain, chemotherapy is the first-line treatment in a child under age 6 while radiation of the optic nerve tumor would be the primary option in an older child. Surgical resection is generally reserved for those patients who are already blind when first seen; for patients with severe proptosis; and for patients whose lesions seem to be threatening the optic chiasm. No clinical trials have been performed to indicate if removal of an apparently unilateral optic nerve glioma is associated with a better visual and neurologic prognosis than no treatment at all.

Most gliomas that infiltrate the optic nerve or chiasm are benign juvenile pilocytic astrocytomas. Rarely, **malignant optic nerve gliomas** occur, almost always in adults. When the tumor initially affects the intracranial optic nerves or chiasm, there is rapidly progressive visual loss associated with optic discs that initially appear normal but that rapidly become atrophic. The visual loss in these cases is often bilateral and simultaneous, but it may initially begin in one eye and thus may be mistaken for retrobulbar optic neuritis, particularly when there is associated pain. When the malignant glioma initially affects the proximal portion of the intraorbital optic nerve, there is acute loss of vision associated with optic disc swelling and the ophthalmoscopic appearance of a central retinal vein occlusion (Fig. 8.9). The prognosis in almost all cases of malignant optic glioma is poor, regardless of treatment with radiotherapy or chemotherapy. Most patients become completely blind within several months after the onset of symptoms, and most die within 6 to 12 months.

Astrocytic hamartomas (mulberry astrocytomas) can infiltrate the optic disc. In most cases, they protrude above or overlie the surface of the affected disc. They initially have a grayish or grayish-pink

Figure 8.9 Malignant optic nerve glioma. The patient was a 67-year-old man with sudden loss of vision in his right eye. Visual acuity was light perception in the eye; the left eye had normal acuity. **A:** The right fundus shows changes consistent with an acute central retinal vein occlusion. **B:** T1-weighted, contrast-enhanced axial MR image shows fusiform enlargement and enhancement of the entire orbital portion of the right optic nerve.

appearance (Fig. 8.10A), but they later develop a glistening, yellow, mulberry appearance (Fig. 8.10B). Although this latter appearance is similar to that of optic disc drusen, drusen are located within the substance of the disc *beneath* the disc vessels (Fig. 8.11A), whereas astrocytic hamartomas overlie the disc (Fig. 8.11B). Astrocytic hamartomas are composed almost entirely of acellular laminated calcific concretions, often interspersed among areas composed of large glial cells. The visual function in an eye with an astrocytic hamartoma of the optic disc is usually normal. Some eyes, however, develop a serous detachment of the retina or vitreous hemorrhage, resulting in variable loss of vision. Seventy percent of astrocytic hamartomas occur in patients with tuberous sclerosis or NF-1.

Figure 8.10 Astrocytic hamartoma of the optic disc. **A:** Before significant calcification, lesion appears as a pinkish gray mass rising above the disc. **B:** When calcification occurs, small globular clusters can be observed within the mass. Eventually, the entire mass may become calcified.

A B

Figure 8.11 Difference in ophthalmoscopic appearance of optic disc drusen and astrocytic hamartoma of the optic disc. **A:** Optic disc drusen are located within the substance of the disc *beneath* the vessels. **B:** Astrocytic hamartomas are located *above* the optic disc, thus obscuring the vessels.

Both **capillary and cavernous hemangiomas** can occur within the substance of the optic disc. In addition, cavernous hemangiomas can develop at any location in the optic nerve and in the optic chiasm. Capillary hemangiomas may be endophytic or exophytic. The endophytic type appears as a circular, reddish, slightly elevated mass internal to the disc vasculature and is represented histologically by a capillary hemangioma lying immediately beneath the internal

limiting membrane (Fig. 8.12). These lesions may be a manifestation of von Hippel–Lindau disease, or they may occur as an isolated phenomenon. The exophytic type of capillary hemangioma is typically seen as blurring and elevation of the disc margin, often associated with a variable degree of serous detachment of the peripapillary sensory retina and a ring of lipid deposition (Fig. 8.13). This lesion is often misdiagnosed as unilateral papilledema or papillitis, but fluorescein

A B

Figure 8.12 Endophytic capillary angiomas. **A:** The lesion appears as an oval, red-orange, slightly elevated mass obscuring the superior portion of the right optic disc. **B:** Fluorescein angiography shows intense staining and leakage from the lesion. (*continued*)

C

D

Figure 8.12 (*continued*) **C:** In another patient, the lesion occupies the majority of the left optic disc. **D:** Fluorescein angiography shows extensive staining and leakage from the majority of the disc.

angiography clearly demonstrates the vascular anomaly, as does ultrasonography.

Cavernous hemangiomas consist of large-caliber vascular channels. When these lesions occur as isolated masses within the orbit, they are well circumscribed and encapsulated. Within the eye, however, their appearance is that of a cluster of small purple blobs located within and above the substance of the optic disc (Fig. 8.14). The blood flow within the vessels in cavernous hemangiomas is extremely slow, indicating that this lesion is more isolated from the general circulation than its capillary counterpart. Cavernous hemangiomas of the optic

disc are usually unilateral, more common in females, and almost always asymptomatic.

Cavernous hemangiomas, unlike capillary hemangiomas, can occur within the retrolaminar, intracanalicular, and intracranial optic nerves, the optic chiasm, or the optic tracts. In some cases, the lesion itself causes slowly progressive loss of vision. In most cases, however, visual loss is rapidly progressive and occurs because of hemorrhage into the surrounding tissue. Up to one-third of patients have episodes of transient visual loss that are erroneously diagnosed as optic neuritis. Cavernous hemangiomas are not associated

Figure 8.13 Exophytic capillary angioma of the optic disc. This lesion appears as diffuse blurring and elevation of the disc, associated with a variable degree of serous detachment of the peripapillary sensory retina and a ring of lipid deposition.

Figure 8.14 Cavernous angioma of the optic disc. Note "cluster of grapes" appearance of lesion.

with von Hippel–Lindau disease, but they are often associated with similar lesions of the skin and brain and may also be associated with anomalies of extra-cranial and intracranial arteries.

Not all vascular lesions within the substance of the optic nerve are benign. Both the orbital and intracranial portions of the nerve can be infiltrated by a malignant **hemangioblastoma**. The typical patient with an optic nerve hemangioblastoma presents with progressive visual loss and evidence of an optic neuropathy that may be anterior or retrobulbar. The affected portion of the optic nerve is enlarged and has a fusiform appearance that mimics an optic nerve glioma on neuroimaging. Only 30% of these lesions are associated with the von Hippel–Lindau disease; however, partial expression of genetic disorders is being documented with increasing frequency, and many of the other lesions associated with von Hippel–Lindau disease may not become apparent for a number of years.

Melanocytomas are intraocular tumors that typically occur within the substance of the optic disc. Clinically, these lesions are elevated masses that are gray to dark black in color and are located eccentrically on the disc (Fig. 8.15). About 90% are 2 disc diameters or less in diameter, and the majority are less than 2 mm in height. Swelling of the disc occurs in about 25% of cases and is thought to be caused by a disturbance of axoplasmic flow secondary to chronic compression. Vascular sheathing may be seen in 30% of eyes, and subretinal fluid is observed in approximately 10% of patients. A nevus may be seen adjacent to a melanocytoma in up to 50% of cases. Visual acuity

Figure 8.15 Melanocytoma of the optic disc. The optic disc is almost completely obscured by an elevated, black mass. The mass is much darker than a malignant melanoma.

remains 20/20 or better in the majority of patients, and nearly all patients retain visual acuity of 20/50 or better. Although few patients are aware of any visual distortion, most have abnormal visual fields, especially blind spot enlargement, arcuate scotomas, and even generalized constriction. Rarely, patients develop an associated central retinal artery occlusion, or ischemic necrosis of the tumor and surrounding neural tissue.

Melanocytomas are benign tumors that do not require therapy. Slight growth may occur over many years in a minority of patients, and malignant transformation is not characteristic. The deep black appearance of melanocytomas generally allows them to be differentiated not only from optic disc swelling but also from other lesions that infiltrate the optic disc, particularly malignant melanomas. Nevertheless, the distinction can be difficult in rare cases, particularly when the lesion is not changing in size or shape.

Secondary Tumors

The most common secondary tumors that infiltrate the optic nerve are metastatic and locally invasive carcinomas and various lymphoreticular malignancies, particularly lymphoma and leukemia.

The optic nerve may be the site of **metastasis** from distant tumors. Metastasis can reach the optic nerve by one of four routes: (1) from the choroid, (2) by vascular dissemination, (3) by invasion from the orbit, or (4) from the CNS. Regardless of the mode of spread, the substance of the nerve is affected more often than the sheath.

Patients with metastases to the optic nerve usually have evidence of an optic neuropathy. The visual loss is usually severe, but relatively normal vision may be present in the early stages. When the metastasis is located in the prelaminar or immediately retrolaminar portion of the optic nerve, the optic disc is usually swollen; a yellow-white mass can be seen to protrude from the surface of the nerve (Fig. 8.16A); and clumps of tumor cells can occasionally be seen in the vitreous overlying the disc. A central retinal vein occlusion occurs in up to 50% of eyes. When the metastasis is to the posterior aspect of the orbital portion of the optic nerve or to the intracanalicular or intracranial portions of the nerve, the optic disc initially appears normal.

The most common metastatic tumors to the optic nerve are adenocarcinomas, primarily because these are the most common metastatic tumors to all parts of the body. In women, carcinomas of the breast and lung are the most common tumors, whereas carcinomas of the lung and bowel are most common in men. Other tumors that can metastasize to the optic nerve include carcinomas of the stomach, pancreas, uterus, ovary, prostate, kidney, and tonsillar fossa. Skin cancers, malignant melanoma, and mediastinal tumors also may metastasize to one or both optic nerves.

A   B

Figure 8.16 Infiltration of the optic disc by secondary malignancies. **A:** Metastatic breast adenocarcinoma in a 47-year-old woman. The entire optic disc is infiltrated by a large mass of yellow-white tissue. Note extension of the tumor beneath the peripapillary retina. **B:** Acute leukemia in a 15-year-old boy. Note elevated white mass obscuring normal optic disc architecture.

Isolated metastases to the optic nerve of intracranial tumors, such as medulloblastomas, may rarely occur.

Contiguous spread of primary tumors from the paranasal sinuses, brain, and adjacent intraocular structures to the optic nerve occurs much less often than does metastasis to the nerve. Because of its close anatomic association with the paranasal sinuses, the optic nerve can be infiltrated or compressed by cancer that arises in the sinuses or the nasopharynx. In most cases, the tumor invades the posterior orbit or cavernous sinus, producing a syndrome that is characterized by loss of vision, diplopia, ophthalmoparesis, and trigeminal sensory neuropathy.

Most patients with metastatic tumor to the optic nerve already have a known diagnosis of a primary carcinoma with other evidence of metastases at the time that visual loss occurs. This makes the diagnosis relatively straightforward, whereas most patients with a tumor that spreads contiguously to the optic nerve are not known to harbor a tumor when they first experience loss of vision. Any person with known cancer in another part of the body, with or without other evidence of metastases, who develops an optic neuropathy should be suspected of having cancer as the cause until proven otherwise. Similarly, any patient with a basal skull tumor who develops an optic neuropathy should be assumed to have spread of tumor to the optic nerve unless there has been previous radiation therapy to the region, in which case the possibility of radiation-induced optic neuropathy must also be considered.

Neuroimaging should be performed in all patients suspected of having infiltration of the optic nerve by cancer. Imaging typically shows an enhancing nerve that may or may not be enlarged. Most metastatic optic nerve tumors show at least a temporary response to radiation therapy.

Meningeal tumor cuffing or direct infiltration of the optic nerve can cause loss of vision in the setting of meningeal spread of carcinoma. This phenomenon is called **carcinomatous meningitis** or **meningeal carcinomatosis**. The frequency of optic nerve involvement in patients with carcinomatosis of the meninges ranges from 15% to 40%. Patients who develop meningeal carcinomatosis with visual loss may do so after the primary lesion, usually lung or breast, has already been diagnosed. In other cases, visual loss may occur coincident with other signs of chronic meningitis or as an isolated finding as the first sign of disease.

Although blindness may begin in one eye, both eyes are usually affected within a short period of time. The optic neuropathy that occurs in the setting of meningeal carcinomatosis is usually associated with a "diagnostic quartet" that consists of (1) headaches typical of raised intracranial pressure, (2) blindness, (3) sluggish or absent pupillary reflexes, and (4) normal-appearing optic discs. In some cases, there is true histopathologic evidence of infiltration of the optic nerve; in other cases, the lesion is more compressive than infiltrative, with malignant cells invading the subarachnoid space surrounding the optic nerve.

Lymphoreticular malignancies, such as leukemia and lymphoma, may infiltrate the optic nerve (Fig. 8.16B). Central nervous system involvement in non-Hodgkin lymphoma (NHL) is unusual, but it occurs in about 10% of cases. Of these, 5% (or a total of 0.5% of patients with NHL) will have infiltration of the optic nerve at some time during the course of their disease. Infiltration of the optic nerve in Hodgkin disease is even less common.

The symptoms and signs of patients with lymphomatous infiltration of the anterior visual system depend on the location and extent of the lesion. In some cases, the visual loss is insidious in onset and slowly progressive, whereas in other cases the visual loss is acute and mimics optic neuritis or ischemic optic neuropathy. The neuroimaging appearance of optic nerve infiltration by lymphoma is nonspecific. The infiltrated structure is enlarged and typically enhances on neuroimaging (Fig. 8.17). **Multiple myeloma, lymphomatoid granulomatosis,** and **Langerhans cell histiocytosis** can all also produce an optic neuropathy, sometimes via infiltration rather than compression of the nerve.

About 4% of children with acute **leukemia** have evidence of optic nerve infiltration. In some of the patients, visual acuity is lost abruptly; in others, there is a gradual progression of visual loss over days, weeks, or months. In still others, the disc appears swollen, but there is no evidence of visual dysfunction. Most patients with leukemic infiltration of the optic nerve are known to have leukemia at the time the visual loss occurs or the patient is found to have asymptomatic disc swelling. Patients can have acute lymphocytic leukemia, acute myelogenous leukemia, monocytic leukemia, erythroleukemia, or chronic lymphocytic leukemia.

Two distinct clinical patterns of infiltration can occur: (1) infiltration of the optic disc and (2) infiltration of the immediate retrolaminar portion of the proximal optic nerve. In leukemic infiltration of the optic disc, the features of the disc are obscured by a whitish fluffy infiltrate that is often associated with true disc swelling and peripapillary hemorrhage (Fig. 8.16B). The visual acuity in such patients is minimally affected unless the infiltration or associated edema and hemorrhage extend into the macula. Infiltration of the proximal optic nerve just posterior to the lamina cribrosa usually produces markedly decreased visual acuity associated with true optic disc swelling. Such patients have a variety of visual field defects, and a relative afferent pupillary defect is invariably present unless the infiltration is bilateral and symmetric. In addition, there are often peripapillary and peripheral retinal hemorrhages. Neuroimaging in such cases typically reveals a diffusely enlarged and enhancing optic nerve.

Figure 8.17 Neuroimaging appearance of infiltration of the right optic nerve, chiasm, and tract by a lymphoma. **A:** T1-weighted MRI, coronal view, shows enlarged right optic nerve (*arrowhead*). **B:** T1-weighted, contrast-enhanced, coronal MR image shows enhancement of the right optic nerve and, to a lesser extent, the left optic nerve (*arrowheads*) just anterior to the optic chiasm. **C:** T1-weighted, contrast-enhanced, axial MR image shows enhancement of anterior portion of the right optic tract (*arrowhead*).

The response of leukemic infiltration of the optic nerve to radiation therapy usually is rapid and dramatic. In almost all cases, visual function returns to normal or near normal, and the disc elevation, if present, resolves. The same results can occur—at least temporarily—in patients with lymphoma (Fig. 8.18).

Figure 8.18 Infiltration of the optic discs mimicking optic disc swelling in a 52-year-old woman with CNS extension of a B-cell lymphoma. **A:** The appearance is similar to papilledema, including Paton lines, suggestive of acquired disc swelling; however, the nerves have a "lumpy-bumpy" appearance suggestive of tumor aggregations within the nerve. **B:** Post-gadolinium MRI showing infiltration of both optic nerves, in a pattern similar to that of an optic nerve sheath meningioma. **C:** Following chemotherapy, both discs appear much improved, with mild residual temporal pallor (OS>OD).

One must consider a number of pathologic mechanisms in addition to infiltration in any patient with acute leukemia and apparent optic disc swelling. Swelling of the optic disc can occur in patients with acute leukemia when central nervous system involvement by the disease results in increased intracranial pressure. Optic disc swelling and neovascularization also occur as a local phenomenon in the setting of the diffuse retinopathy of acute leukemia.

Inflammatory and Infectious Infiltrative Optic Neuropathies

The intraocular, intraorbital, intracanalicular, and intracranial segments of the optic nerve can all be infiltrated by inflammatory and infectious processes. The most common inflammatory process that produces an infiltrative optic neuropathy is sarcoidosis. The most common infectious processes that produce an infiltrative optic neuropathy are syphilis, tuberculosis, and opportunistic fungal infections such as cryptococcosis.

Sarcoidosis

Optic nerve dysfunction probably is the most common neuro-ophthalmologic manifestation of sarcoidosis. The optic nerve may be affected at any time during the course of the disease and may be the site of its initial presentation. Sarcoidosis may affect the optic nerve in several different ways. It may produce papilledema, a compressive anterior or retrobulbar optic neuropathy, an ischemic optic neuropathy, or anterior or retrobulbar optic neuritis. The optic neuritis results from granulomatous infiltration of the optic disc, anterior orbital, posterior orbital, intracanalicular, or intracranial portions of the nerve, or a combination of these. In some cases, more than one process is responsible.

Granulomatous infiltration of the optic disc may or may not be associated with evidence by neuroimaging or ultrasonography of diffuse enlargement of the orbital portion of the optic nerve. The optic disc in such cases usually is markedly elevated, either diffusely or sectorially (Fig. 8.19), and it often has a solid or nodular appearance. There may be dilated vessels resembling neovascularization on the surface of the disc.

The appearance of optic disc infiltration by sarcoid granulomas may mimic that of papilledema, except that the former condition is more often unilateral than bilateral, and it is usually associated with decreased vision, intraocular inflammation, and/or neuroimaging evidence of an intracranial process affecting the base of the skull.

When the proximal portion of the intraorbital optic nerve is infiltrated by granulomatous inflammation in patients with sarcoidosis, the condition typically presents as an acute, subacute, or rarely chronic optic neuritis, with progressive loss of vision and disc

Figure 8.19 Sarcoid granuloma infiltrating the optic disc. Note irregular, lumpy elevation of the disc.

swelling. This condition may be impossible to differentiate clinically from demyelinating optic neuritis and even from certain causes of compressive optic neuropathy, particularly optic nerve sheath meningioma. Even neuroimaging, which shows enlargement and enhancement of the orbital portion of the optic nerve (Fig. 8.20), cannot establish the diagnosis with certainty. In some cases, the diagnosis is made by finding clinical, radiographic, or laboratory evidence of sarcoidosis elsewhere. In other cases, the diagnosis is not confirmed until a biopsy of the nerve or other abnormal tissue is performed.

Because of the predilection of neurosarcoidosis to affect the basal meninges, the intracranial portion of one or both optic nerves and the optic chiasm may occasionally be affected by the disease, producing a variety of patterns of visual loss. In some patients, visual loss is associated with evidence of hypothalamic dysfunction and/or hypothalamic hypopituitarism (particularly gonadotropin failure).

The diagnosis of sarcoidosis when suspected on a seemingly isolated presentation of optic neuropathy can be very challenging. A standard chest radiograph is an essential part of the evaluation at the very least, with likely greater yield obtained by chest CT. Abnormal uptake on gallium scanning, although not specific for sarcoidosis, may reveal areas accessible for biopsy. Conjunctival or lacrimal gland biopsy can establish the diagnosis, especially if the biopsied tissues are clinically affected. Testing for elevated ACE levels, although routinely performed, is of low yield in cases without pulmonary involvement.

The primary treatment of sarcoidosis is with corticosteroids. Most of the neurologic manifestations,

Figure 8.20 Magnetic resonance imaging in patients with sarcoidosis of the optic nerves. **A:** T1-weighted, contrast-enhanced, fat-suppressed MR image, axial view, in a 52-year-old woman with progressive loss of vision in the right eye shows irregular enhancement of the right optic nerve near the apex of the orbit and within the optic canal (*hollow arrows*). The intracranial portions of the optic nerves and the optic chiasm do not enhance and appear normal in size and shape (*solid arrows*). **B:** T1-weighted, contrast-enhanced, fat-suppressed MR image, coronal view, in the same patient shows enlargement and abnormal enhancement of the orbital portion of the right optic nerve (*black arrow*). The left optic nerve is normal in size and does not enhance (*large white arrow*); however, there is mild enhancement of its leptomeningeal sheath (*small white arrows*). A biopsy of the nerve revealed noncaseating granulomas. **C:** T1-weighted, contrast-enhanced, fat-suppressed MR image, coronal view, in another patient with sarcoidosis and progressive bilateral loss of vision with evidence of bilateral optic neuropathies reveals enlargement and abnormal enhancement of the orbital portions of both optic nerves. The right optic nerve is slightly larger than the left. Note mild enhancement of the leptomeningeal sheath of the left optic nerve (*arrow*). **D:** T1-weighted, contrast-enhanced, fat-suppressed MR image, axial view, in the same patient shows enlargement and abnormal enhancement of both optic nerves throughout the orbits, with extension through the optic canal on the right side. (Reprinted with permission from Engelken JD, Yuh WTC, Carter KD, et al. Optic nerve sarcoidosis: MR findings. *AJNR Am J Neuroradiol.* 1992;13:228–230.) (*continued*)

E

Figure 8.20 (*continued*) **E:** Enhancement and thickening of the prechiasmal optic nerves in a patient with subacute bilateral visual loss due to sarcoid. Note characteristic enlargement of the infundibulum.

including optic neuropathy, respond promptly to treatment; however, many patients require chronic therapy. Other agents reported beneficial in the treatment of sarcoid optic neuropathy, either separately or in combination with steroids, include

immunosuppressive drugs such as cyclosporine, azathioprine, methotrexate, and cyclophosphamide, and radiation therapy.

Infectious Disorders

Tuberculosis can infiltrate the optic nerve. In some cases, the tuberculoma is adjacent to the optic nerve and is part of a dense adhesive arachnoiditis that may or may not be separable from the surrounding structures. In other cases, however, the inflammatory tissue actually invades the nerve, making removal impossible. Rarely, a tuberculoma is completely contained within the optic nerve.

Syphilitic gummas may act in a similar fashion. Retrobulbar optic neuritis occurs in patients with syphilis, and gummas within the optic disc also have been described. Viral diseases such as cytomegalovirus and some of the herpes viruses can produce an infiltrative process of the optic nerve.

Invasion of the anterior visual system by cryptococcal organisms in the setting of cryptococcal meningitis is not uncommon, especially in patients with AIDS. Visual loss in such instances may reflect direct optic nerve or chiasmal invasion by the organisms, adhesive constricting arachnoiditis, increased intracranial pressure with papilledema, or a combination of these processes. Visual loss can be sudden, subacute over days, or chronic over a period of months. Presumably, other organisms causing both acute and chronic meningitis cause visual loss in a similar manner.

Traumatic Optic Neuropathies*

9

Classification

Epidemiology

Clinical Assessment

Pathology

Pathogenesis

Pharmacology

Management

Classification

Traumatic optic neuropathy is classically separated into two types of injury: direct and indirect. **Direct** optic nerve injuries result from orbital or cerebral trauma that transgresses normal tissue planes to disrupt the anatomic and functional integrity of the optic nerve, due to a penetrating force that directly collides with the optic nerve. **Indirect** injuries are caused by forces transmitted at a distance from the optic nerve. Normal tissue planes are not transgressed in indirect optic nerve injuries. Instead, the anatomy and function of the optic nerve are compromised by energy absorbed by the nerve at the moment of impact. The classic example of an indirect injury to the optic nerve is that which occurs when blunt trauma to the forehead results in a transmission of force through the cranium to the confined intracanalicular portion of the nerve.

The prognosis of an optic nerve injury depends in part on whether it is direct or indirect. Direct injuries tend to produce severe and immediate visual loss with little likelihood of recovery. Indirect optic neuropathies, on the other hand, are not infrequently associated with visual recovery and may also produce delayed visual loss that occurs several hours to days after the injury.

Optic nerve injuries can also be classified anatomically as optic disc trauma (avulsion), anterior optic neuropathy, or posterior optic neuropathy. An avulsion of the optic nerve as it enters the globe produces

a distinct ophthalmoscopic appearance, consisting of a partial ring of hemorrhage at the optic nerve head. In some cases, the site of the avulsion can be identified (Fig. 9.1A).

Injuries to the proximal portion of the optic nerve within 10 mm of the globe, anterior to where the central retinal vessels penetrate the nerve, produce a variety of disturbances that are immediately apparent in the ocular fundus, including an ophthalmoscopic picture of a central retinal or branch artery occlusion, central retinal vein occlusion, or anterior ischemic optic neuropathy (Fig. 9.2).

In contrast, injuries to the optic nerve posterior to the entrance of the central retinal artery produce no immediate change in the appearance of the ocular fundus. Specifically, the optic disc remains normal in appearance for at least 3 to 5 weeks, following which it becomes pale. The most common site of posterior indirect optic nerve injury is the optic canal.

The intracranial optic nerve is the next most common site of injury. When the intracranial portion of the optic nerve is injured, the field defect is likely to be hemianopic, and bilateral injury is common, as is associated injury to the optic chiasm.

Epidemiology

The type of trauma that produces a traumatic optic neuropathy is usually a deceleration injury of significant momentum. In cases of isolated traumatic optic neuropathy, the force of the impact is typically directed to the ipsilateral forehead or to the midface region. Motor vehicle and bicycle accidents are the most frequent causes, accounting for 17% to 63% of cases. Motorcycle accident victims may be particularly vulnerable to traumatic optic neuropathy, with up to 18% of such accidents resulting in optic nerve dysfunction. Falls are the next most common cause. Traumatic optic neuropathy can also occur in such diverse settings as frontal impact caused by falling debris, assault, stab wounds, gunshot wounds, and following seemingly trivial head trauma. It may also occur from iatrogenic injury, particularly after endoscopic sinus surgery and orbital surgery. Optic nerve injury is often associated with multisystem trauma and serious

*The authors acknowledge the past contributions of Kenneth David Steinsapir to this chapter.

A

B

Figure 9.1 A: Traumatic avulsion of the optic disc. Note ring of hemorrhage around the optic disc. The site of avulsion is clearly visible as a crescentic dark area at the temporal portion of the disc (*arrowhead*). **B:** Traumatic avulsion of left optic nerve with superior branch retinal artery occlusion. (Courtesy of Dr. Jennifer Thorne.)

brain injury. Loss of consciousness occurs in 40% to 72% of patients with traumatic optic neuropathy, and traumatic optic neuropathy occurs in about 1.6% of head trauma cases and in 2.5% of patients with maxillofacial trauma.

Traumatic optic neuropathy that occurs in the setting of orbital hemorrhage defines an important subset of optic nerve injury that does not fit well into the classic delineation of direct and indirect optic nerve injuries. For example, orbital hemorrhage after

A

B

C

Figure 9.2 Traumatic (proximal) anterior optic neuropathy and central retinal vein occlusion. The patient was a 24-year-old man who was struck in the left eye while playing basketball and who immediately noted loss of vision in the eye. Visual acuity was light perception OD and 20/15 OS. **A:** Ophthalmoscopic appearance of the right ocular fundus reveals moderate hyperemic swelling of the optic disc. The retinal veins are moderately dilated, and there are flame-shaped hemorrhages in the peripapillary region. **B:** CT scan, axial view, shows moderate enlargement of the orbital portion of the right optic nerve. **C:** CT scan, coronal view, shows enlargement of right optic nerve compared with left nerve. Note small areas of increased density, consistent with hemorrhage, within the enlarged nerve.

retrobulbar block occurs in 0.44% to 3% of patients. In most cases, the hemorrhage is quickly recognized and readily managed, with little impact on visual outcome unless a direct optic nerve injury has occurred from perforation of the nerve by the retrobulbar needle. Thus, the incidence of traumatic optic neuropathy in the setting of iatrogenic orbital hemorrhage is extremely low.

When retrobulbar hemorrhage occurs in association with blunt trauma to the orbit, the risk of visual loss is much greater. In this setting, blood may be dispersed throughout the orbit, in the subperiosteal space, and in the optic nerve sheath. In other cases, a hematic cyst may form, resulting in optic neuropathy from compression of the nerve by the cyst. Imaging studies can help to localize the hemorrhage in such cases. Orbital emphysema is also a rare cause of optic nerve injury. It can follow orbital fractures, usually after vomiting or nose blowing force air into the orbit, compromising the optic nerve.

Clinical Assessment

Traumatic optic neuropathy is a clinical diagnosis typically made when there is evidence of an optic neuropathy that is temporally related to blunt or penetrating head trauma. The head trauma may have been severe, in which case the patient may be unconscious. In some cases, there is no other evidence of orbital or ocular trauma; in other cases, there is obvious evidence of injury to the eye or orbit, such as periorbital or ocular hemorrhage, ecchymosis, or lacerations.

The clinical evaluation of a patient with visual loss following trauma should begin with a complete history, usually obtained from family, friends, or witnesses to the trauma. It is particularly important, for both medical and legal purposes, to determine if the patient with evidence of visual loss had any visual deficits before the injury. The examination of a patient with a possible traumatic optic neuropathy is limited by numerous patient factors, including the presence or absence of other injuries, the patient's level of consciousness, and the patient's ability or willingness to cooperate with the examiner. Hence, a good history and careful objective examination is critical.

The severity of initial visual loss in patients with traumatic optic neuropathy varies dramatically, from no light perception to 20/20 with an associated field defect. The prevalence of severe initial visual loss from traumatic optic neuropathy probably ranges from 43% to 56%. Visual loss is more likely to be severe in patients with neuroimaging evidence of a fracture of the optic canal, often signifying direct injury to the optic nerve. Delayed visual loss is reported to be as high as 10% in some series. **Color vision**, an excellent

test of optic nerve function, can be assessed at bedside using a red object and/or color plates.

In cases of unilateral traumatic optic neuropathy a **relative afferent pupillary defect** (RAPD) must be present on the side of the presumed optic nerve injury. A patient with a presumed traumatic optic neuropathy who does not have an RAPD either does not have an optic neuropathy at all or has a bilateral optic neuropathy. Furthermore, because patients with 20/20 vision in the setting of an optic neuropathy can have an RAPD, the presence of an RAPD in a comatose or semicomatose patient whose visual acuity cannot be measured cannot be taken as evidence that there is little or no vision in the eye. Only when the pupil does not react at all to direct light but reacts consensually (indicating intact efferent function) can one be certain that the patient has no light perception.

A complete and thorough examination of the eye and ocular adnexa is essential following trauma. Palpation of the orbital rim can identify step-off fractures. Periorbital swelling may mask the presence of proptosis. Resistance to retropulsion of the globe followed by tonometry can rapidly identify an orbit that is tense from a retro-orbital hemorrhage.

Posteriorly, blood in the vitreous may obscure the fundus. Presence of an RAPD in this setting suggests a large associated retinal detachment or traumatic optic neuropathy. Vitreous hemorrhage can be seen in the setting of subarachnoid hemorrhage as well (Terson syndrome). If the patient is neurologically unstable, the treating neurosurgeon or trauma surgeon should be consulted before dilating the eyes. If a dilated examination is performed, proper documentation must occur and only short-acting agents should be used. An adequate **fundus examination** will include assessment of abnormalities of the retinal circulation. Partial and complete avulsion of the optic nerve head produces a ring of hemorrhage at the site of injury or the appearance of a deep round pit (Fig. 9.1). Anterior injuries between the globe and where the central retinal vessels enter the optic nerve produce disturbances in the retinal circulation including venous obstruction and traumatic anterior ischemic optic neuropathy (Fig. 9.2). Hemorrhages in the optic nerve sheath posterior to the origin of the central retinal vessels may leave the circulation of the retina intact, but produce optic nerve head swelling. Frank papilledema may be seen in the setting of raised intracranial pressure in addition to the presence of traumatic optic neuropathy. The presence of choroidal rupture or **commotio retinae** may explain visual loss. Clinical judgment must be exercised to decide if these conditions are consistent with an RAPD.

The presence of decreased visual acuity and an RAPD in the absence of intraocular pathology should suggest a posterior orbital, intracanalicular, or intracranial optic nerve injury. The optic disc in these cases will appear normal for 3 to 5 weeks, after which the disc becomes progressively pale and atrophic. The observation of optic atrophy in a patient with acute head trauma and evidence of an optic neuropathy absolutely indicates that at least some disturbance of the optic nerve was present **before** the trauma and was not caused by it, although patients with a mild asymptomatic compressive optic neuropathy from a slowly expanding intracranial mass can occasionally experience acute loss of vision after seemingly trivial trauma from the effects of the trauma on an already compromised optic nerve.

Whenever possible, some type of **visual field testing** should be performed in the awake cooperative patient with possible traumatic optic neuropathy. The visual field may provide limited information regarding the possible location of optic nerve damage. Within the optic canal, for example, the pial penetrating vessels that provide blood to the optic nerve are subject to shearing forces at the moment of injury. Because the superior portion of the optic nerve is most tightly bound within the canal, the superior pial vessels are thought to be the most susceptible to shearing forces. If this concept is correct, patients with injuries to the intracanalicular portion of the optic nerve that spare some vision should have a visual field defect that is worse inferiorly than superiorly. However, there is no pathognomonic visual field defect that is diagnostic of optic nerve trauma. Altitudinal, central, paracentral, cecocentral, and hemianopic defects can all occur, as can generalized field constriction.

CT scanning permits visualization not only of the optic nerve and adjacent soft tissue in the orbit and neural and vascular structures in the brain, but also of the bony anatomy of the optic canals and paranasal sinuses. CT evidence of a fracture through the optic canal on the side of a traumatic optic neuropathy occurs in about 36% to 67% of cases (Fig. 9.3). The fracture in such cases may injure the optic nerve directly, or it may serve as a marker of the severity of force transferred into the optic nerve.

Although CT scanning is clearly superior to MRI in delineating fractures of bone, MRI is superior to CT scanning in its ability to image soft tissue. The role of MRI in traumatic optic neuropathy has yet to be fully defined. Certainly, MRI is more sensitive in the detection and the evaluation of associated intracranial abnormalities, and it may indeed prove useful in the detection of subtle hemorrhage of the optic nerve or sheath, especially within the optic canal. In general, MRI should be performed only after a metallic intracranial, intraorbital, or intraocular foreign body has been ruled out by CT scanning or conventional radiographs.

Figure 9.3 CT scan appearance (axial view) of an optic canal fracture (*arrow*) in a patient with a traumatic right optic neuropathy.

Pathology

Pathologic examination of the optic nerves from autopsies performed soon after closed head trauma has revealed optic nerve dural sheath hemorrhages in 83% of cases, interstitial optic nerve hemorrhages in 36% of cases (with the hemorrhage being present in the optic canal in two-thirds of these cases), and shearing lesions and ischemic necrosis in 44% of cases (with the intracanalicular optic nerve and the intracranial optic nerves affected 81% and 54% of the time, respectively).

The not uncommon finding of fractures of the sphenoid bone in patients with traumatic optic neuropathy after blunt head trauma is one indication of the substantial force that is transmitted to the optic nerve in such cases. Studies using CT scanning suggest that over 50% of cases of traumatic optic neuropathy are associated with a fracture of the sphenoid bone. Studies using laser interferometry suggest that, whether or not there is a fracture of the optic canal, the forces applied to the frontal bone during a deceleration injury are transmitted to and concentrated in the region of the optic canal. Indeed, the entire force of deceleration is applied to the facial bones over several milliseconds, whereupon elastic deformation of the sphenoid bone results in the direct transfer of force into the intracanalicular portion of the optic nerve. Because the nerve sheath is tightly adherent to the bony canal, the forces cause immediate contusion necrosis of the nerve by disrupting axons and vasculature. The development and location of a fracture in such cases is determined by the elastic limits of the affected bone. Thin bone is more likely to deform, whereas thick bone is inelastic and more likely to

Figure 9.4 Relationship of the optic nerve and the falciform dural fold (also called the falciform ligament). Note that as the nerve exits the optic canal, it is covered by the fold (Falc. Lig.). Ant. Clin., anterior clinoid process; Ant. Root, superior aspect of the optic canal; Car. A., internal carotid artery; CN II, oculomotor nerve; M1, M1 segment of the middle cerebral artery; Rec. A., recurrent artery of Heubner. (From Joo W, Funaki T, Yoshioka F, et al. Microsurgical anatomy of the carotid cave. *Neurosurgery.* 2012;70(2 Suppl Operative):300–311, with permission.)

fracture. Although fractures of the optic canal are not uncommon in patients with traumatic optic neuropathy, direct injury to the nerve by displaced bone fragments is infrequent.

The intracranial optic nerve can also be injured against the falciform dural fold, which overlies the sphenoid plane or where the nerve becomes fixed entering the intracranial opening of the optic foramen (Fig. 9.4). It has been hypothesized that swelling of the optic nerve within the bony canal may make the intracanalicular portion of the nerve susceptible to ischemic injury. However, there is evidence that astrocytic swelling in the optic nerve is less significant than in brain injury, and optic nerve swelling may be less significant than previously thought.

Pathogenesis

Whether direct or indirect, optic nerve injury results in both mechanical and ischemic damage. This damage can result from both primary and secondary mechanisms. **Primary mechanisms** cause permanent injury to the optic nerve axons at the moment of impact. Thus, the primary injury may be caused by laceration of the optic nerve or by shearing forces of deceleration that are transferred to the nerve, particularly within the optic canal, where the nerve is tightly bound.

Secondary mechanisms cause damage to the optic nerve subsequent to the force of impact. These mechanisms include vasoconstriction and swelling of the optic nerve within the confines of the nonexpansile optic canal, leading to worsening ischemia and irreversible damage to axons that may have been spared at the time of the initial injury or that were injured but possessed the potential for recovery immediately following impact. The implication in this concept is that immediate and appropriate intervention after an initial optic nerve injury has the potential to stop secondary injury and preserve vision by salvaging the axons that survived the initial insult.

Ischemia is perhaps the most important feature of secondary injury following trauma. The mechanism of injury is not simply cessation of blood flow. Partial ischemia and reperfusion of transiently ischemic regions generate **oxygen free radicals** resulting in reperfusion damage. **Bradykinin** initiates the release of arachidonic acid from neurons, and the resulting prostaglandins, oxygen free radicals, and lipid peroxides produce a loss of cerebrovascular autoregulation. Other potential mechanisms of injury include thromboxane-induced platelet adhesion and microvascular sludging, other triggers of free radical production, release of excitatory amino acids, and disruption of normal calcium metabolism. In addition, the early phases of CNS injury are characterized by the release of mediators of **inflammation** with resultant acute and chronic inflammatory damage.

Pharmacology

Research in acute spinal cord trauma demonstrates that the pharmacologic actions of very high doses of corticosteroids in this setting are separate and distinct from the actions of steroids in the doses more typically encountered in clinical practice. Experimental studies have demonstrated a biphasic dose response to methylprednisolone in a range of doses much higher than the usual clinical usage. Specifically, in animals with experimental CNS injury and ischemia, there appears to be a distinct pharmacologic benefit of doses of methylprednisolone in the range of 30 mg/kg—15 to 30 times the standard clinical dose. The most important of these effects appears to be as an antioxidant that limits tissue damage caused by oxygen free radicals.

The second National Acute Spinal Cord Injury Study (NASCIS II) was a multicenter, randomized, double-blind, placebo-controlled study. Patients enrolled in the study were randomized to one of three treatment arms within 12 hours of injury. The treatment arms consisted of placebo, naloxone, and methylprednisolone. Naloxone, an opiate receptor partial agonist that is effective in limiting neurologic injury in animals, was administered in an initial bolus of 5.4 mg/kg and then at a continuous infusion rate of 4.0 mg/kg/hr for 24 hours. Methylprednisolone was administered as an initial dose of 30 mg/kg followed by a continuous infusion of 5.4 mg/kg/hr for 24 hours (i.e., about 160 mg/kg or 10 g total over 24 hours).

This study showed that treatment with methylprednisolone within 8 hours of injury at the dose described above resulted in a significant improvement in motor and sensory function compared with either patients who received the placebo or patients treated with naloxone. Patients treated with methylprednisolone more than 8 hours after injury did not demonstrate an improvement in neurologic scores when compared with patients given the placebo. Indeed, subsequent analysis of the NASCIS II data suggested that methylprednisolone treatment given in the manner and dose described above and begun more than 8 hours after injury **was detrimental**.

Management

The management of traumatic optic neuropathy should be guided by the Hippocratic adage to do no harm. There is very little definitive help from the published literature on this subject. For example, it is very difficult to use the retrospective data in the literature to characterize the natural history of traumatic optic neuropathy, given the marked heterogeneity in presentation severity and circumstances. Traumatic optic neuropathy is a complex injury that often has both direct and indirect components and both primary and secondary intracellular and extracellular mechanisms of damage. Without an accurate knowledge of the natural history of traumatic optic neuropathy, determining the beneficial effect of a medical, surgical, or combined approach is very difficult.

At present, no studies validate a particular approach to the management of traumatic optic neuropathy. However, the use of systemic corticosteroids in the management of this condition has become commonplace. The beneficial clinical effect of these agents in the treatment of spinal cord injury provided theoretical rationale for the use of these agents in traumatic optic neuropathy, although the doses used by most authors do not approach those used in the NASCIS II study. In addition, there are fundamental differences between the spinal cord and the optic nerve, so the successful application of high-dose corticosteroids in the treatment of spinal cord injury may not fully generalize to the treatment of optic nerve trauma.

In the International Optic Nerve Trauma Study, recruitment was insufficient for a randomized trial, and it was converted to a comparative, nonrandomized interventional study. A total of 133 patients met criteria for inclusion and analysis. There were three treatment arms: untreated patients, steroid treatment, and surgery with or without steroids. There was no clear benefit for either corticosteroid therapy or optic canal decompression, although a trend toward more favorable outcome was suggested if high-dose steroids were given within the first 8 hours from injury. Indeed, critical review of the traumatic optic neuropathy literature does not provide statistical evidence to conclude that either surgery, corticosteroids, or a combination of corticosteroids and surgery is more beneficial than no treatment.

Mounting evidence, including the International Optic Nerve Trauma Study, raises significant questions regarding the potential benefits of corticosteroids in the treatment of traumatic optic neuropathy. First, there are no statistically valid studies supporting the use of corticosteroids in the treatment of traumatic optic neuropathy. Importantly, analysis of the NASCIS II data demonstrated that methylprednisolone treatment initiated more than 8 hours after spinal cord injury is detrimental.

In addition, there are at least two lines of experimental evidence that suggest methylprednisolone is harmful for injured optic nerves. In one study using a rat optic nerve crush injury, there was a dose-dependent decline in residual axons with increasing doses of methylprednisolone. The body's neuroimmunologic response to trauma may indeed be hindered or suppressed by exogenous administration of steroids. Third, in an experimental model of multiple sclerosis, high-dose methylprednisolone significantly increased apoptotic retinal ganglion cell loss. Given the lack of clinical evidence that corticosteroids are beneficial in the treatment of traumatic optic neuropathy, combined with growing experimental evidence that methylprednisolone may be harmful to the injured optic nerve, clinicians should consider abandoning the routine use of megadose corticosteroids for the treatment of traumatic optic neuropathy.

Surgical intervention for traumatic optic neuropathy also remains empirical. A large percentage of intracanalicular injuries take place at the falciform dural fold, and this is a location that will not benefit from optic canal decompression. However, it is possible that subsets of injuries might benefit from surgical intervention. For example, reduction of bone fragments impinging on the optic nerve is a compelling reason for surgical intervention, especially in cases of delayed visual loss, although these may represent untreatable injuries. The hypothesis that reducing the canal fracture benefits the injured nerve remains untested. The fracture may just be residual evidence of the forces imparted into the nerve at the moment of impact; lifting these fragments of bone may not provide any therapeutic benefit.

Case reports and small series demonstrate visual improvement following evacuation of intraoptic nerve sheath hematomas, or subperiosteal hematomas causing optic nerve embarrassment. These examples provide only limited experience on which to base recommendations for surgery for individual patients.

Intracanalicular optic nerve injury is the most common form of traumatic optic neuropathy. Not surprisingly, decompression of the optic canal is the most commonly reported surgical intervention. Theoretically, opening the canal to provide room for the optic nerve to swell into should be beneficial. However, the International Optic Nerve Trauma Study failed to demonstrate a beneficial effect for surgical decompression. This study had significant limitations and it is possible that the study did not have the power to identify a small beneficial effect for a subset of patients. Consequently, it is difficult to advocate a set of best practices based on this study. Certainly in the case of orbital hemorrhage causing optic nerve compromise, there is little controversy regarding the need to provide immediate surgical relief of the compressive orbitopathy.

It is reasonable to expect that if surgery is to be of benefit, then performing it earlier may decrease secondary axonal loss. An orbitotomy provides the best access for the evacuation of an optic nerve sheath hematoma, reduction of a depressed lateral orbital wall fracture that compromises the optic nerve, or drainage of a subperiosteal hematoma with posterior compression of the optic nerve. An accurate anatomical diagnosis must be made to plan appropriate surgical intervention. Avoidance of surgical intervention on the unconscious patient continues to be a reasonable recommendation until such time as there is clear evidence establishing the value of surgical intervention.

Toxic and Deficiency Optic Neuropathies

10

Etiologic Criteria
  Nutritional Optic Neuropathies
  Toxic Optic Neuropathies

Clinical Characteristics of Nutritional and Toxic Optic Neuropathies

Differential Diagnosis

Specific Nutritional Optic Neuropathies
  Epidemic Nutritional Optic Neuropathy
  Isolated Nutritional Optic Neuropathy

Specific Toxic Optic Neuropathies
  Primary Toxic Optic Neuropathy: Ethambutol
  Demyelinating Optic Neuropathy: Tumor Necrosis
    Factor-alpha Inhibitors
  Pseudotoxic Optic Neuropathy: Amiodarone

Physicians have known for centuries that the anterior visual pathway is vulnerable to damage from nutritional deficiency and chemicals. The resulting disorders share many signs and symptoms, and several appear to have a multifactorial etiology in which both undernutrition and toxicity play a role. In light of these facts, it is reasonable to group them together. It must be emphasized that evidence for the localization of the primary lesions is lacking in many of the so-called toxic and nutritional optic neuropathies. In some cases, the optic nerve axon is the damaged structure; however, in others, such as the ocular toxicity produced by several of the tumor necrosis factor-alpha (TNF-α) inhibitors and toluene, it is the myelin covering the optic nerves, and the resulting optic neuropathy is due to demyelination. In still other cases, the retinal ganglion cells are damaged directly. In addition, there probably is a genetic component to some of the toxic and nutritional optic neuropathies, which explain why two individuals may be exposed to the same substance or be deficient in a particular nutrient and yet one develops a "toxic" or "nutritional" optic neuropathy and the other does not. The genetic component may be chromosomal, mitochondrial, or both.

Etiologic Criteria

Nutritional Optic Neuropathies

In the Western hemisphere, the most common cause of a nutritional optic neuropathy probably is alcohol abuse leading to a diet lacking crucial nutrients, particularly vitamin B_{12} and folate. Other settings include malabsorption syndromes, postbariatric surgery, incorrect vegetarianism, and severe depression. In general, nutritional optic neuropathies develop over months rather than days to weeks. Although some patients with nutritional optic neuropathies show evidence of undernutrition, usually manifested in such obvious forms as weight loss and wasting, many do not do so and appear otherwise perfectly well. Thus, signs such as peripheral neuropathy and hearing loss are useful, when present. Unfortunately, they usually are not.

Identifying the specific nutritional deficiency responsible for an optic neuropathy is very difficult. Undernourished individuals are rarely deficient in only one nutrient; multiple deficiencies are the rule. Even if a specific deficiency is identified in a patient with loss of vision, it does not prove that the deficiency caused the visual loss, nor does recovery when the deficient nutrient is resupplied necessarily establish that the resupplied nutrient effected the cure. With the exception of vitamin B_{12} (which only rarely becomes deficient for dietary reasons), no specific nutrient deficiency has been proved conclusively to cause optic neuropathy in humans. At the present state of knowledge, one can only speculate about which specific deficiencies can cause or contribute to nutritional optic neuropathy.

Toxic Optic Neuropathies

The primary issue in a patient suspected of having a toxic optic neuropathy is whether or not he/she was exposed to a substance that has been proved to damage the optic nerve by the same route of exposure. Visual loss may occur from either acute or chronic intoxication depending upon the agent, and the patient must have symptoms and signs that are consistent with those of a toxic optic neuropathy and typical of those in other patients proved to have suffered loss of vision from the same agent. In most cases, the exposure is via ingestion (e.g., ethambutol), but in some cases the causative agent has been inhaled (e.g., toluene), and in still others implanted (e.g., cobalt-covered prosthesis).

The response of patients to rechallenge is helpful in evaluating the validity of presumed intoxications and in helping to establish the cause of the patient's optic neuropathy. If a patient who has recovered vision following cessation of exposure to a drug or chemical loses vision again when reexposed, the recurrent loss of vision tends to verify the neurotoxic nature of the agent and the toxic etiology of the visual loss. Epidemiologic data, especially those showing correlation of changing disease incidence when and where specific drugs or chemicals are introduced or withdrawn, also can prove useful.

Confirmatory evidence of exposure from laboratory tests or from associated nonvisual symptoms always is desirable although not always possible. Nontoxic disorders must be considered in the diagnosis of these patients and should be ruled out with appropriate investigations. Animal models can help validate the optic nerve toxicity of putative intoxicants, despite such problems as species variation in susceptibility and difficulty in measuring visual function.

Clinical Characteristics of Nutritional and Toxic Optic Neuropathies

Persons of all ages, races, places, and economic strata are vulnerable to the toxic and nutritional optic neuropathies. Certain groups are at higher risk because they are under treatment with drugs, have occupational exposure, or practice habits such as smoking and alcohol consumption. The value of obtaining a thorough history, including dietary intake, exposure to drugs, use of tobacco, and social and occupational background, cannot be overemphasized, and the history must be obtained in an appropriate manner. For example, it is not sufficient to ask the patient if he or she has a normal diet. Rather, one should ask something like "What did you eat for dinner last night?" Depending on the answer, the next question might be "What about the night before that?" or "What about lunch?"

The symptoms and signs of nutritional and toxic optic neuropathy are similar and most closely resemble those of Leber hereditary optic neuropathy (LHON), with the exception of the speed at which vision is lost (see below). Nevertheless, other etiologies, such as primary demyelination and even compression, ischemia, and infiltration must be considered in some cases.

Toxic and nutritional optic neuropathies are not painful. Thus, one should inquire carefully about this symptom because associated ocular or orbital pain suggests some other diagnosis.

Dyschromatopsia is present early and may be the initial symptom in observant patients. Some patients notice that certain colors, such as red, are no longer as bright and vivid as previously. Others experience a general loss of color perception.

Patients with nutritional or toxic optic neuropathies often initially notice a blur, fog, or cloud at the point of fixation, following which the visual acuity progressively declines. The rate of decline can be quite rapid but usually progresses slowly over weeks to months. In most cases, vision decreases to no worse than 20/400, although some substances, such as methanol can cause such severe visual loss that the patient has no light perception in either eye. Nevertheless, in most patients, loss of vision below 20/400 should suggest an etiology other than a nutritional deficiency or a typical toxic process. Bilaterality is the rule, although in the early stages one eye may be affected before the other becomes symptomatic.

Patients with toxic or nutritional optic neuropathies typically have central (Fig. 10.1) or cecocentral (Fig. 10.2) scotomas with sparing of the peripheral visual field (Fig. 10.3). Peripheral constriction and altitudinal visual field loss are rare. Because of the symmetric and bilateral visual impairment in toxic and nutritional optic neuropathies, a relative afferent pupillary defect is not a common finding in affected patients. When the patient is bilaterally blind (e.g., as a consequence of methanol poisoning), the pupillary light response will be absent or weak and the pupils will be dilated; however, in most cases, the pupils have relatively normal responses to light and near stimulation.

In the early stages of nutritional optic neuropathy, the disc is normal or slightly hyperemic. Disc hemorrhages may be present in eyes with hyperemic discs, but they are rare and usually small. Similarly, most patients in the initial stages of toxic optic neuropathy also have normal discs. In both nutritional and toxic optic neuropathies, lack of treatment of the nutritional deficiency or continued exposure to the toxic substance results in the development of bilateral optic disc pallor, particularly temporally, associated with profound thinning or even loss of the retinal nerve fiber layer in the papillomacular bundle (Figs. 10.4 and 10.5).

Differential Diagnosis

When an individual complains of bilateral visual loss that refraction cannot correct and has an otherwise normal examination, there are many diagnostic possibilities in addition to the toxic and nutritional optic neuropathies. Certain maculopathies can present in this guise (see Chapter 2). With time, the fundus will show abnormalities, but until then, optical coherence tomography and/or fluorescein angiography may show structural abnormalities, and multifocal electroretinography will establish the retinal nature of the process.

One always should be alert to the possibility of nonorganic visual loss. The absence of optic disc pallor and retinal nerve fiber layer thinning are important clues when the visual loss is longstanding. In such cases, an OCT of the peripapillary retinal nerve fiber layer is extremely helpful. In addition, whereas the

Figure 10.1 Bilateral central scotomas in a 57-year-old woman with a bilateral toxic optic neuropathy from ethambutol. Her visual acuity was 20/70 OU. Peripheral fields were full.

visual field defects in the toxic and nutritional optic neuropathies are typically central or cecocentral, such defects are exceptional in patients with nonorganic visual loss; in these patients, visual fields usually are constricted (see Chapter 23).

Dominantly inherited (Kjer) and mitochondrially inherited (Leber) optic neuropathies can be confused with a bilateral nutritional or toxic optic neuropathy if no other family members are known to be affected. The confusion is most likely to occur in patients who

Figure 10.2 Bilateral cecocentral scotomas in a 27-year-old woman with a bilateral nutritional optic neuropathy related to chronic alcohol abuse. Her visual acuity was 20/80 OD and 20/100 OS.

Figure 10.3 Kinetic perimetry obtained in the patient whose central fields are seen in Figure 10.2 indicate that the peripheral fields are full. Note the appearance of the scotomas when mapped using this type of perimetry.

are first evaluated late in their course. Dominant optic neuropathy progresses much more slowly than the nutritional and toxic optic neuropathies, and optic disc pallor is an early finding. In LHON, the onset of visual loss is simultaneous and symmetric or nearly so. Thus, this disorder must be considered in any patient in whom a toxic or nutritional optic neuropathy is thought to be present, and appropriate genetic testing may be required in some cases (see Chapter 11). Nevertheless, in general, the visual loss that occurs in LHON generally progresses much more rapidly than the visual loss in toxic or nutritional optic neuropathies. In addition, many cases of LHON are characterized by hyperemia and apparent swelling of the optic discs (almost never associated with peripapillary hemorrhages) and telangiectatic vessels on the optic discs and in the peripapillary region. In such cases, fluorescein angiography, which typically reveals marked leakage of dye from swollen discs of all etiologies, shows no disc leakage.

It can be tragic to mistake a compressive or infiltrative lesion of the optic chiasm for nutritional or toxic optic neuropathy. There are few instances in which one should be so confident of the diagnosis of toxic or nutritional optic neuropathy that neuroimaging is omitted. Cecocentral scotomas and the bitemporal visual field

Figure 10.4 Appearance of the optic discs in a patient with a bilateral toxic optic neuropathy from chloramphenicol. Note that both optic discs are hyperemic and somewhat swollen nasally. There is already mild pallor of the temporal portions of both optic discs, associated with early loss of the nerve fiber layer in the papillomacular bundle of both eyes.

Figure 10.5 Appearance of the optic discs in a patient with longstanding bilateral optic neuropathy in the setting of poor nutrition and alcohol abuse. Note the extent of loss of nerve fiber layer from the papillomacular bundle and marked temporal disc pallor. Visual acuity was 20/400 in both eyes, and the patient had bilateral cecocentral scotomas.

defects of chiasmal disease resemble each other, and there are many examples of bilateral central and even cecocentral scotomas from tumors.

If a demyelinating, inflammatory, or infectious optic neuritis begins simultaneously in both eyes, there may be confusion with the toxic and nutritional optic neuropathies. The visual field defects are similar, but there is pain or disc swelling in greater than 90% of cases of optic neuritis (see Chapter 6). In some cases, magnetic resonance imaging (MRI) will indicate the nature of the lesion. In others, it may be necessary to examine the cerebrospinal fluid and perform specific testing for systemic infections and inflammations.

In most cases, analysis of the symptoms and signs obtained from a detailed history and physical examination will establish the diagnosis of a toxic or nutritional optic neuropathy, but it is prudent to obtain neuroimaging unless one is absolutely confident of the diagnosis. MRI with contrast and special attention to the optic nerves and optic chiasm is the optimum investigation in most cases. In cases of presumed nutritional deficiency, the most common nutrients in which the patient is deficient are vitamin B_{12} and folic acid. The roles of pyridoxine, niacin, and riboflavin deficiency in causing an optic neuropathy are controversial, as these vitamins are apt to be depleted in patients who are generally malnourished, but there is no definitive evidence indicating that such deficiencies play a primary etiologic role in nutritional optic neuropathy. Thus, in the setting of a presumed nutritional optic neuropathy, although it probably is not necessary to obtain vitamin levels other than a serum vitamin B_{12} level and a red blood cell folate level (red blood cell folate is a more accurate indicator of systemic folate

levels than serum folate), it makes sense to enrich the diet of patients with loss of vision and evidence of poor nutrition with all of the water-soluble vitamins in which they might be deficient.

When a specific intoxicant is suspected, one should try to identify the toxin or its metabolites in the patient's tissues or fluids. The advice of a toxicologist is invaluable in such instances. In cases of suspected intoxication, one should attempt to evaluate or obtain information about other persons who have had similar exposure. The resulting information has potential public health implications and can help to validate the toxicity of chemicals not previously recognized as dangerous to the human optic nerve.

Specific Nutritional Optic Neuropathies

Epidemic Nutritional Optic Neuropathy

The most useful observations regarding nutritional amblyopia have come not from sporadic cases encountered in practice, but rather from epidemics during war and famine. Two well-documented epidemics were those that afflicted Allied prisoners of war of the Japanese during World War II and Cubans in the early 1990s.

The symptoms developed in an undernourished population after 4 or more months of food deprivation. Among the prisoners of war, vision loss occurred sooner in those who were undernourished at the time they were first incarcerated. Only a minority of people at risk developed loss of vision, and the occurrence of visual loss did not appear to correlate very well with the severity of malnutrition. In some cases, a superficial keratopathy was a prelude to the visual loss, but visual loss developed both with and without a preceding keratopathy. The visual loss was symmetric and often appeared suddenly. In up to one-quarter of cases the visual nadir was reached in 1 day. Vision plateaued after 1 month in the remainder. At the time of visual loss, many victims also had pain or sensory loss in their extremities. There was a high incidence of bilateral sensorineural hearing loss. The fundi were usually normal at first, but a minority had peripapillary hemorrhages associated with mild optic disc hyperemia and swelling. Optic atrophy was a late development. The visual field defects were central or cecocentral. Most abnormalities could be reversed with improved nutrition. Postmortem examinations on repatriated Allied prisoners found atrophy of the papillomacular bundle and lesions in the fasciculus gracilis of the spinal cord.

In 1992 and 1993, an epidemic of optic neuropathy and peripheral neuropathy similar to that reported among the World War II prisoners occurred in Cuba. More than 50,000 persons were affected with bilateral optic neuropathy, sensory and dysautonomic peripheral neuropathy, sensory myelopathy, spastic paraparesis, or sensorineural deafness in various combinations. Slightly more than half of the affected persons had evidence of optic neuropathy, which occurred as a painless rapid loss of vision in both eyes associated with marked dyschromatopsia, central or cecocentral scotomas, and normal appearing optic discs. Patients who did not recover vision developed temporal pallor of the optic discs associated with marked loss of the nerve fiber layer in the papillomacular bundle. The majority of cases occurred in people between 25 and 64 years old, with a predominance of males being among those with optic nerve disease. Partial and complete recovery occurred following treatment with parenteral and oral vitamins. In addition, subsequent supplementation of the general population with B-complex vitamins and vitamin A coincided with a dramatic decrease in new cases of the condition.

Although the loss of vision in the epidemic cases was undoubtedly caused by malnutrition, it is impossible to identify a specific deficient nutrient that caused either of the epidemics. Malnourished individuals have multiple deficiencies. Clinical and laboratory data make it unlikely that vitamin deficiency was the sole factor. Systematic investigation of Cuban epidemic optic neuropathy patients and controls showed an increased risk associated with cassava consumption and a decreased risk associated with high serum levels of antioxidant carotenoids, ingestion of B vitamins, and ingestion of animal products.

Factors additional to malnutrition must explain the visual loss in these cases and in similar cases in other countries such as Tanzania. Tobacco use, especially cigar use, was a risk factor in Cuba. Physical labor also seemed to be a risk factor among the prisoners of war. In any case, the conclusion that epidemic cases of nutritional optic neuropathy (and probably sporadic cases as well) are the result of some multifactorial etiology is inescapable.

Isolated Nutritional Optic Neuropathy

A 29-year-old woman of East Indian descent with a history of chronic anorexia nervosa presented to the Wilmer Eye Institute of the Johns Hopkins Hospital with a chief complaint of blurred vision of 4 days' duration. She described this "as if water was poured on a painting" and complained of complete darkness in her central visual field, blurred vision peripherally, and inability to read or make out shapes. She denied specific difficulty with night vision. Her height was 60.5 in, and her weight was 57 lb. She had undergone bilateral laser-assisted in situ keratomileusis 18 months prior to evaluation.

The patient had been in her usual state of health until 1 week prior to presentation, when she noted bilateral burning and itching in both eyes. This lasted for 2 days and then resolved spontaneously. Four days prior to presentation, however, she developed progressive blurring of vision in both eyes. Her examination revealed uncorrected distance visual acuity of 20/400 OD and 5/200 OS. The patient was unable to see any figures on the Ishihara color plates with either eye. Visual fields were full peripherally, but there were bilateral central scotomas. Both pupils were reactive to light and near stimulation; there was no relative afferent pupillary defect in either eye. Ophthalmoscopic examination was normal, with no evidence of optic disc pallor or retinal pathology.

The patient was adopted and did not know her biologic family history. She had been diagnosed with anorexia nervosa, purging type, at age 22. Her maximum weight was 175 lb at age 18, and her minimum weight was 55 lb at age 25. She reported three prior admissions for anorexia nervosa at the ages of 22, 23, and 25. On each of these occasions, she presented severely malnourished with a weight of around 50 lb. Her eating disorder behaviors included severe restriction, self-induced vomiting, laxative, and diet pill use. She had a rigid and limited food repertoire consisting of daily intake of five Safeway brand: Table Water crackers (70 cal), 1/8 cup of cooked oatmeal (19 cal), 16 fluid oz of water, 11 oz of Pedialyte (25 cal), and one bottle of wine per day. She was not under the care of a psychiatrist.

In addition to her visual symptoms, a review of systems was significant for 20-lb weight loss over the previous 6 months, extreme fatigue, dysphagia, dyspnea, myalgias, and numbness and tingling of her lower extremities bilaterally. Physical examination was significant for severe cachexia, alopecia, and a gross motor tremor of upper extremities bilaterally. On neurologic examination the patient was oriented to person, place, and time. Cranial nerves III to XII were intact. Muscle strength was 4/5 in all major muscle groups with generalized but no focal weakness. Sensation to fine touch was intact in all extremities; however, reduced vibration sense was noted in both lower extremities. Gait was unstable and slow. There was dysmetria on testing of finger-to-nose, heel-to-shin, and rapid alternating movements.

The patient was diagnosed with visual loss secondary to malnutrition resulting from her anorexia nervosa and alcohol abuse. Her vitamin B_{12} level was normal as was a serum folate level, but red blood cell folate level was markedly reduced. The patient was treated with oral folic acid. Within 2 days, the patient's visual acuity had improved significantly to 20/80 OU. She could now correctly identify the figures on all 10 of the Ishihara color plates with each eye. Visual field testing demonstrated persistent but small central field defects with full peripheral fields.

This case highlights the importance of collecting a detailed dietary history in patients with anorexia nervosa for whom a very restricted food repertoire may lead to visual or neurologic complications that may be partly or wholly reversible with nutritional rehabilitation. This is a special concern in patients with comorbid alcohol abuse who may be at greater risk of nutritional deficiencies due to their substance abuse comorbidity.

As this case also illustrates, the treatment of nutritional optic neuropathy is improved nutrition. Unless the vision loss is extensive, there is an excellent prospect for recovery or at least improvement with such treatment.

Specific Toxic Optic Neuropathies

Table 10.1 lists substances that are known or presumed to be toxic to the human optic nerve. It is not always clear if the association of ingestion of, or exposure to, a particular substance and the subsequent visual loss is fortuitous or cause and effect. The literature is uneven in this regard, and several of the agents are of academic interest only because they are no longer in use. Furthermore, it is often difficult to determine if the underlying disease or its treatment is responsible for the visual loss. In addition, the suspected toxin may not be the only agent to which the patient has been exposed, further confounding the issue of causation. Finally, as noted above, a "toxic" optic neuropathy may be produced by substances that

Table 10.1 Substances Known or Believed to Cause Toxic Optic Neuropathy

Amantadine hydrochloride	Halogenated hydroxyquinolines
Amiodarone	Hexachlorophene
Amoproxan	Infliximab
Arsenicals	Interferon-alpha
Aspidium (male fern)	Iodoform
Cafergot	Iodoquinol
Carbon disulfide	Isoniazid
Carbon tetrachloride	Lead
Catha edulis	Linezolid
Chlorambucil	Methanol (methyl alcohol)
Chloramphenicol	Methyl acetate
Chlorodinitrobenzene	Methyl bromide
Chlorpromazine	Octamoxin
Chlorpropamide	Organic solvents
Cisplatin	Penicillamine
Clioquinol	Pheniprazine
Clomiphene	Plasmocid
Cobalt chloride	Quinine
Cyclosporine	Sildenafil
Dapsone	Streptomycin
Desferrioxamine	Styrene (vinyl benzene)
Dinitrobenzene	Sulfonamides
Dinitrochlorobenzene	Tacrolimus
Disulfiram	Tamoxifen
Elcatonin	Thallium
Emetine	Tobacco
Ergot	Toluene
Ethambutol	Triethyltin
Ethchlorvynol	Trichloroethylene
Ethylene glycol	Vincristine
5-Fluorouracil	

directly attack RGCs, axons, or myelin, or by substances that render the nerve susceptible to other pathophysiologic processes such as ischemia. Examples are illustrated below.

Primary Toxic Optic Neuropathy: Ethambutol

Of all the drugs in wide use, ethambutol is undoubtedly the one most often implicated in toxic optic neuropathy. Experiments in monkeys and rats show that ethambutol intoxication causes an axonal neuropathy with a special predilection for the optic chiasm. Ethambutol is metabolized to a chelating agent, and this has been suggested as somehow responsible for the optic neuropathy. It is interesting in this regard that two other chelators—disulfiram and DL-penicillamine—have been implicated in toxic optic neuropathies.

Human ethambutol intoxication is dose related, with loss of vision most likely to occur in patients receiving 25 mg/kg/d or more. However, vision loss may occur in patients receiving much lower doses. Visual loss rarely occurs until the patient has been receiving the drug for at least 2 months, with 7 months being the average. There is evidence that there is greater susceptibility to intoxication and more severe visual impairment in patients with renal tuberculosis, perhaps because ethambutol depends on the kidneys for excretion.

The loss of vision is bilaterally symmetric and begins insidiously, with dyschromatopsia often the earliest symptom. Central scotomas are the rule, but patients also may develop bitemporal defects or peripheral constriction. The fundi are initially normal, but if the drug is not stopped, vision continues to worsen and optic atrophy develops. Visual acuity, color vision, and visual field usually improve slowly once ethambutol is discontinued; however, some patients, particularly but not exclusively those in whom optic atrophy has already developed, do not experience an improvement in visual function.

Beyond stopping the drug, there is no specific therapy for the toxic optic neuropathy caused by ethambutol. Recommendations regarding the appropriate screening strategy are controversial. Certainly, discontinuation of the drug is indicated at the onset of any symptoms or signs of optic neuropathy.

Demyelinating Optic Neuropathy: Tumor Necrosis Factor-Alpha Inhibitors

TNF-α is a multidimensional cytokine with effects on cellular metabolism, antiviral activities, coagulation processes, growth regulation of cells, and insulin response. It was named based on its ability to stimulate necrosis of malignant tumors but soon was found to be an important mediator of cutaneous inflammation.

It is activated mainly by T-lymphocytes and macrophages during acute inflammation.

TNF-α is known to play a crucial role in the pathogenesis of many chronic inflammatory diseases. Elevated levels of TNF-α have been demonstrated in Crohn disease (CD), psoriasis (Ps), psoriatic arthritis (PsA), and rheumatoid arthritis (RA), suggesting a role for TNF-α in their pathogenesis and providing a rationale for the treatment of these diseases with drugs that inhibit it.

TNF-α blockers have demonstrated efficacy in large, randomized controlled clinical trials, either as monotherapy or in combination with other anti-inflammatory or disease-modifying antirheumatic drugs (DMARDs). A number of TNF-α inhibitors are available for clinical use, including infliximab, adalimumab, etanercept, golimumab, and certolizumab pegol. All of these drugs block the biologic effects of TNF-α although there are some differences in their structure, pharmacokinetics, and mechanisms of action (Fig. 10.6).

Although TNF-α inhibitors are generally well tolerated, all have potential adverse effects, including reports of central nervous system (CNS) demyelinating disorders during treatment with anti-TNF-α agents. Several of these cases have been temporally related to anti-TNF therapy and have resolved when treatment was withdrawn. As far as optic neuropathies associated with anti-TNF-α treatment are concerned, it would appear that they are not "toxic" in the normal sense of the word, but rather due to demyelination stimulated by the agents. Be that as it may, there are in the literature several case reports that suggest a potential for the development of a unilateral or bilateral demyelinating optic neuropathy in

Figure 10.6 Anti-TNF molecules bind to and neutralize the activity of TNF-α. Infliximab and adalimumab are monoclonal antibodies. Infliximab is a mouse/human chimera that joints the variable regions of a mouse antibody to the constant region of human IgG1, and adalimumab is a human IgG1 antibody. Etanercept is a dimeric fusion protein that joins the human p75 TNF receptor to the Fc domain of human IgG1. (Reprinted with permission from: Shukla R, Vender RB. Pharmacology of TNF inhibitors. In: Weinberg JM, Buchholz R, eds. *TNF-alpha Inhibitors*. Switzerland: Birkhäuser Verlag; 2006:23–44.)

Figure 10.7 Bilateral anterior optic neuropathy in a 62-year-old man who had been experiencing painless, slowly progressive blurred vision in both eyes for several weeks. He had been taking amiodarone 800 mg/d for 4 months. His visual acuity was 20/30 OD and 20/100 OS. Note that both optic discs are hyperemic and swollen. There are several small hemorrhages in the peripapillary regions of both fundi and on the surface of the left disc.

patients taking TNF-α inhibitors, some of which are associated with other clinical manifestations and neuroimaging findings consistent with multiple sclerosis. Thus, such agents should be used with caution—if at all—in patients with multiple sclerosis and, as in the case of patients beginning treatment with amiodarone (see below), patients about to be placed on one of the TNF-α inhibitors should be told about the possibility of visual loss and told to contact their ophthalmologist immediately should they experience any visual sensory or neurologic symptoms or signs.

Pseudotoxic Optic Neuropathy: Amiodarone

Amiodarone is an antiarrhythmic agent primarily used to treat atrial or ventricular tachyarrhythmias. The most common ocular side effect is the formation of verticillate, pigmented, corneal epithelial deposits that eventually occur in most patients treated with the drug. Amiodarone has been associated with an optic neuropathy that in many cases is indistinguishable from, and very well may be a nonarteritic anterior

ischemic optic neuropathy (Fig. 10.7). Several features proposed as suggestive of an amiodarone effect are insidious bilateral visual loss, protracted bilateral disc swelling, and potential for recovery when the drug is discontinued.

Amiodarone binds phospholipids and forms complexes that accumulate within many tissues, including the cornea, vascular endothelial cells, retinal ganglion cells, and optic nerve axons. Optic neuropathy thus may result from direct involvement of neural tissues or from vascular compromise (and, hence, be a form of ischemic optic neuropathy).

The available data are insufficient to make firm recommendations regarding a screening protocol for patients treated with amiodarone. Certainly, any patient with visual symptoms during treatment should be promptly evaluated. Amiodarone may be a life-saving treatment and the occurrence of an optic neuropathy is therefore not an absolute contraindication to further treatment. However, in patients who have an optic neuropathy while on amiodarone, discontinuation of amiodarone and treatment with an alternative drug should be considered.

Hereditary Optic Neuropathies

11

Monosymptomatic Hereditary Optic Neuropathies
    Leber Hereditary Optic Neuropathy
    Dominant Optic Atrophy
    Other Isolated Hereditary Optic Neuropathies

Hereditary Optic Atrophy with Other Neurologic or Systemic Signs
    Progressive Optic Atrophy with Juvenile Diabetes
        Mellitus, Diabetes Insipidus, and Hearing Loss
        (Wolfram Syndrome, Didmoad)
    Complicated Hereditary Infantile Optic Atrophy
        (Behr Syndrome)

Optic Neuropathy in Hereditary Degenerative or Developmental Diseases
    Hereditary Ataxias
    Hereditary Polyneuropathies
    Hereditary Optic Atrophy Associated with Diffuse
        White-Matter Disease

The hereditary optic neuropathies comprise a group of disorders in which the cause of optic nerve dysfunction is hereditable as demonstrated by familial expression or genetic analysis. Clinical variability, both within and among families with the same disease, often makes recognition and classification difficult. Previously, classification relied on recognition of similar characteristics and similar patterns of transmission, but genetic analysis now permits diagnosis of the hereditary optic neuropathies in the absence of family history or in the setting of unusual clinical presentations. As a result, the clinical phenotypes of each disease are broader, and it is easier to recognize unusual cases.

The inherited optic neuropathies typically manifest as symmetric, bilateral, and central visual loss. In many of these disorders, the papillomacular nerve fiber bundle is exclusively or primarily affected, with resultant central or cecocentral scotomas. The exact location of initial pathology along the ganglion cell and its axon, and the pathophysiologic mechanisms of optic nerve injury remain unknown. Optic nerve damage usually is permanent and, in many diseases, progressive. Once optic atrophy is observed, substantial nerve injury has already occurred although in rare settings, at least partial recovery can still occur.

In classifying the hereditary optic neuropathies, it is important to exclude the primary retinal degenerations that may masquerade as primary optic neuropathies because of the common finding of secondary optic disc pallor (see Chapter 2).

The inherited optic neuropathies generally are classified by their pattern of transmission. The most common patterns are autosomal dominant, autosomal recessive, and maternal (i.e., mitochondrial). In some of the hereditary optic neuropathies, optic nerve dysfunction is, or at least usually is the only manifestation of the disease. In others, a bilateral optic neuropathy is associated with various, apparently disparate neurologic deficits and/or systemic abnormalities. In some of these disorders, both the visual loss and the nonvisual deficits are static, whereas in others, either or both are progressive. Finally, in some patients, a hereditary optic neuropathy is simply a consequence of the optic nerve being a white-matter tract in a patient with a diffuse white-matter disorder or degeneration.

Monosymptomatic Hereditary Optic Neuropathies

Leber Hereditary Optic Neuropathy

Clinical Features

In this maternally inherited disorder (see below), men become symptomatic more frequently than women, with a male predominance of 80% to 90% in most pedigrees. There is incomplete penetrance, with 20% to 60% of men and 4% to 32% of women with one of the causative genetic mutations experiencing visual loss. Affected females are more likely to have affected children, especially daughters, than unaffected female carriers.

Visual loss in patients with Leber hereditary optic neuropathy (LHON) typically begins simultaneously in both eyes (50%) or initially in one eye, followed days, weeks, months or, very rarely, years after the first eye (50%). Reports of unilateral onset are numerous and likely reflect both instances of true unilateral visual loss and cases in which initial involvement of the contralateral eye is unrecognized by the patient.

Indeed, careful visual field testing in apparently unilateral involvement usually shows a subtle field defect in the contralateral asymptomatic eye. In any event, all patients with LHON eventually experience bilateral and symmetric visual loss. Once visual loss begins, it tends to worsen, reaching a nadir in 3 to 6 months. Visual acuity at the point of stabilization usually is about 20/200 to 20/400. Although vision in some patients deteriorates to hand motions, it is distinctly unusual for a patient to have a reduction to light perception or no light perception, and in such cases, the diagnosis of LHON must be questioned, as it must be in patients whose visual loss is minimal (e.g., 20/40 OU).

The visual loss in patients with LHON is always painless, and it is the absence of pain that is a **major feature** that differentiates LHON from other optic neuropathies, particularly optic neuritis, which occurs in the same general age group (although more often in women than in men, the opposite of LHON) but is associated with pain, often on movement of the eye, in over 90% of cases.

In addition to reduction of visual acuity, color vision is severely affected in patients with LHON, often early in the course but rarely if ever before there is significant loss of acuity. Pupillary light responses may be relatively preserved compared with the responses in patients with optic neuropathies from other causes. Indeed, even patients with apparently unilateral visual loss from LHON tend to have either no relative afferent pupillary defect or a very subtle one. This is another feature that differentiates LHON from other optic neuropathies and is thought to be related to selective sparing of the melanopsin-containing retinal ganglion cells in this disorder (see Chapter 2).

Visual field defects in patients with LHON typically are central or cecocentral. The scotomas may be relative during the early stages of visual loss but rapidly become large and absolute. Rarely, field abnormalities mimicking the bitemporal configuration of chiasmal defects occur.

Many patients with LHON have absolutely normal-appearing optic discs and peripapillary retinas at the time visual loss begins and, thus, may be thought to have either retinal disease or nonorganic visual loss, particularly given their relatively preserved pupillary responses to light stimulation and lack of pain. Others, however, have the triad of: (1) optic disc and circumpapillary telangiectasias, (2) hyperemia and fullness of the optic disc (or discs if visual loss is bilateral) without peripapillary hemorrhages or exudates, and (3) absence of leakage from the disc on fluorescein angiography (distinguishing the LHON optic disc appearance from the truly swollen optic disc) (Fig. 11.1). When present, these findings at the time of visual loss are helpful in suggesting the correct diagnosis, but it must be emphasized that their absence—even during

the period of acute visual loss—does not exclude the diagnosis of LHON. As visual loss progresses in patients with LHON, the optic disc becomes pale, particularly temporally, with loss of nerve fibers that is most pronounced in the papillomacular region, producing a typical picture similar to that of patients with severe toxic or nutritional optic neuropathies (Fig. 11.2; see also Chapter 10).

Visual loss in most patients with LHON remains profound and permanent; however, recovery of central vision may occasionally occur after visual deterioration. Unlike the spontaneous improvement in vision that occurs in patients with optic neuritis within several months after onset, spontaneous visual improvement in patients with LHON (4–30%, depending on the mutation–see below) usually occurs about 1 to 2 years later, typically associated with a partial breakup or, rarely, complete resolution of the central field defects. Recovery usually is bilateral and symmetric, and once it occurs, recurrent visual loss is extremely rare.

Associated Findings

In the majority of patients with LHON, visual dysfunction is the only significant manifestation of the disease; however, some pedigrees have members with associated cardiac conduction abnormalities, such as the pre-excitation syndromes (specifically Wolff–Parkinson–White and Lown–Ganong–Levine) and prolongation of the corrected QT interval. Rarely, such patients experience palpitations, syncope, or sudden death. Minor neurologic abnormalities, such as exaggerated or pathologic reflexes, mild cerebellar ataxia, tremor, movement disorders, muscle wasting, or distal sensory neuropathy, are present in some patients with LHON. In addition, some patients with molecularly confirmed LHON, predominantly women, exhibit symptoms and signs consistent with multiple sclerosis (MS) at the time they begin to experience the typical painless, progressive visual loss typical of LHON. Cerebrospinal fluid (CSF) and magnetic resonance imaging (MRI) findings are characteristic of MS in most if not all of these patients. It therefore is likely that this apparent association of LHON and MS is no greater than the prevalence of the two diseases.

Some pedigrees consist of multiple members who exhibit the clinical features of LHON in addition to more severe neurologic abnormalities, the so-called "Leber plus" syndromes. In addition to the typical bilateral optic neuropathy, these syndromes include: (1) movement disorders, spasticity, psychiatric disturbances, skeletal abnormalities, and acute infantile encephalopathy; (2) dystonia, and lesions of the basal ganglia by neuroimaging; optic neuropathy and myelopathy; and (3) fatal encephalopathy in early childhood. Most of these pedigrees are genetically

Figure 11.1 Leber hereditary optic neuropathy. **A:** Both optic discs in the acute phase of the disorder. Note hyperemic appearance of discs. Peripapillary telangiectatic vessels are present. **B:** Both optic discs photographed with red-free (540 nm) light. Note marked hyperemia of the discs with dilation of small vessels both on the surface of the disc and in the peripapillary region. **C:** Fluorescein angiogram in arteriovenous **(left)** and late **(right)** phases shows dilation of right disc and peripapillary vessels but no leakage of fluorescein dye.

Figure 11.2 Progression to bilateral optic atrophy in a patient with Leber hereditary optic neuropathy. **A:** Both optic discs in acute phase of the disease. Visual acuity is 20/100 in both eyes with large cecocentral scotomas. Telangiectatic vessels are evident adjacent to the inferior margin of both discs. The right disc **(left)** is already pale temporally, and there is atrophy of the papillomacular nerve fiber layer. **B:** Two months after onset of visual loss, visual acuity is 5/200 in the right eye and 8/200 in the left eye. Both discs show moderate pallor, particularly temporally, with loss of nerve fiber layer that is especially evident in the papillomacular region. Previously seen telangiectatic vessels are disappearing. **C:** Six months after onset of visual loss, visual acuity remains 5/200 in the right eye and 8/200 in the left eye. Both discs are pale, particularly temporally. The telangiectatic vessels have completely disappeared. One year after these photographs were obtained, the patient noted gradual, partial return of visual acuity in both eyes to 20/50. Subsequent genetic testing showed evidence of a mutation in the mitochondrial DNA at position 14484.

distinct from those with more classic LHON, with some having more than one of the mutations typically associated with this disorder.

Inheritance and Genetics

All pedigrees clinically designated as LHON have a maternal inheritance pattern; that is, all offspring of a woman carrying the trait will inherit the trait, but only the females can pass the trait on to the subsequent generation. Both the father and the mother contribute to the nuclear portion of the zygote, but the mother's egg is essentially the sole provider of the cytoplasmic contents of the zygote. Therefore, a cytoplasmic determinant is necessary for maternal inheritance, and the only source of extranuclear DNA in the cell is in the intracytoplasmic mitochondria.

Almost every cell in the body contains several hundred intracytoplasmic mitochondria that generate the cellular energy necessary for normal cellular function and maintenance. Those cells in tissues particularly reliant on mitochondrial energy production, such as the central nervous system (CNS), contain more mitochondria than cells with low energy requirements. Each mitochondrion contains 2 to 10 double-stranded circles of DNA, with each circle containing 16,500 base pairs compared with the 3×10^9 base pairs contained within the nuclear genome. Because there are several mtDNAs in each mitochondrion and hundreds of mitochondria per cell, the mtDNA comprises approximately 0.3% of the cell's total DNA.

Mitochondrial DNA codes for all the transfer ribonucleic acids (RNAs) and the ribosomal RNAs required for intramitochondrial protein production. It also codes for 13 proteins essential to the oxidative phosphorylation system. The majority of proteins crucial to normal oxidative phosphorylation function are encoded on nuclear genes, manufactured in the cytoplasm, and transported into the mitochondria. Hence, "mitochondrial disease" can result from genetic defects in either the nuclear or mitochondrial genomes.

If a new mutation occurs in the mtDNA, there will be a period of coexistence of mutant and normal mtDNA within the same cell (**heteroplasmy**). At each cell division, the mitochondrial genotype may drift toward pure normal or pure mutant (**homoplasmy**), or it may remain mixed. The phenotype of the cell (and the tissue the cells comprise) depends on the proportion of mtDNA genotypes and the intrinsic energy needs of the cell. The mutant phenotype may only become apparent when the amount of normal mtDNA can no longer provide sufficient mitochondrial function for cell and tissue maintenance.

The most common point mutation in mtDNA linked to LHON is a single nucleotide substitution at position 11778 in the mtDNA (Fig. 11.3). This region codes for subunit 4 (designated ND4) of complex I

(NADH dehydrogenase) in the respiratory chain. The 11778 mutation is present in many racially divergent pedigrees with LHON, suggesting that it has arisen independently on multiple occasions. Whereas 31% to 89% of European, North American, and Australian LHON pedigrees have the 11778 mutation, greater than 90% of Asian LHON patients are 11778 positive.

In addition to the 11778 mutation, several other point mutations in mtDNA are associated with LHON (Fig. 11.3). The majority are located within genes that also code for proteins comprising complex 1, but most are within subunits other than ND4. For example, a point mutation at mtDNA position 3460 within the gene coding for subunit ND1 of complex I accounts for 8% to 15% of LHON cases worldwide, and a point mutation at position 14484 in the gene coding for the subunit ND6 of complex I accounts for 10% to 15% of LHON pedigrees. The mutations at sites 11778, 3460, and 14484 are designated "primary" mutations for LHON in that they: (1) confer a genetic risk for LHON expression individually; (2) change the coding for evolutionarily conserved amino acids in essential proteins; (3) are found in multiple, different, ethnically divergent pedigrees; and (4) are absent or rare among control pedigrees. In total, they account for about 90% of LHON worldwide. Several other mtDNA mutations may be "primary," but they each account for only a few reported pedigrees. Still other mtDNA mutations have been termed "secondary mutations" because they are found with more frequency among LHON patients than in pedigrees that have no members with LHON, but their pathogenetic significance remains unclear (see Fig. 11.3).

Natural History

Although most patients with LHON, regardless of the mtDNA mutation, experience permanent visual loss, some recover normal or near-normal vision despite impressive optic disc pallor. The potential for improvement appears to be related primarily if not exclusively to the mtDNA mutation.

Among patients with the 11778 mutation, about 4% experience spontaneous recovery, compared with 37% to 65% of patients with either the 14484 or 3460 mutations. Furthermore, the ultimate visual acuities in patients with the 14484 mutation are significantly better than those with the 11778 and 3460 mutations.

Unanswered Questions

Genetic analysis allows a broad view of what constitutes the clinical profile of LHON. Most striking are the number of patients without a family history of visual loss. Some of these singleton cases are women, some are outside the typical age range for LHON, and many do not have the classic ophthalmoscopic appearance.

Figure 11.3 Mitochondrial genome showing the point mutations associated with Leber hereditary optic neuropathy (LHON). Over 90% of all cases of LHON are associated with the three primary mutations located inside the genome, and the other mutations are shown outside the genome. These other mutations vary markedly in their prevalence, degree of evolutionary conservation of the encoded amino acids altered, and frequency among controls. Mutations marked * may be primary, but they each account for only one or a few pedigrees worldwide. Mutations marked *d are primary mutations associated with LHON and dystonia. Mutations marked *m are primary mutations associated with LHON/MELAS overlap syndrome.

Clearly, the diagnosis of LHON should be considered in any case of unexplained painless, unilateral or bilateral optic neuropathy associated with normal or relatively normal pupillary reactions to light stimulation and central or cecocentral scotomas, regardless of age of onset, sex, family history, or funduscopic appearance (unless there is obvious optic disc swelling with peripapillary hemorrhages and/or exudates). Nevertheless, many questions remain unanswered regarding the determinants of phenotypic expression of LHON. For example, does the specific mtDNA mutation dictate particular clinical features? Although pedigrees with the "Leber plus" syndromes demonstrate that certain mtDNA mutations may result in specific disease patterns of Leber-like optic neuropathies with other neurologic abnormalities, few significant clinical differences can be demonstrated among patients positive for the 11778 mutation, patients with other mtDNA mutations, or patients as yet genetically unspecified, although cardiac conduction abnormalities occur most commonly in patients with the 3460 mutation.

Another unanswered question is why not everyone with one of the primary mtDNA mutations becomes symptomatic. Indeed, a mtDNA mutation is present in all maternally related family members of patients with LHON, even though most will never become symptomatic. Thus, a mtDNA mutation may be necessary for phenotypic expression, but it may not be sufficient. Does heteroplasmy among individuals in a pedigree play a role in phenotypic expression? In some families, the mutant mtDNA content enriches from one generation to the next and may be at least partially responsible for phenotypic expression of the disease; however, in most large reviews of molecularly confirmed LHON patients, heteroplasmy is documented in the blood of a minority of affected individuals, and once a person becomes symptomatic, there does not appear to be any clinical difference in disease expression among those who are heteroplasmic and those who are homoplasmic.

Recent work with large numbers of symptomatic LHON patients and asymptomatic carriers indicates that symptomatic patients have increased mitochondrial mass and an increased amount of mtDNA per cell compared with normals. More importantly, carriers of the 11778 mutation who remains asymptomatic have markedly increased mitochondrial mass and increased DNA compared with symptomatic LHON patients. It has therefore been postulated that, in general, the positive effects on oxidative phosphorylation of increased numbers of mitochondria and increased mtDNA per cell "trump" the negative effects of the increased amount of mutated mtDNA.

Yet another unresolved issue relates to the fact that in most patients with LHON, a bilateral optic neuropathy is the sole manifestation. Assuming that some persons are 100% homoplasmic for the causative mtDNA mutation in all of their organs, there is no convincing explanation why visual loss should be the sole manifestation of the disease. Varying tissue energy needs may play some role. The CNS is most reliant on mitochondrial adenosine triphosphate (ATP). Histochemical studies of optic nerve in the monkey and rat show a high degree of mitochondrial respiratory activity within the unmyelinated portion of optic nerve fibers located in the prelaminar portion of the optic nerve and it thus has been postulated that it is this region that is most vulnerable to the mitochondrial dysfunction that is produced by the pathogenic mtDNA mutations.

Genetic factors other than the specific mtDNA mutation and the presence and degree of heteroplasmy also may play a role in expression. Other mtDNA mutations may be present that modify the expression of the LHON causative mutation or that result in other abnormal proteins involved in mitochondrial function. Nuclear-encoded factors modifying mtDNA expression, mtDNA products, or mitochondrial metabolism may be necessary for phenotypic expression of LHON. The male predominance of visual loss in LHON may be explained by a modifying factor on the X-chromosome. Tissue energy utilization and reserve also may determine the timing and extent of visual loss. Mitochondrial energy production decreases with age, and the timing of visual loss in patients at risk for LHON may reflect the threshold at which already reduced mitochondrial function deteriorates to a critical level.

Environmental factors also may play a role in which carriers of the primary LHON mtDNA mutations eventually become symptomatic. Both the internal and external environment of the organism must be considered. Systemic illnesses, nutritional deficiencies, and toxins that stress or directly inhibit the body's mitochondrial respiratory capacity may initiate or increase phenotypic expression of the disease. Anecdotal reports suggest a possible role for tobacco and excessive alcohol use in the expression of visual loss, but large studies on the effects of these agents on patients at risk for LHON have yet to be performed.

Treatment

In light of the possibility for spontaneous recovery in some patients with LHON, especially those with the 14484 and 3460 mutations, anecdotal reports of treatment efficacy must be considered with caution. Attempts to treat or prevent the acute phase of visual loss with systemic steroids, hydroxocobalamin, or cyanide antagonists are ineffective. Other therapies tried are naturally occurring cofactors involved in mitochondrial metabolism or agents with antioxidant capabilities, including coenzyme Q_{10}, idebenone (an analog of coenzyme Q), succinate, vitamin K_1, vitamin K_3, vitamin C, thiamine, and vitamin B_2. The results with all of these agents have not been particularly encouraging with the exception of idebenone, and even this drug has not produced consistent or impressive results. In addition, brimonidine, a topically applied agent with purported neuroprotective effects, was unsuccessful in preventing second eye involvement in a small prospective study. A number of investigators have just begun to attempt gene therapy for patients with both acute and long-standing LHON. The results of such an approach remain to be seen.

In view of the lack of spontaneous recovery in the majority of patients with LHON, the lack of any effective treatment, and the suggestion that environmental stress may determine, at least in part, which carriers of the LHON mtDNA mutations become symptomatic and which do not, nonspecific recommendations to avoid agents or behavior that might stress mitochondrial energy production are reasonable. Thus, we advise our patients at risk for LHON to avoid tobacco use, excessive alcohol intake, and environmental toxins.

The importance of genetic counseling of patients with this disease and their families cannot be overemphasized. It should be explained to males with an LHON mutation, whether or not they are visually symptomatic, that they **will not** pass the mutation or the disease to their children. On the other hand, women with one of the LHON mutations **will** pass the mutation to **all** of their children, both male and female, although, as noted above, not all persons with the mutation (indeed, the minority) will become symptomatic.

Dominant Optic Atrophy

Autosomal-dominant optic atrophy (ADOA), also called Kjer or juvenile optic atrophy, is the most common of the hereditary optic neuropathies, with an estimated disease prevalence in the range of 1:50,000, or as high as 1:10,000 in Denmark.

ADOA is an abiotrophy with onset in the first decade in life. It is difficult for patients and their families to identify a precise onset of reduced vision, but most patients appear to become affected between 4 and 6 years of age. Although some severely affected children develop nystagmus and are found to have decreased vision before beginning schooling, the majority of are unaware of a visual problem and are discovered to have optic atrophy (1) because there is a family history of the condition, (2) as a direct consequence of examination of another affected family member, (3) because they fail a school vision screening examination, or (4)

during a "routine" eye examination. These phenomena attest to the usually insidious onset in childhood, mild degree of visual dysfunction, absence of night blindness, and absence of substantial or dramatic progression (as opposed to LHON, see above).

Visual acuity usually is symmetrically reduced in both eyes. Vision ranges from 20/20 to 20/800, with about 15% of patients eventually developing vision of 20/200 or worse; however, a decline to vision of hand motions or worse is extremely rare.

Patients with ADOA nearly always have a disturbance of color perception. Although the tritanopic defect was once deemed classic in patients with this disorder, a generalized dyschromatopsia, with both blue-yellow and red-green defects, is found most commonly. There is no correlation between the severity of the dyschromatopsia and the visual acuity.

Visual fields in patients with ADOA characteristically show central, paracentral, or cecocentral scotomas. A visual field pattern consisting of bilateral temporal depression, mimicking the field defects of chiasmal compression is not uncommonly demonstrated, especially with automated perimetry; however, the difference between patients with these defects and patients with bitemporal scotomas is that patients with ADOA have bilaterally reduced acuity and color vision, whereas patients with bitemporal hemianopic scotomas do not (one can see 20/20 with half a macula!).

The optic atrophy in patients with ADOA may be subtle, temporal only, or may involve the entire disc (Fig. 11.4). The most characteristic change is a triangular (wedge) excavation of the temporal portion of the disc.

Most patients with ADOA have no neurologic deficits; however, like LHON, some patients have a syndrome called "ODOA Plus," in which bilateral typical ADOA is associated with a variety of deficits, including bilateral hearing loss, external ophthalmoplegia, scoliosis, or a combination of these manifestations (Figs. 11.5 and 11.6). Such patients have specific mutations in their nuclear DNA.

Patients with ADOA typically experience a mild, slow, and insidious progression of visual dysfunction with the visual acuity decreasing, on average, about one line per decade of life. There appears to be no correlation between the rate of visual loss and initial visual acuity nor do members of most pedigrees experience identical rates of progression. Rarely, relatively rapid deterioration of vision occurs after years of stable visual function. Spontaneous recovery of vision is not a feature of this disorder.

Almost all of the pedigrees with ADOA have a mutation of a gene on the telomeric portion of the long arm of chromosome 3 (3q28–29) called the OPA1 gene. To date, more than 200 mutations in the OPA1

Figure 11.4 Dominant optic atrophy. **A:** Right and left optic discs in a patient with 20/40 visual acuity in both eyes, a tritanopic color vision defect, and bilateral, small central scotomas. Note minimal temporal pallor. **B:** Right and left discs of the patient's father. Visual acuity is 20/100 in the right eye and 20/80 in the left eye with severe dyschromatopsia and bilateral central scotomas. The pallor is extensive and is primarily temporal in a "wedge" shape.

gene have been found to cause ADOA. The product of the OPA1 gene is a protein targeted to the mitochondria and appears to exert its function in mitochondrial biogenesis and stabilization of mitochondrial membrane integrity. Most of the OPA1 mutations create a premature stop signal in the instructions for making the protein. As a result, an abnormally small protein, which is produced, is likely to be unstable and broken down quickly. Unlike LHON, individuals with one of the pathogenic OPA1 mutations invariably have bilateral optic atrophy (i.e., there is 100% penetrance). There currently is no treatment for ADOA.

Other Isolated Hereditary Optic Neuropathies

Monosymptomatic inherited optic neuropathies other than LHON and ADOA are extremely rare. **Congenital recessive optic atrophy**, the very existence of which has been questioned, is present at birth or discovered by age 3 to 4 years. Visual loss is severe with near-complete blindness and nystagmus. It appears to be nonprogressive and unassociated with neurologic or systemic abnormalities. Similarly, **X-linked optic atrophy** has been demonstrated in only a few

Figure 11.5 Dominant optic atrophy "Plus." External appearance of a 45-year-old woman with long-standing decreased vision in both eyes, external ophthalmoplegia, bilateral hearing loss, and a bilateral optic neuropathy. Genetic analysis identified a G–>A substitution at nucleotide position 1334 in exon 14 of OPA1 causing an arginine-to-histidine change (R445 H).

families, with male members demonstrating early childhood optic atrophy with slow progression. In one family in whom affected males manifested subtle neurologic abnormalities, linkage was established at Xp11.4–11.2.

Hereditary Optic Atrophy with Other Neurologic or Systemic Signs

As noted above, some patients with hereditary optic neuropathies have other neurologic and/or systemic signs. Like the isolated hereditary optic neuropathies, patients with these disorders have bilateral optic nerve dysfunction; however, the severity varies considerably and although many have central field defects with full peripheral fields, others do not. The classic example of

a hereditary optic neuropathy with other neurologic as well as systemic signs is Wolfram syndrome.

Progressive Optic Atrophy with Juvenile Diabetes Mellitus, Diabetes Insipidus, and Hearing Loss (Wolfram Syndrome, Didmoad)

The hallmark of Wolfram syndrome is the association of juvenile diabetes mellitus and progressive visual loss with optic atrophy, almost always associated with diabetes insipidus and neurosensory hearing loss; hence, the eponym "DIDMOAD," for *d*iabetes *i*nsipidus, *d*iabetes *m*ellitus, *o*ptic *a*trophy, and *d*eafness. The progression and development of this syndrome is variable. Symptoms and signs of diabetes mellitus usually occur within the first or second decade of life and usually

Figure 11.6 Appearance of the optic discs in the patient with dominant optic atrophy "plus" shown in Figure 11.5.

precede the development of optic atrophy; however, in some cases, visual loss associated with optic atrophy is the first evidence of the syndrome. In later stages, visual loss becomes severe. Visual fields show both generalized constriction and central scotomas. Optic atrophy is uniformly severe (Fig. 11.7), and there may be mild to moderate cupping of the disc.

The onsets of hearing loss and diabetes insipidus in this syndrome are, as with the onset of visual loss, quite variable. Both begin in the first or second decade of life and may be severe. Atonia of the efferent urinary tract is present in 46% to 58% of patients and is associated with recurrent urinary tract infections, sometimes with fatal complications. Other systemic and neurologic abnormalities include ataxia, axial rigidity, seizures, startle myoclonus, tremor, vestibular malfunction, central apnea, neurogenic upper airway collapse, anosmia, and gastrointestinal dysmotility. Endocrine manifestations include, but are not limited to short stature and primary gonadal atrophy.

Ophthalmologic and other neuro-ophthalmologic disturbances include ptosis, cataracts, pigmentary retinopathy, iritis, lacrimal hyposecretion, tonic pupils, ophthalmoplegia, convergence insufficiency, vertical gaze

Figure 11.7 Appearance of the optic discs in a 7-year-old child with Wolfram syndrome. The child had poor vision in both eyes as well as juvenile diabetes mellitus, diabetes insipidus, and bilateral hearing loss.

palsy, and nystagmus. Mental retardation may occur, as may psychiatric manifestations. Laboratory abnormalities include megaloblastic and sideroblastic anemia, an abnormal ERG, and elevated CSF protein. Neuroimaging studies and pathologic examinations in some patients with Wolfram syndrome reveal widespread atrophic changes and suggest a diffuse neurodegenerative disorder, with particular involvement of the midbrain and pons. Median age at death is 30 years, most commonly due to central respiratory failure with brain stem atrophy.

Many of the associated abnormalities as well as the histopathologic features of Wolfram syndrome are commonly encountered in patients with presumed mitochondrial diseases, especially those patients with the chronic progressive external ophthalmoplegia (CPEO) syndromes. This has led to speculation that patients with Wolfram syndrome have a unifying pathogenesis in underlying mitochondrial dysfunction. As noted above, inherited mitochondrial dysfunction can result from nuclear or mitochondrial DNA defects because both genomes code for proteins essential for normal mitochondrial function. Nevertheless, most cases of Wolfram syndrome have been classified as sporadic or recessively inherited, with linkage analysis in several families localizing the Wolfram gene to the short arm of chromosome 4 (4p16.1) (WFS1). A phenotypic variant of Wolfram was subsequently linked to a second locus on chromosome 4q22–24 (WFS2). The Wolfram phenotype may be nonspecific and may reflect a wide variety of underlying genetic defects in either the nuclear or mitochondrial genomes. When the syndrome is accompanied by anemia, treatment with thiamine may ameliorate the anemia and decrease the insulin requirement.

Complicated Hereditary Infantile Optic Atrophy (Behr Syndrome)

In this heredofamilial syndrome, commonly referred to as **Behr syndrome**, optic atrophy beginning in early childhood is associated with variable pyramidal tract signs, ataxia, mental retardation, urinary incontinence, and pes cavus. Both sexes are affected, although women are affected more often than men, and the syndrome is usually inherited as an autosomal-recessive trait, although cases with an autosomal-dominance pattern associated with an OPA1 mutation have been described. Visual loss usually manifests before age 10 years, is moderate to severe, and is frequently accompanied by nystagmus. In most cases, the abnormalities do not progress after childhood. Neuroimaging may demonstrate diffuse, symmetric white-matter abnormalities. In several Iraqi Jewish pedigrees of Behr syndrome, 3-methylglutaconic aciduria was identified, although the basic enzymatic defect in these families is as yet unknown. These patients have infantile optic atrophy

and an early-onset extrapyramidal movement disorder dominated by chorea. Approximately half the patients develop spastic paraparesis by the second decade. Clinical findings in some patients with Behr syndrome are similar to those in cases of hereditary ataxia; in fact, Behr syndrome may be a transitional form between simple heredofamilial optic atrophy and the hereditary ataxias. Behr syndrome is likely heterogeneous, reflecting different etiologic and genetic factors.

Optic Neuropathy in Hereditary Degenerative or Developmental Diseases

Hereditary Ataxias

The inherited ataxias represent a group of chronic progressive neurodegenerative conditions involving the cerebellum and its connections. The most common classification of the hereditary ataxias is by pattern of inheritance: autosomal dominant (most common), autosomal recessive, X-linked, and maternal (mitochondrial). Advances in biochemical and genetic analysis reveal a wide variability of clinical signs and neuropathology, even within families, and the overlap of clinical and pathologic phenotypes in disorders now known to be caused by different genetic defects makes diagnostic classification by phenotype often inaccurate. A genomic classification by chromosomal location is available for many of these disorders, and the abnormal gene products involved are under investigation. Optic atrophy is not uncommon among individuals with the hereditary ataxias.

The prototype of all forms of progressive ataxia is **Friedreich ataxia**. The onset of the disease is usually between the ages of 8 and 15 years, almost always before age 25. Characteristic clinical features include progressive ataxia of gait and clumsiness in walking and using the hands, dysarthria, loss of joint position and vibratory sensation, absent lower extremity tendon reflexes, and extensor plantar responses. Common findings include scoliosis, foot deformity, diabetes mellitus, and cardiac involvement. Other manifestations include pes cavus, distal wasting, deafness, nystagmus, eye movement abnormalities consistent with abnormal cerebellar function, and optic atrophy. The course is relentlessly progressive, with most patients unable to walk within 15 years of onset, and death from infectious or cardiac causes usually in the fourth or fifth decades. A later-onset, more slowly progressive form has been described.

Friedreich ataxia is inherited in an autosomal-recessive manner, with the gene defect being localized to the long arm of the chromosome 9 (9q13–21). The majority of cases are homozygous for an intronic, unstable, GAA trinucleotide expansion in a gene designated FRDA/X25 that codes for a protein known as frataxin, a mitochondrial protein that appears to regulate iron levels in the mitochondria. Its absence leads to mitochondrial iron overload and overproduction of reactive oxygen species and cell death.

Optic atrophy occurs in up to 50% cases of Friedreich ataxia, although severe visual loss is uncommon with visual acuity less than 20/80 being unusual. Indeed, many patients are asymptomatic, and the degree of optic disc pallor usually is mild (Fig. 11.8).

The most common of the hereditary ataxias are inherited in an autosomal-dominant pattern. The majority of these are now designated by the term **spinocerebellar ataxia** (SCA), reflecting their predominant pathology in the spinal cord and the cerebellar pathways. A wide range of clinical and pathologic findings can be seen within and among pedigrees. Although originally classified by clinical descriptions within specific families, they are now defined by the genetic loci and specific mutations in these families. Indeed, the same phenotype can be caused by a multitude of different gene defects.

As of 2014, there were at least 60 different genetic loci for the SCAs, but SCA1 (chromosome 6p), SCA2 (chromosome 12q), SCA3 (chromosome 14q and allelic with Machado–Joseph disease), SCA6 (chromosome 19p), and SCA7 (chromosome 3p) account for about 80% of the autosomal dominant ones. Many of the SCAs are caused by mutations involving the expansion of a CAG trinucleotide repeat in the protein coding sequences of specific genes, resulting in a series of glutamines. As with other diseases that involve abnor-

mal repeats, the expanded regions can become larger with each successive generation, resulting in a younger age of onset in each generation (anticipation). Anticipation occurs most often when the disease is inherited from the father.

Clinically, the SCAs are characterized by signs and symptoms attributable to cerebellar degeneration and sometimes other neurologic dysfunction secondary to loss of neurons. Loss of vision usually is mild but may be a prominent symptom, occurring in association with constricted visual fields and diffuse optic atrophy; however, it is not clear in some cases if the primary process is optic nerve in origin or is retinal with secondary optic atrophy.

Hereditary Polyneuropathies

Charcot-Marie-Tooth disease (CMTD), also called hereditary motor and sensory neuropathy actually comprises a genetically and clinically heterogeneous group of inherited disorders of the peripheral nervous system characterized by progressive loss of muscle tissue and touch sensation across various parts of the body. Currently incurable, this disease is one of the most common inherited neurological disorders, affecting about 1 in 2,500 persons. Most forms of CMTD begin between the ages of 2 and 15 years, with the first signs being pes cavus, foot deformities, or scoliosis. There is slowly progressive weakness and wasting, first of the feet and legs and then of the hands. Motor symptoms predominate over sensory abnormalities.

The most common form of CMTD is type 1, a demyelinating neuropathy with autosomal-dominant

Figure 11.8 Mild bilateral optic atrophy in a patient with Friedreich ataxia. The patient was asymptomatic, although her vision was 20/30 OU.

Figure 11.9 Severe bilateral optic atrophy in a child with Krabbe disease.

inheritance, mapped most commonly to the short arm of chromosome 17 (17p11.2) (type 1A), although a few pedigrees with this phenotype are linked to the long arm of chromosome 1 (type 1B). CMTD type 2 is clinically similar, but nerve conductions are of normal velocity, suggesting that the process is neuronal rather than demyelinating. Type 2 can be inherited in an autosomal-dominant (linked to the short arm of chromosome 1) or autosomal-recessive (linked to the long arm of chromosome 8) fashion. Type 3 is the most severe form. When type 3 is inherited in an autosomal-dominant pattern, the linkage is to the same region on chromosome 1 associated with type 1B; when it is autosomal recessive, the linkage is to the same region on chromosome 17 associated with type 1A. There also are X-linked forms of CMTD, both X-linked dominant (linked to defects on the long arm) and X-linked recessive (linked to regions on either the long arm or the short arm).

Many patients with CMTD, particularly those with CMTD type 6, have optic atrophy. Associated visual loss usually is mild, and many patients thus are asymptomatic. Nevertheless, clinical and electrophysiologic testing indicates that up to 75% of patients with CMTD have a subclinical optic neuropathy.

Hereditary Optic Atrophy Associated with Diffuse White-Matter Disease

The optic nerve is a white-matter tract of the brain. Thus, it is not surprising that hereditary disorders of white matter, such as Krabbe disease, Pelizaeus–Merzbacher disease, and adrenoleukodystrophy, involve the optic nerves (Fig. 11.9). In most of these potentially fatal disorders, visual loss is severe because of involvement of the entire visual sensory pathway; in others, however, the visual pathway is relatively spared.

Topical Diagnosis of Optic Chiasmal and Retrochiasmal Lesions

Topical Diagnosis of Optic Chiasmal Disorders
   Visual Field Defects
   Neuro-Ophthalmologic Signs and Symptoms
      Associated with the Optic Chiasmal Syndrome
**Topical Diagnosis of Retrochiasmal Visual
Pathway Disorders**
   Topical Diagnosis of Lesions of the Optic Tract
   Topical Diagnosis of Lesions of the Lateral
      Geniculate Body
   Topical Diagnosis of Lesions of the Optic Radiation
   Topical Diagnosis of Lesions of the Occipital Lobe
      and Visual Cortex

Topical Diagnosis of Optic Chiasmal Disorders

The optic chiasm is one of the most important structures in neuro-ophthalmologic diagnosis (Figs. 12.1 and 12.2). The arrangement of visual fibers in the chiasm accounts for characteristic defects in the visual fields caused by such diverse processes as compression, inflammation, demyelination, ischemia, and infiltration. In addition, damage to neurologic and vascular structures adjacent to the chiasm produces typical additional symptoms.

Visual Field Defects

Although there are many variations in the visual field defects caused by damage to the optic chiasm, the essential feature is a bilateral temporal (bitemporal) defect, the hallmark of damage to fibers that cross within the chiasm. The bitemporal defects may be superior, inferior, or complete, and they may be peripheral, central, or both and may be associated with additional defects related to associated damage to one or both optic nerves anteriorly and/or the optic tracts posteriorly.

From Damage to the Anterior Angle of the Optic Chiasm

Where the optic nerve joins the chiasm, at the anterior angle of the chiasm, its particular fiber anatomy provides an opportunity for anatomic diagnosis. The crossed and uncrossed fibers are separated at this level but are quite compact, and a small lesion affecting either the crossed or the uncrossed fibers may produce a unilateral hemianopic defect. Such a defect is called a "junctional scotoma." In such cases, it is not uncommon to find an **asymptomatic scotoma in the upper temporal field of the opposite** eye (Fig. 12.3). This scotoma results from damage to ventral fibers originating from ganglion cells located inferior and nasal to the fovea that, upon reaching the distal end of the optic nerve, have been thought to loop anteriorly about 1 to 2 mm into the contralateral optic nerve (**Wilbrand's knee**, see Chapter 2). There is now some evidence that Wilbrand's knee is not a normal anatomic structure but rather an artifact that develops when there is atrophy of the optic nerve. Although this may be true, Wilbrand's knee clearly exists from a clinical standpoint; that is, a patient with evidence of an optic neuropathy in one eye and an isolated superior temporal defect in the visual field of the opposite eye has a lesion in the region of the anterior optic chiasm.

From Damage to the Body of the Optic Chiasm

Lesions that damage the body of the optic chiasm characteristically produce a bitemporal defect that may be quadrantic or hemianopic and that may be peripheral, central, or both, with or without so-called "splitting of the macula" (Fig. 12.4). In most cases, visual acuity is normal. When the lesion compresses the chiasm from below, such as occurs with a pituitary adenoma, the field defects are typically superior; however, they often are unequal in the two eyes. In some patients, a suprasellar, infrachiasmatic lesion may elevate the chiasm and optic nerves such that the superior aspect of the nerves is compressed by the dural (falciform) folds extending from the intracranial end of the optic canals, thus producing inferior field defects. Thus, patients with bitemporal field defects that are denser below may not necessarily have a suprasellar, suprachiasmatic process. Having made this point, it certainly is true that suprasellar, suprachiasmatic compressive lesions—such as tuberculum sellae meningiomas, craniopharyngiomas, aneurysms, and dolichoectatic anterior cerebral arteries—tend to damage the superior fibers of the chiasm. The defects in the visual fields in such cases are still bitemporal, but are denser inferiorly or are entirely in the inferior fields rather

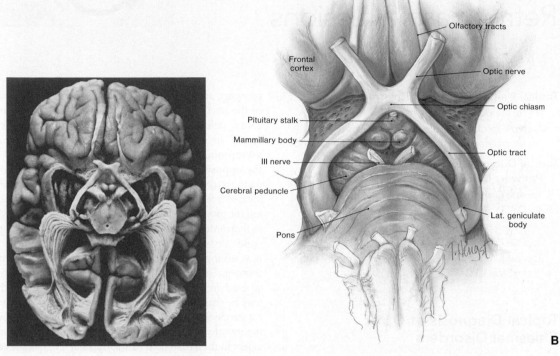

Figure 12.1 Anatomy of the chiasm and postchiasmal visual sensory system. **A:** Appearance of the visual sensory pathway in axial section, viewed from below. Note position of the optic tracts as they originate from the optic chiasm and diverge to end at the lateral geniculate nuclei. (Reprinted with permission from Ghuhbegovic N, Williams TH. *The Human Brain: A Photographic Guide.* Hagerstown, MD: Harper & Row; 1980.) **B:** Artist's drawing of the optic chiasm and optic tracts viewed from below.

Figure 12.2 Artist's drawing of the relationships of the optic nerves and optic chiasm to the sellar structures and third ventricle (III). C, anterior clinoid; D, dorsum sellae.

than the superior fields of both eyes. Papilledema, which is quite unusual in patients with suprasellar, infrachiasmal lesions, is somewhat more common in suprachiasmal lesions because such lesions can extend into and occlude the third ventricle.

Infiltrating tumors, such as gliomas, germ cell tumors, and lymphomas, as well as inflammatory and demyelinating lesions that affect the body of the optic chiasm (e.g., sarcoid, multiple sclerosis), may produce typical bitemporal field defects (Fig. 12.5). In such cases, the field defects may be denser superiorly, inferiorly, or of equal density above and below the horizontal midline.

When trauma damages the optic chiasm, the most common field defect is a complete bitemporal hemianopia. The reason is that in such cases, the chiasm may actually be transected (Fig. 12.6).

From Damage to the Posterior Angle of the Optic Chiasm

Lesions that damage the posterior aspect of the optic chiasm produce characteristic defects in the

Figure 12.3 Anterior optic chiasmal syndrome. Automated static perimetry demonstrates a temporal hemianopia in the field of the right eye. In addition, however, there is a mild but definite superior temporal defect in the field of the left eye (*arrow*).

visual fields: bitemporal hemianopic scotomas. These defects may be superior, inferior, or central in location (Figs. 12.7 to 12.9). When central, such defects may be mistaken for cecocentral scotomas and attributed to a toxic, metabolic, or even hereditary process rather than to a tumor; however, true bitemporal hemianopic scotomas almost always are associated with normal visual acuity and color perception, whereas cecocentral scotomas invariably are associated with reduced visual acuity and acquired dyschromatopsia.

Lesions that damage the posterior aspect of the optic chiasm also may damage one of the optic tracts, thus producing a homonymous field defect that is

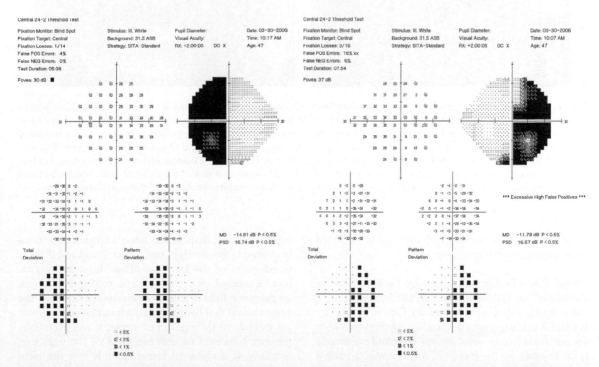

Figure 12.4 Body of the optic chiasm syndrome. Automated static perimetry demonstrates a complete bitemporal hemianopia. The patient's visual acuity was 20/20 OU.

Figure 12.5 Body of the chiasm syndrome associated with a bilateral optic neuropathy in the setting of multiple sclerosis. The patient's visual acuity was counting fingers at 3' OD and 20/100 OS, color vision was diminished in both eyes, and there was a right relative afferent pupillary defect. **A:** Kinetic perimetry at presentation shows a complete temporal hemianopia in the field of vision of the left eye and only a small nasal island in the field of vision of the right eye. **B:** Unenhanced T1-weighted coronal MRI shows an apparently normal optic chiasm. **C:** T1-weighted coronal MRI after intravenous injection of contrast material shows enhancement of the intracranial portions of the optic chiasm. The patient was treated with intravenous corticosteroids and eventually experienced complete resolution of the field defects.

combined with whatever field defect has occurred from damage to the optic chiasm.

Visual Field Defects Caused by Lesions That Damage the Optic Chiasm After Initially Damaging the Optic Nerve or Optic Tract

If there is extension of a lesion from the optic nerve or the optic tract to the optic chiasm, the blind eye usually is on the side of the lesion. If, for example, a patient with a blind right eye exhibits a defect in the temporal field of the left eye, the lesion obviously is on the

right. Similarly, if there has been a left homonymous hemianopia from a right optic tract lesion and if there is extension of the lesion to affect the optic chiasm, blindness develops in the right eye, or if not blindness, an extensive field defect. Conversely, if a lesion of the optic chiasm that has produced a bitemporal hemianopia extends to the right optic nerve, it will eventually produce blindness or near-blindness of the right eye. Similarly, if a chiasmal lesion extends into the right optic tract, there is again blindness or near-blindness of the right eye. In other words, when there is extension

Figure 12.6 Body of the chiasm syndrome after severe head trauma. **A:** Kinetic perimetry demonstrates a complete bitemporal field defect. **B:** Coronal T1-weighted MRI shows transection of the optic chiasm (*arrow*).

of a lesion from an optic nerve or optic tract to the optic chiasm, the blind (or near-blind) eye is always on the side of the original lesion, and when there is extension of a lesion from the optic chiasm to the optic nerve or to the optic tract, the blind (or near-blind) eye is always on the side of the extension of the lesion.

Neuro-Ophthalmologic Signs and Symptoms Associated with the Optic Chiasmal Syndrome

The most frequent symptoms of patients with lesions that damage the optic chiasm are progressive loss of central acuity and dimming of the visual field, particularly in its temporal portion. In addition, bitemporal field defects, whether complete or scotomatous, may produce two other types of visual symptoms. One type consists of a **disturbance of depth perception**. Patients with this symptom have difficulty with near tasks, such as threading needles, sewing, and using precision tools. In such patients, convergence results in crossing of the two blind temporal hemifields. This produces a completely blind triangular area of field with its apex at fixation (Fig. 12.10). The image of an object posterior to fixation falls on blind nasal retinas and thus disappears.

Figure 12.7 Posterior optic chiasmal syndrome in a patient with a craniopharyngioma. Kinetic perimetry demonstrates bilateral temporal paracentral scotomas. The peripheral fields are full. Such field defects result from damage to macular fibers in the posterior portion of the optic chiasm.

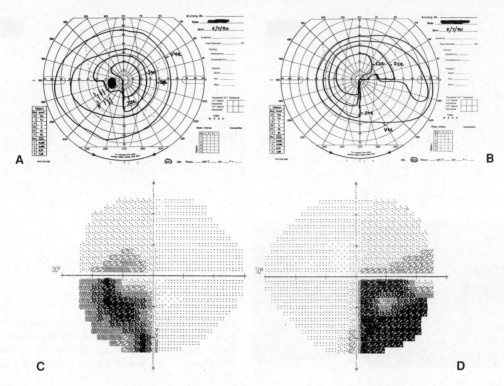

Figure 12.8 Posterior optic chiasmal syndrome. Bitemporal inferior quadrantic scotomas in a patient with a germinoma. **A and B:** Kinetic perimetry shows the scotomatous nature of the field defects. **C and D:** Automated static perimetry demonstrates the dense inferior quadrantic defects in more detail.

Figure 12.9 Posterior optic chiasmal syndrome. Subtle, primarily superior bitemporal hemianopic scotomas in a patient with a pituitary adenoma.

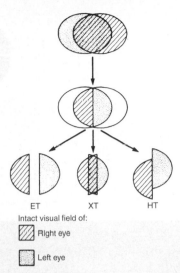

Intact visual field of:

▨ Right eye

☐ Left eye

Figure 12.11 Diagram showing the "hemifield slide phenomena" experienced by patients with bitemporal hemianopias. Patients with a pre-existing exophoria or intermittent exotropia will have overlapping of the intact nasal fields, whereas patients with a pre-existing esophoria or intermittent esotropia will have separation of the nasal hemifields, causing a blind area in the center of the field. Patients with pre-existing hyperdeviations will complain of vertical separation of images crossing the vertical meridian.

☐ Binocular field
▨ Monocular field
■ Blind field

Figure 12.10 Diagram showing the blind triangular area of the binocular visual field that occurs just beyond fixation in patients with complete bitemporal hemianopia. Such patients have intact binocular vision in the triangular area up to fixation and intact uniocular vision temporal and anterior to the triangular blind region.

Patients with bitemporal field defects also may experience diplopia or difficulty reading caused by a horizontal or vertical deviation of images unassociated with evidence of an ocular motor nerve paresis, the **hemifield slide phenomenon**. Such patients have difficulty reading because of doubling or loss of printed letters or words. The problems encountered by these patients result from loss of the normal partial overlap of the temporal field of one eye and the nasal field of the contralateral eye. This overlap normally permits fusion of images and helps stabilize ocular alignment in patients with vertical or horizontal phorias. Because their remaining visual fields represent only the temporal projection from each eye, patients with a bitemporal hemianopia do not have a physiologic linkage between the two remaining hemifields. In such patients, there is loss of fusion, and a pre-existing phoria becomes a tropia, causing diplopia or other sensory difficulties (Fig. 12.11).

Patients with chiasmal syndromes may or may not have ophthalmoscopically apparent nerve fiber layer or optic disc atrophy when first examined; however, when atrophy is present in patients with a complete bitemporal hemianopia unassociated with evidence of a unilateral or bilateral optic neuropathy, the pattern of both retinal nerve fiber layer and optic nerve

atrophy is quite specific. In such cases, degeneration occurs in fibers from peripheral and macular ganglion cells located nasal to the fovea. Axons from **peripheral ganglion cells located nasal to the disc** (and, thus, nasal to the fovea) attain the disc directly, entering its nasal aspect. Fibers from **macular ganglion cells nasal to the fovea but temporal to the disc** (i.e., about half the fibers that comprise the papillomacular bundle) also attain the optic disc directly but enter its temporal aspect. Finally, fibers from peripheral ganglion cells located nasal to the fovea but temporal to the optic disc—which make up a small portion of the superior and inferior arcuate bundles along with a larger number of fibers from peripheral temporal ganglion cells—enter the superior and inferior aspects of the disc. Thus, when there is atrophy of nasal fibers (nasal to both the fovea and disc or nasal to the fovea but temporal to the disc), the normal striations of the nerve fiber layer are lost both nasal and, to a large extent, temporal to the disc in the papillomacular region, and the optic disc shows corresponding atrophy at its nasal and temporal regions with relative sparing of the superior and inferior portions where the majority of spared temporal fibers (subserving nasal field) enter (Fig. 12.12). The optic atrophy occupies a more or less horizontal band across the disc, wider nasally than temporally, so-called "band" or "bow-tie" atrophy.

Figure 12.12 Appearance of the ocular fundus in a patient with a long-standing body of the chiasm syndrome. **A:** Automated static perimetry demonstrates a complete bitemporal hemianopia. **B:** Both optic discs show "band" atrophy with corresponding loss of nerve fibers from ganglion cells located nasal to the fovea. **C:** Artist's drawing of the pattern of optic nerve and retinal nerve fiber layer atrophy in patients with a long-standing complete bitemporal hemianopia.

It is perhaps clinically more useful when atrophy is **absent** in patients with chiasmal (or optic nerve) compression than when it is present. Although patients with significant retinal nerve fiber bundle defects and optic atrophy can have impressive return of both acuity and field when successful decompression is obtained, patients with normal-appearing fundi should have near complete or complete return of visual function. Thus, it is crucial that decompression be carried out as soon as possible in these patients.

Although the presence or absence of optic disc pallor is predictive of visual recovery in patients with chiasmal compression, the thickness of the peripapillary retinal nerve fiber layer (PRNFL) as assessed by optical coherence tomography (OCT) is even more so. The normal average thickness of the PRNFL is about 100 μm. Patients with absolute optic atrophy (i.e., no light perception), whether glaucomatous or nonglaucomatous, have a PRNFL average thickness of 35 to 40 μm. Thus, there is a range of about 65 μm between normal and complete loss. It has been shown that patients with less than 50% reduction in the average thickness of the PRNFL; that is, ≥75 μm, have a high likelihood of regaining both acuity and field after successful decompression. Again, however, patients with more than a 50% reduction in average PRNFL thickness can still experience visual improvement following successful decompression.

Most patients with lesions that affect the optic chiasm have no disturbances of ocular alignment or motility except for the hemifield slide phenomenon (see above); however, some lesions in the parasellar/suprasellar region can damage the ocular motor nerves, causing double vision in addition to visual loss. When the ocular motor nerves are damaged within the cavernous sinus, there also may be pain, evidence of a trigeminal sensory neuropathy, or both, in the territory of the first and/or second divisions of the trigeminal nerve. The third division of the nerve, which does not pass through the cavernous sinus, is not affected by such lesions, and a motor neuropathy thus is never present unless the lesion extends posteriorly. The oculosympathetic fibers also may be damaged by a lesion in the suprasellar or parasellar region, resulting in a postganglionic Horner syndrome characterized by ipsilateral ptosis and a small reactive pupil (see Chapter 15). Horner syndrome often is associated with an ipsilateral abducens nerve palsy because the postganglionic oculosympathetic fibers briefly join the abducens nerve within the cavernous sinus. When both the oculomotor nerve and oculosympathetic fibers are affected, the clinical picture is one of an oculomotor nerve paresis with a small pupil that is normally reactive if the paresis is pupil-sparing or poorly or nonreactive if the paresis involves the pupillomotor fibers. Single or multiple ocular motor nerve pareses

in a patient with a bitemporal field defect suggests a process extrinsic to the chiasm rather than an infiltrative intrinsic lesion.

The unusual phenomenon of **seesaw nystagmus** may occur in patients with tumors of the diencephalon and chiasmal regions (**Video 12.1**). This condition is characterized by synchronous alternating elevation and intorsion of one eye and depression and extorsion of the opposite eye. The cause of seesaw nystagmus is unknown, but it may be related to damage to the interstitial nucleus of Cajal or adjacent structures by the tumor.

Lesions causing a chiasmal syndrome may arise from or extend to the hypothalamus. Patients with this presentation may develop diabetes insipidus and hypothalamic hypopituitarism. Such patients may have excessive fluid intake that may not be obvious unless they are specifically asked how many glasses of water, etc. they drink a day. In addition, prepubertal children may suffer from both growth retardation and delayed sexual development, and young children and infants may have severe failure to thrive (Russell syndrome) and present with severe emaciation.

Topical Diagnosis of Retrochiasmal Visual Pathway Disorders

Unilateral lesions of the visual sensory pathway beyond the optic chiasm—the optic tract, lateral geniculate body (LGB), optic radiation, or striate cortex (see Fig. 12.13A)—produce homonymous visual field defects without loss of visual acuity. When such defects are complete, they do not allow topical diagnosis. In such instances, the clinician must rely on other ocular findings, other symptoms and signs of neurologic disease (or their absence!), and/or on neuroimaging to determine the area and extent of damage as well as the etiology of the lesion.

Homonymous defects in the visual fields characteristically develop slowly when they are caused by compression and rapidly when they are caused by hemorrhage, ischemia, or inflammation. Regardless of the cause, however, such defects include complete homonymous quadrantanopias and hemianopias, incomplete homonymous quadrantanopias and hemianopias with varying degrees of congruity, and homonymous paracentral scotomas.

Almost 90% of patients with isolated homonymous hemianopia have occipital lobe lesions, usually caused by vascular disease in the territory of the posterior cerebral arteries, whereas patients with lesions of the postchiasmal visual pathway anterior to the occipital cortex may or may not have neurologic symptoms and/or signs (see below). In some cases, a relative afferent pupillary defect (RAPD) on the side

Figure 12.13 A 65-year-old man developed headache, sleepiness, personality changes, memory difficulties, right hemiparesis, and difficulty seeing to the right. **A:** Visual fields reveal an incongruous right homonymous hemianopia. **B and C:** CT scans, axial views, before (**B**) and after (**C**) the administration of intravenous contrast reveal an enhancing lesion with surrounding edema in the region of the left optic tract, diagnosed ultimately as lymphoma.

of the hemianopia in the absence of evidence of an optic neuropathy or other cause for the defect helps localize the location of the lesion to the contralateral optic tract, whereas asymmetric responses to optokinetic (OKN) stimulation with the poorer responses observed when targets are moved toward the side opposite the hemianopia (i.e., toward the side of the lesion) generally indicate a lesion of the optic radiations in the parietal lobe (see below). In all cases, however, neuroimaging, preferably MRI, should be used to verify or determine the location and etiology of a homonymous hemianopia.

Topical Diagnosis of Optic Tract Lesions

Although lesions affecting the optic tracts are infrequent, they are of great importance because they are located in the first region beyond the optic chiasm where lesions produce a homonymous visual field defect (Fig. 12.13). The causes are varied and include tumors, vascular processes, demyelinating disease, and trauma (Figs. 12.14 and 12.15).

As noted above, patients with optic tract lesions often have a specific finding that permits the determination of the location of the lesion on clinical grounds

Figure 12.14 A 40-year-old man noted a "black spot" in front of both eyes that gradually worsened over 2 weeks. Visual acuities were normal, but there was a trace right relative afferent pupillary defect. **A:** Visual fields show a highly incongruous right homonymous defect. **B and C:** T2-weighted (**B**) and fluid-attenuated inversion recovery (**C**) MRI sequences reveal multiple white-matter lesions consistent with demyelinating disease, including a large plaque in the left optic tract (*arrows*).

A

Figure 12.15 A 7-year-old girl presented with precocious puberty and was found to have a suprasellar mass with hydrocephalus. **A:** Coronal, T1-weighted MRI without gadolinium. **B:** Axial, T1-weighted MRI without gadolinium. **C:** Axial, T1-weighted MRI with gadolinium. **D:** Visual field testing reveals an incomplete, incongruous, right homonymous inferior quadrantanopia, consistent with damage to the left optic tract. Biopsy showed findings diagnostic of craniopharyngioma.

B

C

D

alone. All patients with a complete or near-complete homonymous hemianopia caused by an isolated optic tract lesion (i.e., no evidence of an associated optic neuropathy) have an RAPD in the eye contralateral to the side of the lesion (i.e., the eye on the side of the hemianopia and that has a temporal field defect). This occurs because (1) the temporal visual field is considerably larger than the nasal field. Therefore, there are more crossing nasal fibers than noncrossing temporal fibers; (2) the pupillomotor fibers within the visual sensory pathway hemidecussate in the optic chiasm along with or as part of the visual axons; and (3) the pupillomotor fibers are present within the optic tract for most of its extent. Because the temporal visual field is 60% to 70% larger than the nasal field, there is a disparity with respect to light input from the two eyes to the mesencephalic pupillary center. A complete lesion of one optic tract thus preferentially reduces input from the contralateral eye, and the result is an RAPD unassociated with any evidence of an optic neuropathy or retinopathy.

Another pupillary phenomenon that sometimes can be elicited in patients with lesions of the optic tract that produce a complete or nearly complete homonymous hemianopia is pupillary hemiakinesia (aka hemianopic pupillary reaction or Wernicke pupil). Because the pupillary afferents are present in this section of the visual system, light that is projected onto the "blind" retinal elements (subserving the nasal visual field in the ipsilateral eye and the temporal visual field in the contralateral eye), results in either no pupillary reaction or a markedly reduced reaction. However, when light is projected onto the intact retinal elements (subserving the temporal visual field in the ipsilateral eye and the nasal visual field in the contralateral eye), a normal pupillary reaction is observed. This phenomenon is best observed with a bright, very focused beam of light, such as that from a slit lamp biomicroscope.

Optic tract lesions do not cause loss of visual acuity nor do they affect color vision unless they also damage the optic chiasm or the intracranial portions of one or both optic nerves. Thus, patients with lesions confined to an optic tract that produce a complete or near-complete homonymous hemianopia have normal visual acuity and color vision, and they have no sensation of reduced light brightness in the eye despite an RAPD. On the other hand, when lesions of the optic tract also damage the ipsilateral optic nerve or chiasm, reduced visual acuity, dyschromatopsia, and an RAPD are present on the side of the lesion.

Patients with a complete or nearly complete homonymous hemianopia from an optic tract lesion eventually develop a characteristic pattern of optic atrophy. There is a "band" of horizontal pallor of the optic disc in the eye contralateral to the lesion (with

temporal field loss) (i.e., bow-tie atrophy; see above). This pattern of optic nerve atrophy is caused by atrophy of retinal nerve fibers originating from ganglion cells nasal to the fovea and is identical with that seen in both eyes of patients with complete bitemporal field loss from chiasmal syndromes. At the same time, however, there is generalized pallor of the optic disc in the eye on the side of the lesion, associated with significant loss of nerve fiber layer details in the superior and inferior arcuate regions that comprise the majority of fibers subserving the nasal visual field and originating from ganglion cells temporal to the fovea (Fig. 12.16).

Not all patients with optic tract lesions have a complete homonymous hemianopia. Many patients have a complete or incomplete homonymous quadrantanopia or an incomplete hemianopia. Such field defects usually are quite incongruous and also may be scotomatous (Fig. 12.14). Indeed, the optic tract is one of only two locations in the postchiasmal pathway in which homonymous scotomas routinely occur; the occipital lobe is the other (see below).

Patients with optic tract lesions often have neurologic manifestations in addition to homonymous visual field defects because lesions that damage the optic tract also may damage adjacent neural structures. Neurologic deficits that may occur in patients with lesions of the optic tract include hypothalamic symptoms and signs and a contralateral hemiparesis or hemiplegia.

Topical Diagnosis of Lesions of the Lateral Geniculate Body

Lesions affecting the LGB are much less common than those that affect other parts of the afferent visual sensory pathway but can be caused by a number of different processes, including vascular disease, neoplasms, inflammation, demyelination, and trauma.

Lesions of the LGB may cause incongruous or congruous homonymous field defects that are unlike any others caused by lesions of other parts of the postchiasmal visual sensory pathway. The specific pattern relates to the unique anatomy and the blood supply of the LGB. The dorsal region of the LGB subserves macular function, the lateral aspect of the LGB subserves the superior visual field, and the medial aspect subserves the inferior field (Fig. 12.17). Although the intricate retinotopic organization of the LGB may result in the production of relative defects, incongruous defects, and even (theoretically) monocular defects, vascular lesions are more likely to respect specific anatomic boundaries within the LGB and produce homonymous sector defects that are, in fact, quite congruous, with abruptly sloping borders. Two specific patterns of relatively congruous

Figure 12.16 Hemianopic optic atrophy in a patient with a left homonymous hemianopia from a right optic tract lesion. **A:** The right optic disc **(left)** has somewhat diffuse, temporal atrophy from loss of nerve fibers from ganglion cells temporal to the fovea. The left optic disc **(right)** shows band atrophy from loss of nerve fibers from ganglion cells nasal to the fovea. **B:** Red-free (540 nm) photographs showing the pattern of atrophy of the right and left optic discs. Note band pattern of atrophy of the left disc **(right)**. **C:** Inferior temporal peripapillary retina of right eye **(left)** shows relative absence of the arcuate nerve fibers, whereas there is relative preservation of the inferior arcuate fiber bundle in the left eye **(right)**. Similar findings were present in the superior temporal peripapillary retinas of the right and left eyes.

Figure 12.17 Anatomy and visual field representation in the lateral geniculate body (LGB). **A:** Artist's drawing shows that the superior and inferior areas of the visual field are represented in the lateral and medial regions of the LGB, respectively, whereas the central field is represented in the center of the LGB. **B:** Artist's drawing of the blood supply of the LGB shows that the medial and lateral regions of the LGB (representing the superior and inferior areas of the visual field) are supplied by the distal anterior choroidal artery (ACA), whereas the center of the LGB (representing the central field) is supplied by the lateral choroidal artery (LCA).

homonymous field defects can occur, most often attributable to focal disease of the LGB caused by infarction in the territory of two specific arteries. Ischemia or other damage in the territory of the lateral choroidal artery typically causes a **congruous homonymous horizontal sectoranopia** (Figs. 12.18 and 12.19). Ischemia in the region of the LGB supplied by the distal portion of the anterior choroidal artery results in loss of the upper and lower homonymous sectors in the visual fields of the two eyes, producing a **congruous homonymous quadruple sectoranopia** (Figs. 12.20 and 12.21).

Because the pupillomotor fibers leave the optic tract to ascend in the brachium of the superior colliculus, the pupillary reactions in patients with LGB lesions are normal (unless the lesion also damages the optic tract or the brachium)—there is neither a contralateral RAPD nor a hemianopic pupillary phenomenon; however, the visual axons from retinal ganglion cells first synapse in the LGB. Thus, sectoral or hemianopic atrophy of the retinal nerve fiber layer and optic disc occurs in patients with lesions of the LGB

that damage the incoming axons. Such defects, when associated with acquired homonymous field defects, whether congruous or incongruous, must be taken as evidence of optic tract or LGB damage in all cases.

Patients with lesions of the LGB frequently have neurologic symptoms and signs consistent with damage to the ipsilateral thalamus or pyramidal tract. Thalamic damage may result in gross impairment of sensation on the side of the body opposite the lesion, or there may be a complaint of pain of central origin that is referred to the opposite side of the body. Damage to the pyramidal tract causes contralateral hemibody weakness.

Topical Diagnosis of Lesions of the Optic Radiation

The optic radiation is that part of the postchiasmal visual sensory pathway that begins in the LGB and transmits visual information to the striate cortex. It may be damaged by lesions in several different locations, including the internal capsule, temporal lobe, and parietal lobe.

Figure 12.18 Left homonymous quadruple sectoranopia from damage to the right lateral geniculate body in the territory of the distal anterior choroidal artery. **A:** Kinetic perimetry shows left-sided superior and inferior defects with sparing of the central field in both eyes. **B:** Automated static perimetry shows the field defects in more detail.

Lesions of the Internal Capsule

Efferent projection fibers from and afferent projection fibers to the cerebral cortex traverse the subcortical white matter where they form a radiating mass of fibers, the corona radiata, that converges toward the brainstem (Fig. 12.22). In the rostral brainstem, the fibers form the **internal capsule**, a broad but compact fiber band that is bordered medially by the thalamus and caudate nucleus and laterally by the lenticular nucleus. The afferent fibers comprise the thalamocortical radiations in the posterior limb of the internal capsule. The efferent bundles include the corticospinal and corticobulbar tracts in the anterior limb, the frontopontine tract from the prefrontal and precentral regions of the cerebral cortex in the anterior limb, the temporoparietopontine tract from the temporal and parietal lobes in the posterior limb, and the optic radiation, which begins in the LGB and occupies only a small region of the capsule because it does not proceed to the brainstem. The internal capsule thus is composed of all fibers, afferent and efferent, that go to, or come from, the cerebral cortex. The most posterior component of the internal capsule is the optic radiation.

Interruption of the optic radiation within the internal capsule is characterized by a contralateral, usually complete, homonymous hemianopia that typically is associated with contralateral hemianesthesia from damage to adjacent thalamocortical fibers in the posterior limb of the internal capsule. Other ocular

Figure 12.19 MRI in the patient whose visual fields are shown in Figure 12.18. There is a hyperintense and enhancing lesion affecting the right lateral geniculate body (*arrow*). The findings are consistent with a cavernous angioma that has bled.

Figure 12.21 MRI in the patient whose visual fields are shown in Figure 12.20 demonstrates a well-circumscribed lesion involving the left lateral geniculate body (*arrow*).

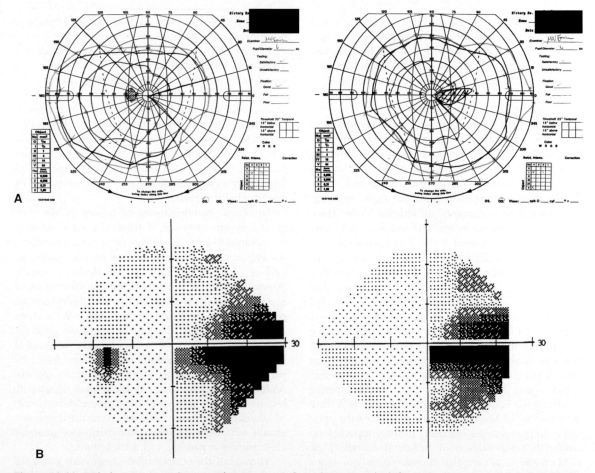

Figure 12.20 Right homonymous horizontal sectoranopia from damage to the left LGB in the territory of the lateral choroidal artery. **A:** Kinetic perimetry shows right-sided wedge-shaped loss of the central field in both eyes. **B:** Automated static perimetry shows the wedge-shaped field defects in more detail.

Figure 12.22 Specimen showing the corona radiata and internal capsule, and their relationship to the optic tract. The internal capsule and corona radiata have been exposed by removal of the corpus callosum, caudate nucleus, and diencephalon. Note that the fibers of the basis pedunculi pass adjacent to the optic tract. CR, corona radiata; IC, internal capsule; BP, basis pedunculi; OT, optic tract. (Reprinted with permission from Ghuhbegovic N, Williams TH. The Human Brain. *A Photographic Guide.* Hagerstown, MD: Harper & Row; 1980.)

findings in lesions of the internal capsule include a transient deviation of the eyes to the side of the lesion in many instances and weakness of the frontalis and orbicularis oculi on the contralateral hemiplegic side in a minority of cases. Vascular causes predominate.

Lesions of the Temporal Lobe

Temporal lobe lesions, most often tumors and abscesses, may damage the optic radiation. In addition, various surgical procedures, such as those to treat temporal lobe seizures, may result in homonymous field defects that often are asymptomatic.

The most anterior aspect of the optic radiation does not extend to the tip of the temporal lobe. Thus, the most anterior portion of the temporal lobe may be damaged or removed without the production of any visual field defect; however, the amount of temporal lobe that may be removed without a resulting field defect is extremely variable. It would appear that about 3 cm of anterior temporal lobe can be removed in most patients without interruption of visual fibers to the extent that a field defect is produced. Once the lobe is sectioned 3 cm or more posterior to the tip, however, most patients will develop a homonymous field defect. In most cases, the homonymous defect is incomplete and either is confined to the superior quadrants or is denser above (Fig. 12.23), reflecting the anatomy of Meyer loop—the portion of the optic radiation that courses anteriorly in the temporal lobe around the temporal horn of the lateral ventricle (Figs. 12.1Left and 12.24) and that consists entirely of axons subserving the superior visual fields of the two eyes (Fig. 12.24). With lesions located or temporal lobecto-

mies beyond 8 cm, almost all patients have a complete homonymous hemianopia.

Patients with temporal lobe lesions that produce a homonymous visual field defect also may experience visual hallucinations. The hallucinations are typically of the formed type and consist of both animate (e.g., people, animals) and inanimate (e.g., flowers, trees, buildings) objects. They are often seen in color and are always in the affected homonymous hemifield on the side contralateral to the lesion. Visual hallucinations caused by temporal lobe lesions may be pleasurable or frightening to the patient and may be accompanied by auditory hallucinations.

Nonvisual manifestations of lesions of the temporal lobe are common. If there is a mass lesion of the temporal lobe, headache may be a prominent accompaniment. Bilateral lesions of the transverse gyri of Heschl can cause cortical deafness, usually associated with aphasia; unilateral lesions may cause a disturbance of hearing and sound discrimination contralateral to the lesion. If the lesion is in the dominant temporal lobe, the patient may have difficulty memorizing a series of spoken words, whereas if the lesion is in the nondominant temporal lobe, the patient may exhibit various forms of auditory agnosia. Auditory hallucinations or illusions may occur with lesions of either temporal lobe. Severe disturbances of language can result from lesions in the dominant, usually left, temporal lobe. Disturbances of memory are common in patients with such lesions.

Tumors of the temporal lobe frequently cause seizures. These seizures typically are characterized by transient changes in emotions, mood, and behavior

Figure 12.23 Visual field defect in two patients with temporal lobe lesions. **A:** In a patient with a cystic astrocytoma occupying much of the left temporal lobe. **Left and Center:** Automated static perimetry demonstrates a right incomplete, somewhat incongruous homonymous hemianopia, denser above. **Right:** MRI shows the large cystic lesion. **B:** In a patient who suffered penetrating trauma to the left temporal lobe *(asterisk)*. **Left and Center:** Automated static perimetry demonstrates a right incomplete incongruous homonymous hemianopia, denser above. Note that the gray scale suggests that the field defect is a homonymous quadrantanopia but the pattern deviation shows that the defect in the field of the left eye extends well below the horizontal midline. **Right:** MRI shows the tract of the penetrating instrument *(asterisk)*. Note that the lesion is not quite 3 cm posterior to the temporal lobe tip.

and are associated with motor automatisms—so-called complex partial seizures or psychomotor epilepsy. If the lesion is situated anteriorly and affects the uncinate gyrus, either directly or through pressure, so-called "uncinate fits" occur that are characterized by an aura of unusual taste or smell, followed by abnormal motor activity of the mouth and lips, during which the patient is not in contact with his or her surroundings.

Lesions of the Parietal Lobe

Lesions in the parietal lobe may produce ocular symptoms that have value in topical diagnosis. Homonymous hemianopias affecting primarily the lower fields

are caused by damage to the optic radiation in the superior parietal lobe (Fig. 12.25). Such defects usually are more congruous than those produced by lesions of the temporal lobe. Because the entire optic radiation passes through the parietal lobe, large lesions may produce a complete homonymous hemianopia.

Neuro-ophthalmologic features suggesting a lesion in the parietal lobe include an incomplete and relatively congruous (or mildly incongruous) homonymous hemianopia that is denser below than above, conjugate movements of the eyes to the side opposite the lesion on forced lid closure (Cogan sign), and an abnormal OKN response when the target is moved toward the side of the lesion.

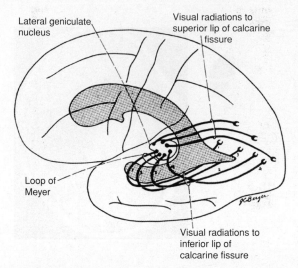

Lateral geniculate nucleus

Visual radiations to superior lip of calcarine fissure

Loop of Meyer

Visual radiations to inferior lip of calcarine fissure

Figure 12.24 Artist's drawing shows the pathway of the optic radiation. Note that the inferior fibers subserving the superior visual field sweep forward and pass around the temporal horn of the lateral ventricle whereas the superior fibers proceed directly back to the occipital cortex.

The abnormal response results from damage to the fiber pathway responsible for ipsilateral pursuit in the parietal lobe. When these fibers are damaged, patients have poor pursuit toward the side of the lesion. This deficit can be brought out by rotation of an OKN drum or horizontal movement of an OKN stripe in one direction and then in the other, necessitating repetitive rapid pursuit movements in the direction of drum/stripe movement followed by refixation saccades in the opposite direction (**Video 12.2**).

A disturbance of fixation reflexes sufficient to interfere with reading ability may develop before the appearance of other symptoms. This disturbance is sometimes manifest during visual field testing, during which the patient cannot maintain central fixation despite repeated instructions to do so, an apparent understanding of the instructions, and an apparent willingness to comply. Other types of visual disturbances caused by lesions in the parietal lobe include visual neglect, visual agnosia, and difficulties with word recognition.

Patients with parietal lobe lesions and homonymous visual field defects often are unaware of their visual deficits. This phenomenon is more likely to occur when the underlying abnormality is in the nondominant cerebral hemisphere (usually the right parietal lobe), but it also can occur in patients with dominant parietal lobe lesions. In other patients, the primary visual pathways may be unaffected or minimally affected, but the patient neglects the contralateral visual field.

The parietal lobe is the principal sensory area of the cerebral cortex, and its postcentral convolution

is of particular importance. The patient may complain of numbness but more commonly has complex problems of sensory integration that can be demonstrated using tests of tactile discrimination, position sense, stereognosis, and visual-spatial coordination. Irritative lesions of the postcentral convolution cause sensory Jacksonian seizures that begin contralateral to the lesion at the part of the body that corresponds to the focus of excitation. Tingling or numbness spreads to other adjacent parts of the body according to the order of their representation in the cortex. Lesions in the dominant parietal lobe can cause aphasia (usually fluent), apraxia, agnosia, acalculia, and agraphia. A lesion in the dominant parietal lobe involving the angular gyrus may produce the Gerstmann syndrome (finger agnosia, right–left disorientation, agraphia, and acalculia) associated with a right homonymous hemianopia. Lesions in the nondominant parietal lobe may cause impaired constructional ability, dyscalculia, and, most commonly, inattention or neglect. Indeed, left spatial neglect after a right hemisphere lesion may accentuate the left hemianopia, hemianesthesia, and hemiplegia, and thus contribute to poor recovery.

Topical Diagnosis of Lesions of the Occipital Lobe and Visual Cortex

Most lesions affecting the occipital lobe are vascular or traumatic in origin, with tumors, abscesses, demyelinating, and toxic disorders of white matter occurring much less frequently. Lesions of the central and posterior occipital lobe cause field defects that are homonymous and congruous, whereas lesions of the anterior occipital lobe may cause contralateral monocular defects (see below).

Unilateral Lesions of the Central and Posterior Occipital Lobe

Field defects seen with lesions of the central and posterior occipital lobe are always homonymous and almost always extremely congruous (Fig. 12.26). The phenomenon of sparing of the macula is often seen in such cases (see below). Lesions of the tip of the occipital lobe (the occipital pole) produce defects that tend to be scotomatous; however, unlike the homonymous scotomas that occur in some patients with optic tract lesions (see above), the homonymous scotomas produced by occipital tip lesions are exquisitely congruous (Figs. 12.26 and 12.27)

Unilateral Lesions of the Anterior Occipital Lobe

Because the temporal field of each eye is larger than the nasal field, the fibers subserving that portion of the peripheral temporal field that has no nasal correlate must be unpaired throughout the postchiasmal

Figure 12.25 Visual field defects in two patients with lesions of the parietal lobe. **A:** In a patient with a glioblastoma of the left parietal lobe. **Left and Center:** Automated static perimetry demonstrates a right incomplete incongruous homonymous hemianopia, denser below. **Right:** MRI shows a large lesion in the left parietal lobe surrounded by peritumoral edema. The scan also shows moderate hydrocephalus with subependymal edema. **B:** In a patient with a glioblastoma multiforme in the right parietal lobe. **Left and Center:** Automated static perimetry demonstrates a left incomplete incongruous homonymous hemianopia, denser below. **Right:** MRI shows the lesion, which is associated with peritumoral edema.

portion of the visual sensory pathway. Damage to these unpaired peripheral fibers produces a monocular defect in the extreme temporal visual field. This field defect is crescentic in shape, and its widest extent is in the horizontal meridian, where it extends from 60 degrees out to approximately 90 degrees. Because of the peculiar shape of the defect, patients with the defect are said to have the **temporal crescent (or half-moon) syndrome** (Fig. 12.28). Although lesions in any part of the chiasmal or postchiasmal visual pathway theoretically could produce a temporal crescent defect, for practical purposes such a defect occurs only with lesions of the most anterior portion of the striate cortex, whereas lesions of the posterior striate cortex

may actually spare all or part of the temporal crescent (Fig. 12.29).

Two important, if basic, facts should be kept in mind when considering the temporal crescent syndrome. First, monocular peripheral temporal visual field defects are caused most often by retinal lesions, not by intracranial ones. Thus, the nasal retinal periphery should be carefully examined ophthalmoscopically in patients with a presumed temporal crescent syndrome. Second, because these defects begin approximately 60 degrees from fixation, central field testing (i.e., that performed using most automated static perimetry programs) will not detect such defects (see Chapter 1).

Figure 12.26 Visual field defects in two patients with occipital lobe lesions. **A:** In a patient with an acute infarct in the right occipital lobe. **Left and Center:** Automated static perimetry demonstrates a left congruous inferior homonymous quadrantanopia. **Right:** MRI shows a lesion of the right occipital lobe associated with edema but no mass effect. **B:** In a patient with a small infarct in the left occipital lobe. **Left and Center:** Automated static perimetry demonstrates small left congruous inferior homonymous scotomas. **Right:** MRI shows location of the lesion (*arrow*).

Macular Sparing

In an otherwise complete or near-complete homonymous hemianopia, when a portion of the affected central field of each eye is preserved, there is said to be "macular sparing." In such cases, the zone of preserved visual field ranges from a few degrees to almost 10 degrees in extent (Fig. 12.30). Macular sparing is seen most often in patients with lesions of the striate cortex; however, it may occur with lesions in any part of the postgeniculate pathway.

The etiology of macular sparing as it applies to lesions of the striate cortex is controversial. Three theories have been proposed to explain the phenomenon: (1) an artifact of testing, (2) bilateral representation of the macula, and (3) incomplete damage to the visual sensory pathway.

There is no doubt that some cases of apparent macular sparing are caused by inaccurate fixation. It is impossible for even otherwise normal persons to obtain perfect fixation, and physiologic movements of the fixing eye, so slight that they cannot be detected by ordinary means, probably account for at least 1 to 2 degrees of deviation of the vertical meridian about the central area.

Histochemical studies demonstrate that, to some extent, a small portion of each macula probably has representation in each occipital lobe. There is a small area of nasotemporal overlap on either side of the vertical meridian in which some axons from ganglion cells temporal to the fovea cross within the chiasm, whereas some axons from ganglion cells nasal to the fovea remain uncrossed. However, the mere presence

Figure 12.27 Exquisitely congruous right homonymous scotomas in a patient with a small infarct at the tip of the left occipital pole.

of an overlap does not necessarily have any clinical visual consequences.

In fact, most clinically obvious cases of homonymous hemianopia with macular sparing occur in the setting of incomplete damage to the visual sensory pathway, usually the occipital lobe, and are related to a residual intact area of the pathway. The unique dual blood supply of the occipital cortex from the posterior cerebral and middle cerebral arteries provides a mechanism for this partial damage. Thus, in patients with homonymous hemianopia and substantial macular sparing, not only is the location of the lesion almost always the occipital lobe, but the pathogenesis almost always is posterior cerebral artery territory infarction.

Bilateral Occipital Lobe Lesions

Bilateral lesions of the occipital lobes may occur simultaneously or consecutively. In addition, because such lesions are neurologically asymptomatic except as regards the visual system, patients with unilateral lesions that cause an homonymous field defect may not be aware of the defect until it is called to their attention (e.g., during a routine ocular examination or after the patient is involved in a motor vehicle accident) or until they experience a similar event on the opposite side, producing a more extensive visual deficit.

A double homonymous hemianopia may occur from a single event. In a majority of these cases, there is complete visual loss at the onset (i.e., cortical blindness)

Figure 12.28 Loss of the temporal crescent in a patient with an infarct in the right anterior occipital lobe. Kinetic perimetry demonstrates a full peripheral field in the right eye **(right)**, but there is loss of the far temporal field (the temporal crescent) in the left eye **(left)**.

Figure 12.29 Sparing of the temporal crescent in a patient with an infarct in the left occipital lobe. **A:** Automated static perimetry demonstrates a left congruous homonymous inferior quadrantanopia. Note that there is no indication that the defect in the left eye is scotomatous because the perimeter is only testing the temporal field out to 24 degrees. **B:** Kinetic perimetry demonstrates a right inferior homonymous quadrantic defect that spares almost all of the far peripheral field of the left eye (the temporal crescent).

that usually is transient, lasting minutes to days, followed by some degree of clearing in one or both homonymous hemifields. Affected patients have similarly shaped visual field defects on corresponding sides of the vertical midline for each eye, equal, usually normal visual acuity for each eye, normal pupils and fundi, and full ocular motility unless there is a coexisting brainstem lesion. The majority of these patients have vascular causes of their visual loss.

Much more commonly, bilateral homonymous hemianopia occurs from consecutive events, invariably vascular in nature. In such cases, the patient experiences an often asymptomatic acute incomplete homonymous field defect or a complete homonymous hemianopia with retention of normal vision with or without sparing of the macula. At a later time, varying from weeks to years, the patient develops a sudden homonymous hemianopia on the opposite side, again with or without macular sparing. After this second event, the patient may be blind or severely visually impaired.

Whether simultaneous or sequential, bilateral occipital lobe disease—whether from infarction, compression, inflammation, infection, or trauma—may result in a variety of bilateral homonymous visual field defects. First, there may be complete blindness.

Figure 12.30 Macular sparing. A 28-year-old woman suffered a persistent visual field defect after an unusually severe migraine attack. **A:** Full-threshold 60-degree visual fields using a Humphrey Field Analyzer show that the central 15 degrees of the left hemifield are intact. In the **inset,** the visual fields mapped at the tangent screen show that the field defect bisects the blind spot representation of the left eye. **B:** T1-weighted parasagittal MRI through the right occipital lobe shows an arteriovenous malformation involving the anterior portion of the right calcarine cortex. The posterior margin of the lesion is situated 31 mm from the occipital tip, marking the approximate location of the representation of the left eye's blind spot. The calcarine (*curved arrow*) and parieto-occipital (*straight arrow*) sulci are indicated. (Reprinted with permission from Horton JC, Hoyt WF. The representation of the visual field in human striate cortex. *Arch Ophthalmol.* 1991;109:816–824.)

Second, there may be a complete hemianopia on one side and an incomplete, congruous hemianopia on the other (Fig. 12.31). Third, there may be a homonymous hemianopia on one side and a quadrantanopia on the other (Fig. 12.32). Fourth, there may be a bilateral homonymous hemianopia with bilateral macular sparing (Fig. 12.33). In this setting, there is a markedly constricted visual field associated with normal or near-normal visual acuity and the patient may be thought to have bilateral optic nerve or retinal disease

or may even be thought to have nonorganic visual field loss because the pupils react relatively normally to light stimulation. Fifth, there may be bilateral homonymous scotomas with or without macular sparing (Fig. 12.34). Finally, a "crossed-quadrant" homonymous defect results when patients develop bilateral quadrantic defects that affect the superior occipital lobe above the calcarine fissure on one side and the inferior occipital lobe below the fissure on the other side. Such defects are sometimes called "checkerboard" fields and occur

Figure 12.31 Visual fields in a patient who experience bilateral simultaneous infarcts in the occipital lobes, left more extensive than right. Kinetic perimetry demonstrates a complete right homonymous hemianopia and an incomplete, congruous right homonymous hemianopia.

Figure 12.32 Visual fields in a 75-year-old woman with hypertension and poorly controlled diabetes mellitus type 1 who had no previous ocular complaints until she experienced sudden loss of vision to the right side. A: Automated static perimetry demonstrates a complete right homonymous hemianopia and an incomplete congruous left superior homonymous quadrantanopia. B: MRI reveals bilateral occipital lobe infarcts, acute on the left and old (and inferior to the calcarine fissure) on the right.

Figure 12.33 Visual fields in a 67-year-old man who suffered extensive trauma to both occipital poles and subsequently complained of "tunnel vision." He had 20/20 visual acuity OU, normal pupillary reactions to light stimulation, and normal-appearing ocular fundi. He initially was thought to have nonorganic visual loss. **A:** Kinetic perimetry demonstrates marked constriction of the fields of both eyes that, in fact, is due to bilateral homonymous hemianopias with macular sparing. Note the symmetry of the spared field on the right and left sides. **B:** Amsler grid testing in the same patient.

quite infrequently, almost always after consecutive rather than simultaneous infarctions (Figs. 12.35 and 12.36).

In addition to the homonymous defects described above, trauma, infarction, and, rarely, tumors affecting both occipital lobes may produce bilateral superior or inferior **altitudinal** field defects (Fig. 12.37). Although vascular damage can produce either superior or inferior defects, traumatic injury (most commonly from bullet wounds) usually causes only bilateral inferior altitudinal defects, probably because damage to the lower portions of the occipital lobes, which would produce bilateral superior altitudinal defects, often results in laceration of the dural sinuses or torcular herophili, with almost uniformly fatal results.

Cortical Blindness and Cerebral Blindness

The term "cortical blindness" indicates loss of vision in both eyes from damage to the striate cortex. "Cerebral blindness" is a more general term indicating blindness from damage to any portion of both visual pathways posterior to the LGBs. Thus, cortical blindness is a form of cerebral blindness.

The essential features of cerebral (and thus also cortical) blindness are: (1) loss of vision in both eyes; (2) retention of the reflex constriction of the pupils to illumination and to convergence movements (the near response); (3) integrity of the normal structure of the eyes as verified with the ophthalmoscope (except for patients who are blind from prenatal or perinatal injury); and (4) retention of full extraocular

Figure 12.34 A 40-year-old man suffered occipital head trauma with a depressed skull fracture and visual complaints. Visual acuity was 20/20 in both eyes. **A:** Kinetic perimetry reveals exquisitely congruous bilateral homonymous scotomas. **B:** CT scan, axial view, reveals a right occipital pole lesion, but axial MRI (**C**) confirms bilateral occipital pole involvement.

Figure 12.35 Crossed-quadrant (checkerboard) hemianopia. These field defects occurred suddenly in a 70-year-old woman with basilar artery disease. Note the quadrantic defects in the right upper field and the left lower field with the narrow congruous isthmus near fixation. Also note sparing of the left temporal crescent.

Figure 12.36 Axial CT scan in the patient whose fields are shown in Figure 12.35 shows bilateral occipital lobe infarcts. Note that the right-sided infarct is situated above the calcarine fissure in the superior occipital lobe, whereas the left-sided infarct is below the calcarine fissure in the inferior occipital lobe.

movements unless there is also damage to ocular motor structures.

Some authors stipulate that patients with bilateral postgeniculate visual loss should be said to have cerebral or cortical blindness only if visual acuity is light perception or no light perception. Others modify this definition to add that any level of visual acuity is possible with cerebral blindness as long as the visual acuity is equal in the two eyes (assuming there is no superimposed abnormality of the anterior visual pathways).

Hypoxia or anoxia involving the occipital lobes is the main cause of cerebral blindness (Fig. 12.38). Such damage is, of course, bilateral. Most commonly, an infarct in the posterior cerebral artery territory is initially unrecognized, but this previously silent hemianopia contributes to complete cortical blindness when a contralateral lesion occurs. The most common mechanism for the infarction is cerebral embolism from either the heart or the more proximal vessels of the vertebrobasilar system. Prolonged hypotension can cause cerebral blindness from bilateral watershed infarctions at the parieto-occipital junctions.

Cerebral blindness is observed under many circumstances other than infarction, as shown in Table 12.1. The mechanism of injury underlying the cerebral blindness caused by these events or substances is not always known, but vascular insufficiency plays a role in many of them.

In certain situations, cerebral blindness is transient. This is particularly true in patients who experience temporary vascular insufficiency in the vertebrobasilar system, in hypertensive syndromes following restoration of normal blood pressure, after removal of many of the toxic agents listed in Table 12.1, and after trauma. Children are more likely to experience recovery from cerebral blindness than adults, regardless of the underlying cause. On rare occasions, transient cerebral blindness may follow seizures or be an ictal manifestation. Because focal lesions may be responsible for ictal amaurosis, we believe that MRI should be performed in all cases. We would also emphasize that complete recovery from ictal or postictal blindness can occur even if the blindness lasts for several days.

It is not unusual for patients with cortical blindness to be unaware of their defect. This denial of blindness is called **anosognosia** or **Anton syndrome**. The syndrome also occurs rarely in patients with blindness from causes other than occipital lobe disease, such as cataracts, retinopathies, or optic atrophy. The explanation for Anton syndrome is unclear and may be different in different cases. It is probable that in many patients with cerebral or cortical blindness, there are

A

B

Figure 12.37 Visual field defects in an 81-year-old man who experienced the acute onset of complete visual loss, followed by clearing superiorly. **A:** Automated static perimetry demonstrates bilateral inferior altitudinal defects. The examination revealed intact visual acuity, normal pupillary reactions to light stimulation, and normal-appearing ocular fundi other than mild macular drusen. **B:** Axial **(left)** and coronal **(right)** MRI shows bilateral occipital infarcts.

lesions in various areas of the brain responsible for the recognition and interpretation of visual images. In such patients, denial of blindness is caused not by the lesion in the primary visual pathway but by another lesion in another region of the brain. In other patients, denial of visual loss may reflect an emotional or psychiatric response, or it may represent a memory disorder.

Other Visual Features of Occipital Lobe Damage

Some patients with homonymous hemianopia, especially those with a vascular occlusion in the occipital lobe, report phosphenes in the blind visual field, particularly early in the course of their disorder. Many of the visual field defects in these patients resolve

substantially, suggesting that the phosphenes may be viewed as a prognostically favorable symptom. Visual association areas bordering damaged primary cortex may be the source of these visual symptoms when they are released from normal inhibitory inputs from primary visual cortex.

Lesions of the Extrastriate Cortex with Defects in the Visual Field

It has been proposed that a lesion in extrastriate cortex; that is, Brodmann areas 18 and 19, can cause a homonymous defect in the visual field. Indeed, not only may a lesion of V2/V3 be sufficient to create a visual field defect, but such lesions may be the principle cause of quadrantic defects that strictly respect the horizontal meridian.

Figure 12.38 Axial CT scan **(left)** and MRI **(right)** in a patient who experienced bilateral blindness when steroids were tapered after he underwent surgery to remove a basal skull meningioma. The patient initially had no light perception in either eye despite normal pupillary responses to light stimulation and normal-appearing ocular fundi. He also had Anton syndrome, indicating to the nursing staff and his doctors that he could see but on assessment not being able to identify any objects presented to him, to find food on his plate, or to identify anyone with whom he came into contact unless they spoke. He subsequently regained some appreciation of movement of objects presented in his left homonymous hemifield (Riddoch phenomenon).

Dissociation of Visual Perceptions

In Chapter 13 of this text, we discuss the topographic diagnosis of disorders of visual processing distal to the primary visual cortex. Because many of these disorders result from lesions in the extrastriate cortex of the occipital lobes, it is worth mentioning a few of the more prominent syndromes here.

The human visual cortex is specialized with respect to specific functions. For example, an area in the lingual and fusiform gyri of the prestriate cortex corresponds to area V4 in the monkey and subserves the perception of color. Lesions in this region may spare the visual field but produce acquired dyschromatopsia in the contralateral hemifield. The area of functional specialization for visual motion is localized to the temporoparieto-occipital junction, a region corresponding to area V5 in the monkey. Lesions in this region, especially when bilateral, may cause a selective deficit in the perception of visual movement without a visual field defect and without impairment of nonvisual movement perception (i.e., movement perceived by acoustic or tactile stimulation).

In some patients, damage to an occipital lobe can cause a complete homonymous hemianopia to nonmoving objects with retention of the ability to detect moving objects within the blind hemifield—this is static–kinetic dissociation, also called the **Riddoch phenomenon**. Such dissociation may have prognostic significance because it usually means that some degree of recovery can be expected to occur. Static–kinetic dissociation is not a pathologic phenomenon that is purely limited to the occipital lobe. It also may occur in patients with lesions of the optic nerves and chiasm, as well as in patients with retrochiasmal visual pathway damage that spares the occipital lobes. In fact, normal individuals perceive moving objects better than static objects of the same size, shape, and luminance. This explains, at least in part, why static perimetry is more sensitive than kinetic perimetry in identifying a subtle visual field defect.

The Riddoch phenomenon is one form of a general category of visual phenomena designated as "blindsight." Some patients with extensive damage to the occipital lobes appear to retain a rudimentary form of vision involving the perception of visual stimuli other than just moving objects. Most patients are not consciously aware of this ability to look, point, detect, and discriminate without truly "seeing." In many cases, blindsight is most likely a result of islands of preserved area 17. However, in some cases, blindsight is a genuine phenomenon that reflects nonstriate visual pathways, such as a direct geniculoextrastriate cortical projection

Table 12.1	Circumstances of Cerebral Blindness

Acute intermittent porphyria
Bacterial endocarditis
Blood transfusions
Cardiac arrest
Cerebral angiography
Correction of hyponatremia
Creutzfeldt–Jakob disease
Diseases of white matter
  Adrenoleukodystrophy
  Metachromatic leukodystrophy
  Pelizaeus–Merzbacher disease
  Progressive multifocal leukoencephalopathy
  Schilder disease
Electroshock
Epilepsy
Exposure to or ingestion of toxins
  Carbon monoxide
  Cisplatin
  Cyclosporin
  Ethanol
  Interferon
  Lead
  Mercury
  Methamphetamine
  Methotrexate
  Nitrous oxide
  Tacrolimus (FK506)
  Vincristine
  Vindesine
Hypoglycemia
Infectious and neoplastic meningitis
Mitochondrial encephalopathy, lactic acidosis, and
  stroke-like episodes (MELAS)
Neoplasm
Malignant hypertension
Subacute sclerosing panencephalitis
Sudden elevation or reduction in intracranial pressure
Syphilis
Toxemia of pregnancy
Trauma
Uremia
Ventriculography

and a retinocollicular projection that reaches extrastriate cortical visual areas via the pulvinar nucleus.

Another way in which visual perceptions may be dissociated is in the syndrome of unilateral inattention or neglect. Patients with this defect may appear to have normal visual function if tested in routine fashion because they are able to correctly perceive objects in each hemifield with either eye. However, when two test objects are presented simultaneously in the right and left hemifields of each eye, the patient perceives only the test object in the hemifield ipsilateral to the lesion. This phenomenon, called **visual extinction**, can occur following damage to the parietal or occipito-parietal cortex as well as to several different regions of

the brain, reflecting the complex integrated network that exists for the modulation of directed attention within extrapersonal space.

Nonvisual Symptoms and Signs of Occipital Lobe Disease

Except with regard to the visual system, lesions of the occipital lobe usually are asymptomatic; however, many patients with occipital infarctions experience acute pain of the head, brow, or eye ipsilateral to the lesion. This presumably reflects the dual trigeminal innervation of the posterior dural structures and the periorbital region. Patients with homonymous hemianopia may also complain of disturbances of equilibrium, a sense that their body is swaying toward the side of the hemianopia. This so-called "visual ataxia" may reflect unopposed tonic input of vision from the intact hemifield rather than any true vestibular impairment or neglect.

If the posterior cerebral artery is occluded proximally, patients with an infarct in the occipital lobe also may develop hemiplegia from damage to the posterior internal capsule or cerebral peduncle, language dysfunction from damage to posterior parietal and temporal structures, and symptoms indicating damage to the ipsilateral thalamus. In addition, because the condition ordinarily is seen in patients with severe atherosclerosis, there may be other evidence of vertebrobasilar insufficiency, including ocular motor abnormalities referable to the rostral brainstem. Patients who develop a bilateral homonymous hemianopia in this setting may be more severely impaired than patients with blindness from bilateral retinal or optic nerve disease. Such patients present major problems as regards rehabilitation.

Tumors of the occipital lobe may cause nonvisual manifestations by virtue of their mass effect. Headache is the most common symptom, occurring in up to 90% of patients. Other symptoms and signs include nausea and vomiting, ataxia, hallucinations that usually are unformed (e.g., flashing lights, geometric shapes), seizures, and mental status changes. Many of these symptoms are nonlocalizing and related to increased intracranial pressure.

Treatment and Rehabilitation for Homonymous Hemianopia

Spontaneous recovery of homonymous visual field defects occurs in some patients, typically within 3 to 6 months after brain injury. Despite a certain amount of plasticity even in the adult cerebral cortex, patients with visual field defects have a consistently poor rehabilitation outcome. The exact anatomic location of the lesion causing the homonymous hemianopia does not appear to affect the functional outcome; however, the greater the number of associated neurologic deficits, the more difficult the rehabilitation and the poorer the functional performance. Contributing further to poor functional improvement is the advanced age of most of these patients, a factor associated even in normal individuals with progressive cognitive, sensory, and motor deficits. Finally, neglect, especially in patients with nondominant hemisphere lesions, also interferes with the rehabilitation process.

Several techniques may assist in the treatment and rehabilitation of patients with homonymous hemianopia. These techniques generally have one of two objectives: (1) to improve use of the existing field, or (2) to expand the existing field.

With respect to improving the use of the existing field, patients who normally read from left to right and who have difficulty reading because of a left homonymous hemianopia can be provided with a "reading screen"—a black screen with an adjustable opening that helps them find the beginning of each line. The same benefit, however, can be achieved with a ruler or other straight-edged object positioned under each line of text or by having the patient place a finger at the beginning of the line of text so that he/she can use proprioception to determine where to look. For patients who normally read from left to right and who have difficulty reading because of a right homonymous hemianopia, there is an "inversion telescope" that enables readers to read from right to left. Again, however, the same benefit may be achieved by placing a finger at the right edge of the text.

Another technique used to help a patient with a homonymous hemianopia use his/her existing field is explorative saccadic training (EST). This method uses a laptop computer with a software program that generates a random array of digits (0–9, 12-pt Ariel font). The digits are distributed with equal probability in the blind and seeing hemifields, and the patient must move the computer cursor over a predefined digit. Once the cursor passes over the digit, the program generates a sound, and the digit turns to a red dollar sign. It has been shown that EST improves saccadic behavior, natural search, and scene exploration in the direction of the blind hemifield and that this improvement is associated with subjective improvement in various activities of daily living.

Yet another technique said to improve the use of the existing field in patients with a homonymous hemianopia is "attention training." This method uses an instrument that has two horizontal arrays, one above the other, of different-colored lights, with an equal number of lights on each side of a fixation point. Initially, one light turns on, and the patient is told to find the light that is on using eye movements, head movements, or both. Once the patient masters this task, two lights are turned on simultaneously and the patient is told to identify the light that is furthest from the center. The benefit of this type of training is as yet unproven and the results may be no better than what the patient would do normally over time.

Figure 12.39 Monocular sector Fresnel press-on prisms for treatment of a complete homonymous hemianopia. These prisms, which are placed above and below the horizontal, are effective at all gaze angles and have been shown to be extremely helpful, particularly in patients without other neurologic deficits.

A final method of helping patients with a homonymous hemianopia use their existing field is placement of monocular sector Fresnel press-on prisms. These prisms, which are placed above and below the horizontal (Fig. 12.39), are effective at all gaze angles and have been shown to be extremely helpful, particularly in patients without other neurologic deficits.

Some investigators believe that patients with an incomplete, relative homonymous hemianopia can experience expansion of their seeing field by so-called visual restoration therapy (VRT). VRT is based on the presumed plasticity in the CNS, even in adults, and the belief that stimulating visual neurons that are adjacent to an area of damage and that are alive but not functioning normally will induce these neurons either to function normally again or to take over the role of the adjacent dead neurons. Using this technique, investigators have reported expansion of a seeing field by 5 to 10 degrees; however, there appears to be no correlation between subjective improvement in vision or ability to perform activities of daily living and improvement in the degree of field expansion or whether or not the field even expands. Indeed, some believe that the so-called field expansion is really an artifact due to changes in fixation induced during training. If VRT works at all, it works best in an otherwise intact, motivated patient with a relative homonymous visual field defect and good central vision. It is not likely to be helpful in a patient with unrealistic expectations, who has other neurologic deficits, particularly ipsilateral neglect, who has poor visual acuity, and/or who has an absolute field defect.

In summary, there is no perfect method for visual rehabilitation in a patient with a homonymous field defect, regardless of whether the defect is isolated or associated with other neurologic defects. Nevertheless, there are some relatively simple methods that can be used to help such individuals.

Central Disorders of Visual Function*

13

Segregation of Visual Inputs

Blindsight and Residual Vision

Cerebral Achromatopsia

Prosopagnosia and Related Disturbances
   of Object Recognition

Acquired Alexia

Disorders of Motion Perception (Akinetopsia)

Balint Syndrome and Related Visuospatial
   Disorders

Positive Visual Phenomena
   Visual Perseveration
   Visual Hallucinations
   Release Hallucinations (Charles Bonnet Syndrome)
   Visual Seizures
   Migrainous Hallucinations
   Other Types of Hallucinations
   Visual Distortions (Dysmetropsia)

Tests of Higher Visual Function

Glossary of Cerebral Visual Deficits

This chapter addresses aspects of behavior disorders caused by damage to the visual cortex and white matter connections. These conditions are often referred to as "central disorders of vision," "cerebral disorders of vision," or "higher disorders of vision." The understanding of these disorders continues to improve with the development of new techniques for measuring visual dysfunction, imaging the behaving brain, rehabilitating visual dysfunction in patients with brain damage, and even creating visual sensations in the blind with prostheses to stimulate visual cortex.

Vision was once thought to be primarily a serial (or hierarchic) process in which visual signals were altered or enhanced at successive way stations from retina to brain until an image of the physical world somehow emerged at the level of conscious experience. It has subsequently become clear that serial processing is

only one of several mechanisms used by the brain to process visual signals. The primate visual system also uses parallel processing, beginning in the retina. Different types of retinal ganglion cells are specialized to transduce different types of physical signals and give rise to different channels. There is cross talk between these channels at several levels from the retina to the cortex, and there also are feedforward and feedback connections between early and late stages of the visual sensory system. Instead of just serial processing, visual functions are explained in terms of multiple interactions among specialized brain regions in the same hemisphere and across the corpus callosum. Central disorders of vision thus can be interpreted as a consequence of disturbing the processing in different sectors or pathways in a complex interconnecting network.

Segregation of Visual Inputs

The functional segregation of visual inputs in the primate visual system is well documented (Figs. 12.38 and 13.1). Retinal information is communicated to cortical neurons through a set of pathways that appear specialized to convey a particular class of visual information. For example, the **parvocellular** or P-pathway, named for its connections to simian striate cortex (area V1) via parvocellular layers 3 to 6 of the lateral geniculate body (LGB), is characterized by color opponency and slow-conducting axons that convey sustained signals. This pathway has strong projections to secondary areas such as V4 and inferior temporal (IT) cortex, located in the inferior occipital lobe and adjacent temporo-occipital regions. These regions, along the ventral or temporal cortical pathway (the "what" pathway), are presumed to play a role in the perception of color, luminance, stereopsis, and pattern recognition. In contrast, the **magnocellular** or M-pathway is characterized by large, fast-conducting axons that convey information about more transient visual signals. This pathway connects to areas in visual association cortex, including the middle temporal (MT) and medial superior temporal (MST) areas. These regions, located along the dorsal or parietal cortical pathway (the "where" pathway), are thought to

*The authors acknowledge the past contributions of Matthew Rizzo and Jason J. S. Barton to this chapter.

analyze the spatial location and movement of objects in the panorama (Fig. 13.1).

Analyses of data from a large number of patients with focal lesions of the visual cortex and its connections support the general concept of separate dorsal

Figure 13.1 Parallel pathways for visual function in the cerebral cortex of the nonhuman primate. Borders between visual areas are indicated by fine dashed lines. The superior temporal sulcus has been opened to show areas that are normally out of sight. The medial hemisphere is not shown. The lower panel shows a flow diagram from area V1 (primary visual cortex) to the parietal pathway that includes area MT and the temporal pathway that includes area V4. The visual information encoded by neurons varies greatly among these different areas. The human brain is likely to respect a similar organization. 7a, Brodmann area 7a. AIT, anterior inferotemporal area (d, dorsal subdivision; v, ventral subdivision). CIT, central inferotemporal area (d, dorsal subdivision; v, ventral subdivision). DP, dorsal parietal area. FST, fundus of the superior temporal area. LIP, lateral intraparietal area. MST, medial superior temporal area. MT, middle temporal area. PIT, posterior inferotemporal area (d, dorsal subdivision; v, ventral subdivision). STP, superior temporal polysensory area. V1, visual area 1 (striate cortex). V2, visual area 2. V4, visual area 4. VIP, ventral intraparietal area. VOT, ventral occipitotemporal area. VP, ventral posterior area. (Reprinted with permission from Maunsell JHR. The brain's visual world: Representation of visual targets in cerebral cortex. *Science*. 1995;270:765–769.)

and ventral processing pathways as a framework for interpreting human clinical disorders. For example, damage to the inferior visual cortex and adjoining temporal regions impairs pattern recognition and learning, producing agnosia for objects and faces (prosopagnosia) or inability to read despite previous literacy (alexia). It can also reduce color perception in the contralateral field—cerebral achromatopsia. By contrast, damage to the superior visual cortex and the adjacent parietal cortex produces disorders of spatial-temporal analysis—inability to judge location, distance, orientation, size, or motion of objects, as well as marked disturbances of visually guided eye and hand control. Balint syndrome is a striking example.

Each of these major divisions probably has functional subdivisions. Furthermore, although the dorsal and ventral visual cortices are associated with different, behaviorally separable functions, there is growing evidence that these two major divisions also have overlapping functions.

Blindsight and Residual Vision

Some patients with lesions of area V1 causing a homonymous field defect perform better than chance on simple forced-choice detection tasks or on localization tasks measuring the accuracy of finger pointing or eye movements toward targets presented in the defective field of vision. Some of these patients deny any conscious experience of the objects they reportedly localize or detect and are thus said to have **blindsight**. This phenomenon is distinct from residual vision that may arise from a small population of spared neurons in V1, and precise anatomic analysis and clinical assessment are needed to ensure that this category of poor visual function is not mistaken for blindsight.

The dominant hypothesis in blindsight research is that the phenomenon represents residual function in a visual pathway parallel to the retino-geniculo-calcarine system. The initial candidate was an alternative pathway involving the superior colliculus, but more recent data implicate areas V5/MT. However, it has been difficult to completely exclude a contribution from residual activity of a small population of neurons in V1. In humans, a complete lesion is nearly impossible to confirm antemortem. Thus, research in nonhuman primates using fMRI before and after a permanent and complete surgical lesion of V1 has been conducted, and results indicate persistent albeit weak activation of V4 with presentation of stimuli in the lesioned hemifield. Further experiments are needed to confirm and expand these findings.

There are also explanations of blindsight that do not invoke parallel pathways. Blindsight may simply reflect a testing phenomenon known as **criterion shift** in which patients tend to use fairly conservative criteria when asked to respond Yes or No during a detection task but use more relaxed criteria when forced to choose an alternative (i.e., guess) in a discriminatory paradigm. Furthermore, studies that attempt to determine if hemianopic patients have blindsight must eliminate all potential testing artifacts, including inadequate fixation, light scatter, nonvisual cues, and nonrandom presentation of targets.

Even if blindsight does exist, it is clear that visual discriminations in blind hemifields are less accurate and more variable than those in normal hemifields. However, the range of visual function demonstrated in patients with either blindsight or residual vision is impressive, including perception of spatial location and discrimination of form, orientation, color, and motion. No clear pattern of visual abilities that are preserved or destroyed has emerged in such patients. The variability in blindsight profiles may have an anatomic basis in the inevitable variability of naturally occurring human lesions. Most lesions of striate cortex also involve some extrastriate regions, but the degree and the areas affected differ from one patient to the next. The fact is, not all patients with cortical field defects have blindsight. Why some patients have blindsight and others do not is unclear. Its presence or absence may reflect differences in lesion anatomy, but this is not proven. Some studies have found that blindsight was present only in patients with hemianopia occurring in childhood, a period of presumably greater neural plasticity, but other studies have not confirmed this impression. A requirement for childhood onset is inconsistent with reports that training in older patients can lead to blindsight. If blindsight truly exists, it is uncommon.

Cerebral Achromatopsia

Cerebral achromatopsia, also called central achromatopsia, is an uncommon defect of color perception caused by damage to the visual cortex. Some patients with this condition complain that colors look dull, wrong, or less bright, whereas others report that their world is completely colorless and that objects appear only in shades of gray, like in old black and white movies. Although the term "cerebral achromatopsia" is sometimes used to include all degrees of cerebral color deficits, we believe that this term is best reserved for the most severe cases and that the term **cerebral dyschromatopsia** should be used in cases where there is residual color sensation.

Either cerebral achromatopsia or cerebral dyschromatopsia may be a presenting symptom or may evolve during recovery from cortical blindness. The most common setting is vertebrobasilar ischemia affecting the posterior cerebral arterial blood supply to the occipital lobes. Other causes of achromatopsia include herpes simplex encephalitis, cerebral metastases, recurrent focal seizures, and dementia with visual cortical involvement. Transient achromatopsia may also occur as part of the aura of migraine.

Anatomic and functional imaging studies indicate that color is processed by a large network of structures, including V1, V2, V3, V4 (the most emphasized), and IT. Nevertheless, the lesions causing cerebral achromatopsia are rather restricted and usually affect the ventromedial sectors of the occipital lobe in the lingual and fusiform gyri (Fig. 13.2). Lesions of the middle third of the lingual gyrus or the white matter immediately behind the posterior tip of the lateral ventricle

Figure 13.2 Magnetic resonance imaging in a patient with cerebral dyschromatopsia. Nonenhanced sagittal T1-weighted images show bilateral lesions in the visual cortices. The lesion of the right hemisphere (**R**) is responsible for the left homonymous hemianopia. The lesion of the left hemisphere (**L**) is located below the calcarine fissure in the inferior visual association cortex in regions thought to process color. (Reprinted with permission from Rizzo M, Nawrot M, Blake R, et al. A human visual disorder resembling area V4 dysfunction in the monkey. *Neurology.* 1992;42:1175–1180.)

are said to be critical. Bilateral lesions are necessary for complete achromatopsia; unilateral right or left occipital lesions may produce a hemiachromatopsia.

Common accompaniments of cerebral achromatopsia include superior homonymous quadrantanopia, visual agnosia, and acquired alexia. The **quadrantanopia** may be complete or incomplete; but in either case, the achromatopsia affects the remaining inferior quadrants of the visual fields on the side opposite the lesion (i.e., on the same side as the visual field defect). **Visual agnosia**—the inability to recognize previously familiar objects or to learn the identity of new objects by sight alone despite adequate visual sensory abilities—is also seen in patients with cerebral achromatopsia, particularly in patients with bilateral lesions. The syndrome in such patients includes **prosopagnosia** in which the agnosic defect is most striking for faces; and **topographagnosia** or topographic disorientation in which patients tend to get lost in familiar visual surroundings, partly because of an inability to recognize previously familiar local landmarks. Some patients have **pure alexia**, also known as alexia without agraphia, the acquired inability to read in previously literate individuals (see below). Defects of visual memory and even generalized amnesia can accompany cerebral achromatopsia, depending on the extent of the lesion into more anterior and mesial structures in the temporal lobes.

One should be cautious in interpreting the verbal report of a patient with cerebral achromatopsia. Assessment of color naming and associations should be conducted independently of color perception testing. This allows the best opportunity to distinguish cerebral achromatopsia and dyschromatopsia from color anomia, agnosia, and related defects of language and memory. Using matching tasks in addition to naming tasks is crucial.

Color anomia is often part of a more general anomia in aphasic patients, but there are instances in which color naming is disproportionately affected. These cases tend to occur with left occipital lesions and are associated with a complete right homonymous hemianopia, rather than just the upper quadrantanopia seen with cerebral achromatopsia. One possible mechanism in such cases is an interhemispheric disconnection syndrome associated with right homonymous hemianopia and pure alexia. Because of the complete right homonymous hemianopia, visual input to language areas in the left hemisphere must arise from the right visual cortex. However, a concurrent lesion of the splenium of the corpus callosum interrupts this process. Affected patients can perceive colors yet not name them (color anomia) and may also see letters but not be able to read them (pure alexia). Preserved tactile naming in such patients suggests preservation of callosal fibers anterior to those required for reading

and color naming. Color anomia, together with pure alexia, can also occur without a callosal lesion when there is damage near the posterior aspect of the occipital horn on the left, interrupting connections from both visual fields to language areas.

Prosopagnosia and Related Disturbances of Object Recognition

Visual agnosia is an inability to recognize familiar objects, despite adequate visual perception attention, intellect, and language. **Prosopagnosia** is a restricted form of visual agnosia characterized by the impaired ability to recognize familiar faces or to learn to recognize new faces. It is a specific functional disorder with a specific neuroanatomic basis. Prosopagnosia may actually cover a spectrum of deficits, with individual patients varying in the degree of perceptual versus memory dysfunction or even having disconnections between the two processes. Furthermore, abnormal face recognition may be part of more generalized perceptual, cognitive, or memory problems. We will reserve the term "prosopagnosia" for cases in which the facial recognition deficit is disproportionately more severe than other associated deficits.

Patients with prosopagnosia are usually aware of their difficulty and complain of the social embarrassment of not recognizing acquaintances. When they do recognize others, it is often by reliance on specific facial features or paraphernalia (e.g., a hairstyle, glasses, beards and mustaches, a missing tooth, or a particular scar) that bypass the need for an overall analysis of the shape of the face. They may also use nonfacial visual cues, such as gait and posture, or nonvisual cues, such as voice. The context of the encounter is also important. For example, patients with prosopagnosia may be able to recognize hospital staff but are unable to recognize the same persons when they meet them later on the street. Persons with childhood onset of prosopagnosia and, occasionally, persons with onset in adulthood may be ignorant of their deficit.

Despite abnormal recognition of familiar faces, many patients with prosopagnosia can accurately discriminate among unfamiliar faces, even with varying lighting conditions or facial views (i.e., Benton Facial Recognition Test [BVRT]). However, patients with prosopagnosia may require much more time than normal to arrive at correct judgments, suggesting that they use an inefficient and abnormal route for processing face information.

Some individuals with prosopagnosia can judge the age, gender, and emotional expression of faces they cannot recognize, and some even lip-read. Again, prosopagnosics may use different perceptual processes from those used by normal individuals to make such judgments. For example, a patient with prosopagnosia might rely on wrinkles to tell age, whereas normal individuals can still make age judgments in the absence of such local features. Other prosopagnosic patients, usually those with more pervasive perceptual dysfunction, are impaired with respect to judgments about facial age, sex, emotional expression, and the direction of the person's gaze, the last item being an important social signal.

An important theoretical issue is whether the prosopagnosic defect is specific for faces or also affects perception of other objects. Some patients have difficulty distinguishing types of objects, such as makes of cars, flowers, food, and coins. They also have trouble identifying previously familiar items, such as buildings, handwriting, and personal belongings or clothing. These cases imply that in prosopagnosia, impaired facial recognition may simply be the most prominent manifestation of a more general recognition or perceptual problem. On the other hand, some patients can distinguish nonface objects relatively well despite severe prosopagnosia. Specific tests of face versus object recognition appear to confirm this dissociation.

Although patients with prosopagnosia deny familiarity with and cannot identify known faces, some patients retain covert (i.e., nonconscious) recognition of these faces at a variety of levels. Investigators have shown two main phenomena: **Covert familiarity,** in which the patient is able to distinguish previously familiar but unrecognized faces from completely unknown faces, and **covert semantic knowledge,** in which the patient retains information about name, occupation, and other facts associated with a face.

Patients with prosopagnosia usually have difficulty recognizing faces of people with whom they were familiar before the start of the illness (retrograde prosopagnosia) as well as people whom they meet after the onset of the condition (anterograde prosopagnosia). Some patients have slightly better recognition of people long known to them, whereas others have only anterograde prosopagnosia. Prosopagnosia historically has been segregated into two main forms: **Apperceptive prosopagnosia,** in which there is a failure to form a sufficiently accurate facial percept; and **associative prosopagnosia,** in which there is an inability to match an accurate percept to facial memories.

In most cases of prosopagnosia, the lesion is in the inferior temporo-occipital cortex, usually in the lingual and fusiform gyri (Fig. 13.3). In occasional cases, the lesion appears to be located in the more anterior temporal cortex. All autopsied cases of prosopagnosia have **bilateral** lesions, often symmetric, presumably affecting homologous regions of both hemispheres. However, the position of the left-sided lesion can be more variable. A left-sided hemispheric lesion or a lesion of the splenium of the corpus callosum might disconnect a right hemispheric locus for facial recognition from visual input of the right hemifield, with critical effects in cases with left homonymous hemianopia. Furthermore, reports of neuroimaging showing apparently unilateral right temporo-occipital lesions have accumulated. The type of face perception deficits caused by unilateral as opposed to bilateral cerebral lesions may differ. It has been suggested that apperceptive types of prosopagnosia occur with damage to right ventral and dorsal temporo-occipital areas, whereas bilateral ventral temporo-occipital lesions result in an associative or dysmnesic form.

Almost all patients with prosopagnosia have other visual deficits. Visual field defects are frequent, the most common being left homonymous hemianopia, left superior homonymous quadrantanopia, bilateral superior quadrantanopia, or combinations of these. The visual field defect, achromatopsia or hemiachromatopsia, and topographagnosia often form a common tetrad with prosopagnosia. Nevertheless, cases of prosopagnosia associated with normal color vision exist, showing that prosopagnosia and achromatopsia are dissociable. Visual object agnosia is said to be absent in some patients with prosopagnosia and present, though proportionately milder, in others.

A frequent finding in patients with prosopagnosia is impaired visual memory. In some of these patients, the memory deficit also affects verbal material. Other patients with prosopagnosia also have simultanagnosia, palinopsia, visual hallucinations, constructional difficulties, and left hemineglect. Hemisensory deficits or hemiparesis occur in some patients with unilateral right-sided lesions, although in some of these cases, the motor and sensory findings are related to other lesions. Pure alexia (see below) can occur in some patients with prosopagnosia.

The most common lesions causing prosopagnosia are posterior cerebral artery infarctions and, less often, viral encephalitis. The predominance of these conditions may be related to their potential to inflict bilateral damage, although the neuroimaging in some cases shows only a unilateral lesion. Other unilateral lesions, such as tumors, hematomas, abscesses, and surgical resections, are less frequently reported.

Impaired facial recognition can occur as part of the generalized dementia in Alzheimer disease, in Parkinson disease, and rarely in elderly patients with bilateral or unilateral right temporal lobar degeneration. The last disorder is one of the focal progressive atrophies, others of which affect the frontal, parietal, or left temporal lobes possibly related to Alzheimer or Pick disease.

Developmental prosopagnosia also has been described. Patients with this condition usually are not aware that they have problems with face recognition until they experience social difficulties related to the impairment. In addition to problems with

Figure 13.3 Location of bilateral lesions in three patients with prosopagnosia. Axial template drawings with shaded areas representing the lesions of three patients with prosopagnosia. Bilateral damage, greater on the left than the right, is present in all three cases. (Reprinted with permission from Damasio AR, Damasio H, van Hoesen GW. Prosopagnosia: Anatomic basis and behavioral mechanisms. *Neurology.* 1982;32:331–341.)

facial recognition, these patients have difficulty judging facial age, sex, and expressions. They also perform facial matching tasks very slowly, suggesting a perceptual process differing from normal. In some cases, developmental prosopagnosia is present in other family members, possibly as an autosomal-dominant trait, and coexists with the Asperger syndrome of autism. The prevalence of prosopagnosia among all autistic individuals is unknown, as are the effects of the face perception disorder on other aspects of psychosocial development.

Acquired Alexia

Acquired alexia is the loss of efficient reading for comprehension, despite adequate visual acuity. Reading is a complex behavior involving perception of form, spatial attention, ocular fixation, scanning saccadic eye movements, and linguistic processing. Not surprisingly, many types of cerebral or visual dysfunction can disrupt the reading process. Although other clinical signs may overshadow the difficulty, impaired reading is sometimes the chief complaint. The severity of reading difficulty can range from a mild defect with slow reading and occasional errors, which may only be identified by comparison with normal controls matched for educational level, to a complete inability to read even numbers and letters. Thus, "dyslexia" is the more appropriate term in most cases, and it is used in this manner (and not to describe a learning disorder) in this chapter. Analysis of not only the severity but also the type of reading errors can help differentiate among the various forms of reading impairment and their causes.

Most syndromes of alexia can be explained by the disconnectionist theories. The left angular gyrus stores the visual representation of words necessary for reading and writing. Therefore, disconnecting the visual inputs of both hemispheres from the left angular gyrus could disrupt reading but leave writing intact—that is, pure alexia.

The key feature of **pure alexia (alexia without agraphia, or word blindness)**, is a dramatic dissociation between the ability to read and the ability to write. Patients with this condition can write fluently and spontaneously, but having done so are unable to read what they have just written. The severity varies from a slow, laborious reading of words one letter at a time (letter-by-letter reading; spelling alexia) to complete inability to read words or letters (global alexia) and sometimes even numbers or other symbols. Covert reading ability can be detected in at least some patients with pure alexia. These patients have aspects of preserved reading ability of which they are not aware.

Lesions causing pure alexia are almost always located in the left hemisphere, most commonly in the inferior temporo-occipital region (Fig. 13.4). A visual word forming area (VWFA) has been identified in this area by fMRI. The majority of lesions are caused by infarction within the vascular territory of the left posterior cerebral artery, but other causes include primary and metastatic tumors, arteriovenous malformations, hemorrhage, herpes simplex, encephalitis, and a rare focal posterior cortical dementia.

One popular explanation of pure alexia is that it is a disconnection of visual information from linguistic

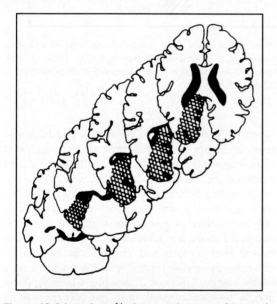

Figure 13.4 Location of lesions causing pure alexia, right homonymous hemianopia, and color dysnomia. Template drawings of axial CT images, combined from five patients, show lesions affecting the left medial and lateral occipital lobes, medial temporo-occipital lobe and paraventricular white matter, and forceps major, sometimes extending into the splenium proper. (Reprinted with permission from Damasio AR, Damasio H. The anatomic basis of pure alexia. *Neurology.* 1983;33:1573–1583.)

processing centers. Visual information from the right hemifield is either absent in cases with right hemianopia, or it is interrupted in its course through left extrastriate centers to the reading center in the left angular gyrus. Callosal pathways transmitting visual information from visual association cortex of the right hemisphere to homologous regions in the left hemisphere are interrupted by a lesion in the splenium, forceps major, or periventricular white matter surrounding the occipital horn of the lateral ventricle. Thus, words in the left hemifield also cannot access the left angular gyrus. Similarly, other visual information is isolated, causing an associated anomia for colors and objects.

Associated signs with pure alexia are common. There is often a right homonymous field defect, usually a complete homonymous hemianopia but sometimes only a superior quadrantanopia, in which case there may also be a right hemiachromatopsia. Pure alexia cannot be attributed to the field defect, however, because pure alexia can occur without a field defect, and many patients with a right homonymous hemianopia that splits (i.e., does not spare) the macula do not have pure alexia. Although associated dyschromatopsia is generally restricted to the right homonymous hemifield, naming of colors in the whole field may be abnormal. Anomia is not necessarily restricted to the visual modality but can include objects perceived by touch, implying some nonvisual language disturbance from extension of the lesion outside the visual association cortex. Verbal memory deficits and visual agnosia can occur. Some authors describe a form of optic ataxia (see below) in which the dominant right hand has difficulty with purposeful movements to objects in the nondominant left visual field.

Pure alexia without a homonymous hemianopia occurs in some patients with lesions of the white matter underlying the angular gyrus. Indeed, degeneration of the inferior longitudinal fasciculus, which connects the VWFA and the occipital cortex, has been described in a patient with pure alexia after resection of a small epileptogenic focus. Studies of similar patients may help to define these pathways in additional detail.

Although some cases of pure alexia may be a visual agnosia from left extrastriate damage, at least some cases do represent a true visual–verbal disconnection. For example, pure alexia can occur with the combination of a splenial lesion and a left geniculate nuclear lesion causing a right homonymous hemianopia; there is no damage to striate or extrastriate cortex in such patients. These cases demonstrate that disconnection is sufficient to cause pure alexia.

The disconnection hypothesis involves two deafferentations of the left angular gyrus: The disconnection of right hemispheric vision and the disconnection or destruction of left hemispheric vision. Each of these can occur independently and is called a **hemi-alexia**.

In left hemi-alexia, reading is impaired in the left hemi-field only because of isolated damage to the posterior corpus callosum or callosal fibers elsewhere. Right hemi-alexia occurs when a lesion of the left medial and ventral occipital lobe spares other visual functions in the right field.

Left **hemiparalexia** is a rare syndrome attributed to damage to the splenium of the corpus callosum. The reading pattern in patients with this condition is similar to that in patients with left hemineglect, in that substitution and omission errors occur for the first letter of words. However, these patients do not have evidence of hemineglect, and although patients with left hemineglect usually have a right hemispheric (usually parietal) lesion and an associated left homonymous hemianopia, some of the patients with left hemiparalexia have left occipital lesions and a right homonymous hemianopia (Fig. 13.5). Patients with left hemiparalexia may have other signs of callosal disconnection, such as inability to name objects felt by the nondominant (left) hand, left-hand agraphia, and inability to duplicate the unseen movements of one hand by the other.

A combination of impaired reading and writing constitutes **alexia with agraphia**. This syndrome is usually associated with lesions of the left angular gyrus, although lesions of the adjacent temporoparietal junction have also been implicated. In patients with left parietal lesions, alexia with agraphia may be accompanied by acalculia, right-left disorientation, and finger agnosia, the other elements of **Gerstmann syndrome**.

In some rare cases, there is relative preservation of oral and auditory language functions, although more often there are other elements of aphasia.

Another form of alexia and agraphia is described as an accompaniment of Broca aphasia (nonfluent aphasia), which is caused by lesions of the dominant (left) inferior frontal lobe. These patients have difficulty reading aloud and writing, attributable to their problems with all forms of expressive language output. However, comprehension of text is also often impaired in such patients, despite relatively preserved comprehension of auditory language. In contrast with the letter-by-letter reading in pure alexia, these patients are better at occasionally grasping a whole word even though they are unable to name the letters of the word. Thus, this type of alexia with agraphia sometimes is called **literal alexia** or "letter blindness." These patients also have impaired comprehension of syntactic structure, just as their speech output often demonstrates a significant impairment of syntax called **agrammatism**. The underlying mechanism is unknown. Gaze paresis and difficulty in maintaining verbal sequences have been proposed but not proven. It may be that this frontal alexia is a variant of deep dyslexia, a type of central dyslexia (see below).

Some patients with visual field defects have reading problems despite normal or near-normal visual acuity and may be described as having **hemianopic dyslexia**. This condition results from inability to see letters in the central 3 degrees of the blind hemifield and not from a failure to recognize or process the written

Figure 13.5 Neuroimaging in a patient with left hemiparalexia. **A** to **C**: Axial T2-weighted MRI at three successive levels from a 40-year-old woman who underwent embolization of a left medial parieto-occipital arteriovenous malformation. After the procedure, she had a right homonymous hemianopia, left unilateral tactile dysnomia, and alien hand syndrome on the left. During reading, she missed the letters on the left side of words even though she had an intact left homonymous hemifield and no left hemineglect. The images show changes consistent with infarction in the left ventral–caudal splenium (*arrowhead,* level B) and medial occipital lobe (levels A and B), with sparing of the rostral splenium (*arrowhead,* level C). (Reprinted with permission from Binder JR, Lazar RM, Tatemichi TK, et al. Left hemiparalexia. *Neurology.* 1992;42:562–569.)

information. Reading speed is markedly reduced in such patients and may be refractory to compensatory training efforts.

Disturbances of attention can also cause a number of so-called peripheral dyslexias. Simultanagnosia, in which perception of single items is adequate but perception of several objects simultaneously is impaired, has been implicated in **attentional dyslexia**. Patients with this condition read single words normally but not several words together. They also identify single letters but not the letters in a word. Attentional dyslexia occurs from lesions in the left temporo-occipital junction and the left parietal lobe. Its diagnosis rests upon the difference between reading of single versus multiple words and the presence of simultanagnosia for other visual items besides words.

Subtle acquired dyslexic deficits occur in addition to the more overt disturbances described above. Many of these deficits occur in association with other aphasic features and thus could be classified as aphasic alexias; however, they can occasionally occur as isolated deficits. These reading defects are sometimes labeled **central dyslexias** because they reflect dysfunction of central reading processes rather than "peripheral" attention or visual deficits.

Disorders of Motion Perception (Cerebral Akinetopsia)

Akinetopsia (cerebral akinetopsia) is the term used to describe complete loss of movement perception from an acquired cerebral lesion. Although akinetopsia requires bilateral cerebral lesions, subtle and generally asymptomatic disturbances of motion perception can occur with unilateral cerebral lesions.

Motion perception plays many roles in vision. One is the perception of moving objects in the environment. Because objects usually occupy only a small part of the visual field, motion relative to the stationary background enhances their perception. Object motion guides limb-reaching movements and smooth-pursuit eye movements, and it influences saccadic accuracy. In addition to object motion, information about self-motion can be obtained from motion perception. As the observer moves or turns the head or eyes, the image of the entire visual environment moves in the opposite direction. Thus, motion of large portions of the visual field usually implies self-motion rather than motion of an external object. This large-field motion generates optokinetic responses that complement the vestibulo-ocular reflex in stabilizing sight during head- or self-motion. Information about object identity is also available from visual motion.

PET scanning studies performed in normal humans during motion perception show activation in the lateral occipital gyri at the junction of Brodmann areas 19 and 37. This motion-selective area is most consistently related to the conjunction of the anterior limb of the IT sulcus with the lateral occipital sulcus. Other areas activated during motion perception include V1, V2, and the dorsal cuneus, which may correspond to V3 in nonhuman primates. Cerebellar activation also occurs with directed rather than random motion (Fig. 13.6). Functional MRI signal changes in lateral temporo-occipital cortex correlate with motion aftereffects. Both motion perception and pursuit-related signals are present in lateral temporo-occipital cortex. Magnetic stimulation can be used to create temporary dysfunction within specific cortical areas. Stimulation over lateral temporo-occipital cortex impairs motion direction discrimination but not form discrimination in the contralateral hemifield and, to a lesser degree, in the ipsilateral hemifield.

There are few clinical tests of motion perception. Smooth pursuit eye movements and optokinetic nystagmus can be observed and measured, but only laboratory studies with large, animated displays simulating environmental motion allow accurate investigation and characterization of these problems.

Cerebral akinetopsia appears to require bilateral lesions affecting the lateral temporo-occipital cortex. However, multiple but unilateral infarcts of the right parietal lobe and parieto-occipital junction may also give akinetopsia. The cause in one well-described case was sagittal sinus thrombosis with bilateral infarctions involving the lateral aspects of Brodmann areas 18, 19, and 39 (lateral occipital, MT, and angular gyri). In another well-studied case, acute hypertensive hemorrhage resulted in bilateral lesions in the lateral temporo-occipital regions.

Patients with motion perception deficits may have other abnormalities caused by lesions of the lateral temporo-occipital area. Perception of form may be abnormal, as may be object recognition, spatial vision, and stereopsis. Hemianopias of various degrees are more often left-sided, reflecting the right brain predominance of the causative lesions.

Balint Syndrome and Related Visuospatial Disorders

In 1909, Balint described a triad of visual defects in a man with bilateral parieto-occipital lesions (Fig. 13.7). The most significant deficit was an inability to perceive together at any one time the several items of a visual scene, which Balint interpreted as a "spatial disorder of attention." Other terms used to describe this deficit subsequently included "visual disorientation" and "simultanagnosia" (an inability to interpret the totality of a picture scene despite preservation of ability

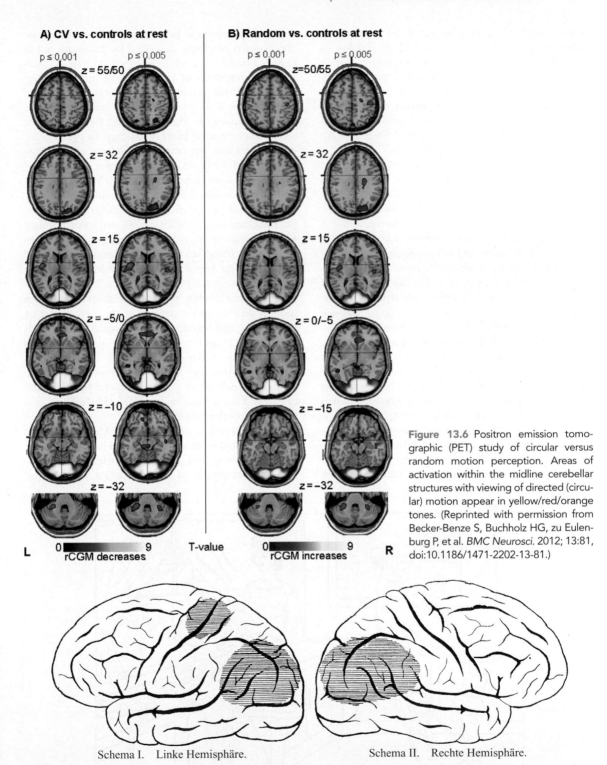

Figure 13.6 Positron emission tomographic (PET) study of circular versus random motion perception. Areas of activation within the midline cerebellar structures with viewing of directed (circular) motion appear in yellow/red/orange tones. (Reprinted with permission from Becker-Benze S, Buchholz HG, zu Eulenburg P, et al. *BMC Neurosci.* 2012; 13:81, doi:10.1186/1471-2202-13-81.)

Schema I.   Linke Hemisphäre.   Schema II.   Rechte Hemisphäre.

Figure 13.7 Drawing of the locations of the major lesions in the case described by Balint in 1909, as pictured on lateral views of the hemispheres. The views are idealized and do not convey the full extent of the pathology. The surface of the brain was actually atrophic. Not seen in this view are several lesions of potential importance to the patient's behavior presentation. These included lesions of the posterior white matter in which optic radiations travel on both sides, and of the pulvinar, a critical structure for visuospatial integration in primates. (Reprinted with permission from Balint R. Seelenlahmung des "Schauens," optische Ataxie, räumliche Störung der Aufmerksamkeit. *Monatschr Psychiatr Neurol.* 1909;25:51–181.)

to apprehend individual portions of the whole). The patient described by Balint also had an inability to move the eyes voluntarily to objects of interest despite unrestricted eye rotations, the so-called "psychic paralysis of gaze," "spasm of fixation," or "acquired ocular apraxia." The third deficit present in the patient described by Balint was a defect of hand movements under visual guidance despite normal limb strength and position sense, termed "optic ataxia."

Among the many reported causes of the so-called **Balint syndrome** are cerebrovascular disease (especially watershed infarctions as in Balint original case), tumor, trauma, Creutzfeldt–Jakob disease, and degenerative conditions such as Alzheimer disease.

Simultanagnosia is best understood as an inability to report all the items and relationships in a complex visual display despite unrestricted head and eye movements. A suitable screening tool is the Cookie Theft Picture from the Boston Diagnostic Aphasia Examination or any similar picture containing a balance of information among the four quadrants (Fig. 13.8). The patient's report can be correlated with a checklist of the items in the picture. Because verbal fluency is assumed, these tools should not be used in severely aphasic patients. It is also crucial to exclude or at least be aware of poor visual acuity or impaired visual fields. For example, objects may seem to vanish into a central scotoma, paracentral scotoma, or a hemianopia, causing symptoms that mimic simultanagnosia.

Balint syndrome may not occur in isolation. Affected patients often have a number of other devastating defects in behavior, and the three classic components originally described by Balint are not as closely bound as is often assumed. Moreover, individual components of the syndrome appear to represent relatively broad categories comprising other more specific defects. Furthermore, Balint syndrome does not appear to have a specific neuroanatomic significance because bilateral damage to the parieto-occipital regions can cause other defects, and damage elsewhere in the brain can cause similar clinical disorders. It is probably best to consider Balint syndrome a variety of combined deficits from lesions of the dorsolateral visual association cortices, which include the putative human area MT complex and its projections to the parieto-occipital cortex. Damage to these areas and to the cortices surrounding the angular gyrus and parietal insular cortex can disturb multiple aspects of spatial and temporal processing, including the perception of visual motion, perceptions of structure from motion and dynamic stereopsis, the perception of egomotion, and coordination of visual (eye-centered) and vestibular (gravity-centered) coordinate systems that orient us in the physical world. Bilateral lower quadrantanopias may also occur from damage to the primary visual cortex lining the dorsal banks of the calcarine fissure (human area V1), thus adding to a patient's overall problem.

The observations of Balint on what he called "optic ataxia" sparked interest in the neural basis of visually guided **reaching and grasping**. Reaching and grasping external objects is a fundamental activity that

Figure 13.8 The "Cookie Theft Picture" from the Boston Diagnostic Aphasia Examination. This picture contains a balance of information among the four quadrants. The patient is asked to describe the events depicted in the picture.

demands the coordination of several different nervous system functions. To accomplish this task, the brain transforms a target's visual coordinates to body-centered space, plans a hand path and trajectory (the sequence of hand position and velocity to target), and computes multiple joint torques, especially about the shoulder and elbow. It also specifies the necessary limb segment orientations from among many possibilities, activates appropriate muscle groups, and inhibits others to meet those specifications.

Reaching can be separated into two different phases. In the transport phase of reaching, the hand is moved toward an object whose position is determined by vision or memory. In the acquisition phase, grasp formation depends on somatosensory and visual information on the limb and target, familiarity with the target, and perhaps on predetermined motor programs. These two phases mature at different rates, may be controlled independently before becoming coordinated, and can be dissociated by focal brain lesions. Posterior parietal damage may affect neurons coding eye position in the head and stimulus location on the retina that, together with neurons in motor and premotor cortex, permit hand movements to visual targets in a body-centered coordinate system.

In "optic ataxia" as described by Balint, patients reportedly reach as if blind toward targets they nevertheless can see and describe. Limb strength and position sense are normal; however, there is severe visual sensory loss and poor visuospatial perception, and patients may even appear demented because of their extensive bilateral lesions. Inability to reach and grasp targets in these cases is often multifactorial, including V1-type visual field defects, defective visual attention, and inability to locate targets with the eyes. Indeed, in screening for optic ataxia, the examiner should verify that the patient has foveated the target for a reach before making any observations on limb movement control. Another possible cause of defective reaching is abnormal sensorimotor transformation, an inability to transform the visual coordinates of external objects to appropriate limb coordinates for generating accurate reaches.

Lesions in the right inferior and superior parietal lobules, as in Balint's original case, are likely to produce visuomotor difficulty in reaches conducted with the left hand to both visual fields (hand effects) and with both hands to the left visual fields (field effects). Subsequent studies of patients with defective reaching have demonstrated lesions in the inferior parietal lobule, the occipitotemporal region, or both. Distance and direction errors may be dissociable, especially with lesions of the inferior posterior parietal cortex, suggesting that localization of a target with reaching movements depends on a network of structures in the visual association cortex.

Positive Visual Phenomena

Cerebral lesions that affect vision usually create deficits in the visual fields—that is, **negative phenomena**. On occasions, however, they create **positive phenomena,** in which false visual images are seen. These false visual images can be classified as visual perseverations, hallucinations, and distortions (dysmetropsia).

Visual Perseveration

Visual perseveration is the persistence, recurrence, or duplication of a visual image. It is a rare complaint in patients with cerebral lesions. Several varieties exist: Palinopsia—the perseveration of a visual image in time; cerebral diplopia or polyopia—the perseveration of a visual image in space; and illusory visual spread—the contents or surface appearance of an object spread beyond the spatial boundaries of the object.

The content of visual hallucinations is often imagery created de novo, or sometimes from the distant past (experiential hallucinations), but the palinopsic illusion contains elements of a more recently viewed scene or even one that is still being viewed. There are at least two forms of **palinopsia**, an immediate and a delayed type. With the **immediate type** of palinopsia, an image persists after the disappearance of the actual scene, usually fading after a period of several minutes. This type of palinopsia bears some similarity to the normal phenomenon of an afterimage experienced after prolonged viewing of a bright object. With the **delayed type** of palinopsia, an image of a previously seen object reappears after an interval of minutes to hours, sometimes repeatedly for days or even weeks. Some patients have both immediate and delayed types of palinopsia.

A perseverated image can assume almost any location in the visual field. It may persist in the same retinal location as the original image, which is usually at the fovea, and thus move as the eyes move, much as a normal afterimage does. Sometimes, the image is translocated into a coexistent visual field defect and indeed can be a transient feature in the evolution of cerebral homonymous field defects. In other cases, the image is multiplied across otherwise intact visual fields. On rare occasions, the location of palinopsic images is contextually specific, as when patients report that after viewing a face on television, everyone else in the room has the same face as the person on television, or that the sign over one shop reappears on the boarding over other shops. Although some of these cases may represent a complex form of palinopsic polyopia, others may also be consistent with a constant foveal or perifoveal perseverative image that repeatedly manifests itself when the context is appropriate.

A wide range of other symptoms can accompany palinopsia. An associated homonymous visual field defect is almost always present and may be a complete hemianopia, incomplete hemianopia, superior quadrantanopia, or inferior quadrantanopia. There may be other spatial illusions, such as metamorphopsia, macropsia, and micropsia. Less frequently, ventral stream deficits occur, such as topographagnosia, prosopagnosia, and achromatopsia.

The natural history of palinopsia is variable. In some patients, palinopsia is a transient phase in either the resolution or progression of a visual field defect and lasts from days to months, eventually resolving. Other cases of palinopsia persist for months or even years. Anticonvulsant medication may prove helpful in prolonged cases.

The pathophysiologic mechanisms of palinopsia are unclear. The main hypotheses include (1) a pathologic exaggeration of the normal afterimage; (2) a seizure disorder; (3) hallucinations; and (4) psychogenic. It is likely that different mechanisms account for similar palinopic phenomena in different patients.

In etiologic investigations, drug-induced palinopsia must be considered first. Intoxication with hallucinogens such as mescaline, lysergic acid diethylamide (LSD), and 3,4-methylenedioxymethamphetamine (Ecstasy) can cause palinopsia, sometimes permanently. Isolated reports assert that palinopsia and other visual illusions may occur with prescribed medication, such as clomiphene, interleukin 2, and trazodone, or with abnormal metabolic states such as nonketotic hyperglycemia. Palinopsia can also occur in psychiatric conditions, such as schizophrenia and psychotic depression. Once intoxication and psychiatric conditions are excluded, visual perseveration almost always indicates a cerebral lesion.

The localizing value of palinopsia is not clear. Most studies find a predominance of right parieto-occipital lesions in patients with palinopsia, although left hemispheric lesions may be under-represented because of aphasia. There are also reports of medial occipital and temporo-occipital lesions verified by neuroimaging and autopsy results.

Patients with **cerebral polyopia** see two or more copies of a single object simultaneously. This form of visual perseveration is described much less frequently than is palinopsia. It occurs with monocular viewing, distinguishing it from the binocular diplopia caused by misalignment of the eyes. Cerebral polyopia can generally be differentiated from monocular polyopia caused by ocular abnormalities such as uncorrected or miscorrected refractive errors, corneal opacities, and cataract, because the images of cerebral polyopia are all seen with equal clarity, do not resolve during viewing with a pinhole, and are unchanged in appearance whether the patient is viewing binocularly or monocularly with either eye. Some patients experience cerebral polyopia only in certain positions of gaze, causing confusion with binocular diplopia until the monocular nature of the polyopia is recognized. Some patients see only two images; others see dozens.

Cerebral polyopia is most commonly encountered after parietal lobe or parieto-occipital region strokes. It can occur as a transient phase in the recovery from cortical blindness secondary to strokes or traumatic injury. Other reported causes of cerebral polyopia include encephalitis, multiple sclerosis, and tumors. Cerebral polyopia rarely occurs in isolation and is usually associated with other problems such as homonymous visual field defects, difficulties with visually guided reaching, cerebral achromatopsia or dyschromatopsia, object agnosia, fluctuations in the visual image, and abnormal visual afterimages.

Patients with **illusory visual spread** see the contents or surface appearance of an object spread beyond the spatial boundaries of the object. Thus, wallpaper patterns spread beyond the surface of the wall, and cloth patterns spread from a shirt to the wearer's face. Illusory visual spread may occur in isolation or may be a feature of palinopsic images.

Visual Hallucinations

Hallucinations are perceptions without external stimulation of the relevant sensory organ. They are common in patients with dementia or confusional states secondary to metabolic insults, including alcohol withdrawal, where they form the predominant type of hallucination. Drugs reported to cause hallucinations include digoxin, bupropion, ganciclovir, vincristine, cyclosporine, lithium, lidocaine, itraconazole, dopaminergic agonists, and baclofen withdrawal. Visual hallucinations can occur in patients with a variety of psychiatric disorders. In such cases, they are usually accompanied by hallucinations in other sensory modalities (especially auditory) and by other signs of mental illness.

Isolated visual hallucinations in persons with intact cognition and mental function are often a sign of underlying neurologic or ophthalmologic disease. Isolated visual hallucinations can be separated into three main pathophysiologic groups (1) release hallucinations, (2) visual seizures, and (3) migraine.

Release Hallucinations (Charles Bonnet Syndrome)

Bilateral simultaneous or sequential visual loss from any cause can result in visual hallucinations. These are often called **release hallucinations** because it is thought that they arise from, or are "released" in, visual cortex that is no longer receiving the incoming visual sensory impulses that usually filter out nonvisual stimuli. Release visual hallucinations usually occur in patients with visual acuity in the better eye of 20/60 or worse. Any type of visual loss, whether ocular or cerebral in origin, can lead to release hallucinations. When the disease-causing visual loss is ocular and occurs first in one eye and then in the other, hallucinations usually do not develop until the second eye loses vision.

Some series report that up to 57% of patients with a variety of causes of visual loss have release hallucinations. In fact, the true incidence of release hallucinations may be much higher because of reluctance on the part of affected patients to tell their physicians that they are experiencing hallucinations, for fear of being labeled "crazy." Patients with release hallucinations are mentally lucid; the majority are aware that the visions are not real; and, in general, they are not distressed by them. Notable is the absence of other sensory hallucinations.

Release hallucinations can be classified as simple (unformed) or complex (formed) (Fig. 13.9). Simple

Figure 13.9 Appearance of both simple and complex hallucinations. Drawing by a patient with occipital lobe damage showing his most frequent hallucinations. Note that some are complex (*above*), whereas others are simple (*middle and below*). (Reprinted with permission from Anderson SW, Rizzo M. Hallucinations following occipital lobe damage: The pathologic activation of visual representations. *J Clin Exp Neurol.* 1994;16:651–663.)

hallucinations consist of brief flashes or points of light, colored lines, shapes, or patterns (phosphenes). Complex hallucinations contain recognizable objects and figures, such as flowers, animals, and humans, with a potential for bizarre, dreamlike imagery of considerable detail and clarity, including dragons and angels. Sometimes the vision is a recognizable image from the patient's past, such as a deceased friend or relative. Simple hallucinations are at least twice as common as complex ones. In most series, complex hallucinations account for 10% to 30% of release hallucinations.

Some authors reserve the term "Charles Bonnet syndrome" for the association of visual loss with complex formed hallucinations. However, some patients have simple hallucinations initially and later experience complex ones. A similar progression in visual hallucinatory content is reported in normal people subjected to sensory deprivation. Furthermore, the type of hallucination does not correlate with an anatomic location and thus lacks diagnostic value.

There must be other contributing factors besides visual loss in the development of release hallucinations, because they do not develop in all patients with visual loss. Older age may be one risk factor, but even patients as young as 10 years can have release hallucinations. Social isolation is another potential factor, thought to act by accentuating the sensory deprivation of visual loss.

In the brain, visual experience is represented by patterns of coordinated impulses within the visual cortex. These patterns are generated by sensory stimuli and represent the current experience of the individual; however, the brain can generate these neural patterns spontaneously and, in fact, does so during sensory deprivation from either imposed isolation or pathologic denervation. These spontaneous neural patterns could correspond to hallucinations. A similar explanation has been invoked for the phantom-limb phenomenon after amputation and presumably also underlies other release phenomena, such as musical hallucinations in cases of deafness. Supporting evidence for the analogy with sensory deprivation includes the fact that these hallucinations tend to occur when patients are alone or inactive, and in the evening or night when the lighting is poor.

Release hallucinations may be brief, with each episode lasting a few seconds or minutes, or nearly continuous. Hallucinations most often follow the onset of visual loss by several days or weeks, but the delay can be longer. That loss of vision triggers the hallucinations is supported by the observation that release hallucinations disappear in patients whose vision subsequently improves. In many patients, release hallucinations last for a few days to a few months and then spontaneously disappear even though visual function remains stable. In others, however, the hallucinations persist for years or even decades.

Although release hallucinations do not bother many patients, a sizable minority is quite bothered and finds them highly disturbing. Unfortunately, there is no proven effective treatment for such patients. Moving socially isolated patients into a more stimulating environment may lessen the hallucinations, and anticonvulsant drugs may improve the hallucinations but not consistently.

Visual Seizures

Visual seizures are not common in patients with epilepsy. When they do occur, they can be confused with migraine and release hallucinations. Much of the confusion related to the localizing value of the visual content of hallucinations stems from failure to distinguish between release hallucinations and true visual seizures. The content of release hallucinations is highly variable and independent of the site of pathology, whereas the content of visual seizures may have more localizing value. Older human stimulation experiments found that simple flashes of light and colors resulted from electric activity in striate cortex, whereas stimulation of visual association cortex in areas 19 and temporal regions resulted in complex formed images. A similar distinction probably holds for epileptic visual hallucinations (Fig. 13.10). Nevertheless, temporal lobe lesions can occasionally produce simple unformed hallucinations, and occipital lesions can produce complex hallucinations. In the latter setting, spread of ictal activity into extrastriate cortex probably is responsible for the complex character of the hallucinations. Hence, the content at the onset of a visual seizure has the most localizing value.

The association with other ictal phenomena or a homonymous visual field defect may be helpful in identifying visual seizures from a cerebral lesion. Accompanying head or eye deviation (usually but not always contralateral) and rapid blinking are common accompaniments of occipital seizures. Other features that also strongly support ictal origin are signs of more distant spread of seizure activity, such as confusion, dysphasia, tonic–clonic limb movements, and the automatisms of complex partial seizures. Because routine scalp electroencephalographic leads often do not localize an occipital focus accurately, suspicion of such a focus usually requires intracranial electrodes for confirmation.

Although a variety of pathologies in the visual cortex may be associated with visual seizures, one syndrome requiring emphasis is **benign childhood epilepsy with occipital spike–waves**. This idiopathic epilepsy syndrome begins between 5 and 9 years of age and ceases spontaneously in the teenage years. Seizures are characterized by blindness and/or hallucinations of both simple and complex types, and it

Figure 13.10 Visual illusions of occipital lobe epilepsy as perceived by four different patients. (Reprinted with permission from Panayiotopoulos CP. Elementary visual hallucinations in migraine and epilepsy. *J Neurol Neurosurg Psychiatry.* 1994;57:1371–1374.)

may progress to motor or partial complex seizures. Some children develop nausea and headache following the visual seizure, leading to an erroneous diagnosis of migraine. The diagnosis is established by occipital spike–waves occurring during eye closure on electro-encephalography.

Migrainous Hallucinations

A variety of visual phenomena can occur in migraine. In migraine with visual aura (classic migraine), the visual phenomena generally precede the headache, whereas in migraine aura without headache (acephalgic migraine), visual phenomena occur alone. Photopic images are most common in both settings and are described as spots, wavy lines, or shimmering of the environment similar to heat waves over a road on a hot day. The scintillating scotoma is a blind region surrounded by a margin of sparkling lights, which often slowly enlarges over time and which may move across the visual field or expand concentrically from a small point to distort some or all of the field of vision of both eyes. In some patients, the sparkling margin can be discerned as a zig-zag pattern of lines oriented at 60 degrees to each other, usually in one hemifield and on the leading edge of a C-shaped scotoma (Fig. 13.11). This is the fortification spectrum or teichopsia (from the Greek word *teichos,* meaning "town wall"), which is so-named because of the resemblance of the zig-zag margin to the ground plan of town fortifications in Europe. There may be several sets of zig-zag lines in parallel, often shimmering or oscillating in brightness. They may be black and white or vividly colored. These zig-zag lines begin near the center of the field and expand toward the periphery with increasing speed over a period of about 20 minutes, with both the speed and the size of the lines increasing with retinal eccentricity. The relation of speed and size to eccentricity is predicted by the cortical magnification factor, which is a measure of the area of visual field represented in a given amount of striate cortex as a function of retinal eccentricity. This suggests that migrainous hallucinations are generated by a wave of neuronal excitation spreading from posterior to anterior striate cortex at a constant speed, leaving a transient neuronal depression that causes the temporary scotoma in its wake. It is also hypothesized that the zig-zag nature of the lines reflects the sensitivity to line orientation of striate cortex and the pattern of inhibitory interconnections within and among striate columns.

Other Types of Hallucinations

Hallucinations associated with lesions of the mesencephalon, so-called **peduncular hallucinations** (or peduncular hallucinosis), are rare. They have many similarities to the complex release hallucinations

Figure 13.11 Photographic negative of a migraine phosphene protocol. The scintillating phosphene was progressing through the lower quadrant and part of the upper quadrant of the left visual hemifield. Thirteen drawings were made between 2 and 29 minutes after the phosphene first appeared near the center of the visual field. To evaluate the distance between the phosphene and the center of the visual field, several radii were drawn across the protocol. The angular distance from the fovea center, computed in degrees of visual angle, is indicated by circles. Circles and radii were added to the sheet after the observations were made. Observation distance = 34 cm. (Reprinted with permission from Grüsser O–J. Migraine phosphenes and the retino–cortical magnification factor. *Vision Res.* 1995;35:1125–1134.)

associated with visual loss. They can be continuous or episodic, with detailed formed imagery, such as flying birds, dogs, roaring lions, crawling snakes, gangsters with knife wounds, and men herding cattle. These hallucinations are not stereotyped and vary from one episode to the next. In some cases with thalamic rather than midbrain infarcts, the hallucinations are from events in the patient's past. Many patients with peduncular hallucinations realize that the hallucinations are not real. Similar hallucinations occur for sounds, and some patients have multimodality hallucinations, involving vision, touch, sound, and even the sense of body posture.

The most frequently described etiology of peduncular hallucinations is infarction involving the substantia nigra pars reticulata and its connections to the pedunculopontine nucleus, and/or the reticular formation and the ascending reticular activating system. Peduncular hallucinations are almost invariably associated with inversion of the sleep–wake cycle—that is, diurnal somnolence and nocturnal insomnia. Other associated signs from damage to adjacent structures in the midbrain include unilateral or bilateral oculomotor nerve palsy, hemiparkinsonism, hemiparesis, and gait ataxia. In cases caused by infarction, the hallucinations can resolve, but they usually persist indefinitely, although the episodes may become shorter.

Rare patients experience **hallucinations with eye closure**. Causative settings include drug toxicity from atropine and probably lidocaine, infection with high fever, and after major surgery. It has been proposed that they are similar to hypnagogic hallucinations, suggesting a disturbance in sleep–wake cycle mechanisms.

Visual Distortions (Dysmetropsia)

Illusions about the spatial aspect of visual stimuli can be separated into three main categories: (1) micropsia—the illusion that objects are smaller than in reality; (2) macropsia—the illusion that objects are larger than in reality; (3) metamorphopsia—the illusion that objects are distorted.

Micropsia is the most common of the visual distortions and has the largest variety of possible etiologies. Convergence-accommodative micropsia is a normal and physiologic phenomenon in which an object at a set distance appears smaller when the observer focuses at near rather than far, even though there is no change in the retinal angle covered by the object and no change in its spatial relations to the surroundings. It is unusual for accommodative micropsia to be a source of complaints.

Psychogenic micropsia is the subject of extensive psychoanalytic interpretations, with the most prevailing theory being that it occurs in patients who are literally trying to "distance" themselves from environments fraught with conflict.

Retinal micropsia occurs when the distance between photoreceptors is increased. The micropsia usually occurs in foveal vision and is caused by macular edema. There may be associated metamorphopsia if the receptor separation is irregular. Visual acuity is also reduced in such cases. Causes of macular edema and micropsia include central serous chorioretinopathy, diabetic retinopathy, severe papilledema, and retinal detachment. The condition may resolve or persist for years.

Cerebral micropsia, in contrast to retinal micropsia, is always binocular. Unusual variants include hemimicropsia, which occurs in the hemifield contralateral to the cerebral lesion. Given the small number of cases, the localization value of cerebral micropsia is uncertain. Temporo-occipital lesions are present in some cases, with either medial or lateral involvement. One survey of over 3,000 adolescent students revealed that complaints of episodic micropsia or macropsia were not rare, occurring in 9%. Some occurred in the hypnagogic state or during fever, and there was a correlation with a history of migraine. Indeed,

Figure 13.12 Drawing of cerebral micropsia by a child with migraine. The child stated that during some of her attacks, other children (*right*) appeared unusually small to her (*left*). (Reprinted with permission from Hachinski VC, Porchawka J, Steele JC. Visual symptoms in the migraine syndrome. *Neurology.* 1973;23:570–579.)

micropsia occurs not infrequently in migraine, particularly in childhood, and migraine is probably the most common setting in which cerebral micropsia is encountered (Fig. 13.12).

Macropsia is much less frequently described than micropsia. Retinal macropsia can occur in the late scarring stage of macular edema, and it can be a side effect of the drug zolpidem. Cerebral macropsia can rarely occur during seizures. Cerebral hemimacropsia was reported in a patient with a left occipital tumor and also in a patient with a right occipital infarct. As noted above, both micropsia and macropsia occur episodically in children and seem to correlate with childhood migraine.

Ocular causes of **metamorphopsia** are far more common than cerebral causes. Most often, the metamorphopsia occurs from retinal pathology causing traction, such as epiretinal membrane, and in such cases, it often coexists with micropsia. As with retinal micropsia, metamorphopsia from ocular disease is usually monocular. In those rare cases in which it is binocular, the distortions are almost never identical in the two eyes. Metamorphopsia is most often tested using an Amsler grid.

Cerebral metamorphopsia occurs in some patients during seizures. Other reported causes include right parietal glioma, right parietal arteriovenous malformation, medial posterior cerebral artery infarction, a transient stage in the development of cortical blindness, and even brainstem lesions.

Tests of Higher Visual Function

Chapter 1 of this text contains detailed descriptions of the standard vision tests used to measure the visual abilities in patients. However, standard vision and

Figure 13.13 Tests of higher visual function. A plate (number 22/30) from the Hooper Visual Organization Test (HVOT). The patient is required to identify each of the 30 items on the plate from their cut-up rearranged line drawings. This test is memory dependent, in that it depends on the history of exposure of the patient to the items on the plate.

screening tools generally do not provide a measure of higher-order visual functions, nor are they meant to do so. Basic categories of higher visual function tests include tests of:

1 **Reading,** such as the reading subtest of the Wide Range Achievement Test and Chapman–Cook Speed of Reading Test.
2 **Visual recognition,** such as the recognition of famous faces, the Boston Naming Test, and the Visual Naming Test from the Multilingual Aphasia Examination.
3 **Mental imagery,** such as the Hooper Visual Organization Test (Fig. 13.13).
4 **Visual perception,** such as the Facial Recognition Test and Judgment of Line Orientation.
5 **Visual attention,** such as the Cookie Theft Picture (see Fig. 13.8), and the line bisection task.
6 **Visuoconstruction,** such as drawing to dictation and copy (Fig. 13.14), writing to dictation copy and spontaneously, and the 3D Block Construction Test.
7 **Visual memory,** such as the Benton Visual Retention Test (BVRT) and relevant sections of the Wechsler Memory Scale (WMS).

Glossary of Cerebral Visual Deficits

Agnosia (also known as **associative agnosia**). The inability to recognize previously familiar objects despite adequate perception. Objects are effectively stripped of their meanings.

Figure 13.14 Tests of higher visual function. **A:** The Rey–Osterreith Complex Figure. **B:** Defective copy of this figure by a patient with frontotemporal dementia.

Alexia without agraphia (also known as **pure alexia** or **acquired dyslexia**). The acquired inability to read in previously literate individuals. Should not be confused with developmental dyslexia.
Anosognosia. Failure to recognize one's own impairment (see Anton syndrome).
Anton Syndrome. The denial of cerebral blindness.
Apperceptive agnosia. Failure to identify previously familiar objects due to impaired perception.
Balint syndrome. Simultanagnosia, ocular apraxia, and optic ataxia.
Blindsight. Residual vision in the fields of a putative striate scotoma; redefined more broadly as a "visual capacity in a field defect in the absence of acknowledged awareness."
Central (paracentral) scotoma. A visual field defect at (or near) the fixation point.
Cerebral achromatopsia (also known as **central achromatopsia**). An uncommon defect of color perception caused by damage to the visual cortex and connections.

The term achromatopsia implies complete color loss. The term dyschromatopsia should be used when there is some sparing of color sensation.

Cerebral akinetopsia. Defective processing of visual motion cues due to cerebral lesions. The ability to perceive motion direction, shape from motion, and other "higher-order" motion processes may be impaired.

Cerebral blindness. Bilateral loss of vision from bilateral damage to the optic radiations or striate cortex. Cortical blindness (see below) is a form of cerebral blindness.

Color agnosia. Inability to identify colors despite preserved ability to discriminate among colors.

Color anomia. Inability to name colors despite adequate color perception and recognition.

Cortical blindness. Inability to see following bilateral damage to the visual cortex. Affected patients generally have considerable damage that extends well beyond V1. Cortical blindness is a specific form of cerebral blindness (see above).

Foveal (macular) sparing. A homonymous hemianopia in which 2 to 10 degrees of the central vision are preserved on the affected side.

Foveal (macular) splitting. A homonymous hemianopia that includes the entire foveal representation on the affected side.

Keyhole vision (cerebral tunnel vision). Homonymous hemianopias may be bilateral (double homonymous hemianopia) leading to a severe loss of peripheral vision; if there is bilateral foveal sparing, a tunnel or keyhole of vision remains around fixation.

Macropsia. The illusion that objects are larger than in reality.

Metamorphopsia. The illusion that objects are distorted.

Micropsia. The illusion that objects are smaller than in reality.

Ocular apraxia (also called **psychic paralysis of gaze** or **spasm of fixation**). An inability to move the eyes to objects of interest despite unrestricted ocular rotations.

Optic ataxia. A defect of hand movements under visual guidance despite adequate limb strength, position sense, and coordination.

Palinopsia. Persistence of visual afterimages of an object despite looking away.

Prosopagnosia. Inability to recognize previously familiar faces or to learn new faces despite adequate perception. This is a restricted form of (associative) agnosia.

Scotoma. An area of blindness surrounded by intact vision. The physiologic blind spot is a scotoma.

Simultanagnosia (simultagnosia). This is often equated with Balint's "spatial disorder of attention," an inability to interpret the totality of a picture scene despite preservation of ability to apprehend individual portions of the whole.

Examination of the Pupils and Accommodation*

Assessment of Pupillary Size, Shape, and Function
  History
  Examination
  Pharmacologic Testing

Assessment of Accommodation, Convergence, and the Near Response
  History
  Examination

Assessment of Pupillary Size, Shape, and Function

Assessment of the pupils requires a precise history and careful examination and may be followed by pharmacologic testing.

History

Patients are often not aware of any abnormality of pupil size. A spouse, friend, or physician may bring the abnormality to attention. The pupil abnormality may be intermittent or episodic. Dating the onset of the pupillary abnormality may be aided by reviewing photographs with the aid of a magnifying lens, although digital photography has made this technique less useful.

Symptoms associated with abnormalities of pupillary size and shape include light sensitivity, difficulty focusing while adjusting to changing lighting conditions, or blurred vision. Complaints of blurry vision are typically nonspecific.

Important past medical history includes a history of previous infections, trauma, operations (particularly in the neck), or migraine. Occupational history may be important. Farmers or gardeners may be exposed to plants or pesticides that produce pupillary dilation or constriction. Physicians, nurses, or other health professionals may work with or have access to topical dilating or constricting substances. Medication history may be important as opiates may cause pupil constriction, and anticholinergics used in inhalers for asthmatics may cause pupillary dilation.

Examination

Slit lamp examination of the anterior segment is essential in patients with a pupillary abnormality. It may reveal a corneal injury that could affect pupillary size or anterior chamber inflammation that may be associated with ciliary spasm and miosis. Examination of the iris should include assessment of the iris sphincter for small traumatic tears and transillumination of the iris for defects. In addition, by placing a wide beam at an angle to the iris and turning the light off and on, the light reflex can be assessed for segmental defects, such as occur in eyes with tonic pupils or aberrant regeneration of the oculomotor nerve.

Pupil measurements may be performed using a hand-held pupil gauge, hand-held pupil camera, or infrared video pupillometry. The hand-held pupil gauge is held next to the eye to determine pupil size in both light and darkness. Pupil gauges consist of a series of solid or open circles or half circles with diameters that increase by 0.2 mm in steps (Fig. 14.1). Infrared video pupillometry is perhaps the most accurate method of assessing the size of the pupil. An infrared video pupillometer permits observation of pupils not only in lighted conditions but also in total darkness. Commercial infrared devices are available and supplant pupil photography but have not been adopted widely.

During clinical evaluation, the examiner should first assess the size of the pupils. The examiner should determine if the pupils are equal. If they are not equal, the examiner should determine whether the difference in size is greater in light or darkness. Other questions that should be answered pertain to whether the pupils constrict with the same velocity, whether they redilate equally with the same velocity, and how the pupillary reaction to light compares to the pupillary reaction to near. Finally, the examiner must assess whether a relative afferent pupillary defect is present.

Assessing Pupillary Size
The diameter of both pupils should be estimated or measured in light, using either normal room light or

---

*The authors acknowledge the past contributions of Kathleen B. Digre to this chapter.

Figure 14.1 Pupil gauges. The best gauges measure in 0.5-mm steps.

a hand-held light source. The diameter of the pupils should then be assessed in darkness, using the dimmest room light in which the examiner can still see the edge of the pupil. Finally, the pupillary size should be assessed during near stimulation using an accommodative target to achieve maximum constriction of the pupils.

Measurements of the pupil in light and dark should determine if **anisocoria**, a difference in the pupils of 0.4 mm or more, is present. A substantial percentage (20%) of the normal population has clinically detectable anisocoria, referred to as "physiologic anisocoria." Anisocoria may be produced by damage to the iris sphincter or dilator muscles or to their nerve supply. The amount of anisocoria may be affected by illumination. For example, a greater degree of anisocoria is present in darkness than in light in patients with physiologic anisocoria or Horner syndrome. Anisocoria can also be affected by the degree of accommodation, by fatigue, and by sympathetic drive.

Testing the Pupillary Reaction to Light

When testing the reaction of a pupil to light shined in the eye—the **direct pupillary light reaction**—it is important to have a quiet and dimly lit room. The patient must be fixating on a distant target to eliminate any effect of accommodation on pupillary size.

The light source used to illuminate the pupils should be bright enough to produce a maximum rate of con-

striction and redilation. If the light source is too bright, a prolonged contraction lasting several seconds will occur, making determination of the normal light reflex difficult. It may be helpful to use a dim secondary light source to provide oblique illumination of the pupil in some cases as this technique increases visualization of darkly pigmented irides. Pupil visualization with very dark irides also may be enhanced having the patient look up while the light is directed forward; this technique moves the corneal light reflex away from the axis of the pupil (Fig. 14.2, and **Videos 14.1** and **14.2**).

The light source should be directed straight into the eye for a few seconds and then moved downward away from the eye to eliminate the stimulation. The pupil response should be assessed during this maneuver, which should be repeated several times. The normal response to a bright light is a contraction called "pupillary capture." "Pupillary escape," on the other hand, is a phenomenon in which the pupil initially constricts and then slowly redilates and returns to its original size. Pupillary escape most often occurs on the side of a diseased optic nerve or retina and in normal persons tested with a low-intensity light source. The initial size of the pupil is important in assessing both pupillary capture and pupillary escape. A larger pupil is more likely to show pupillary escape, whereas a smaller pupil is more likely to show pupillary capture.

The latency and speed with which a pupil constricts to light and redilates after light stimulation can be

Figure 14.2 Comparison of the oblique illumination technique and upgaze pupil testing technique. **A:** The normal method of testing the pupillary light reaction is with the patient looking straight ahead and the examiner aiming the light directly at the center of the cornea. **B:** One way to try to see the pupillary light reaction better in a patient with dark irides is to have the patient look straight ahead and aim the light upward from below. **C:** An even better way to see the pupillary light reaction in a patient with dark irides is to have the patient look up and shine the light from directly in front of the patient. (Reprinted with permission from Hsu JL, Weikert MP, Foroozan R. Modified upgaze technique for pupil examination. *J Neuroophthalmol.* 2010;30(4):344–346.) See also **videos 14.1** and **14.2**.

assessed using pupillography. The use of pupillography to record waveforms of pupillary constriction and dilation is generally limited to research, although commercial pupillographic devices have been developed.

When light is shined in one eye, the contralateral pupil constricts as well in a **consensual light response**. The consensual light response is assessed using a light source for illumination of the pupil of one eye and a dimmer light source that is held obliquely to the side of the contralateral eye being observed. The consensual pupillary response should be approximately equal in both velocity and extent to the direct response, because the pupillary decussation in the midbrain is about 50% to each eye.

Testing the Pupillary Near Response

The near response, a component of the near triad that also includes accommodation and convergence, should be tested in a room with light that is adequate for the patient to fixate an accommodative target. A nonaccommodative target, such as a pencil, may not be a sufficient stimulus to produce a proper near response even in a normal person. The near response should not

be induced by having the patient look at a bright light stimulus, because the light itself may produce pupillary constriction. One can document the light and near response with photographs or pupillometry (Fig. 14.3).

Assessment of Pupillary Dilation

Dilation of the pupils occurs in a variety of settings. Most often, the pupils dilate after they have constricted to light or near stimulation. In patients with certain retinal and, less often, optic nerve disease, they may actually dilate when light is shined in one eye (paradoxical pupillary response). Reflex pupillary dilation can also be elicited by sudden noise or by pinching the back of the neck.

When assessing pupillary dilation, the examiner should look specifically for dilation lag. This phenomenon is present when there is more anisocoria 4 to 5 seconds after pupillary constriction to light than there is 15 seconds after pupillary constriction. Dilation lag typically occurs in patients with a defect in the sympathetic innervation of the pupil (i.e., Horner syndrome), although it also occurs in some normal subjects.

Dilation lag may be tested by observing both pupils simultaneously in a very dim light after a bright light

Figure 14.3 Use of a smartphone camera to document size of the pupils in light and darkness in a normal subject. **A:** In room light without any other stimulation. **B:** In room light during stimulation with a bright light. **C:** In room light during stimulation with an accommodative target. Note associated convergence.

has been turned off. Normal pupils return to their widest size within 12 to 15 seconds, with most of their dilation occurring in the first 5 seconds. Pupils that show dilation lag may take up to 25 seconds to return to maximum size in darkness with most of the dilation occurring about 10 to 12 seconds after the light goes out. Infrared pupillography may help identify the phenomenon as well, although some systems allow only one eye to be viewed at a time.

Testing for Light-Near Dissociation

A dissociation between the pupillary response to light stimulation and the pupillary response to near stimulation (light-near dissociation) occurs in patients with a variety of disorders (see Chapter 15). In almost all cases, the pupillary reaction to light is impaired, whereas the pupillary response to near is normal or almost normal. Thus, light-near dissociation should be considered in any patient with an impaired pupillary light reaction. Essentially all cases of light-near dissociation in which there is a normal pupillary reaction to light and a poor pupillary response to near are caused by lack of effort on the part of the patient during attempted near viewing.

Testing for a Relative Afferent Pupillary Defect

When a patient has an optic neuropathy in one eye or an asymmetric bilateral optic neuropathy, covering one eye and then the other reveals that the pupil of the normal eye constricts when it is uncovered and the abnormal eye is covered, whereas the pupil of the abnormal eye dilates when it is uncovered and the pupil of the normal eye is covered (Fig. 14.4). The abnormal pupil is often called a "Marcus Gunn pupil." The term "relative afferent pupillary defect" is preferred because it describes the nature of the pupillary abnormality.

The **swinging flashlight test** (Fig. 14.5), which accentuates differences in the pupillary response to light, is probably the most valuable clinical test of optic

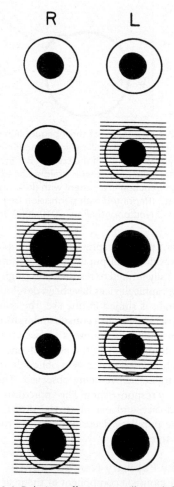

Figure 14.4 Relative afferent pupillary defect in the left eye demonstrated by the alternate cover test as described by Kestenbaum. The left pupil dilates (as does the right) when the left eye is uncovered and the right eye is covered. (Redrawn from HS Thompson. Pupillary signs in the ophthalmologic diagnosis of optic nerve disease. *Trans Ophthalmol Soc UK.* 1976;96(3):377–381.)

R   L

Figure 14.5 Relative afferent pupillary defect in the left eye demonstrated using the swinging flashlight test. The pupils constrict when the light is shined directly into the right eye; however, when the flashlight is swung back to the left eye, both pupils dilate. (Redrawn from HS Thompson. Pupillary signs in the ophthalmologic diagnosis of optic nerve disease. *Trans Ophthalmol Soc UK.* 1976;96(3):377–381.)

nerve dysfunction available to the general physician. The patient focuses on a distant target in a darkened room, and a light is swung back and forth multiple times to bring out the best response.

The swinging flashlight test should be performed with a bright hand light in a darkened room to maximize the amplitude of the pupillary movement and make it easier to see a small RAPD. Using too bright a light will produce an afterimage that may keep the pupils small for several seconds, obscuring the pupillary dilation in the abnormal eye. The patients must fixate on a distant target during testing to prevent miosis that occurs in the near response. In patients with ocular misalignment (i.e., strabismus or displacement of the globe by an orbital or intracranial process), care must be taken to shine the light along the visual axis. The light should cross from one eye to the other fairly rapidly but should remain on each eye for 3 to 5 seconds to allow pupillary stabilization. Thus, there are really two parts of the pupillary response that must be observed during the swinging flashlight test: (1) the initial pupillary constriction response and (2) the pupillary escape that is observed for 2 to 5 seconds after the light meets the pupil. Most examiners vary the rate at which they move the light from eye to eye. There is often an optimum swing rate that brings out an RAPD and that varies among patients.

Some authors recommend moving the light from one pupil to the other before the latter can escape from the consensual response to bring out an afferent defect. However, **the light should never be left longer on one eye than on the other**. This might tend to create a RAPD in the eye with the longer light exposure, because the longer the light is kept on the eye, the more pupillary dilation occurs as the eye adapts to the light.

In addition, if the retina becomes bleached in one eye and not in the other, a small RAPD will be produced. Special care must be taken to keep retina bleach equal, especially when measuring with neutral density filters greater than 1.2 log units in density (see below).

Finally, the swinging flashlight test can be performed as long as there are two pupils, even when one pupil is nonreactive and dilated or constricted from neurologic disease, iris trauma, or topical drugs. Recall that as the light is shifted from the normal to the abnormal eye, the total pupillomotor input is reduced. Thus, the efferent stimulus for pupillary constriction is reduced in *both* eyes so that both pupils dilate. In performing the swinging flashlight test, one tends to observe only the pupil that is being illuminated; however, the opposite pupil is responding **in an identical fashion**. Thus, if one pupil is mechanically or pharmacologically nonreactive, one can simply perform a swinging flashlight test observing only the reactive pupil. If the abnormal eye is the eye with a fixed pupil, the pupil of the normal eye will constrict briskly when light is shined directly in it and will dilate when the light is shined in the opposite eye. If the abnormal eye is the eye with the reactive pupil, the pupil will constrict when light is shined in the opposite eye and dilate when the light is shined directly in it. This is extremely helpful in attempting to determine if a patient with an oculomotor nerve paresis or traumatic iridoplegia also has an optic neuropathy or retinal dysfunction.

The swinging flashlight test can be further refined in patients in whom a unilateral optic neuropathy is suspected but who do not seem to have a RAPD when a standard swinging flashlight test is performed. In such patients, the use of a neutral density filter with a transmission of 0.3 log units often permits the detection of the defect (Fig. 14.6). The test is performed as follows. The filter is first placed over one eye, and the swinging flashlight test is performed. The filter is then placed over the opposite eye, and the swinging flashlight test is repeated. If there is truly no defect in the afferent system in either eye, placing the filter over either eye will simply induce a slight but symmetric RAPD in the eye covered by the filter, from reduction in the amount of light entering the system through that eye. On the other hand, if one eye already has a mild RAPD, placement of the filter over that eye will further reduce the amount of light entering the system through that eye, thus increasing the previously inapparent defect and causing it to become recognizable; placement of the filter over the opposite (normal) eye will simply balance the afferent defect in the opposite eye, and there will be no significant asymmetry in pupillary responses to light.

One can quantify the RAPD using graded neutral density filters that are calibrated in percent transmittance. After determining that a RAPD is present, the examiner balances the defect by adding successive neutral density filters in 0.3 logarithmic steps over the **normal** eye while performing the swinging flashlight test until the defect disappears (Fig. 14.7). The most useful neutral density filters are those ranging in transmission from 80% (0.1 log unit) to 1% (2.0 log units) (Fig. 14.8).

To reach the endpoint of the test, the examiner should "overshoot the endpoint"—that is, produce a RAPD in the normal (covered) eye. The examiner should then rebleach the retina of that eye and perform the swinging flashlight test with another filter at the next lower amount. Several "rules of thumb" in measuring the RAPD for various conditions are found in Table 14.1.

There is some correlation between the severity of an RAPD and the size of the peripheral field defects detected with kinetic perimetry using a Goldmann perimeter. There is less convincing evidence of a correlation between the pupillary response and field defects in the central field detected using static perimetry.

Tests used to detect a RAPD, particularly the swinging flashlight test, are sensitive tests for optic nerve dysfunction; however, they represent only one type of test used to determine whether a patient has an optic neuropathy, and, if so, what the degree of severity of the optic nerve dysfunction is.

Figure 14.6 The use of neutral density filters to bring out a relative afferent pupillary defect (RAPD). A previous swinging flashlight test has failed to demonstrate a convincing RAPD. A 0.3 log unit neutral density filter is placed over the right eye and a swinging flashlight test is performed. The filter is then placed over the left eye and the test is repeated. If there is a subtle optic neuropathy in the left eye, placing the filter in front of that eye will reduce the light stimulation even further, and there will now be a RAPD during the swinging flashlight test. When the filter is placed in front of the right eye, however, the reduced brightness in the right eye will tend to balance the reduced brightness in the left eye (from the optic neuropathy), and no RAPD will be seen.

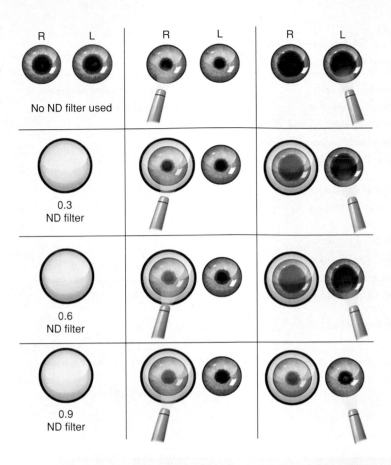

Figure 14.7 Quantification of the relative afferent pupillary defect (RAPD) using neutral density filters and the swinging flashlight test. Neutral density filters of increasing density are placed in front of the normal eye in a patient with a contralateral RAPD, and a swinging flashlight test is performed until the RAPD disappears. In this case, the RAPD is balanced with a 0.9 log unit filter.

Figure 14.8 The equipment needed to quantify or bring out a relative afferent pupillary defect includes a bright handheld light source, a pupil gauge, and a set of photographic neutral density filters in 0.3, 0.6, 0.9, and 1.2 steps.

Table 14.1 Expected RAPD in Various Situations—"Rules of Thumb"

Condition	Expected RAPD in Log Units	Comment
Optic neuritis	0.3 to over 3 log units	If no RAPD, suspect bilateral disease
Optic tract	0.4–0.6 contralateral eye	Look for temporal visual field defect
Pretectal lesion	Contralateral RAPD without VF loss	
Visual field defect	Correlates with Goldmann/Humphrey	
Amblyopia	Less than 0.5 log units	If greater than 1.0 log unit, look for other disease
Anisocoria	0.1 log unit for every 1 mm	Test in light
Macular disease	Better than 20/200, no more than 0.5	Worst macular disease less than 1.0 log unit
Central serous	Less than 0.3 log units	
Central retinal vein occlusion	Ischemic 0.9–1.2 log units	
Central retinal vein occlusion	Nonischemic <0.6 log units	
Retinal detachment	1 quad 0.3; 2 quad 0.6; macular 0.9; complete 2.0	
Retinitis pigmentosa	0.3 log units or less	
Cataract	None	If dense, expect RAPD in opposite eye
Patching; dark adaptation	Up to 1.5 log units in unoccluded eye	Maximum RAPD in 30 min; reverses in 10 min
Glaucoma	Varies	Corresponds with retinal rim
Nonorganic visual loss	None	

Pharmacologic Testing

If a judgment is to be made about the dilation or constriction of the pupil in response to a drop of some drug in the conjunctival sac, then whenever possible one pupil should be used as an internal control (Table 14.2). Thus, if the condition is unilateral, the drug should be placed in both eyes so that the responses of the two eyes can be compared. When the condition is bilateral, no such comparison is possible, but an attempt should be made to make certain that the observed response is indeed caused by the instilled drug. In such cases, the drug may be placed in one eye only so that the responses of the medicated and unmedicated eyes can be compared.

Other problems can occur when performing pharmacologic testing of the pupil using topical drugs. The drug may be outdated and thus more or less potent; the patient may develop sufficient tearing that the strength

Table 14.2 Pharmacologic Testing in Diagnosing Common Pupil Conditions

Agent	Purpose	Dose (%)	Time (min)	Lighting	Measure
Dilute pilocarpine	Supersensitivity testing	0.625	30	Dim light or darkness	Change in pupil diameter
Pilocarpine 2%	Pharmacologic pupil blockade	2	40	Darkness	Change in pupil diameter
Cocaine	To demonstrate sympathetic defect	10	60	Light	Postcocaine anisocoria
Hydroxyamphetamine	To detect postganglionic sympathetic defect		50–60	Light	Absolute dilation OU or anisocoria >1 mm or change in anisocoria >1 mm
Apraclonidine	To demonstrate sympathetic defect	0.5	45	Light	Reversal of anisocoria

of the drug is altered by dilution or washed out of the inferior conjunctival sac before it can be absorbed; the patient may squeeze the eyes tightly during instillation of the drug, thus preventing a sufficient amount of drug from being placed in the inferior conjunctival sac. One must also consider individual variations in the action of the drug on patients of different ages or with different-colored irides. Determining the results of pupillary testing can also be difficult depending on the initial size of the pupil.

Assessment of Accommodation, Convergence, and the Near Response

Accommodation may be too great, too little, or too slow. Disturbances of the other two components of the near response—convergence and pupillary miosis—may manifest themselves as overactive or impaired.

History

While the symptoms of patients with disturbances of accommodation tend to be nonspecific, some aspects of the history may be important. Patients with accommodative insufficiency, for instance, usually complain of blurred vision at near and not in the distance. Patients with the most common problem with accommodation, presbyopia, may report that the farther away they hold an object, the better they can see it. Frequently, presbyopia and other accommodative insufficient states can be precipitated with medications having anticholinergic effects.

Accommodative excess or spasm is typically associated with clear vision at near but poor distance vision. In addition, these patients often complain of brow ache. When convergence is affected in addition to accommodation, other symptoms may be present. Convergence excess is often associated with diplopia in the distance, blurring of vision, oscillopsia, or pain. On the other hand, convergence insufficiency is associated with trouble reading, diplopia at near, blurred vision that clears when either eye is covered, and pain or discomfort during near tasks.

In patients with spasm of the near reflex, symptoms are related to dysfunction of all three components. Such patients have accommodative spasm (up to 8 to 10 diopters), extreme miosis, and strabismus caused by convergence.

Examination

General Principles

Accommodation is the ability of the lens to change its refractive power to keep the image of an object clear on the retina. The primary stimulus for accommodation

is blur, and most tests of accommodation depend on producing or eliminating blur. Stimuli for accommodation besides blur, including chromatic aberration and perceived nearness, may also be used to test accommodation.

Accommodation is part of a complex triad that maintains clear near vision: the **near response** (also called the **near reflex**). Even though the components of the near response—accommodation, convergence, and pupillary miosis—normally work in concert during near viewing, each component can be tested separately. For example, one can weaken the stimulus to accommodation with plus lenses or strengthen the stimulus to accommodation with weak minus lenses without stimulating convergence or miosis. One can use weak base-out prisms to stimulate convergence without changing accommodation. Under certain conditions, one can test accommodation without inducing pupillary constriction. Even in presbyopia, in which accommodation fails, convergence and miosis continue. Furthermore, if one paralyzes accommodation with drugs, convergence remains intact.

The **near point of accommodation** (NPA) is the point closest to the eye at which a target is sharply focused on the retina. Accommodation is measured by the **accommodative amplitude**—the power that the lens can vary from the nonaccommodative state to full accommodation. This power is measured in units called **diopters**. A diopter (D) is the reciprocal of the fixation distance. For example, 1 meter is 1 D; 0.5 m is 2 D; 0.33 m is 3 D; etc. The **range of accommodation** is the distance between the farthest point an object is in clear sight and the nearest point at which the eye can maintain clear vision.

Convergence is a vergence adduction movement that increases the visual angle to permit single binocular vision during near viewing. Convergence can be voluntary but need not be; that is, no stimulus needs to be present to elicit it. It is also reflexive and a comovement in the near response. Accommodation and convergence are related; a unit change in one normally causes a unit change in the other. Convergence may be separated into four subtypes: tonic convergence, accommodative convergence, fusional convergence, and voluntary convergence.

The eyes normally tend to diverge. Keeping the eyes straight thus requires increased tone in the medial rectus muscles. This tone is **tonic convergence**.

Accommodative convergence is the amount of convergence elicited for a given amount of accommodation. The relationship between accommodation and convergence is usually expressed as the ratio of accommodative convergence in prism diopters to accommodation in diopters: the AC/A ratio. Because accommodation decreases with age, the AC/A ratio increases with age.

Fusional convergence is convergence that is stimulated not by changes in accommodation but by disparate retinal images. It is thought to "fine tune" normal convergence.

Voluntary convergence is measured by determining the near point of convergence (NPC)—the nearest point to which the eye can converge. It is closer to the eyes than the NPA and, in general, does not deteriorate with age as the NPA does. The NPC is usually 10 cm or less.

The pupil constricts when changing fixation from distance to near—this is **miosis**. This movement can occur in darkness, is slower than the light reflex, and is maintained as long as the near reaction is maintained. Miosis improves the range through which an object is seen clearly without any change in accommodation, called the **depth of field**. In patients with presbyopia, pupil size continues to decrease even when accommodation has reached its maximum.

In testing accommodation and the near vision response, the above relationships must be remembered. Furthermore, one must remember that accommodation is never measured or tested in an absolute sense, but rather in response to how it changes under certain testing conditions.

There are few if any neuro-ophthalmologic conditions, which result in disturbed accommodation, and clinical testing of accommodative amplitudes and ranges is rarely indicated.

Convergence

Total convergence is usually measured by testing the NPC. This is done by asking the patient to fixate on an accommodative target held 33 cm from the eyes. The target is then moved toward the nose, with the patient being instructed to try to keep the target in focus. The end point of the test is when the patient reports horizontal diplopia or one of the inward turning eyes is observed to turn suddenly outward. The distance at which this occurs can be determined with a millimeter ruler placed alongside the patient's nose. In normal persons, the NPC is usually between 5 and 10 cm. An NPC greater than 30 cm indicates convergence insufficiency.

Another way to determine whether or not convergence is normal is to perform a cover–uncover test while the patient is reading. This is helpful only if the patient has full versions and no previous strabismus.

Disorders of Pupillary Function and Accommodation*

Disorders of Pupillary Function
 Efferent Abnormalities: Anisocoria
 Afferent Abnormalities
 Light-Near Dissociation
 Disturbances during Seizures
 Disturbances in Coma
 Disturbances in Disorders of the Neuromuscular
  Junction
 Drug Effects
 Structural Defects of the Iris

Disorders of Accommodation
 Accommodation Insufficiency and Paralysis
 Accommodation Spasm and Spasm of the Near
  Reflex

Disorders of Lacrimation

**Generalized Disturbances of Autonomic
 Function**

Disorders of Pupillary Function

The value of observation of pupillary size and motility in the evaluation of patients with neurologic disease cannot be overemphasized. In many patients with visual loss, an abnormal pupillary response is the only objective sign of organic visual dysfunction.

Efferent Abnormalities: Anisocoria

Efferent disturbances of the pupil are usually unilateral and thus produce a difference in the size of the pupils called **anisocoria**. When assessing the pupils, one should always attempt to determine if anisocoria is present. If anisocoria is present, there is often something wrong with one or both irides or with the innervation of the iris muscles. Accordingly, once anisocoria is found, the examiner should determine not only if anisocoria is more noticeable in dim or bright illumination, but also which pupil has abnormal reactivity

and/or dilation. Specific pupil examination techniques are discussed in Chapter 14. Causes of anisocoria are described below and are outlined in Table 15.1.

Physiologic Anisocoria (Simple Anisocoria, Central Anisocoria, Benign Anisocorla)

In dim light, at least 20% of the normal population has an anisocoria of 0.4 mm or more at the moment of the examination. In room light, this number drops to about 10%. This form of anisocoria, called **physiologic anisocoria**, is rarely more than 0.6 mm, but it may be as much as 1.0 mm (Fig. 15.1). The anisocoria is almost the same in light and in dark, but there is a tendency for it to decrease in light, perhaps because the smaller pupil reaches the zone of mechanical resistance first, giving the larger pupil a chance to catch up. Other terms for physiologic anisocoria are "simple anisocoria," "central anisocoria," and "benign anisocoria."

In a patient with physiologic anisocoria, the amount of pupillary inequality may vary. Physiologic anisocoria may be observed in prior pictures, even back to infancy or early childhood. The anisocoria seldom reverses.

Horner Syndrome

When the sympathetic innervation to the eye is interrupted, the retractor muscles in the eyelids are weakened, allowing the upper lid to droop and the lower lid to rise. The dilator muscle of the iris is weakened, allowing the pupil to become smaller, and vasomotor and sudomotor control of parts of the face may be lost. This combination of ptosis, miosis, and anhidrosis is called **Horner syndrome** (Fig. 15.2, **Video 15.1**).

Clinical Features. The affected eye often looks small or sunken in patients with Horner syndrome. The upper eyelid is slightly ptotic because of paralysis of the sympathetically innervated smooth muscle (Müller muscle) that contributes to the position of the opened upper eyelid. This **ptosis** is sometimes so slight or so variable that it escapes attention. Similar smooth muscle fibers in the lower eyelid also lose their nerve supply in Horner syndrome. Thus, the lower lid is usually slightly elevated, producing an "upside-down

*The authors acknowledge the past contributions of Aki Kawasaki to this chapter.

Table 15.1	Causes of Anisocoria

More Anisocoria in Darkness

Simple (physiologic) anisocoria

Inhibition of the sympathetic pathway
- Horner syndrome
- Pharmacologic (dapiprazole, thymoxamine)

Stimulation of the sympathetic pathway
- Tadpole pupils
- Intermittent dilation of one pupil caused by sympathetic hyperactivity
- Pharmacologic (cocaine, eye-whitening drops, adrenergic drugs)

Pharmacologic stimulation of the parasympathetic pathway (eserine, organophosphate esters, pilocarpine, methacholine, arecoline)

More Anisocoria in Light

Damage to the parasympathetic outflow to the iris sphincter muscle
- Oculomotor nerve paresis
- Tonic pupil syndromes (including Adie)
- Intermittent dilation of one pupil caused by inhibition of the parasympathetic pathway

Trauma to the iris sphincter

Acute glaucoma siderosis

Pharmacologic inhibition of the parasympathetic pathway (atropine, scopolamine)

A

B

C

Figure 15.2 Horner syndrome in two patients. **A:** Congenital right Horner syndrome. Note associated heterochromia iridis and minimal ptosis. **B:** Spontaneous left Horner syndrome showing upper eyelid ptosis and lower eyelid elevation. **C:** Anisocoria better demonstrated with eyelids manually raised. **Video 15.1**: Infrared pupillography in a patient with left Horner syndrome. Starting in darkness, anisocoria is present but of small magnitude. With light, both pupils show brisk constriction, and anisocoria is accentuated when the light is turned off because of dilation lag in the affected eye (Courtesy of Randy H. Kardon, MD.)

ptosis," further narrowing of the palpebral fissure, and an **apparent enophthalmos**.

The palsy of the iris dilator muscle in Horner syndrome allows the iris sphincter to constrict, producing **miosis.** If the dilator muscle is stimulated (e.g., after an adrenergic eye drop is used), the pupil will dilate widely. Endogenous catecholamines can produce a similar phenomenon if the iris dilator muscle is supersensitive because of denervation. This "paradoxical pupillary dilation" is caused by denervation supersensitivity of the dilator muscle to circulating adrenergic substances.

In Horner syndrome, the weakness of the dilator muscle is most apparent in darkness. The anisocoria is greater in the dark and almost disappears in light. The anisocoria of Horner syndrome is diminished in bright light because the normal action of both sphincters tends to make the two pupils more nearly equal.

Paresis of the dilator muscle in Horner syndrome can be detected in several ways. When the lights are turned out, the Horner pupil dilates more slowly than

Figure 15.1 Physiologic (simple) anisocoria in a teenage male with a history of migraine headache; right pupil is 0.3 mm larger than left. Both pupils reacted normally to light and near stimulus.

the normal pupil (**dilation lag**). A sudden noise will produce an increased sympathetic discharge to the dilator muscle resulting in a transient increase in anisocoria. When looking for dilation lag in a patient with anisocoria that may be caused by Horner syndrome, it is helpful to interject a sudden noise just after the lights go out.

Depigmentation of the ipsilateral iris is not usually seen in patients with an acquired Horner syndrome, but it is a typical feature of congenital Horner syndrome. Nevertheless, it rarely can occur after injury to the sympathetic nervous system in adults.

Characteristic vasomotor and sudomotor changes of the facial skin occur on the affected side in some patients with Horner syndrome. The best known of these is loss of sweating (**anhidrosis**). In a warm environment, the skin on the affected side will feel dry, whereas the skin on the normal side will be damp. The postganglionic sympathetic sudomotor fibers for the face, after synapsing at the superior cervical ganglion, follow the external carotid artery to the face, whereas the sympathetic fibers to the eye travel via the carotid plexus of the internal carotid artery, carrying only a few sweat fibers for the skin of the forehead. Thus, anhidrosis occurs only in patients with a central or preganglionic Horner syndrome, never with a postganglionic Horner syndrome.

After acute, preganglionic sympathetic denervation, the temperature of the skin rises on the side of the lesion because of loss of vasomotor control and consequent dilation of blood vessels. Acutely, there may be some flushing and some conjunctival hyperemia, epiphora, and nasal stuffiness.

Diagnosis. It is important to differentiate a Horner syndrome from physiologic anisocoria. The diagnosis of Horner syndrome can be made by pharmacologic testing. The **cocaine test** remains the "gold standard" test and is based on the failure of cocaine to dilate a sympathetically denervated pupil. Cocaine blocks the reuptake of norepinephrine into the sympathetic nerve endings. In a normal eye, a 10% solution of cocaine causes dilation of the pupil, often to 8 mm or more, within about 45 minutes. However, a sufficient quantity of norepinephrine does not accumulate at the receptors of effector cells unless norepinephrine is continually being released by action potentials within the sympathetic nerves to those cells, which do not occur when there is sympathetic denervation of the pupillary dilator muscle (Fig. 15.3).

The first drop of topical cocaine stings briefly until the anesthetic effect occurs. Peak effect is attained in 40 to 60 minutes. There are no apparent psychoactive effects from a 10% solution of cocaine, but metabolites of the drug can be found in the urine in 100% of patients after 24 hours and in 50% at 36 hours.

Figure 15.3 Response of Horner pupils to cocaine. **A:** Right Horner syndrome associated with Raeder paratrigeminal neuralgia in a 65-year-old man. **B:** Photo taken 45 minutes after conjunctival instillation of two drops of a 10% cocaine solution in each eye. The left pupil is dilated, whereas the right pupil remains unchanged.

Cocaine affects only the sympathetic system, not the parasympathetic system. If the patient is observed while seated in a lighted room, the pupils may appear not to have responded to the cocaine because the light tends to produce pupillary constriction. The patient must be brought into the examination room and the lights dimmed, at which time the pharmacologic dilation of one or both pupils can easily be appreciated.

The odds of an anisocoria being caused by an oculosympathetic palsy increase with the amount of anisocoria measured 45 minutes after the instillation of 10% cocaine into both eyes. It is not necessary to compare the before and after measurements; a post-cocaine anisocoria of 0.8 mm is sufficient to diagnose a Horner syndrome.

Testing with apraclonidine, either 0.5% or 1% solution, takes advantage of the denervation hypersensitivity of the affected pupil and results in pupillary dilation and eyelid elevation on the affected side. Unlike phenylephrine, which should dilate both pupils but may have a greater effect on the Horner syndrome eye, apraclonidine affects only the abnormal eye. Apraclonidine is a weak alpha-1 adrenergic agonist with its primary action being on alpha-2 receptors. In normal eyes, apraclonidine either has no effect on the pupil or causes slight miosis by alpha-2 stimulation and inhibition of norepinephrine release. However, both because the Horner syndrome pupil is supersensitive to alpha-1 stimulation and norepinephrine release already is minimal, the alpha-1 activity predominates and the Horner

Figure 15.4 Response of Horner pupils to apraclonidine. **A:** Right Horner syndrome after neck trauma in a 52-year-old woman. **B:** Photo taken 40 minutes after topical application of 0.5% apraclonidine solution in both eyes. Note the reversal of both ptosis and anisocoria.

pupil dilates. Similarly, the upper eyelid elevates slightly relative to the fellow eye (Fig. 15.4). Both anisocoria and ptosis may reverse (with the normal eye now showing miosis and a "droopy" upper eyelid) at 30 to 45 minutes after drop instillation, although in some cases observation at 60 minutes is needed to confirm the findings.

Because apraclonidine is a standard ophthalmic solution and is much easier to obtain in most outpatient settings than medical cocaine, it has supplanted cocaine testing in most clinical situations. The time after onset to the appearance of supersensitivity must be taken into account when interpreting the apraclonidine test. Positive tests have been described as soon as 36 hours after a known event causing the Horner syndrome, but supersensitivity may not develop at the same rate in all patients. A negative apraclonidine test, when clinical suspicion for Horner syndrome is high, should be repeated several days later; cocaine testing 1 to 2 days later also may be considered.

Localization. Regardless of the site of the lesion in the long sympathetic pathway, all patients with Horner syndrome have a similar ptosis and miosis. It is, however, clinically important to separate the pathway into three major divisions: the central (first-order), the preganglionic (second-order), and the postganglionic (third-order) neurons.

Central Horner Syndromes. The **central** (first-order) neuron begins in the ipsilateral hypothalamus and extends to the ciliospinal center of Budge and Waller in the intermediolateral gray column of the spinal cord at C8–T1 (Fig. 15.5). The path may actually be polysynaptic, but it seems to stay lateral in the brainstem and cervical cord. Thus, Horner syndrome caused by damage to the central neuron is almost always unilateral. There is no pharmacologic test that identifies a central-neuron Horner syndrome; so the clinician must put localizing weight on the associated clinical signs. For example, lesions of the hypothalamus that cause an ipsilateral Horner syndrome are often associated with a contralateral hemiparesis, and some of these patients also have a contralateral hypesthesia.

Another neurologic syndrome characterized in part by a central Horner syndrome is **Wallenberg syndrome**. This condition, which is caused by damage to the lateral medulla, is also characterized by ipsilateral impairment of pain and temperature sensation over the face, limb ataxia, and a bulbar disturbance causing dysarthria and dysphagia. Contralaterally, pain and temperature sensation are impaired over the trunk and limbs. Lateropulsion, a compelling sensation of being pulled toward the side of the lesion, is often a prominent complaint of patients with Wallenberg syndrome and is also evident in the ocular motor findings.

The occurrence of a unilateral Horner syndrome and a contralateral trochlear nerve paresis indicates involvement either of the trochlear nucleus on the side of the Horner syndrome or of the ipsilateral fascicle before its decussation. However, not all patients with a first-order neuron Horner syndrome have other neurologic manifestations. Patients with cervical spondylosis, for example, may have no symptoms or signs of spinal cord disease. Such patients may present only with a Horner syndrome and perhaps some neck pain.

Preganglionic Horner Syndromes. The **preganglionic** (second-order) neuron exits from the ciliospinal center of Budge and passes across the pulmonary apex (see Fig. 15.5). It then turns upward, passes through the stellate ganglion and goes up the carotid sheath to the superior cervical ganglion, near the bifurcation of the common carotid artery.

The ptosis and miosis of a preganglionic Horner syndrome are nonspecific, but the distribution of anhidrosis is characteristic. The entire side of the head, the face, and the neck down to the clavicle are usually involved.

Malignancy is a common cause of a preganglionic Horner syndrome. The most common tumors, not surprisingly, are lung and breast cancer, but Horner syndrome is usually not an early sign of these tumors. Tumors that spread behind the carotid sheath at the C6 level may produce a preganglionic Horner syndrome associated with paralysis of the phrenic, vagus, and recurrent laryngeal nerves: the "Rowland Payne

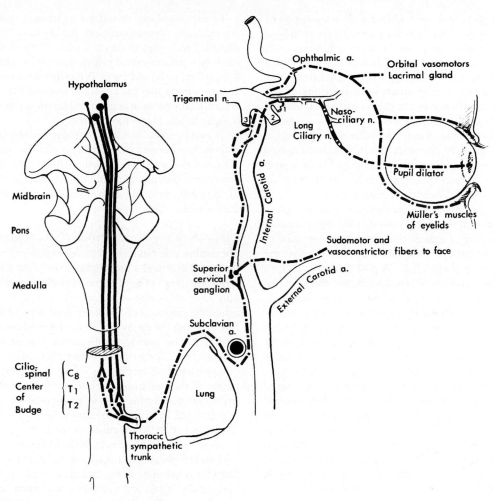

Figure 15.5 The oculosympathetic pathway. Note location of central (first-order), preganglionic (second-order), and postganglionic (third-order) neurons. (Reprinted with permission from Glaser JS. *Neuro-Ophthalmology.* 1st ed. Hagerstown, MD: Harper & Row; 1978:173.)

syndrome." Benign tumors in this region, such as schwannoma of the sympathetic chain, as well as thyroid gland enlargement as in goiter, can also produce a preganglionic Horner syndrome.

A preganglionic Horner syndrome can be caused by accidental or surgical injury (e.g., disc herniation at C8 or T1, trauma to the brachial plexus, pneumothorax, coronary artery bypass surgery, or insertion of a pacemaker). The preganglionic neuron can also be transiently blocked by an epidural anesthetic that flows the wrong way or by an interpleural anesthetic that soaks through the pleura at the pulmonary apex to reach the stellate ganglion. Chest tubes, vascular catheters, and stray bullets can directly injure the preganglionic sympathetic nerves.

Postganglionic Horner Syndromes. The **postganglionic** (third-order) neuron of the sympathetic pathway to the iris dilator muscle extends from the superior

cervical ganglion behind the angle of the mandible and up along the internal carotid artery, where it is called the "carotid plexus" or the "carotid nerve." Within the cavernous sinus, the sympathetic fibers leave the internal carotid artery, join briefly with the abducens nerve, and then leave it to join the ophthalmic division of the trigeminal nerve, entering the orbit with its nasociliary branch. The sympathetic fibers in the nasociliary nerve divide into the two long ciliary nerves that travel with the lateral and medial suprachoroidal vascular bundles to reach the anterior segment of the eye and innervate the iris dilator muscle. The fibers pass through but do not synapse within the ciliary ganglion.

Lesions that affect the postganglionic third-order sympathetic neuron may be extracranial or intracranial. Extracranial lesions damage the cervical sympathetics in the neck, whereas intracranial lesions damage the sympathetic chain at the base of the skull, in the carotid canal and middle ear, or in the region of the cavernous sinus. It is very unusual for an orbital lesion to produce an isolated Horner syndrome.

Lesions of or along the internal carotid artery are a common cause of a postganglionic Horner syndrome. Both traumatic and spontaneous **dissections of the internal carotid artery** can produce sudden ipsilateral face and neck pain associated with a postganglionic Horner syndrome. Raeder paratrigeminal neuralgia, the name given to a headache syndrome characterized by persistent trigeminal pain associated with a post-ganglionic Horner syndrome, likely represents unrecognized carotid dissection in many patients.

A postganglionic Horner syndrome may be caused by tumors, inflammatory lesions, and other masses in the neck. Any neoplasm that extends or metastasizes to the cervical lymph nodes may also damage the cervical sympathetic chain. A postganglionic Horner syndrome, paralysis of the tongue, anesthesia of the pharynx, and dysphagia, all on the same side, may indicate a tumor of the nasopharynx or jugular foramen.

Tumors, aneurysms, infections, and other lesions in the cavernous sinus may produce a postganglionic Horner syndrome. In many of these cases, there is associated ipsilateral ophthalmoplegia as well as pain or dysesthesia of the ipsilateral side of the face caused by involvement of one or more ocular motor nerves and the trigeminal nerve within the sinus. Because the abducens nerve and oculosympathetic nerves are briefly joined in the cavernous sinus, an abducens palsy and a postganglionic Horner syndrome occurring together without other neurologic signs should immediately suggest a cavernous sinus lesion.

Cluster headache manifests as intense, unilateral lancinating or dysesthetic pain, usually lasts 30 to 120 minutes, and often occurs at night. Affected patients often have an associated sympathetic palsy, and there is ipsilateral nasal stuffiness. Typically, the Horner syndrome persists after the headache resolves. Other ischemic conditions, such as giant cell arteritis, can cause a postganglionic Horner syndrome.

A middle fossa mass encroaching on Meckel cave and on the internal carotid artery at the foramen lacerum can also produce a postganglionic Horner syndrome associated with pain. Other lesions at the base of the skull, including a basal skull fracture, can produce a similar clinical picture.

Differentiating Localizations. The **hydroxyamphetamine test** can be used to differentiate between a postganglionic and a preganglionic or central Horner syndrome (Fig. 15.6). This test should be performed only after a cocaine or apraclonidine test has established the diagnosis of a Horner syndrome or in a setting in which the diagnosis of Horner syndrome is not in doubt. The hydroxyamphetamine test should not be performed for 24 to 48 hours after ether cocaine or apraclonidine testing, to allow the corneas and pupils to recover from the effects of the drug. The hydroxyamphetamine test is performed by placing two drops of hydroxyamphetamine hydrobromide 1% (Paredrine) in the lower cul-de-sac of each eye, and the pupils are assessed in a dim light about 45 minutes later. Hydroxyamphetamine releases stored norepinephrine from the adrenergic nerve ending, producing variable but usually significant mydriasis in normal subjects.

Figure 15.6 Response of Horner pupils to hydroxyamphetamine. **A:** Left Horner syndrome in a 55-year-old man with an apical lung tumor. **B:** At 45 minutes after conjunctival instillation of two drops of 1% hydroxyamphetamine solution in each eye, both pupils are dilated, indicating an intact postganglionic neuron (i.e., a preganglionic Horner syndrome).

When the lesion causing a Horner syndrome is in the **postganglionic neuron,** the nerve endings themselves are destroyed, there are no stores of norepinephrine to release, and hydroxyamphetamine thus has no mydriatic effect. If the lesion is in the **preganglionic or central neuron,** the pupil will dilate fully and may even become larger than the opposite pupil, presumably because of upregulation of the postsynaptic receptors on the dilator muscle. False-negative results may occur within the first week after the Horner syndrome has developed, before the stores of norepinephrine at the presynaptic terminals have been depleted. Thus, a smaller pupil that fails to dilate to cocaine and/or enlarges with apraclonidine and subsequently does not dilate after topical administration of hydroxyamphetamine or a similar substance is likely to be caused by a lesion of the postganglionic sympathetic neuron.

Acquired Horner Syndrome in Children. While an acquired Horner syndrome in childhood is sometimes associated with neoplasia, including spinal cord tumors, embryonal cell carcinoma, neuroblastoma, and rhabdomyosarcoma, this association is quite rare. A Horner syndrome in childhood is usually *not* associated with a tumor and is often an isolated finding of no significance. Other causes of an acquired Horner syndrome in childhood include traumatic brachial plexus palsy, intrathoracic aneurysm, and thrombosis of the internal carotid artery. If old photographs clearly indicate that a Horner syndrome in a child is acquired, it is recommended to begin further evaluation with CT scanning or MRI of the chest.

Congenital Horner Syndrome. Congenital Horner syndrome is an uncommon disorder. In its fully developed form, the syndrome consists of ptosis, miosis, facial anhidrosis, and hypochromia of the affected iris. Injury to the brachial plexus at birth is responsible for many of these cases (Fig. 15.7), but some cases occur in association with congenital tumors, and others occur after viral infections.

Most patients with congenital Horner syndrome can be separated into one of three groups: patients with evidence of obstetric trauma to the internal carotid artery sympathetic plexus, patients without a history of birth trauma but with a lesion that is clinically and pharmacologically localized to the superior cervical ganglion, and those with evidence of surgical or obstetric injury to the preganglionic sympathetic pathway.

The first group of patients tends to have had substantial perinatal head trauma as a result of difficult forceps deliveries. Clinically, such patients have obvious ptosis and miosis with generally intact facial sweating. Pharmacologic testing is consistent with a postganglionic lesion.

Figure 15.7 Horner syndrome (**top**) associated with injury of the right brachial plexus at birth. Note the underdeveloped right arm and forearm (**bottom**).

In the second group of patients, pharmacologic testing also is consistent with a postganglionic lesion but such patients have facial anhidrosis, indicating a lesion proximal to the separation of the sudomotor fibers with the external carotid artery. The causes of such a lesion could include an embryopathy directly involving the superior cervical ganglion, damage to the vascular supply of the superior cervical ganglion, or transsynaptic dysgenesis of the superior cervical ganglion following a defect located more proximally in the sympathetic pathway.

The third group of patients has suffered trauma to the preganglionic oculosympathetic pathway. Injuries include trauma to the brachial plexus and surgery in the thoracic region. Although patients in this group should have a preganglionic Horner syndrome, some have pharmacologic testing consistent with a postganglionic lesion, presumably indicating transsynaptic degeneration occurring in the postganglionic neuron following preganglionic injury (Fig 15.8A).

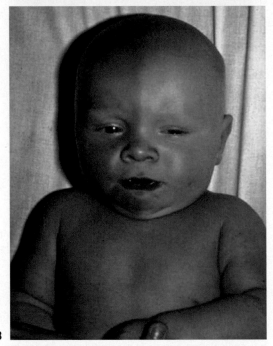

Figure 15.8 Facial coloration changes in Horner syndrome patients. **A:** Lack of facial flushing and sweating due to transsynaptic degeneration of sympathetic fibers in a patient who underwent extensive resection of a right cavernous sinus tumor. She also had complete ptosis and ophthalmoplegia from damage to cranial nerves 3, 4, and 6. **B:** Atropinic flushing in a child with a congenital left Horner syndrome. Note that the atropinic flush is present only on the side of the face opposite the Horner syndrome.

Parents of infants with congenital Horner syndrome sometimes report that the baby develops a hemifacial flush when it is nursing or crying. It is likely that the hemifacial flushing seen in infants is on the side opposite the Horner syndrome and is simply the normal response, which appears more obvious because of the impaired facial vasodilation on the side of a congenital Horner syndrome.

When a child has unilateral ptosis and ipsilateral miosis, and there is doubt as to whether or not a sympathetic defect is present, a cycloplegic refraction can sometimes unexpectedly answer the question by producing an atropinic flush. This reaction only occurs when there is an intact sympathetic innervation to the skin and thus is absent on the side of the Horner syndrome (Fig. 15.8B).

A child with Horner syndrome and very blue eyes will not develop visible iris heterochromia, but most children with Horner syndrome have paler iris on the affected side. This occurs whether the lesion is preganglionic or postganglionic because of anterograde transsynaptic dysgenesis. When the sympathetic pathway is interrupted in the preganglionic neuron, the next distal ganglion—the superior cervical ganglion—does not develop normally. There are fewer cells in the ganglion and less norepinephrine stores to release with hydroxyamphetamine. This results in impaired development of iris melanophores, causing hypochromia of the iris stroma.

Pharmacological testing in children under age 2 should be approached cautiously, as systemic absorption of cocaine may increase blood pressure or heart rate, and apraclonidine crosses the blood–brain barrier in this age group and can produce CNS depression.

Sympathetic Hyperactivity

Sympathetic hyperactivity occurs in a number of settings in which the pupils are affected. In such cases, there may be anisocoria that is more obvious in darkness than in light.

A **tadpole pupil** is an intermittent and benign phenomenon in which the pupil of one eye becomes distorted for a minute or two. The pupil is pulled in one direction like the tail of a tadpole. It may be caused by repeated bursts of sympathetic innervation, an irritation that eventually causes loss of fibers and a Horner syndrome. This condition is distinct from the **episodic unilateral mydriasis** that occurs in some young patients during a typical migraine attack, although there is some similarity.

Some patients who sustain trauma to the low cervical or high thoracic spinal cord experience episodes of unilateral pupillary dilation associated with unilateral sweating; this syndrome was described in the early eighteenth century by the French military surgeon Francois Pourfour du Petit and bears his name. Pharmacologic testing in such patients suggests that the mydriasis is caused by episodic sympathetic irritation.

Pharmacologic Stimulation of the Iris Sphincter

Almost all cases of acute anisocoria in which one pupil is nonreactive are caused by pharmacologic blockade of the iris sphincter muscle. In such cases, the anisocoria is worse in light than in darkness because the affected pupil cannot constrict. In rare instances, however, a pharmacologic agent, such as an organophosphate used in pesticides, may produce anisocoria by stimulating rather than blocking the parasympathetic system, thus producing a nonreactive, **miotic** pupil. In such cases and in other cases of pharmacologic stimulation of the ocular parasympathetic pathway, a 1% solution of tropicamide will dilate the larger, reactive pupil but will fail to dilate the small, nonreactive pupil.

Pharmacologic Stimulation of the Iris Dilator

Topical cocaine placed in the nose for medical or for other reasons can back up the lacrimal duct into the conjunctival sac. Most eye-whitening drops that contain sympathomimetic components are too weak to dilate the pupil, but if the cornea is abraded (e.g., by a contact lens), enough of the oxymetazoline or the phenylephrine may get into the aqueous humor to dilate the pupil. Other adrenergic drugs given in a mist for pulmonary therapy may escape around the edge of the face mask and condense in the conjunctival sac, causing pupillary dilation that is more evident in darkness than in light.

More Anisocoria in Light

Damage to the Parasympathetic Outflow to the Iris Sphincter Muscle.

The final common pathway for pupillary reactivity to light and near stimulation begins in the mesencephalon with the visceral oculomotor nuclei, continues via the oculomotor nerve to the ciliary ganglion, and reaches the iris sphincter through the short ciliary nerves. Lesions that affect this parasympathetic pathway can produce absolute paralysis of pupillary constriction. The pupil is then dilated and nonreactive, and all constrictor reflexes are absent. In many cases, all parasympathetic input to the eye is damaged simultaneously so that accommodation is also lost. This combination of iridoplegia and cycloplegia is often called **internal ophthalmoplegia** to distinguish it from the external ophthalmoplegia that occurs when the extraocular muscles are paralyzed in the setting of normal pupillary responses.

Topical diagnosis of paralysis of the iris sphincter is simplified when signs of an oculomotor nerve palsy are present. In the setting of ptosis and paralysis of the superior, inferior, and medial rectus muscles, as well as the inferior oblique muscle, a nonreactive, dilated pupil is but a part of the classic picture of a lesion of the oculomotor nerve. This chapter provides a brief overview of oculomotor nerve disease causing anisocoria. For additional considerations and details, please see Chapter 18. However, isolated iris paralysis can be a difficult diagnostic problem. One must consider lesions of the mesencephalon, the oculomotor nerve, the ciliary ganglion, the short ciliary nerves, and the eye itself.

Damage to the Edinger–Westphal Nuclei.

Lesions of the rostral mesencephalon almost never produce an isolated unilateral, nonreactive, dilated pupil. When there is isolated damage to the Edinger–Westphal nuclei, bilateral pupillary abnormalities are the rule. In addition, most lesions in this region that produce pupillary abnormalities also affect other parts of the oculomotor nucleus, causing ptosis, ophthalmoparesis, or both.

Damage to Pupillomotor Fibers in the Oculomotor Nerve.

Because the fibers emerging from the Edinger–Westphal nucleus are among the most rostral in the oculomotor group (Fig. 15.9), it is possible for a fascicular lesion to damage just the fibers serving pupillary function, thus producing a unilateral, dilated, nonreactive pupil. This occurs exceptionally rarely. The separate bundles of the oculomotor nerve exit the mesencephalon merge to form the oculomotor nerve in the subarachnoid space. The pupillary fibers are superficial and migrate from a superior medial position to the inferior part of the nerve (Fig. 15.10). Thus, the pupillomotor fibers are subject to injury from noxious CSF processes such as basal meningitis as well as compressive lesions including cerebral aneurysms and tumors. Isolated pupil abnormality without oculomotor dysfunction is rarely seen with compressive lesions. Intrinsic lesions of the oculomotor nerve in the subarachnoid space can produce an oculomotor nerve paresis that begins with a dilated pupil. Such lesions include schwannomas and angiomas.

Damage to the Ciliary Ganglion and Its Roots in the Orbit: Tonic Pupil

Damage to the postganglionic parasympathetic innervation of the intraocular muscles produces a characteristic syndrome. Initially, there may be an isolated internal ophthalmoplegia. Later, one or more of the following abnormalities may be observed: a poor pupillary reaction to light that can be seen to be a regional palsy of the iris sphincter by slit lamp biomicroscopy, paresis of accommodation, cholinergic supersensitivity of the denervated muscles, a pupillary response to near stimuli that is unusually strong and tonic, and a slow and tonic redilation after constriction to near stimuli.

Pupils that react in this manner are called **tonic pupils** (Fig. 15.11). The lesions that produce them damage the ciliary ganglion or the short ciliary nerves in the retrobulbar space or in the intraocular,

Figure 15.9 Position of the pupillomotor fibers in the fascicle of the human oculomotor nerve. Note that the fibers destined to innervate the iris sphincter muscle (*P*) are located rostral and medial to the fibers that innervate the extraocular muscles and the levator palpebrae superioris (*LP*). *IO*, inferior oblique; *IR*, inferior rectus; *MR*, medial rectus; *SR*, superior rectus; *MRa, MRb,* and *MRc*, subnuclei serving medial rectus function in the oculomotor nuclear complex; *CCN*, central caudal nucleus. (Reprinted with permission from Ksiazek SM, Slamovits TL, Rosen CE, et al. Fascicular arrangement in partial oculomotor paresis. *Am J Ophthalmol.* 1994;118:97–103.)

suprachoroidal space (Fig. 15.12). The slowness and tonicity of the pupillary movement is caused by aberrant regeneration of ciliary nerves into the iris sphincter. Tonic pupils can be separated into three categories: local, neuropathic, and the Holmes–Adie syndrome.

Local Tonic Pupil. Acute internal ophthalmoplegia followed by the development of a tonic pupil occurs from a variety of inflammations, infections, and infiltrative processes that affect the ciliary ganglion in isolation or as part of a systemic process. Disorders that can cause a **local** tonic pupil include herpes zoster, chickenpox, measles, diphtheria, syphilis (both congenital and acquired), sarcoidosis, scarlet fever, pertussis, smallpox, influenza, sinusitis, Vogt–Koyanagi–Harada syndrome, rheumatoid arthritis, viral hepatitis, choroiditis, primary and metastatic choroidal and orbital tumors, blunt injury to the globe, and penetrating orbital injury. Siderosis from an intraocular iron foreign body apparently damages the nerves more than the sphincter muscle and may produce an iron mydriasis. Various ocular or orbital surgical procedures, including retinal reattachment surgery, inferior oblique muscle surgery, orbital surgery, optic nerve sheath fenestration, photocoagulation, transconjunctival cryotherapy, transscleral diathermy, and retrobulbar injections of alcohol can

cause a local tonic pupil, as can inferior dental blocks with local anesthesia. Ischemia of the ciliary ganglion or short ciliary nerves from migraine, giant cell arteritis, and other vasculitides also can cause a tonic pupil.

Neuropathic Tonic Pupil. **Neuropathic tonic pupils** occur in patients in whom a tonic pupil is part of a generalized, widespread, peripheral or autonomic neuropathy that also involves the ciliary ganglion, the short ciliary nerves, or both. In some cases, there is evidence of both a sympathetic and a parasympathetic disturbance. Diseases that produce this syndrome include syphilis, chronic alcoholism, diabetes mellitus, some of the spinocerebellar ataxias, Guillain–Barré syndrome (GBS), and the Miller Fisher variant of GBS. Other systemic diseases involving autonomic nervous system dysfunction that may be associated with a tonic pupil are acute pandysautonomia, Shy–Drager syndrome, and Ross syndrome (hyporeflexia, progressive segmental hypohidrosis, and tonic pupil). Patients with systemic lupus erythematosus may develop tonic pupils in association with a more generalized autonomic neuropathy, as may patients with Sjögren syndrome, in whom the pupillary disturbance may even be the first sign of the disorder. Tonic pupils can also develop in patients with systemic amyloidosis, hereditary sensory neuropathy, a paraneoplastic syndrome,

Figure 15.10 Course of preganglionic autonomic nerve fibers from the brainstem to the ciliary ganglion in humans. A sagittal reconstruction of the brainstem with the course of the oculomotor nerve is shown at top. The corresponding locations of the preganglionic autonomic fibers for pupillo-constriction and accommodation within the right (**R**) and left (**L**) oculomotor nerves are shown in *black* in coronal sections through slices at 1 (emergence from the brainstem), 2 (midpoint in the subarachnoid space), 3 (at the point where the third nerve enters the dura), and 4 (in the anterior cavernous sinus where the fibers have entered the anatomical inferior division of the third nerve). The autonomic fibers are located superiorly as the oculomotor nerve exits the brainstem and then come to lie more medially as the oculomotor nerve passes toward the orbit. *A*, dorsal, and *B*, ventral side of brainstem; *P*, pons; *M*, medulla; *EW*, Edinger–Westphal nucleus; *IIIn*, somatic portion of third nerve nucleus; *III*, third nerve; *ID*, inferior division of third nerve; *SD*, superior division of third nerve; *NCilV*, nasociliary branch of the fifth nerve; *CG*, ciliary ganglion; *Sym*, sympathetic route; *m*, medial; *l*, lateral. (Reprinted with permission from Kerr FWL, Hallowell OW. Location of pupillomotor and accommodation fibers in the oculomotor nerve: experimental observations on paralytic mydriasis. *J Neurol Neurosurg Psychiatry.* 1964;27:473–481.)

and hereditary motor–sensory neuropathy (Charcot–Marie–Tooth disease).

Holmes–Adie Tonic Pupil Syndrome. The **Holmes–Adie tonic pupil syndrome** (also called Adie syndrome) consists of unilateral or bilateral tonically reacting pupils developing in otherwise healthy persons and in patients with unrelated conditions. Most of these patients also have a disturbance in deep tendon reflexes, but they have no evidence of local ocular or orbital disease or of generalized peripheral or autonomic nervous system dysfunction.

Adie syndrome is not common. It nearly always occurs as a sporadic entity, although it can be familial. Most patients are between 20 and 50 years of

Figure 15.11 Tonic pupil syndrome. About 4 months earlier, this 38-year-old man noted that his right pupil was larger than his left pupil. **A:** In the dark looking in the distance, both pupils are dilated and relatively equal in size. **B:** In bright light, the right pupil does not constrict, whereas the left pupil constricts normally, producing a marked anisocoria. **C:** In room light looking in the distance, there is a moderate anisocoria. **D:** During near viewing, however, both pupils constrict. The right pupil constricted much slower than the left and redilated slowly.

age when the condition is noticed. Seventy percent of cases occur in women and 30% in men. Adie syndrome is unilateral in about 80% of cases. When the condition is bilateral, the onset is occasionally simultaneous but usually occurs in separate episodes months or even years apart.

Most patients with Adie syndrome have visual complaints including photophobia, blurred near vision, an enlarged pupil, and headaches. Over time, the dilated pupil becomes smaller, and accommodation improves; however, many patients continue to have difficulty focusing. If, some years later, the other eye is similarly affected, as occurs in about 4% of cases per year, it seems to produce far fewer symptoms and may in fact pass unnoticed.

It may also be confused with a pharmacologically induced mydriasis and cycloplegia until a slit lamp examination is performed, at which time segmental contractions of the iris sphincter are observed. These

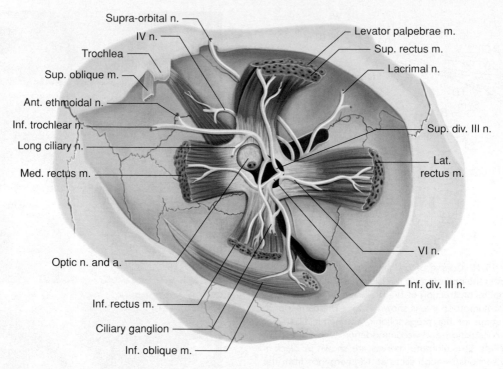

Supra-orbital n.
IV n.
Trochlea
Sup. oblique m.
Ant. ethmoidal n.
Inf. trochlear n.
Long ciliary n.
Med. rectus m.

Levator palpebrae m.
Sup. rectus m.
Lacrimal n.
Sup. div. III n.
Lat. rectus m.

Optic n. and a.
Inf. rectus m.
Ciliary ganglion
Inf. oblique m.

VI n.
Inf. div. III n.

Figure 15.12 View of the posterior orbit showing the relationship of the optic nerve to the ocular motor nerves and extraocular muscles. Note the location of the ciliary ganglion. (Redrawn from Wolff E. *Anatomy of the Eye and Orbit.* 6th ed. Philadelphia, PA: WB Saunders, 1968.)

segmental contractions or "vermiform movements" are observed in all forms of tonic pupil, including Adie syndrome, whereas a pharmacologic anticholinergic blockade always paralyzes the **entire** sphincter. Segmental palsy of the iris sphincter is a critical diagnostic observation. Almost every Adie pupil that has any reaction to light (about 90%) has such a segmental palsy of the sphincter.

In most patients with Adie syndrome, the accommodative paresis resolves over several months. In some patients, however, aberrant regeneration within the ciliary muscle produces an accommodative paresis that may persist until presbyopia develops and diminishes the symptoms.

Hyporeflexia or areflexia is present in a substantial number of patients with Adie syndrome. The most likely explanation is that the responsible lesion is located centrally within the spinal cord. Indeed, pathologic studies in a few patients with Adie syndrome report atrophic changes in the dorsal columns. It thus seems most likely that degeneration of cell bodies in the dorsal columns similar to that which occurs in the ciliary ganglion is responsible for the loss of deep tendon reflexes that occur in the majority of patients with Adie syndrome.

The tonic pupil of patients with Adie syndrome is supersensitive to acetylcholine and similar substances, including pilocarpine. For example, conjunctival administration of two drops of a 0.1% solution of pilocarpine causes intense miosis in most tonic pupils (Fig. 15.13), whereas such solutions do not generally cause any change in the size of normal pupils. Unfortunately, the clinical utility of the **denervation supersensitivity test** for a tonic pupil is limited because the pupils of many patients with oculomotor nerve palsies constrict about as much as Adie pupils to weak solutions of pilocarpine.

Denervation supersensitivity in Adie pupil parallels the phenomenon seen in Horner syndrome with the sympathetic system. If the diagnosis of a tonic pupil is uncertain, it is certainly appropriate to test for cholinergic supersensitivity. We use a 0.0625% pilocarpine solution, prepared in a syringe from one part commercially available 1% pilocarpine and 15 parts normal saline. The sphincter should not be considered supersensitive unless it becomes the smaller of the two medicated pupils.

Five features of Adie syndrome change over time: the accommodation paresis seems to recover; the pupillary light reaction does not recover and may become even weaker, deep tendon reflexes tend to become increasingly hyporeflexic, the affected pupil gradually becomes smaller, and there is a tendency for patients with unilateral Adie syndrome to develop a tonic pupil in the opposite eye with time.

A

B

Figure 15.13 Postganglionic supersensitivity in the tonic pupil syndrome. **A:** A right tonic pupil in a 36-year-old woman. **B:** At 45 minutes after conjunctival instillation of two drops of 0.1% pilocarpine solution in each eye, the right pupil is constricted and nonreactive. The left pupil remains unchanged and normally reactive.

The etiology of Adie syndrome remains obscure. Both pharmacologic studies and pathologic studies indicate that the ciliary ganglion, short ciliary nerves, or both are the location of the lesion that produces Adie syndrome.

The explanation for why the light reflex is so much more severely impaired than the near vision constriction is that the near-vision reaction is not so much **spared** as it is **restored**. Fibers originally destined for the ciliary muscle resprout randomly, with some of the fibers reaching the iris sphincter and causing a miosis every time the ciliary muscle is stimulated. In addition, pupillomotor fibers to the iris sphincter muscle constitute only about 3% of the total number of postganglionic neurons that leave the ciliary ganglion; the rest innervate the ciliary muscle. Thus, when the ciliary ganglion is injured, there is a greater chance of survival for cells or fibers that serve accommodation than for those that innervate the iris. When the new collateral fibers sprout, the probability is much greater that these new fibers arise from accommodative elements than from those that originally innervated the iris. These new fibers now innervate both the ciliary muscle and the iris, and the pupil once again constricts when the patient looks at a near object (Fig 15.14).

Damage to the Iris Sphincter

Tears in the iris sphincter or in the iris base may occur from blunt trauma to the eye. Such damage may produce a nonreactive or poorly reactive irregularly dilated pupil that may be mistaken for the dilated pupil of an oculomotor nerve palsy. In most cases, iris tears or dialysis are easily observed using a standard or portable slit lamp. Other signs suggesting damage to the eye include scattered pigment on the anterior iris stroma, pigment on the anterior lens capsule (Vossius ring), focal cataract, choroidal rupture, commotio retinae, and retinal hemorrhages.

Pharmacologic Blockade with Parasympatholytic Agents

A dilated, nonreactive pupil can be caused by topical administration of one of several parasympatholytic agents, many of which are described below in the section on drug effects. It should be emphasized that pharmacologic mydriasis is extreme, usually more than 8 mm. Because an acute tonic pupil may have a somewhat similar appearance, it is necessary to be able to distinguish between these two entities. In addition, although a dilated pupil from oculomotor nerve involvement is rarely widely dilated and is nearly always associated with other signs of oculomotor nerve dysfunction, clinicians occasionally become concerned that a dilated, nonreactive pupil may be the earliest sign of an acute oculomotor nerve palsy. A 1% solution of pilocarpine can be used to differentiate a pupil that is dilated from pharmacologic blockade of the iris sphincter cells from a pupil that is dilated from neurologic damage to the parasympathetic pathway from the brainstem to the iris sphincter. A pupil that is dilated from pharmacologic blockade will be unchanged or poorly constricted by a topical solution of pilocarpine strong enough to maximally constrict the opposite pupil (Fig. 15.15), and a tonic pupil will constrict to even weaker solutions of pilocarpine because of denervation supersensitivity (see above) and should certainly constrict to 1% pilocarpine. A pupil that is dilated from oculomotor nerve dysfunction will also constrict maximally after instillation of pilocarpine.

Anisocoria That May Be More Obvious in Darkness or in Light

When some normal persons look in extreme lateral gaze, the pupil on that side becomes larger than the pupil on the opposite side, which becomes smaller. This phenomenon is called **Tournay phenomenon**. It is of no clinical significance.

Figure 15.14 Misregeneration theory as it pertains to the findings in the tonic pupil syndrome. **Above:** Before injury, most of the fibers in the ciliary ganglion are destined for the ciliary muscle to produce accommodation. **Below:** Following injury, it is more likely that a regenerating postganglionic fiber will be one for accommodation; however, many of these fibers send branches or collaterals to the iris, producing pupillary constriction during attempted accommodation convergence. In this drawing, postganglionic fiber 1, for accommodation, has not been injured; fibers 2 and 5, also accommodative, have regenerated, sending sprouts to both the ciliary muscle and the iris sphincter; fiber 3, for pupillary constriction, has sent a sprout to the ciliary muscle via the remaining nerve sheath of fiber 4, which has been damaged; fiber 6, for pupillary constriction, has been destroyed and has not regenerated. Thus, accommodation and pupillary constriction will occur primarily on attempted accommodation convergence.

Figure 15.15 Pharmacologically dilated pupil. **A:** Nonreactive, dilated left pupil in a 25-year-old woman complaining of headache and blurred vision. **B:** At 45 minutes after conjunctival instillation of two drops of 2% pilocarpine in each eye, the left pupil is unchanged, whereas the right pupil is markedly constricted. The patient subsequently admitted to recent scopolamine patch use and was presumed to have inadvertently touched the left eye after handling the patch.

Transient unilateral dilation of the pupil occurs in otherwise healthy young adults in association with blurred vision and headaches (Fig. 15.16). No other signs of oculomotor nerve palsy are present in these patients, and neuroimaging studies, including cerebral arteriography, show no intracranial abnormalities. Such patients were once thought to have a variant of ophthalmoplegic migraine, and it was believed that damage to efferent pupillomotor fibers along the oculomotor nerve or in the orbit were responsible; however, some patients demonstrate sympathetic hyperactivity of the iris rather than parasympathetic weakness.

Thus, the first step in determining the management of a patient with a headache and a unilateral dilated pupil is to determine, by assessing the reactivity of the pupils to light and the amount of accommodative amplitude if the anisocoria is caused by parasympathetic or sympathetic dysfunction. If sympathetic hyperactivity is present, no further assessment is necessary. Although some patients with parasympathetic insufficiency may require angiography to exclude an aneurysm, the availability of increasingly sensitive

A   B

Figure 15.16 Intermittent unilateral pupillary dilation in a young woman during a severe migraine headache. **A:** During the migraine attack, the left pupil is dilated and poorly reactive. Accommodation is normal, however, suggesting that the dilation is caused by sympathetic hyperactivity rather than parasympathetic hypoactivity. **B:** Between attacks, the pupils are isocoric.

neuroimaging tests, such as standard MRI, MR angiography, and CT angiography, allows such patients to be evaluated in a noninvasive manner, and, if the studies are negative, to be followed for either resolution of pupillary dilation or development of other signs of oculomotor nerve dysfunction.

Transient unilateral pupillary dilation occurs in some healthy persons unassociated with headache, and this phenomenon may also be caused by parasympathetic interruption or sympathetic irritation. Such episodes may last minutes, hours, or even weeks, and they may recur for several years. In some patients, the pupillary dilation is associated with evidence of loss of accommodation in the affected eye, thus implicating a parasympathetic process; however, in others, there is other evidence of autonomic dysfunction, including labile blood pressure and erythromelalgia of the neck and thorax. These features, along with normal accommodation, suggest hyperactivity of the sympathetic system. Thus, episodic unilateral pupillary mydriasis, whether or not it is associated with headache, may be caused by parasympathetic hypofunction or sympathetic hyperfunction.

Differentiation of Anisocoria

From a practical standpoint, anisocoria that is more evident in darkness than in light indicates that the iris sphincter muscles and the parasympathetic pathway that constricts them are intact. There is more dilation in darkness of one pupil than the other because both pupils constrict to light stimulation, but one pupil dilates more in darkness than the other. Anisocoria that is more evident in light than in darkness indicates a defect of the ocular parasympathetic pathway, the iris sphincter muscles, or both. This permits a relatively straightforward approach to the patient with anisocoria, using the reaction of the pupils to light stimulation as the initial differentiating feature (Fig. 15.17).

If there is a good light reaction in both eyes, the patient almost always has either physiologic anisocoria or a Horner syndrome. These two entities are then differentiated using the cocaine or apraclonidine test. If testing indicates that the patient has a Horner syndrome, the hydroxyamphetamine test may be performed on another occasion at least 24 hours later to differentiate a central or preganglionic Horner syndrome from a postganglionic Horner syndrome.

If there is a poor light reaction in one or both eyes, the patient has a defect of the parasympathetic system or the iris sphincter muscle. The iris should be examined using a slit lamp biomicroscope to determine if there is a sphincter tear or other iris damage and to see if there is any evidence of a segmental palsy of the iris sphincter or vermiform movements. If there is no evidence of iris damage, a 1% solution of pilocarpine can be used to distinguish between a pharmacologically blockaded pupil and a neurogenic cause. If the results of the test indicate neurogenic anisocoria, but there is no other evidence of an oculomotor nerve paresis, a 0.1% solution of pilocarpine can be used at another time to detect denervation supersensitivity of the parasympathetic system that most often occurs in association with a tonic pupil syndrome. Alternatively, one can begin with a 0.1% solution of pilocarpine to test for denervation supersensitivity. If neither pupil constricts, a 1% solution of pilocarpine can then be used at the same sitting.

Afferent Abnormalities

The Relative Afferent Pupillary Defect

The relative afferent pupil defect (RAPD) is one of the most important objective signs in ophthalmology. It may be the only evidence of organic afferent visual sensory system dysfunction in a patient who complains of visual loss in one or both eyes but who has a normal ocular fundus.

Figure 15.17 Flow chart indicating steps that should be taken to differentiate among causes of anisocoria.

Most patients with a unilateral or pathologically asymmetric bilateral **optic neuropathy**, regardless of the cause, have a RAPD (Fig. 15.18). Patients with **glaucoma** have a RAPD only if the glaucoma is unilateral or asymmetric, and patients with **optic disc drusen** have a RAPD only when there is associated visual field loss in one eye only or asymmetrically in both eyes. If visual acuity is 20/200 or better and is caused by **macular disease,** such as macular degeneration, any RAPD will usually be 0.5 log units or less. Indeed, it is difficult to produce a RAPD greater than 1.0 log units with a lesion confined to the macula. Central serous maculopathy, which can clinically mimic an optic neuropathy, produces a minimal RAPD, usually 0.3 log units or less. A RAPD can occur in a patient with a **retinal detachment.** Each quadrant of a fresh, bullous retinal detachment produces about 0.3 log of RAPD, and when the macula detaches, the RAPD increases by about another 0.7 log units. A RAPD can be produced by a **central retinal vein occlusion** (CRVO), particularly when it is an ischemic occlusion. About 90% of nonischemic

CRVOs are associated with a RAPD that is 0.3 log units or less, and none have a RAPD larger than 0.9 log units. In contrast, over 90% of ischemic CRVOs are associated with a RAPD of 1.2 log units or more, and none have a RAPD smaller than 0.6 log units.

In **anisocoria**, the eye with the smaller pupil has a relatively shaded retina, and when less light strikes one retina during the swinging flashlight test it can look like a RAPD. This asymmetry only becomes clinically significant when one pupil is very small or when the anisocoria is large (2 mm or more). In suppression **amblyopia**, a small RAPD can often be seen in an amblyopic eye. It is generally less than 0.5 log units, and the number does not correlate well with the visual acuity. An eye that is **occluded** becomes increasingly dark-adapted and light-sensitive during the first 30 minutes of occlusion. This can temporarily produce up to 1.5 log units of a false RAPD in the unpatched eye.

A unilateral **cataract,** even one that is very dense and brunescent, produces little or no RAPD. This may be partly because of the dark-adapted retina behind

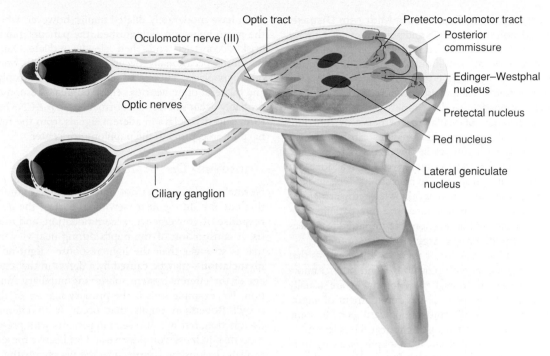

Figure 15.18 Diagram of the path of the pupillary light reflex.

the cataract and partly because the beam of light coming through the pupil is diffused by the cataract to cover a broader area of retinal than normal. Indeed, a unilateral, white, opaque cataract routinely seems to produce a small RAPD in the opposite eye.

A complete or nearly complete lesion of the **optic tract** not only produces a contralateral homonymous hemianopia, it also produces a definite RAPD (0.3 to 1.8 log units) in the contralateral eye—the eye with the temporal field loss. This is partly because there are more crossed than uncrossed fibers in the chiasm and also because there are more crossed than uncrossed fibers in the midbrain hemidecussation of the pupillary pathways.

Most patients with homonymous hemianopias do not have a RAPD unless the lesion affects the contralateral optic tract. An exception is the patient with a **postgeniculate congenital homonymous hemianopia**. In such cases, the RAPD is on the side opposite the lesion (on the side of the hemianopia) and results from transsynaptic degeneration of the optic tract ipsilateral to the lesion. Such patients also have bilateral, hemianopic retinal and optic nerve atrophy.

A unilateral lesion in the **pretectal nucleus or in the brachium of the superior colliculus** will damage the pupillary fibers coming from the ipsilateral optic tract. This can produce a contralateral RAPD without any loss of visual acuity or color vision and without any visual field defect, although the RAPD may occasionally be associated with an ipsilateral or contralateral trochlear nerve paresis. In addition, lesions that

involve the lateral geniculate body or the proximal portion of the retrogeniculate pathway may be associated with a contralateral RAPD not from involvement of that pathway but from involvement of the adjacent intercalated neurons between the visual pathway and the pupillomotor centers in the pretectum.

Neither nonorganic loss of visual acuity nor nonorganic constriction of the visual field in one eye ever produces a RAPD. In contrast, the vast majority of patients with monocular neurogenic loss of the visual field do have a RAPD. Thus, the absence of this sign in a patient with monocular loss of vision and no evidence of a refractive error, opacified media, or small macular lesion should suggest a nonorganic process. If a patient with a suspected unilateral optic neuropathy, regardless of the cause, has no RAPD, either the patient does not have an optic neuropathy or the patient has a bilateral optic neuropathy.

Some normal subjects show a persistent but small RAPD in the absence of any detectable pathologic disease. The RAPD in such cases is quite small, usually 0.3 log units or less, and variable in degree.

Wernicke Pupil

When the optic chiasm is bisected sagittally, the nasal halves of each retina become insensitive to light so that there is not only a bitemporal hemianopia, but also a bitemporal pupillary hemiakinesia. Light falling on the nasal retina of either eye will fail to produce pupillary constriction.

Poorly Reacting Pupils from Midbrain Disease

Dilated, nonreactive pupils and pupils that react poorly to both light and near stimuli may be produced by damage to the afferent input to the visceral oculomotor nuclei or by damage to the nuclei and their efferent fiber tracts. The precise location of such lesions is almost impossible to determine unless there is associated evidence of ocular motor nerve dysfunction. A variety of pupillary abnormalities can be detected in patients with tumors in the pineal region. Some patients have markedly impaired light reactions but relatively intact responses to near stimuli (classic light-near dissociation), whereas others have impairment of both light and near reactions, and rare patients have relatively intact light reactions but impaired responses to near stimuli (inverse Argyll Robertson pupils).

Dilated, nonreactive or poorly reactive pupils that occur in patients with pinealomas and other tumors that damage the dorsal mesencephalon are usually bilateral and may precede the development of supranuclear paralysis of conjugate upward gaze. In some cases, there may initially be light-near dissociation.

Bilateral, dilated, nonreactive pupils rarely occur in isolation when caused by damage to the rostral oculomotor nuclear complex. Lesions that produce these changes must be located in the periaqueductal gray matter near the rostral end of the aqueduct. Vascular, inflammatory, neoplastic, and demyelinating diseases that affect this area almost always produce associated signs, including nuclear ophthalmoplegia, paralysis of vertical gaze, loss of convergence, exotropia, ptosis, and other defects of ocular movement.

Paradoxical Reaction of the Pupils to Light and Darkness

Patients with congenital stationary night blindness, congenital achromatopsia, blue-cone monochromatism, and Leber congenital amaurosis often exhibit a "paradoxical" pupillary response characterized by constriction in darkness. In a lighted room, such patients often have moderately dilated pupils; however, when the room lights are extinguished, the patients' pupils briskly constrict and then slowly redilate. Such responses occasionally occur in patients with optic disc hypoplasia, autosomal-dominant optic atrophy, and bilateral optic neuritis. These pupillary responses probably occur not from abnormalities in the CNS but from selective delays in afferent signals from the retinal photoreceptors to the pupillomotor center.

Light-Near Dissociation

Normal pupils constrict not only from light stimulation but also during near viewing as part of the **near response** of convergence, accommodation, and miosis. A constriction of the pupils during near-viewing that is stronger than the light response—**light-near dissociation**—may be caused by a defect in the afferent or the efferent system subserving pupillary function. For example, this is the primary feature of the Argyll Robertson pupils that occur from efferent dysfunction, but it is also seen in patients with pregeniculate blindness, compressive and infiltrative mesencephalic lesions, and damage to the parasympathetic innervation of the iris sphincter.

Argyll Robertson Pupils

The characteristic features of this syndrome as first described are (1) retinas sensitive to light, (2) pupils unresponsive to light, (3) normal pupillary constriction during accommodation and convergence for near objects, and (4) very small pupils (Fig. 15.19, **Video 15.2**). The Argyll Robertson pupil is widely accepted as being almost pathognomonic of neurosyphilis.

Argyll Robertson pupils are typically small and dilate poorly in darkness. An additional important feature is irregularity of the pupil. In the fully developed Argyll Robertson pupil, there is complete loss of pupillary constriction. Although constriction of the pupils to near stimulation often appears normal, the

Figure 15.19 Argyll Robertson pupils in a patient with neurosyphilis. **A:** Small irregular pupils in light. **B:** Further constriction with accommodative effort. **Video 15.2: light-near dissociation in the same patient.**

reaction usually is slightly impaired. Argyll Robertson pupils are usually bilateral and symmetric.

The site of the lesion responsible for the production of Argyll Robertson pupils is the region of the sylvian aqueduct in the rostral midbrain. In this location, the damage interferes with the light reflex fibers and the supranuclear inhibitory fibers as they approach the visceral oculomotor nuclei, but it spares the fibers subserving pupillary constriction for near-viewing.

The "complete" Argyll Robertson syndrome may be observed in patients with diabetes mellitus, chronic alcoholism, encephalitis, multiple sclerosis, age-related and degenerative diseases of the CNS, some rare midbrain tumors, and, rarely, in systemic inflammatory diseases, including sarcoidosis and neuroborreliosis. However, a patient with Argyll Robertson pupils should still be assumed to have neurosyphilis until proven otherwise.

Mesencephalic Lesions

Pressure on the dorsal mesencephalon may produce Parinaud syndrome (also called the sylvian aqueduct syndrome or dorsal midbrain syndrome). This syndrome of the rostral midbrain in the region of the posterior commissure consists of supranuclear paralysis of upward gaze (often worse for saccades than pursuit), lid retraction, accommodation difficulties, convergence-retraction nystagmus on attempted upward gaze, and disturbances of pupillary function. The pupils in such patients are typically large, fail to constrict to light or do so very poorly, and yet react well to near stimuli (Fig. 15.20). Such pupils may be the first sign of a pineal or other tumor that compresses or infiltrates the dorsal midbrain or of hydrocephalus, particularly that caused by aqueductal stenosis or a blocked shunt.

Lesions of the Afferent Pathway

Lesions of the visual sensory pathway from the retina to the point at which the pupillomotor fibers exit impair the light reaction but spare the near response. If the patient is blind from optic nerve disease, for example, there will be no reaction of the pupil in the blind eye to direct light stimulation, but the near reaction may be well preserved when tested using proprioception as a stimulus.

Aberrant Regeneration After Damage to the Innervation of the Iris Sphincter

In some patients who have damage to the innervation of the iris sphincter, the light reaction is not truly "spared," rather it is restored by aberrant regeneration of damaged fibers. This phenomenon occurs in the setting of aberrant regeneration after structural damage to the **preganglionic** oculomotor nerve. Fibers headed for extraocular muscles or the ciliary muscle may be diverted into the iris sphincter, which is such

A

B

Figure 15.20 Pupillary light-near dissociation in a patient with a dysgerminoma producing a dorsal midbrain syndrome. In a dimly lighted room, both pupils were large and slightly anisocoric. **A:** When a bright light is shined in either eye, both pupils constrict sluggishly and incompletely. **B:** When the patient is asked to look at an accommodative target, both pupils constrict briskly and extensively. The patient also had difficulty with upward gaze. **Video 15.3A: Lack of light response in another patient with the dorsal midbrain syndrome; Video 15.3B: Brisk near response.**

a small muscle that only a few of these fibers are sufficient to make the iris sphincter contract. Although such pupils are often called "tonic" pupils, two cardinal features of the tonic pupil—a slow sustained contraction to near effort and a slow redilation after constriction—are absent.

Disturbances During Seizures

Some patients, most of them children, experience unilateral, transient pupillary mydriasis during and after seizures. In most instances, the seizures are of the petit mal type. The mechanism of the pupillary dilation that occurs during and following seizure activity appears to be a combination of interruption of parasympathetic impulses and irritation of the sympathetic system.

Not all patients with pupillary disturbances during a seizure have dilation of the pupils. Some experience ictal unilateral or bilateral pupillary constriction, with and without ptosis.

Disturbances in Coma

Coma is a state of unarousable psychologic unresponsiveness in which the patient lies with eyes closed. Patients in coma show no psychologically understandable response to external stimuli or inner needs. Causes of coma include supratentorial lesions, infratentorial lesions, and diffuse brain dysfunction from a variety of inflammatory, infectious, degenerative, and metabolic processes. The prevalence of pupillary abnormalities in comatose patients is high and may, in some instances, help in the initial understanding and localization of the process.

Cerebral lesions that cause coma may produce primary abnormalities of pupillary size and reactivity. For example, damage to the **hypothalamus**, especially in the posterior and ventrolateral regions, may produce an ipsilateral central Horner syndrome. Downward displacement of the hypothalamus with unilateral Horner syndrome is often the first clear sign of incipient transtentorial herniation. Damage to the **diencephalon**, particularly during rostral–caudal brainstem deterioration caused by supratentorial lesions, produces symmetrically small but briskly reactive pupils.

Lesions of the dorsal tectal or pretectal regions of the **mesencephalon** interrupt the pupillary light reflex but may spare the response to near stimuli (light-near dissociation). The pupils are either in midposition or slightly dilated and are round. Mesencephalic lesions in the region of the oculomotor nerve nucleus nearly always damage both sympathetic and parasympathetic pathways to the eye. The resulting pupils are usually slightly irregular and unequal. They are midpositioned and nonreactive to light stimuli.

Lesions of the tegmental portion of the **pons** may interrupt descending sympathetic pathways and produce bilaterally small pupils. In many cases, especially those with pontine hemorrhage, the pupils are pinpoint, presumably from a combination of sympathetic interruption and parasympathetic disinhibition.

The pupillary fibers within the **peripheral oculomotor nerve** are particularly susceptible when uncal herniation compresses the nerve against the posterior cerebral artery or the edge of the cerebellar tentorium. In these instances, pupillary dilation may precede other signs of ocular motor nerve paralysis, and such patients may present with nonreactive, dilated, or oval pupils.

Supratentorial lesions produce neurologic dysfunction by two mechanisms: primary cerebral damage and secondary brainstem dysfunction from displacement, tissue compression, swelling, and vascular stasis. Of the two processes, secondary brainstem dysfunction is the more threatening to life. It usually presents as one of two main patterns. Most patients develop signs of bilateral diencephalic impairment: **the central syndrome**. In this syndrome, pupillary, ocular motor, and respiratory signs develop that indicate that diencephalic, mesencephalic, pontine, and, finally, medullary function are being lost in an orderly rostral–caudal fashion. Other patients develop signs of uncal herniation with oculomotor nerve and lateral mesencephalic compression, either ipsilaterally or contralaterally: **the uncal syndrome**.

In patients in deep coma, the state of the pupils may become the single most important criterion that clinically distinguishes between metabolic and structural disease. Pupillary pathways are relatively resistant to metabolic insults. Thus, the presence of preserved pupillary light reflexes despite concomitant respiratory depression, caloric unresponsiveness, decerebrate rigidity, or motor flaccidity suggests **metabolic coma**. Conversely, if asphyxia, drug ingestion, or pre-existing pupillary disease can be eliminated as a cause of coma, the absence of pupillary light reflexes in a comatose patient strongly implicates a structural lesion rather than a metabolic process.

Disturbances in Disorders of the Neuromuscular Junction

Despite being of neuroectodermal origin, the iris musculature may be affected by systemic myopathies and by generalized disorders of the neuromuscular junction. Although most investigators describe no pupillary abnormalities in patients with **myasthenia gravis**, rare patients with ocular myasthenia gravis have anisocoria, sluggishly reactive pupils, or both that show fatigue on prolonged light stimulation. This dysfunction **is not clinically significant** and should not confuse the diagnosis.

Botulism is a life-threatening disease that occurs from the effects of the toxin produced by one of several strains of the organism, *Clostridium botulinum*. In most instances, the source of the botulism is oral ingestion of the toxin in spoiled foods. Nearly all patients who develop botulism have multiple symptoms and signs of cholinergic dysfunction, including dilated, poorly reactive or nonreactive pupils, paresis of accommodation, ptosis, and ophthalmoplegia.

Drug Effects

Drugs That Dilate the Pupils

Parasympatholytic (Anticholinergic) Drugs. The pharmacology of the parasympathetic innervation of the iris is illustrated in Figure 15.21.

Sympathomimetic (Adrenergic) Drugs. The pharmacology of the sympathetic innervation of the iris is illustrated in Figure 15.22.

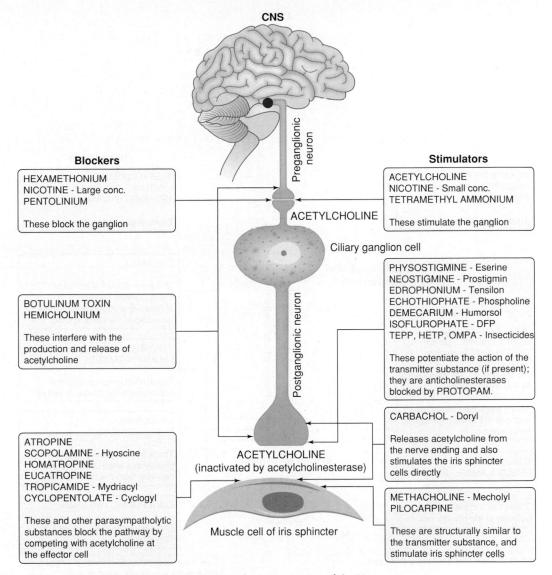

CNS

Blockers

Preganglionic neuron

Stimulators

HEXAMETHONIUM
NICOTINE - Large conc.
PENTOLINIUM

These block the ganglion

ACETYLCHOLINE

ACETYLCHOLINE
NICOTINE - Small conc.
TETRAMETHYL AMMONIUM

These stimulate the ganglion

Ciliary ganglion cell

PHYSOSTIGMINE - Eserine
NEOSTIGMINE - Prostigmin
EDROPHONIUM - Tensilon
ECHOTHIOPHATE - Phospholine
DEMECARIUM - Humorsol
ISOFLUROPHATE - DFP
TEPP, HETP, OMPA - Insecticides

These potentiate the action of the
transmitter substance (if present);
they are anticholinesterases
blocked by PROTOPAM.

BOTULINUM TOXIN
HEMICHOLINIUM

These interfere with the
production and release of
acetylcholine

Postganglionic neuron

CARBACHOL - Doryl

Releases acetylcholine from
the nerve ending and also
stimulates the iris sphincter
cells directly

ATROPINE
SCOPOLAMINE - Hyoscine
HOMATROPINE
EUCATROPINE
TROPICAMIDE - Mydriacyl
CYCLOPENTOLATE - Cyclogyl

These and other parasympatholytic
substances block the pathway by
competing with acetylcholine at
the effector cell

ACETYLCHOLINE
(inactivated by acetylcholinesterase)

Muscle cell of iris sphincter

METHACHOLINE - Mecholyl
PILOCARPINE

These are structurally similar to
the transmitter substance, and
stimulate iris sphincter cells

Figure 15.21 The pharmacology of the parasympathetic innervation of the iris.

Drugs That Constrict the Pupils

Parasympathomimetic (Cholinergic) Drugs. The pharmacology of the parasympathetic innervation of the iris is illustrated in Figure 15.21.

Sympatholytic (Antiadrenergic) Drugs. The pharmacology of the sympathetic innervation of the iris is illustrated in Figure 15.22.

Structural Defects of the Iris

Congenital. Aniridia is a congenital abnormality in which the iris appears clinically to be absent (Fig. 15.23A). In almost all cases, histologic or gonioscopic examination reveals small remnants of iris tissue. The condition is usually bilateral and may occur as a hereditary condition or as a sporadic phenomenon. When the condition is hereditary, it is usually transmitted in an autosomal-dominant fashion; however, rare cases of recessive transmission occur. Patients with aniridia usually have poor visual acuity and other ocular abnormalities, including nystagmus, glaucoma, cataracts, ectopia lentis, corneal degeneration, and optic nerve or macular hypoplasia or aplasia. Systemic abnormalities found in patients with aniridia include polydactyly, oligophrenia, cranial dysostosis, malformations of the extremities and external ears, hydrocephalus, cerebellar ataxia, and mental retardation. The most important association, however, is with the childhood cancer Wilms tumor.

CNS

C-8
T-1
T-2

Preganglionic neuron

Blockers

HEXAMETHONIUM
NICOTINE - Large conc.
PENTOLINIUM

These block the ganglion

ACETYLCHOLINE

Stimulators

ACETYLCHOLINE
NICOTINE - Small conc.
TETRAMETHYL AMMONIUM

These stimulate the ganglion

Superior cervical
ganglion cell

COCAINE

This potentiates the action of
the transmitter substance
(if present) probably by preventing
rebinding at the nerve ending

Postganglionic neuron

GUANETHIDINE - Ismelin
BRETYLIUM - Darenthin
RESERPINE
∝ METHYLDOPA - Aldomet
M A O INHIBITORS

These block the sympathetic
pathway at the postaganglionic
never ending.

TYRAMINE
OH-AMPHETAMINE - Paredrine

These release norepinephrine
(if present) from the nerve ending

REBIND

NOREPINEPHRINE

EPHEDRINE
PHENYLEPHRINE-Neo-Synephrine

These stimulate the dilator cells
directly; but also release norepinephrine from the nerve ending

DIBENZYLINE
PHENTOLAMINE - Regitine
TOLAZOLINE - Priscoline

These block the sympathetic
pathway at the effector cell

COMT**

EPINEPHRINE - Adrenalin

This stimulates the iris dilator
cells directly

Muscle cell of iris dilator

** COMT - catechol 0-methyl transferase

* These sympathomimetic amines are structurally
similar to the transmitter substance.

Figure 15.22 The pharmacology of the sympathetic innervation of the iris.

A **coloboma** is a full-thickness defect that may be limited to the iris tissue or may be part of a larger defect that involving the ciliary body, choroid, and optic disc (see Fig. 15.23B). Coloboma of the iris may be transmitted either as a dominant or a recessive trait.

Misplaced or **ectopic pupils** (corectopia, ectopia pupillae) are usually bilateral and symmetric. They are typically displaced up and out from the center of the cornea. Such displacement of the pupils may be isolated but is frequently associated with ectopia lentis, congenital glaucoma, microcornea, ocular coloboma, albinism, external ophthalmoplegia, and high myopia (see Fig. 15.23C).

Persistent pupillary membrane remnants are vestiges of the embryonic pupillary membrane that can be seen as thread-like bands running across the pupillary space and attaching to the lesser circle of the iris (see Fig. 15.23D). These remnants do not interfere with pupillary movements, and they do not have clinical significance.

In true **polycoria**, the extra pupil(s) has a sphincter muscle that contracts on exposure to light. In fact, most additional pupils are actually just holes in the iris without a separate sphincter muscle. This **pseudo-polycoria** may be a congenital disorder, such as an iris coloboma or persistent pupillary membrane, or it may

Figure 15.23 Iris anomalies that may simulate neurologic pupillary abnormalities. **A:** Aniridia. Note associated upward lens dislocation. (Courtesy of Dr. Irene H. Maumenee.) **B:** Typical iris coloboma. (Courtesy of Dr. Irene H. Maumenee.) **C:** Acquired corectopia in iridocorneal–endothelial adhesion syndrome. (Courtesy of Dr. Harry A. Quigley.) **D:** Persistent pupillary membrane. (Reprinted with permission from Gutman ED, Goldberg MF. Persistent pupillary membrane and other ocular abnormalities. *Arch Ophthalmol.* 1976;94:156–157.) **E:** Pseudopolycoria from iridocorneal–endothelial adhesion syndrome. (Courtesy of Dr. Harry A. Quigley.) **F:** Heterochromia iridis in a patient with congenital Horner syndrome. Note that the lighter iris is the abnormal iris.

be part of one of several syndromes characterized by mesodermal dysgenesis. More commonly, pseudo-polycoria occurs as an acquired disorder from direct iris trauma, including surgery, photocoagulation, ischemia, and glaucoma, or as part of a degenerative process such as the ICE syndrome (see Fig. 15.23E).

Congenital miosis, which is usually bilateral, is characterized by extremely small pupils that react

slightly to light stimuli and dilate poorly after instillation of sympathomimetic agents. The anomaly appears to result from congenital absence of the iris dilator muscle. Congenital miosis may be an isolated phenomenon, or it may be associated with other ocular abnormalities, including microcornea, iris atrophy, myopia, heterochromia iridis, and anterior chamber angle deformities.

Congenital mydriasis is a unilateral or bilateral disorder that may be difficult to distinguish from aniridia unless a careful ocular examination is performed. There appear to be numerous causes of congenital mydriasis. It may occur as an isolated phenomenon or in association with developmental delay and has been reported in a patient with Waardenburg syndrome.

The color of the iris depends upon the pigment in the iris stroma. In albinism, there is failure of mesodermal and ectodermal pigmentation. Consequently, the iris has a transparent, grayish-red color and transilluminates readily. In a number of congenital and acquired conditions, the iris of one eye differs in color from the iris of the other eye. In other instances, one iris is entirely normal, and a part of the iris in the opposite eye has a different color than the rest of the iris surrounding it (iris bicolor). These abnormalities, collectively called **heterochromia iridis**, may occur as: (1) an isolated congenital anomaly; (2) in association with other ocular abnormalities, such as iris or optic disc coloboma; (3) in association with systemic congenital abnormalities, as in patients with Waardenburg syndrome, congenital Horner syndrome, or incontinentia pigmenti; or (4) from an acquired ocular condition (see Fig. 15.23F).

Acquired. **Iritis** or **iridocyclitis** in its acute stages produces swelling of the iris, miosis, and slight reddening of the circumcorneal tissues. The miosis of iritis results from the release of substance P, which produces miosis through interaction with a specific receptor in the iris sphincter muscle. In patients with intraocular inflammation, dilation of the pupil with mydriatics may be difficult because of adhesions between the iris and the lens (posterior synechiae). These adhesions in chronic iritis may distort the shape of the pupil. They may also fix the pupil in a dilated position.

Ischemia of the anterior segment of the globe can produce iridoplegia. Transient dilation of the pupil may occur during an episode of monocular amaurosis associated with carotid occlusive disease, migraine, giant cell arteritis, or Raynaud disease. This unilateral pupillary change is *not* caused by the blindness but by the hypoxic process that affects the entire eye, including the iris sphincter. If the whole globe is ischemic (as in angle-closure glaucoma), iris ischemia will relax the iris sphincter and dilate the pupil. Chronic ischemia of the anterior segment of the globe results in neovascularization of the chamber angle and the surface of the iris (rubeosis iridis), producing iris atrophy, ectropion of the pigment layer at the pupillary margin (ectropion uveae), glaucoma, and immobility of the iris.

Very few **tumors** affect the iris, but those that do can cause irregularity of the iris border, anisocoria, and an abnormally reactive pupil. Leiomyoma, malignant melanoma, and lymphoma can all present in this fashion.

Spastic miosis is a constant and immediate result of **trauma** to the globe and occurs immediately after blunt trauma to the cornea or perforating injury to the eye. The constriction of the pupil is profound but usually transient and often followed by iridoplegia. Dilation of the pupil frequently occurs after concussion of the globe and is often followed by paralysis of accommodation after the initial intense miosis has resolved. The frequent absence of detectable pathologic change suggests that the effect may occur from injury of the fine nerves of the ciliary plexus. In other cases, tears in the iris or rupture of the iris sphincter may be identified using slit lamp biomicroscopy with transillumination, and a traumatic, peripheral iridodialysis may be present, with resultant distortion of the normally round pupil.

Iris **atrophy** may be caused by inflammation, ischemia, or trauma. It may be circumscribed or diffuse and may involve the anterior border layer, the stroma and sphincter muscle, the anterior epithelium and dilator muscle, the posterior pigmented epithelium, or a combination of these structures.

Some patients experience an irreversible mydriasis and pupillary immobility after an otherwise uncomplicated keratoplasty or uneventful cataract extraction. This **postoperative mydriasis** or "atonic pupil" probably results from direct damage to the iris sphincter muscle during surgery.

Disorders of Accommodation

Abnormalities of accommodation are usually acquired, although congenital anomalies do occur. Acquired disturbances of accommodation occur most frequently as part of the normal aging process (presbyopia); however, disturbances of accommodation may also occur in otherwise healthy persons, in persons with generalized systemic and neurologic disorders, and in persons with lesions that produce a focal interruption of the parasympathetic (and, rarely, the sympathetic) innervation of the ciliary body. Finally, accommodation may be voluntarily disrupted.

Accommodation Insufficiency and Paralysis

Congenital and Hereditary Accommodation Insufficiency and Paralysis
Congenital defects are a rare cause of isolated lack of accommodation. The ciliary body is, however, defective in a number of congenital ocular anomalies. In most cases, vision is so defective that the inability to accommodate is never noted by either the patient or the physician. Aniridia and choroidal coloboma cause obvious defects of the ciliary body, but ciliary aplasia

also occurs in well-formed eyes in which the iris is intact and reacts normally to light.

Acquired Accommodation Paresis

Isolated Accommodation Insufficiency. Accommodation insufficiency may be separated into two groups: static insufficiency and dynamic insufficiency.

Patients with **static insufficiency** of accommodation have normal ciliary body innervation and normal innervational impulses, but there is an inadequate response of either the lens or the ciliary muscle. A majority of patients in this group suffer from presbyopia. Static accommodation insufficiency usually occurs gradually as changes occur in either the lens or the ciliary body. In some cases, however, there is sudden loss of accommodation that does not recover. Patients with static accommodation insufficiency require appropriate spectacle correction.

Patients with **dynamic insufficiency** have inadequate parasympathetic impulses required to stimulate the ciliary musculature. Patients with isolated dynamic accommodation insufficiency have normal pupillary size and reactivity. The diagnosis of dynamic accommodation insufficiency is made by measurements of accommodation that are found to be below the minimum for the age of the patient. Such patients often have associated convergence insufficiency. The symptoms of dynamic accommodation insufficiency are asthenopia, tiring of the eyes sometimes associated with brow ache, irritation and burning of the eyes, blurred vision particularly for near work, inability to concentrate, and photophobia. Dynamic insufficiency of accommodation usually occurs in asthenopic persons who become ill with some unrelated condition, although it may also occur suddenly in otherwise healthy individuals. As a general rule, accommodation recovers once the patient's illness is successfully treated.

The management of dynamic accommodation insufficiency is treatment of the underlying illness, after which the patient's symptoms often disappear. If accommodation insufficiency remains, the prescription of convex (plus) lenses is indicated, regardless of the patient's age. In patients with an associated convergence insufficiency, convergence exercises or base-out prisms added to the patient's near correction may be of benefit.

Accommodation Insufficiency Associated with Primary Ocular Disease

Inflammatory conditions (iridocyclitis), glaucoma in young patients, choroidal metastases, ocular trauma (including surgery), and other primary ocular processes may damage the ciliary body or its innervation. Recognition of these entities avoids unnecessary investigations for more widespread disorders.

Accommodation Insufficiency Associated with Neuromuscular Disorders

Some diseases produce myopathic changes in the smooth muscle fibers of the ciliary body. Isolated ocular involvement of this type is rare, however.

Myotonic dystrophy frequently produces degenerative changes in the lens, the region of the ora serrata, and the anterior chamber angle. Because other smooth muscle dysfunction occurs in such patients, the ciliary muscle also may be affected.

Myasthenia gravis rarely may cause defective accommodation, and this may be the first symptom of the disorder.

Accommodation paralysis is a common and early sign of **botulism.** In some cases, it is the initial sign of nervous system involvement, usually heralding the onset of complete internal and external ophthalmoplegia and various bulbar palsies. It persists for as long as a year, if the patient survives.

Tetanus can produce accommodation paralysis. In most cases, the accommodation paralysis occurs in the setting of generalized ophthalmoparesis.

Accommodation Insufficiency Associated with Focal or Generalized Neurologic Disease

Accommodation paresis may be caused by both focal and generalized neurologic disorders that interrupt the innervation of the ciliary body. In some cases, focal lesions of the oculoparasympathetic pathway produce characteristic abnormalities of accommodation combined with disturbances of pupillary function, ocular motility, or both. In other instances, the parasympathetic innervation to the ciliary body is interrupted as part of the overall involvement of the nervous system.

Accommodation may become paretic in both eyes from lesions of the parasympathetic nuclei in the midbrain (e.g., following encephalitis). The pupils may or may not be affected. Vague visual complaints resulting from an abnormality of accommodation can be one of the earliest symptoms of pressure on the **dorsal mesencephalon,** either from hydrocephalus or from an extrinsic mass lesion such as a pineal tumor. Multiple sclerosis, Guillain–Barré syndrome, and ischemia can all cause accommodation paralysis through their effects on the mesencephalon. In most patients, there are other signs of mesencephalic dysfunction.

Acute neurologic dysfunction of the hemispheres may cause accommodation insufficiency. The lesions that can produce this phenomenon include acute ischemic **stroke** and **hematoma**; thus far, reported cases are confined to the left cerebral hemisphere.

Wilson's disease is a hereditary disorder of copper metabolism that is characterized by a progressive degeneration of the CNS associated with hepatic cirrhosis. Ocular findings in patients with Wilson disease include a peripheral corneal ring of copper deposition involving Descemet membrane (Kayser–Fleischer ring), copper pigment under the lens capsule, and various ocular motor disturbances. Paresis of accommodation is common in such patients.

Most patients with **tonic pupil syndromes** initially have an accommodative paresis. In most cases of tonic pupil syndrome, particularly in Adie syndrome, the accommodation insufficiency shows marked improvement over several months; however, because of denervation supersensitivity of the ciliary body, some patients have persistent tonic accommodation, and others have persistent fluctuations in accommodation.

Accommodation Insufficiency Associated with Systemic Disease

Children and adults may develop transient accommodation paresis following various systemic illnesses. In such cases, the accommodation paresis often appears to occur as an indirect complication of the systemic disorder rather than from direct damage to the ciliary body or its innervation. There are, however, certain systemic diseases that produce accommodation insufficiency through direct effects on the ciliary body and lens or on their innervation.

In patients who develop **diphtheria**, accommodative paralysis is usually bilateral and often occurs during or after the third week following the onset of infection. Patients typically have normal pupillary responses to light but almost no movement of the pupil during attempted near-viewing.

Transient loss of accommodation may occur in patients with **diabetes mellitus**, particularly in the young. It develops in 14% to 19% of new diabetics in all age groups, but in 77% of patients under 30 years of age who also have refractive changes. Although the accommodation paresis may develop in patients with uncontrolled diabetes, it usually occurs after treatment has begun. Hyperopia and accommodation weakness develop concurrently within a few days after the patient's blood glucose has been lowered and then gradually return to normal over 2 to 6 weeks. Either metabolic or neurologic mechanisms can be responsible for accommodation paresis in a patient with this disease.

Accommodation Insufficiency Associated with Trauma to the Head and Neck

Symptoms of difficulty with focusing at near and at far, commonly associated with headache and pains about the eyes, are common complaints in patients who have experienced cerebral concussion or craniocervical extension injuries. These vague and ill-defined complaints are most prominent during the first weeks or months after injury. The persistence of such complaints for many months or even years is most common in patients who are seeking compensation for their injury through litigation. An organic basis for

these complaints is difficult, if not impossible, to establish. Theoretically, any cerebral injury could impair the highly complex neurophysiologic system involved in the coordination of the near response.

Accommodation Insufficiency and Paralysis from Pharmacologic Agents

Some pharmacologic agents that produce pupillary mydriasis after ocular instillation also produce cycloplegia, including atropine, scopolamine, homatropine, eucatropine, tropicamide, cyclopentolate, and oxyphenonium. None of these agents ever causes persistent paralysis of accommodation after discontinuation.

When cycloplegic agents or related substances are incorporated in medications that are taken internally or applied to the skin, there may be sufficient absorption to produce paresis of accommodation. In such cases, there is never complete paralysis of accommodation, and recovery begins shortly after the medication is discontinued.

Accommodation Paralysis for Distance: Sympathetic Paralysis

Lesions of the cervical sympathetic outflow may produce a defect that prevents the patient from accommodating fully from near to far, but most reports describe an **increase** in accommodative amplitude on the side of the Horner syndrome. Accommodation paresis for distance may also occur periodically in patients with Raeder paratrigeminal neuralgia.

Accommodation Spasm and Spasm of the Near Reflex

Accommodation Spasm Associated with Organic Disease

Accommodation crises or spasms produce an increase in myopia or pseudomyopia. This increase in myopia is often associated with convergence and miosis—that is, a **spasm of the near reflex**. In rare instances, these spasms are caused by or associated with a variety of diverse organic ocular motor and neurologic diseases, such as hepatic encephalopathy, neurosyphilis, ocular inflammation, Raeder paratrigeminal syndrome, cyclic oculomotor palsy, coma, and myasthenia gravis.

Patients with both primary and secondary **aberrant reinnervation of the oculomotor nerve** have pupillary disturbances, and such patients may also have aberrant reinnervation of the ciliary body. Accommodation in these patients may thus be increased, compared with a normal age-matched population.

Accommodation Spasm Unassociated with Organic Disease

Many young persons, when undergoing a noncycloplegic refraction, consistently accept overcorrecting concave (minus) lenses. When the same patients undergo a cycloplegic refraction, they are found to be emmetropic or at least significantly less myopic than they appeared to be when not cyclopleged. Such persons are exhibiting an increase or "spasm" of accommodation. In some patients, the accommodation spasm may be significant, as much as 10 D, and may persist for several years. Accommodation spasm of such magnitude is often associated with excessive convergence that produces a variable esotropia with miosis.

Spasm of accommodation occurs most often in patients who are malingering or who have conversion hysteria. In these patients, it usually occurs as intermittent attacks of accommodative spasm, convergence, and miosis—spasm of the near reflex. The degree of accommodation and convergence spasm in such

patients is variable; however, miosis is always present and impressive (Fig. 15.24).

Spasm of the near reflex may be associated with headache, photophobia, defective vision for near and distance, inability to concentrate, and diplopia with bilateral or unilateral limitation of horizontal eye movements. The observation of **miosis** in a patient with apparent unilateral or bilateral limitation of abduction and severe myopia (8 to 10 D) is crucial in arriving at the correct diagnosis. This miosis generally resolves as soon as either eye is occluded with a hand-held occluder or patch. In addition, despite apparent bilateral abduction weakness with both eyes open, such patients usually show full abduction in each eye when the opposite eye is patched and ductions are tested directly. Refraction with and without cycloplegia will establish the presence of pseudomyopia.

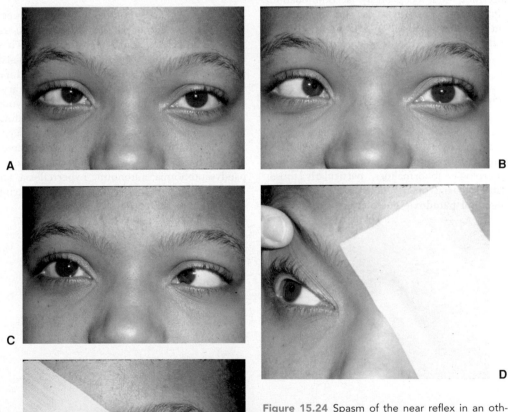

Figure 15.24 Spasm of the near reflex in an otherwise healthy 15-year-old woman. **A:** In primary position, the eyes are esotropic, and the pupils are constricted. **B:** On attempted left gaze, the left eye does not abduct, and both pupils become even smaller. **C:** On attempted right gaze, the right eye does not abduct, and both pupils become smaller. **D:** With the left eye patched, the right eye abducts fully on oculocephalic testing, and the pupil dilates. **E:** With the right eye patched, the left eye abducts fully on oculocephalic testing, and the pupil dilates.

The management of patients with spasm of the near reflex depends on the setting in which it occurs. Some patients require only simple reassurance that they have no irreversible visual or neurologic disorder. For others, psychiatric counseling is appropriate. In some patients, symptomatic relief may be achieved with a cycloplegic agent and bifocal spectacles or reading glasses. Glasses with an opaque inner third of the lens can be used to treat some patients with spasm of the near reflex. These glasses are designed to occlude vision when the eyes are esotropic, thus interrupting the convergence spasm.

Accommodation Spasm from Pharmacologic Agents

Most of the cholinergic agents that are mentioned in the earlier section of this chapter concerning pharmacologically induced miosis also produce an increase in accommodation and, occasionally, accommodation spasm. Pilocarpine, physostigmine, and the organophosphate esters produce the most accommodation, whereas the effect of aceclidine on accommodation is minimal.

Disorders of Lacrimation

Tear secretion may be altered by supranuclear lesions as well as by lesions along the pathway from the brainstem to the lacrimal gland. In most cases, there are other neurologic abnormalities, particularly those that relate to facial or trigeminal nerve function. The **congenital paradoxic gustolacrimal reflex** is a rare phenomenon that may be associated with congenital absence of ocular abduction or Duane syndrome on the involved side. Occasional patients with small vestibular schwannomas report **excessive lacrimation** on the side of their deafness. This symptom may only be apparent during meals. Inappropriate tearing with chewing (crocodile tears) may develop in patients with lesions affecting the gasserian ganglion and the greater superficial petrosal nerve, in which aberrant regeneration of masseter fibers occurs. Abducens dysfunction also may be seen, and patients with an apparently isolated abduction deficit should have tearing function evaluated in addition to ocular motor and sensory testing.

Generalized Disturbances of Autonomic Function

Pupillary and accommodation abnormalities may occur as part of generalized dysfunction of various portions of the autonomic nervous system. These disorders include, but are not restricted to, familial dysautonomia (Riley-Day syndrome); congenital familial sensory neuropathy with anhidrosis; hereditary anhidrotic ectodermal dysplasia; neural crest syndrome; congenital cholinergic nervous system dysfunction; tonic pupils, areflexia, and progressive segmental hypohidrosis (Ross syndrome); primary acquired autonomic dysfunction (Shy–Drager syndrome); acute pandysautonomia; autonomic hyperreflexia; and the Miller Fisher variant of Guillain–Barré syndrome (ophthalmoplegia, ataxia, and areflexia).

Examination of Ocular Motility and Alignment*

History
  Diplopia
  Visual Confusion
  Blurred Vision
  Vestibular Symptoms: Vertigo, Oscillopsia, and Tilt
Examination
  Fixation and Gaze-Holding Ability
  Range of Eye Movements
  Ocular Alignment
  Performance of Versions

History

A careful history should always precede a complete examination of the ocular motor system. Patients with ocular motor disorders may complain of a number of visual difficulties, including diplopia, visual confusion, blurred vision, and the vestibular symptoms of vertigo, oscillopsia, or tilt.

Diplopia

Because misalignment of the visual axes causes the image of an object of interest to fall on noncorresponding parts of the two retinas, usually the fovea of one eye and extrafoveal retina of the other eye, a sensory phenomenon occurs that is usually interpreted as **diplopia**, the visualization of an object in two different spatial locations. Diplopia may be horizontal, vertical, torsional, or a combination of these.

Diplopia that results from ocular misalignment disappears with either eye closed—it is a **binocular** phenomenon. Binocular diplopia is almost never caused by intraocular disease, although it may occur in rare patients in the setting of a monocular macular lesion, such as a subretinal neovascular membrane or epiretinal membrane formation. The pathophysiology of binocular diplopia with uniocular disease may represent the establishment of rivalry between central and

peripheral fusion mechanisms, as seen in the dragged fovea diplopia syndrome.

Diplopia that persists with one eye closed, **monocular diplopia**, is rarely caused by neurologic disease. In almost all cases, it is produced by local ocular phenomena, including uncorrected astigmatism or other refractive errors, corneal and iris abnormalities, cataract, and macular disease. Most patients with this type of monocular diplopia recognize a difference in the intensity of the two images that they see and may be described as a "ghost image" that overlaps the clear image. A pinhole will typically eliminate this form of diplopia, making it a useful test in patients suspected of monocular diplopia due to anterior segment or refractive abnormalities.

Cases of monocular diplopia and polyopia are occasionally reported in patients with central nervous system (CNS) disease. Patients with "cerebral polyopia" generally see each image with equal clarity and many copies of the same image. In addition, the monocular diplopia in these patients is always seen with either eye covered. Such patients usually have lesions in the parieto-occipital region and associated visual field defects. The mechanism of cerebral diplopia–polyopia is unknown.

For patients with true binocular diplopia, the eyes are presumably misaligned, and the examiner should ascertain if the diplopia is horizontal, vertical, or oblique; better or worse in any particular direction of gaze; intermittent or constant; different when viewing at distance or near; or affected by head posture.

Visual Confusion

In patients with misalignment of the visual axes, the maculae of the two eyes are simultaneously viewing two different objects or areas, interpreted as existing at the same point in space. This sensory phenomenon is called **visual confusion**. Patients with visual confusion complain that the images of objects of interest are superimposed on inappropriate backgrounds.

Blurred Vision

Misalignment of the visual axes does not always produce diplopia or visual confusion. In some patients, the images of an object seen by noncorresponding parts of the retina are so close together that the patient

---

*The authors acknowledge the past contributions of Mark S. Borchert to this chapter.

does not recognize two distinctly separated images but instead complains that the vision is blurred when both eyes are open. In such patients, the blurred vision clears completely if **either eye** is closed.

Blurred vision that resolves with one but not either eye closed usually suggests a primary visual sensory disturbance. Blurred vision that does not resolve with either eye closed also usually occurs from visual sensory disease but may also occur in some patients with oscillopsia, disorders of saccades (e.g., saccadic oscillations such as ocular flutter), and in patients with impaired pursuit leading to disordered tracking.

Vestibular Symptoms: Vertigo, Oscillopsia, and Tilt

Patients with disorders that affect the vestibular system may complain of disequilibrium or unsteadiness, symptoms that reflect imbalance of vestibular tone. A common complaint of patients with vestibular imbalance (disease of vestibular organ, nerve, or brainstem nuclei) is **vertigo**, the illusory sensation of motion of self or of the environment. Vertigo usually reflects a mismatch among vestibular, visual, and somatosensory inputs concerning the position or motion of one's body in space. It is best to evaluate the vestibular sense alone by asking the patient about the perceived direction of self-rotation with the **eyes closed**, thus eliminating conflicting visual stimuli.

Oscillopsia is an illusory to-and-fro movement of the environment that may be horizontal, vertical, torsional, or a combination of these directions, caused by an instability of fixation, typically of neurologic origin. When oscillopsia is produced or accentuated by head movement it is usually due to vestibular imbalance. Oscillopsia is rarely present when ocular motor dysfunction is congenital (e.g., congenital or latent nystagmus).

A third group of vestibular symptoms include the perception of **tilt**: static rotation of the perceived world or the body. These complaints usually reflect a disturbance of the otolith organs from either peripheral or central causes. When dealing with such patients, as with patients who complain of vertigo, the examiner should ask about the perception of the position of the body relative to the earth vertical, with the eyes closed to eliminate conflicting visual stimuli.

Examination

The examination of the ocular motor system generally consists of the assessment of (1) fixation and gaze-holding ability, (2) range of monocular and binocular eye movements, (3) ocular alignment, and (4) performance of versions (saccades, pursuit). In addition, depending on the findings of the basic examination,

it may be appropriate to test the vestibulo-ocular and optokinetic reflexes to differentiate between supranuclear and nuclear or infranuclear disorders.

Fixation and Gaze-Holding Ability

Principles

In a normal, awake person, the eyes are never absolutely still. Fixation is interrupted by three distinctive types of miniature eye movements including microsaccades, continuous microdrift, and microtremor. Square-wave jerks—spontaneous, horizontal saccades of about 0.5 degrees, followed about 200 msec later by a corrective saccade and occurring at a rate of less than 9 per minute—can also be observed during fixation in most normal individuals.

When no efforts are being made toward ocular fixation or accommodation, the eyes are said to be in a "physiologic" position of rest. With total ophthalmoplegia, there is usually a slight divergence of the visual axes, and this position usually also occurs during sleep, deep anesthesia, and death.

Technique

In patients complaining of intermittent diplopia, visual confusion, or strabismus, tests of sensory fusion (e.g., stereoacuity) and fixation should be performed before the eyes are dissociated by tests of monocular visual function (e.g., visual acuity, color vision, visual fields).

Range of Eye Movements

Principles

To discuss eye movements, it is necessary to have a frame of reference against which any movement may be quantified. Accordingly, the **primary** position of the eyes is arbitrarily designated as that position from which all other ocular movements are initiated or measured.

All movements of the globe around the hypothetical center of rotation can be analyzed in terms of a coordinate system with three axes perpendicular to each other and intersecting at the center of rotation (Fig. 16.1). The Y axis is equivalent to the visual axis; the Z axis is vertical (around which the eye rotates horizontally); and the X axis is horizontal (around which the eye rotates vertically).

Rotations of either eye alone without attention to the movements of the other eye are called **ductions**. Horizontal rotation is termed **adduction** if the anterior pole of the eye is rotated nasally and **abduction** if the anterior pole of the eye is rotated temporally. Vertical rotation is called **elevation** if the anterior pole of the eye rotates upward and **depression** if it rotates downward.

Rotation around either the horizontal or vertical axis places the eye in a **secondary** position of gaze. In achieving this position, there is no rotation of the globe around the Y axis (i.e., there is no torsion). The

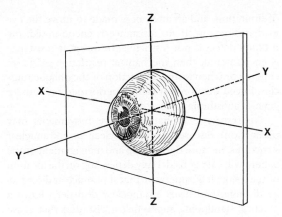

Figure 16.1 The axes of rotation of the eye. The Y axis corresponds to the line of sight when the eye is in the primary position, looking straight ahead.

oblique positions of gaze are called **tertiary** positions. They are achieved by a simultaneous rotation around the horizontal and vertical axes. When an eye moves obliquely out of primary position, the vertical axis of the globe tilts with respect to the X and Z axes.

True ocular torsion is defined by the direction of the rotation around the Y axis (i.e., the visual axis) relative to the nose. If the 12 o'clock region of the limbus rotates toward the nose, the movement is called **intorsion** (incycloduction; incyclotorsion). If the same area rotates away from the nose, the movement is called **extorsion** (excycloduction; excyclotorsion).

Torsion occurs mainly as part of the involuntary compensatory eye movements that take place during head tilt. In this setting, the torsion movements are called **countertorsion** or **counter rolling**. **Dynamic countertorsion** occurs during head tilt and reflects the semicircular canal-induced torsional vestibulo-ocular reflex (VOR). **Static countertorsion** persists at a given angle of any head tilt, but the amount of rotation is minor compared with that which occurs from dynamic countertorsion. Static countertorsion reflects a tonic otolith–ocular reflex. Each utricle influences

both eyes in both directions but primarily controls tilt to the contralateral side.

The actions of the extraocular muscles are typically discussed in terms of individual antagonist pairs and have primary, and potentially secondary, and tertiary actions (see Table 16.1). Normal eye movements are binocular. Such movements are called **versions** if the movements of the two eyes are in the same direction and **vergence** movements if they are in opposite directions (i.e., divergence or convergence). For practical purposes, the extraocular muscles of each eye work in pairs during both versions and vergence movements, with one muscle of each eye contracting (the **agonist**) while its opposing muscle relaxes (the **antagonist**). The three agonist–antagonist muscle pairs for each eye are the medial and lateral rectus muscles, the superior and inferior rectus muscles, and the superior and inferior oblique muscles. Whenever an agonist muscle receives a neural impulse to contract, an equivalent inhibitory impulse is sent to the motor neurons supplying the antagonist muscle so that it will relax. This is called **Sherrington law of reciprocal innervation**.

For the eyes to move together to produce a horizontal version, the lateral rectus of one eye and the medial rectus of the opposite eye must contract together. These muscles constitute a **yoke pair**. The other two yoke pairs are the superior rectus muscle of one eye and the inferior oblique muscle of the other eye, and the superior oblique muscle of one eye and the inferior rectus muscle of the other eye. Implicit in the concept of a yoke pair is that such muscles receive equal innervation so that the eyes move together, which forms the basis of **Hering law of motor correspondence**.

Techniques

When testing the range of ocular movement, the examiner should ask the patient to follow a target through the full range of movement, including the cardinal (or diagnostic) positions of gaze. The eyes are tested individually with one eye covered and together with both eyes open. The normal range of movements

Table 16.1	**Actions of the Extraocular Muscles**		
Extraocular Muscle	**Primary**	**Secondary**	**Tertiary**
Medial rectus	Adduction	None	None
Lateral rectus	Abduction	None	None
Superior rectus	Elevation	Incyclotorsion	Adduction
Inferior rectus	Depression	Excyclotorsion	Adduction
Superior oblique	Incyclotorsion	Depression	Abduction
Inferior oblique	Excyclotorsion	Elevation	Abduction

is fairly stable throughout life for all directions except upgaze. Normal abduction is usually 50 degrees; adduction, 50 degrees; and depression, 45 degrees. Limitation of upward gaze in an older individual may simply be age-related and not necessarily a new, pathologic process.

When the range of motion is limited, it is necessary to determine if the limitation is mechanical, and if not, whether the disturbance is supranuclear or peripheral.

Several tests may be used to determine if a mechanical restriction of ocular motion is present. Mechanical limitation of motion (such as that seen in patients with thyroid ophthalmopathy or orbital floor fracture with entrapment) can be inferred if intraocular pressure increases substantially when the patient attempts to look in the direction of gaze limitation.

Mechanical limitation of motion can more reliably be detected with **forced duction** testing. In such tests, an attempt is made to move the eye forcibly in the direction(s) of gaze limitation while the patient is attempting to look in that direction (Fig. 16.2). After adequate topical anesthesia, the conjunctiva is grasped with a fine-toothed forceps near the limbus on the side opposite the direction in which the eye is to be moved. The patient is instructed to try to look in the direction

Figure 16.2 Forced duction testing. After the eye has been anesthetized with topical proparacaine and cocaine, the conjunctiva just posterior to the limbus is grasped with a fine-toothed forceps at a point opposite the direction of limitation. An attempt is then made to rotate the eye in the direction of limitation. If no mechanical limitation is present, the eye can be moved fully into the direction of limitation (*solid black arrow*). If mechanical limitation is present, the eye will resist attempts to rotate it into the field of limitation (*dashed black arrow*).

of limitation, and an attempt is made to move the eye in that direction. If no resistance is encountered, the motility defect is not restrictive; however, if resistance is encountered, then mechanical restriction exists. In children or when testing restriction of the oblique muscles, forced duction test can be performed only under general anesthesia.

Nonrestrictive limitation of eye movements may occur from disease of supranuclear or infranuclear structures. Because the workup and management of the patient will vary considerably depending on the location of the lesion, it is imperative that supranuclear disorders be distinguished from infranuclear disorders. From a practical standpoint, supranuclear disorders that cause abnormalities in the range of eye movements usually result from lesions of the cerebral hemispheres or the brainstem premotor structures, whereas infranuclear disorders may be caused by lesions of the brainstem, ocular motor nerves, or the extraocular muscles themselves. In all cases, stimulation of the vestibular apparatus can be used to assess the integrity of the peripheral ocular motor pathways either by **oculocephalic testing** (**the doll's head maneuver**) or by **caloric testing**.

In the oculocephalic test, the awake patient is asked to fixate on a target straight ahead while the head (or the entire body) is rotated from side to side and up and down. A normal response consists of a conjugate eye deviation in the direction away from head or body rotation such that the eyes remain stable with respect to space despite the head movement. Normal responses during oculocephalic testing indicate that the nuclear and infranuclear ocular motor structures are intact and capable of being stimulated by an intact vestibular system. This test can also be used in unconscious patients and with nonorganic limitation of gaze to show that a full range of eye movement can be elicited.

The vestibular system may also be stimulated by caloric irrigation. This test is performed in the light, with the patient in a supine position and the head flexed 30 degrees. This places the lateral (horizontal) semicircular canals in a nearly vertical position allowing the thermal stimulus to induce maximal convection currents in the endolymph. Up to 200 mL of warm (44°C) or cold (30°C) water is infused into the external canal using a small tube fitted onto a syringe. In the awake patient, a normal response consists of conjugate nystagmus, with the slow phase toward the side of cold water irrigation (or away from the side of warm water irrigation) and the fast phase away from the side of cold water irrigation (or toward the side of warm water irrigation). The nystagmus occurs because an initial slow-phase movement of the eyes produced by stimulation of the vestibular system is followed by a refixation movement (quick phase or saccade). If the induced nystagmus is consistently less when one ear is irrigated, regardless of the stimulus temperature, a peripheral vestibular disturbance is present on that side. If the nystagmus is consistently greater in one direction, regardless of which ear is stimulated, the patient has a directional preponderance of the vestibular system that may occur with central or peripheral vestibular lesions and is otherwise nonlocalizing.

In comatose patients with intact nuclear and infranuclear ocular motor structures and an intact vestibular system, a normal response is simply a tonic, conjugate ocular deviation toward the side of cold water irrigation and away from the side of warm water irrigation. There are no significant refixation movements because all horizontal quick phases are generated by the paramedian pontine reticular formation (PPRF), which is not functioning in such patients. Absence of the VOR by either oculocephalic or caloric stimulation in comatose patients is consistently associated with poor outcome.

In some patients with paresis of upward gaze, **Bell phenomenon** may be helpful in differentiating an infranuclear from a supranuclear lesion. Bell phenomenon consists of outward and upward rolling of the eyes when forcible efforts are made to close the eyelids against resistance. The presence of this movement in persons who cannot voluntarily elevate their eyes usually indicates that brainstem pathways between the facial nerve nucleus and that portion of the oculomotor nucleus responsible for ocular elevation are intact and, thus, that an upward gaze paresis is supranuclear in origin. Absence of a Bell phenomenon has less diagnostic usefulness because about 10% of normal subjects do not have this facio-ocular movement.

Ocular Alignment

Principles

When the eyes are not aligned on the same object, **strabismus** is present. The strabismus may be congenital or acquired and may be caused by central or peripheral dysfunction. In some persons, particularly those with isolated congenital strabismus, the amount of ocular misalignment is unchanged regardless of the direction of gaze or of which eye is fixating the target. This type of strabismus is termed **comitant** or **concomitant**. When the amount of an ocular deviation changes in various directions of gaze, with either eye fixing or both, the strabismus is said to be **incomitant** or **noncomitant.** Congenital comitant strabismus is occasionally associated with other neurologic dysfunction and acquired comitant strabismus may be a sign of intracranial disease. In addition, comitant strabismus may appear in otherwise normal children and adults, as well as in persons with neurologic or systemic disease, from **decompensation** of a pre-existing phoria. Nevertheless, most instances of neuropathic or myopathic strabismus are of the incomitant variety.

Primary and Secondary Deviations

Any patient with a manifest deviation of one eye (heterotropia) will fixate a target with only one eye at a time. During viewing with that eye, the visual axis of the opposite (nonfixing) eye will be deviated a certain amount away from the target. Patients with a comitant strabismus have the same amount of deviation of the nonfixing eye regardless of the eye that is fixing or the field of gaze. Most patients with incomitant (and especially paralytic) strabismus tend to fix with the nonparetic eye if visual acuity is equal in the two eyes. In these patients, the deviation of the nonfixing eye is called the **primary** deviation. When such patients are forced to fix the same target with the paretic eye, the deviation that results, the **secondary** deviation, is always greater than the primary deviation (Fig. 16.3).

When the paretic eye is fixating a target, it is held in an orbital position farther in the direction of action of the paretic muscle than when the nonparetic eye is fixating the same target. This results in a secondary deviation that is greater than the primary deviation simply because of the change in eye position toward the direction of action of the paretic muscle when the paretic eye is forced to take up fixation. The innervation to both muscles in the yoke pair is increased in that direction as predicted by Hering law, and this increased innervation is more effective in the nonparetic muscle. However, the innervation is not increased any more than if the nonparetic eye is forced to take up fixation in eccentric gaze to achieve the same final orbital position.

Past-Pointing and Disturbances of Egocentric Localization

Patients with paralytic strabismus often have anomalies of spatial localization called **past-pointing** or **false orientation.** If a patient is asked to point at an object in the field of action of a paretic muscle while the paretic eye is fixating, the patient's finger will point beyond the object **toward** the field of action of the paretic muscle. During this test, it is important that the hand be covered or that the patient point rapidly toward the object so as to avoid visual correction of the error of localization while the hand is still moving toward the object.

Head Turns and Tilts

Patients with strabismus commonly turn or tilt the head to minimize diplopia. Head turns are frequently associated with paresis of the horizontal extraocular muscles, with the turn being toward the side of the weakness. Similarly, patients with vertical extraocular muscle paresis may carry their head flexed or extended. Some patients adopt a head posture that actually increases the distance between the two images, allowing one of the images to be more easily ignored.

Head tilts are most commonly observed in patients with paresis of the oblique muscles, particularly the

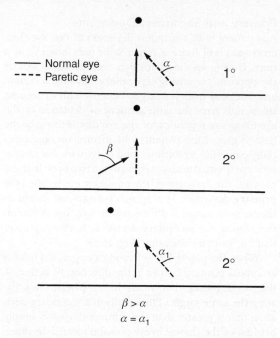

Figure 16.3 The principle of primary and secondary deviations. **Top:** When the normal eye fixes on a target directly ahead, the paretic eye deviates from the primary position by a certain amount (α). This is called the primary deviation. **Middle:** When the paretic eye fixes on a target in primary position, the normal eye also deviates from primary position by a certain amount (β), but this secondary deviation of the normal eye when the paretic eye is fixing is greater than the amount of deviation of the paretic eye when the normal eye is fixing ($\beta > \alpha$). **Bottom:** Although the common explanation of primary and secondary deviation is based on Hering law of equal innervation to yoke muscles, some authors believe that the secondary deviation is greater than the primary deviation in paretic strabismus because when the paretic eye is fixing in primary position it is forced farther into its field of limitation. If the paretic eye were fixing on an object in the opposite direction, the deviation of the eye from primary position (α_1) would be the same as if the normal eye were fixing on an object straight ahead ($\alpha = \alpha_1$). Thus, although Hering law is maintained, the explanation for primary and secondary deviations is based upon the position of the eyes within the orbit and not upon which eye is fixing.

superior oblique. With an acquired superior oblique palsy, for example, the face is usually turned away from the paretic eye, the chin is down slightly, and the head is tilted toward the side opposite the paretic muscle. This permits fusion of images.

Techniques

Ocular alignment may be tested subjectively or objectively, depending on the circumstances under which the examination is performed and the physical and mental state of the patient.

Subjective Testing

When a patient is cooperative, subjective testing of diplopia reliably indicates the disparity between retinal images. The simplest subjective tests of ocular alignment use colored filters to dissociate the deviation and to emphasize and differentiate the images so that the patient and the observer can interpret them. A fixation light is used to provide the image. A red filter held over one eye suffices in most cases; however, the addition of a green filter over the opposite eye gives better results. The use of complementary colored filters, one over each eye, produces maximum dissociation of images because there is no part of the visible spectrum common to both eyes.

The red filter is always placed over the patient's right eye, and all questions posed to the patient relate to the relationship of the red image with respect to the white (or green) image. The patient is first asked if he or she sees one or two lights. If the patient sees two lights, he or she is then asked what color they are. After the appropriate answer, the patient is asked if the red light is to the right or left of the other light and if it is above or below the other light.

It should be remembered that the image of an object is always displaced in the *opposite* direction to the position of the eye (Fig. 16.4). Thus, if an eye is exotropic, the patient will have **crossed** diplopia, and (with a red filter over the right eye) the patient will see the red image to the *left* of the other image. Similarly, if the patient has an esotropia, the red image will be seen to the *right* of the other image (**uncrossed** diplopia). If the patient has a vertical deviation of the eyes, the eye that is higher will see the image of an object *below* that of the opposite eye.

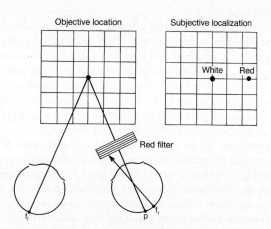

Figure 16.4 The principle of diplopia tests. A red filter is placed in front of the right eye, and the patient fixes a single light in the distance. If the eyes are misaligned, the light is imaged on the fovea of one eye (f_l) and the nonfoveal retina (p) of the opposite eye. The patient thus sees two images, white and red, in different locations in space.

Once a patient indicates that there is a clear separation of images when he or she is fixing on a light held straight ahead, the examiner can determine the area of maximum vertical separation, horizontal separation, or both, by having the patient look at a light held in the eight other cardinal positions of gaze.

In addition to the use of filters placed over one or both eyes, one can place a red Maddox rod over one eye and have the patient fixate on a white light. The "rod" is, in fact, a set of small half-cylinders aligned side by side in a frame in such a way that when the eye views a light through the cylinders, the image seen is that of a line perpendicular to the cylinder axis. Thus, if one views a white light with one eye covered by a red Maddox rod, the images will be those of a red line and a white light. The Maddox rod can be placed in such a manner as to produce a vertical, horizontal, or oblique line. Persons who are orthophoric see the line pass through the light. When the rod is oriented to produce the image of a vertical line, patients with a horizontal strabismus will see the line to the left or right of the light. When the rod is oriented so that a horizontal line image is produced, patients with a vertical strabismus will see the line above or below the light (Fig. 16.5).

Torsional misalignment of the eyes (e.g., superior oblique palsy) can be tested with two Maddox rods, one over each eye. This is best performed using a trial lens frame. If both rods are oriented so as to produce a horizontal line image, an eye with torsional dysfunction will see the line as oblique, rather than horizontal. The patient is then asked to rotate the rod until the line is perceived as horizontal. By this method, the amount of torsion can be measured and followed.

Other subjective techniques to assess ocular misalignment may be used in which two test objects rather than one are presented to the patient in such a way that each object is viewed with only one eye (Fig. 16.5). The patient is then required to place the two objects in such a fashion that they appear to be superimposed. The objects only appear superimposed when their images fall on the fovea of each eye. Misalignment of the foveae results in the patient placing the objects in different locations in space. The eyes are differentiated and dissociated in various ways. Each eye may be presented with a different target, or complementary colors may be placed into the visual field, either directly or by projection, with each eye being provided with a corresponding colored filter. These **haploscopic** tests include the use of a major amblyoscope, and the Hess screen and Lancaster red green tests (Fig. 16.6).

Objective Testing
Corneal Light Reflex. The simplest objective method of determining ocular alignment is the use of a hand light to cast a reflection on the corneal surfaces of both eyes in the cardinal positions of gaze. If the images

Figure 16.5 A: Image from the paretic (deviated) eye is projected in the direction of action of the paretic muscle. **B:** Maddox rod in front of eye, right eye, for patient with a right hypertropia. (Courtesy of David S. Zee, and modified from Figure 10_01 in Leigh and Zee, The Neurology of Eye Movements, 5th edition, with permission.)

Figure 16.6 The principle of haploscopic tests. Red and green test objects are used, and the patient has a red filter placed in front of one eye and a green filter in front of the other eye.

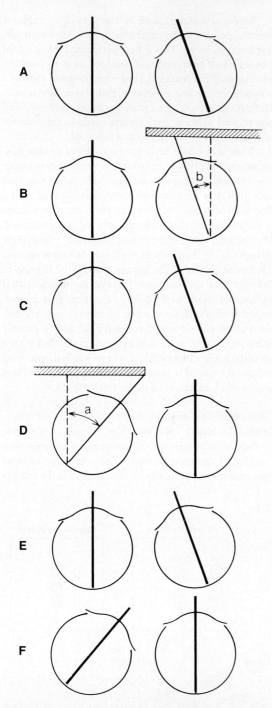

from the two corneas appear centered, then the visual axes are usually correctly aligned. If the light reflexes are not centered, one can estimate the amount of misalignment based on the apparent amount of decentration of the light reflex (the **Hirschberg test**). With the fixation light held 33 cm from the patient, 1 mm of decentration equals 7 degrees of ocular deviation.

Alternately, prisms can be placed over either of the eyes until the light reflexes appear centered (the **Krimsky test**). In general, prisms are placed over the fixing eye; however, in circumstances where the nonfixing eye is so eccentric or has incomplete ductions that centration of the light reflex is impossible or requires excessive prism over the fixing eye, holding the prism over the fixing eye results in a measurement of the deviation only in eccentric gaze. This is essentially the same as measuring the secondary, rather than the primary, deviation. In such cases, centering of the light reflex, and thus measurement of the deviation, can be achieved by placing the prism directly in front of the deviated eye.

A number of conditions other than a heterotropia may cause decentration of the corneal light reflex and must be considered to interpret correctly tests based on centration of the light reflex. The **angle kappa** is defined as the angle between the visual line (the line connecting the point of fixation with the fovea) and the pupillary axis (the line through the center of the pupil perpendicular to the cornea). The angle is measured at the center of the pupil. It is considered positive when the light reflex is displaced nasally, and negative when the light reflex is displaced temporally. A positive angle kappa may simulate an exodeviation, and a negative angle kappa may simulate an esodeviation.

Cover Tests. The most precise, objective methods of measuring ocular alignment are the **cover tests**. Although these tests require that the patient be able to fixate a target with either eye, they generally require less cooperation than do the subjective tests described above. The three types of cover tests used by most clinicians are the single-cover test, the cover–uncover test, and the alternate-cover (cross-cover) test.

In the **single-cover test**, the patient fixates an accommodative target at 33 cm (near target) or 6 meters (distant target). An opaque occluder is placed in front of one eye, and the examiner observes the opposite eye to see if it moves to take up fixation of the target (Fig. 16.7).

Figure 16.7 The single-cover and cover–uncover tests. In both tests, one eye is covered at a time; however, in the single-cover test, one eye is covered, and the opposite eye is observed. In the cover–uncover test, one eye is covered, and the behavior of that eye is observed when the cover is removed. **A:** Initially, with both eyes viewing, the left eye is fixating the target, and the right eye is esotropic. **B:** When the right eye is covered, no movement of the left (uncovered) eye is observed. **C:** Nor is any movement of the right eye observed when the cover is removed. **D:** When the left eye is covered, the right eye moves outward to take up fixation. Note that the deviation of the normal eye under cover (the secondary deviation, *a*) is greater than that of the paretic eye under cover (primary deviation, *b*). When the cover is removed, either **(E)** the left eye again takes up fixation, or **(F)** the paretic right eye continues to fixate.

If the patient has a manifest ocular deviation (**heterotropia**), the previously nonfixing eye will be observed to change position to take up fixation when the fixing eye is covered. On the other hand, when the nonfixing eye is covered, no movement of the fixing eye will be observed (because it is already fixing on the target).

In the **cover–uncover test**, the patient fixates on an accommodative target, and one eye is occluded. The behavior of that eye is then observed as the cover is removed (see Fig. 16.7). The direction of any deviation and the speed and rate of recovery to binocular fixation are noted.

If no movement of the uncovered eye is observed when the cover–uncover test is performed, an **alternate-cover test** may be used to detect a latent deviation of the eyes (**heterophoria**). Instead of occluding one eye and then taking the occluder away, first one eye and then the other is alternately occluded. The cover should remain in front of each eye long enough to allow the patient to take up fixation with the uncovered eye. This test prevents fusion and dissociates the visual axes. Any movement of either uncovered eye suggests that although the eyes are straight during binocular viewing, loss of fusion (i.e., by the alternate occlusion of the two eyes) results in a deviation of whichever eye is covered (Fig. 16.7).

The importance of distinguishing between heterophorias and heterotropias cannot be overemphasized because patients with heterophorias have binocular central fusion, whereas patients with heterotropias do not.

If either the cover–uncover or alternate-cover tests detect evidence of ocular misalignment, prisms can be used to neutralize the movement and thereby measure the deviation, whether it is a heterotropia or heterophoria. Prisms are placed in front of either eye such that the apex of the prism is oriented in the direction of the deviation, and the prism strength is altered until the deviation is no longer observed.

Head Tilt Test. When there is a vertical ocular deviation, it is often helpful to perform cover tests with the head tilted first toward one side and then toward the other. This test is useful primarily in the diagnosis of superior oblique palsy because patients with this disorder consistently show a hypertropia of the involved eye when the head is tilted toward the involved side. Patients with skew deviation (Chapter 18) will also typically present with a head tilt.

When a patient with a trochlear nerve palsy tilts the head toward the affected side, intorsion of that eye should occur to keep the vertical meridian perpendicular to the horizon. This intorsion is usually about 10 degrees and is produced by the otolith–ocular reflex, resulting in synergistic contractions of the superior rectus and superior oblique muscles. If the superior oblique muscle is paretic, its secondary action (depression) is also impaired. The superior rectus muscle is therefore the only means by which the eye can be intorted, and its main action (elevation), is unopposed resulting in worsening of the hypertropia with head tilt toward the involved eye (detailed discussion in Chapter 18).

Direct Observation of the Fundus. A final objective method of determining ocular torsion is direct observation of the ocular fundus. The normal fovea is generally located about 7 degrees below center of the optic disc (range, 0 to 16 degrees) or along a horizontal line originating from a point between the middle and lower thirds of the optic disc. When an eye is extorted, the foveal reflex rotates below this plane, whereas intorsion results in upward rotation of the reflex (Fig. 16.8). The amount of torsion can be determined using a variety of ophthalmoscopic and photographic methods.

Performance of Versions

Versions may be tested by examining the saccadic, pursuit, vestibular, and optokinetic systems.

Clinical Examination of Saccades
Saccadic eye movements are examined clinically by instructing the patient to alternately fixate upon two targets—usually the examiner's finger and nose. Saccades in each direction can be examined in each field of gaze in both the horizontal and vertical planes. The examiner must determine if the saccades are (1) promptly initiated (latency), (2) of normal velocity, and (3) accurate (metricity).

Saccadic latencies can be appreciated by noting the time it takes the patient to initiate the saccade and may be reduced in diffuse cortical or brainstem injury as well as ocular motor apraxia. Abnormal voluntary saccadic velocities may be accentuated by using a handheld drum or tape with repetitive patterns, and often indicate a paralytic process. Larger amplitude attempts should be requested of the patient, to accentuate any abnormalities.

Disorders of saccadic accuracy—such as **saccadic dysmetria**—can be inferred from the direction and size of corrective saccades that the patient must make to ultimately acquire the fixation target. Because saccades as small as 0.5 degrees can be easily identified during clinical observation, minimal degrees of saccadic dysmetria can be easily appreciated during the clinical examination. The occasional under- or overshoot is physiologic—the cerebellum adapts to correct the dysmetria. Smaller amplitude attempts allow dysmetria if present, to be revealed on examination more readily.

Clinical Examination of Pursuit
Patients with isolated deficiency of smooth pursuit do not usually complain of visual symptoms because

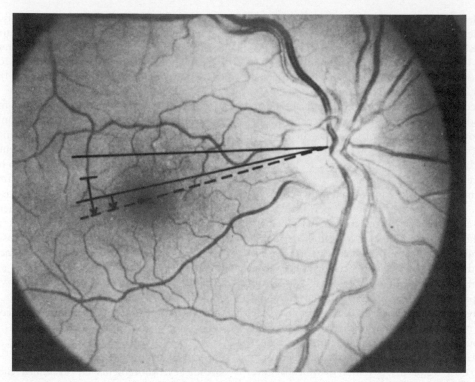

Figure 16.8 Torsion of the ocular fundus. Photograph of an extorted right fundus, direct view, with a *dashed line* drawn from the center of the optic disc through the fovea. The normal angular range of the fovea from the center of the disc is shown by the two *solid lines*. The amount of extorsion can be measured in degrees from the center of the normal range (*long arrow*) or from the limit of the normal range (*short arrow*). (Courtesy of Dr. David L Guyton.)

they can track moving objects with a series of saccades. Only very demanding tracking tasks (e.g., playing tennis, baseball, or intense reading) may cause patients with impaired pursuit to report difficulties. The vision of normal subjects deteriorates during tracking of targets moving at velocity; hence, complaints of inability to track fast-moving objects may not signify a disorder of smooth pursuit.

To test the pursuit system, the examiner should ask the patient to track a small target, such as a pencil tip held a meter or more from the eyes, with the head held still. The target should initially be moved at a low, uniform velocity. Pursuit movements that do not match the target velocity result in corrective saccades. If these are "catch-up" saccades, then the pursuit gain is low. If pursuit gain is too high, then "back-up" saccades are observed. Small children, uncooperative patients, or persons thought to have nonorganic blindness may be tested with a slowly rotating large mirror held before their eyes.

Although hand-held drums or tapes with repetitive targets do not truly test the optokinetic system, they do stimulate pursuit and may be useful in the detection of pursuit asymmetries and other abnormalities of the pursuit system.

The smooth-pursuit system can also be assessed using the VOR. The VOR normally generates eye movements that compensate for angular displacement of the head and maintain the visual axes "on target." If one observes a slowly moving target by moving the head, so that the target remains stationary relative to the head, the eye movements generated by the VOR are inappropriate and must be suppressed. The ability of a patient to suppress (or cancel) the VOR can be evaluated by using a central fixation target that moves in the same direction and at the same velocity as the head. Patients often do this best by fixating their thumbnail with their arm outstretched while being rotated in the examination chair. When suppression of the VOR and pursuit are compared in normal human subjects similar frequency response curves are obtained leading to the hypothesis that suppression of the VOR depends directly on information derived from the smooth-pursuit system. This hypothesis is supported by the clinical observation that patients with impaired smooth pursuit also have abnormal suppression of the VOR. Deficits in VOR suppression, however, are nonlocalizing, as they may also occur with either cerebral or cerebellar disease.

Clinical Examination of the Vestibular and Optokinetic Systems

The clinical methods used to test the vestibular system (oculocephalic and caloric testing) are described above. Although the optokinetic system can be tested in the laboratory (see below), the system cannot be tested as part of a routine clinical examination. As noted above, so-called "optokinetic" hand-held drums and tapes actually assess the smooth-pursuit system, not the optokinetic system.

The Vestibulo-ocular Reflex

The oculocephalic and caloric tests that are performed in patients with apparent limitation of eye movement primarily test the function of the semicircular canals of the vestibular system. More extensive testing is usually directed toward determining gain, phase, and balance. Rotation tests give more accurate and reproducible results than do caloric tests. The gain of the VOR may be obtained by measuring the peak eye velocity in response to a velocity step (e.g., sudden sustained rotation at 60 degrees per second) in darkness. This is usually done in vestibular laboratories equipped with servo-controlled chairs and

eye-monitoring equipment, although portable systems for this purpose are available. Utilizing the VOR to generate conjugate eye movements allows the examiner to differentiate between a supranuclear and nuclear disorder. If the VOR is able to overcome a deficit of gaze, then the disorder is most likely supranuclear since the final motor pathways controlled by cranial nerve nuclei must be intact.

The Optokinetic System

The hand-held "optokinetic" drums or tapes that are used to elicit smooth movements primarily test the pursuit system. True optokinetic testing requires a stimulus that fills the field of vision. A common technique is to have the patient sit inside a large, patterned optokinetic drum that is rotated around the patient. A true optokinetic stimulus induces a sensation of self-rotation. Another method of eliciting a true optokinetic response is rotation of an individual at a constant velocity in the light for over 1 minute. The sustained nystagmus that results is caused by purely visual stimuli (the vestibular response having died away); however, it is still difficult to separate its pursuit and optokinetic components.

Supranuclear and Internuclear Ocular Motor Disorders*

17

Ocular Motor Syndromes Caused by Lesions of the Medulla
Wallenberg Syndrome (Lateral Medullary Infarction)
Syndrome of the Anterior Inferior Cerebellar Artery
Syndrome of the Superior Cerebellar Artery
Skew Deviation and the Ocular Tilt Reaction

Ocular Motor Syndromes Caused by Lesions of the Cerebellum
Location of Lesions and their Manifestations
Etiologies

Ocular Motor Syndromes Caused by Lesions of the Pons
Lesions of the Internuclear System: Internuclear Ophthalmoplegia
Lesions of the Abducens Nucleus
Lesions of the Paramedian Pontine Reticular Formation
Combined Unilateral Conjugate Gaze Palsy and Internuclear Ophthalmoplegia (One-and-a-Half Syndrome)
Slow Saccades from Pontine Lesions

Ocular Motor Syndromes Caused by Lesions of the Mesencephalon
Sites and Manifestations of Lesions
Neurologic Disorders that Primarily Affect the Mesencephalon

Ocular Motor Abnormalities and Disease of the Basal Ganglia
Parkinson Disease
Huntington Disease

Ocular Motor Syndromes Caused by Lesions in the Cerebral Hemispheres
Acute Unilateral Lesions
Persistent Deficits Caused by Large Unilateral Lesions
Focal Lesions
Abnormal Eye Movements and Dementia

Ocular Motor Manifestations of Seizures
Eye Movements in Stupor and Coma

Ocular Motor Manifestations of Some Metabolic Disorders

Effects of Drugs on Eye Movements

Supranuclear ocular motor disorders can be caused by lesions in the brainstem (excluding the cranial nerve nuclei or fascicles), cerebellum, or cerebral hemispheres. Internuclear ocular motor disorders, by definition, are caused by damage to brainstem pathways that coordinate the movements of the two eyes. In this chapter, we discuss the features and causes of supranuclear and internuclear ocular motor disorders.

Ocular Motor Syndromes Caused by Lesions of the Medulla

The medulla contains a number of structures that are important in the control of eye movements: vestibular nuclei, perihypoglossal nuclei, medullary reticular formation, inferior olive, and restiform body (inferior cerebellar peduncle) (Fig. 17.1). The perihypoglossal nuclei consist of the nucleus prepositus hypoglossi (NPH), which lies in the floor of the fourth ventricle, the intercalatus nucleus, and the nucleus of Roller. These nuclei have rich connections with other ocular motor structures. The NPH and the adjacent medial vestibular nucleus (MVN) are of critical importance for holding horizontal positions of gaze (the neural integrator). These structures also participate in vertical gaze holding, although more rostral structures, especially the interstitial nucleus of Cajal (INC), provide the primary tonic contribution for vertical and torsional eye movements. Lesions of the paramedian structures of the medulla often produce nystagmus— commonly upbeat, but sometimes horizontal with a gaze-evoked component.

Lesions of the **inferior olivary nucleus** (ION) or its connections may produce the **oculopalatal myoclonus syndrome (oculopalatal tremor)**. It is thought to occur due to an interruption in the Guillain– Mollaret triangle, which connects the red nucleus to

*The authors acknowledge the past contributions of David S. Zee— to this chapter.

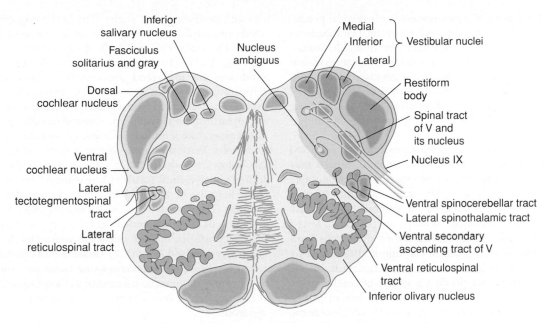

Inferior
salivary nucleus

Fasciculus
solitarius and gray

Nucleus
ambiguus

Medial
Inferior
Lateral

Vestibular nuclei

Dorsal
cochlear nucleus

Restiform
body

Spinal tract
of V and
its nucleus

Nucleus IX

Ventral
cochlear nucleus

Lateral
tectotegmentospinal
tract

Lateral
reticulospinal tract

Ventral spinocerebellar tract
Lateral spinothalamic tract

Ventral secondary
ascending tract of V

Ventral reticulospinal
tract

Inferior olivary nucleus

Figure 17.1 Schematic drawing of the medulla oblongata. The specific neural structures that are commonly damaged in Wallenberg syndrome are shaded.

the ipsilateral ION (via central tegmental tract), to the contralateral dentate nucleus (via inferior cerebellar peduncle), back to the red nucleus (via superior cerebellar peduncle). This condition usually develops weeks to months after a brainstem or cerebellar infarction, although it may also occur with degenerative conditions or posttrauma (diffuse axonal injury). The delay in presentation occurs due to chronic deafferentation of the ION, which leads to a vacuolar degenerative hypertrophy and resulting disordered control of the ION (see Fig. 17.2). The term **myoclonus** is misleading, because the movements of affected muscles are to-and-fro and are approximately synchronized, typically at a rate of 2 to 4 cycles/sec.

Figure 17.2 Hypertrophy of the right inferior olivary nucleus in a patient with oculopalatal tremor (myoclonus). **Left:** At time of presentation with pontine hemorrhage from a cavernoma (not visualized), shows normal medullary anatomy. **Right:** Seven months later, at time of presentation with oculopalatal tremor showing enlargement of right ION.

A majority of cases present with vertical pendular oscillations that often have a vertical and torsional component. The oscillations can resemble seesaw nystagmus but lack the alternation in elevation seen in the latter. These oscillations are associated with rhythmic undulations of the soft palate (see **Video 17.1**). Relatively high-dose gabapentin (1,200 to 2,400 mg daily) is commonly tried to improve the eye movements.

Occasionally, acute disease processes are restricted to the **vestibular nuclei**. For example, vertigo may be the sole symptom of an exacerbation of multiple sclerosis (MS) and of brainstem ischemia. Nystagmus caused by disease of the vestibular nuclei may be purely horizontal, vertical, or torsional. Mixed patterns also may occur. Moreover, nystagmus from a central vestibular lesion can mimic that caused by peripheral vestibular disease. Dolichoectasia of the basilar artery may produce a variety of combinations of central and peripheral vestibular syndromes. Microvascular compression of the vestibulocochlear nerve may also give rise to paroxysmal vertigo.

Wallenberg Syndrome (Lateral Medullary Infarction)

Typically, lesions of the vestibular nuclei also affect neighboring structures, especially the cerebellar pedun-cles and perihypoglossal nuclei. The best recognized syndrome involving the vestibular nuclei is caused by a lateral medullary infarction (Wallenberg syndrome) (see Fig. 17.1). The typical findings of Wallenberg syndrome are **ipsilateral** impairment of pain and temperature sensation over the face, central Horner syndrome, limb ataxia, and a bulbar disturbance causing dysarthria and dysphagia. **Contralaterally**, pain and temperature sensation are impaired over the trunk and limbs. Vertical diplopia due to a skew deviation (see below) may also occur, often with an altered subjective visual vertical (ocular tilt reaction). The facial nerve may also be affected if the infarct extends more rostrally. The disorder is most commonly caused by occlusion of the ipsilateral vertebral artery; occasionally, the posterior inferior cerebellar artery (PICA) is selectively involved (Fig. 17.3). Dissection of the vertebral artery (either spontaneous or traumatic, such as following chiropractic manipulation) is occasionally the cause. Rarely, demyelinating disease produces this syndrome.

Lateropulsion, a compelling sensation of being pulled toward the side of the lesion, is often a prominent complaint of patients with Wallenberg syndrome and is also evident in the ocular motor findings. If the patient is asked to fixate straight ahead and then gently close the lids, the eyes deviate conjugately toward the side of the lesion. This is reflected by the corrective

Figure 17.3 Neuroimaging of Wallenberg syndrome. On left, T2-weighted FLAIR MRI, axial view, of a man presenting with acute findings of Wallenberg syndrome—characterized in part by lateropulsion of saccades toward the right side, a skew deviation with the right eye being hypotropic, and the ocular tilt reaction—shows a hyperintense area consistent with an infarct on the right side of the medulla. The DWI image of the same patient on right shows that the infarct is relatively acute. (Courtesy of Carlos Torres, MD.)

Figure 17.4 Lateropulsion of saccades in a patient with a left Wallenberg syndrome. **A:** On attempted leftward gaze, the patient overshoots the target and must make a corrective saccade. **B:** On attempted rightward gaze, the patient makes a series of hypometric saccades. **C** and **D:** On attempted upward and downward gaze, the eyes move obliquely to the left and must make several refixation movements back to center. (Redrawn from Kommerell G, Hoyt WF. Lateropulsion of saccadic eye movements. Electro-oculographic studies in a patient with Wallenberg's syndrome. *Arch Neurol.* 1973;28:313–318.)

saccades that the patient must make on eye opening to reacquire the target. Lateropulsion may even appear with a blink.

Saccadic eye movements are also affected by lateropulsion (Fig. 17.4). Horizontally, saccades directed toward the side of the lesion usually overshoot the target, and saccades directed away from the side of the lesion undershoot the target; this is referred to as **ipsipulsion** of saccades and should be differentiated from the **contrapulsion** of saccades that occurs with infarcts from occlusion of the superior cerebellar artery (SCA). Quick phases of nystagmus are similarly affected in Wallenberg syndrome, so saccades directed away from the side of the lesion are smaller than those directed toward the lesion. On attempting a purely vertical refixation, the patient produces an oblique saccade directed toward the side of the lesion. Corrective saccades then bring the eyes back to the target.

When present, spontaneous **nystagmus** in Wallenberg syndrome is usually horizontal or mixed horizontal–torsional with a small vertical component. In primary position, the slow phase is directed toward the side of the lesion ("beats toward the better ear"), although it may reverse direction in eccentric positions, suggesting coexistent abnormalities of the gaze-holding mechanism. Lid nystagmus (synkinetic lid twitches with horizontal quick phases) can also occur. The **ocular tilt reaction** (OTR) commonly occurs in Wallenberg syndrome, including a **skew deviation**, with an ipsilateral hypotropia. There is a conjugate yet asymmetric degree of cyclotorsion of both eyes— the higher eye incyclotorts, while the hypotropic eye excylotorts more significantly. Some patients show ipsilateral head tilt (toward the lower eye). The skew deviation and head tilt arise from imbalance in pathways mediating otolith responses (Fig. 17.5). The

Ocular Tilt Reaction (OTR) PATHWAY
Utricle - Vestibular Nuclei – MLF - III, IV - INC

Wallenberg
Laby/VIII N.

IPSI TILT
EYE LOWER
on side of
lesion

Medial
longitudinal **INO**
fasciculus
CONTRA TILT
EYE HIGHER on
side of lesion

- Vertical deviation, comitant, lower eye on side of lower ear
- Head tilt toward side of lower eye (and ear)
- Ocular counterroll (torsion), top poles toward the lower eye (and lower ear)

A

Figure 17.5 A: Ocular tilt reaction consists of vertical misalignment (skew deviation), conjugate cyclotorsion, and head tilt. The otolith–ocular pathway is shown in red. A lesion prior to the decussation (posterior skew) results in an ipsilateral hypotropia, while an anterior lesion (midbrain, rostral pons) produces an ipsilateral hypertropia. The higher eye is always incyclorted, in contrast to a fourth nerve palsy (Illustration courtesy of David S. Zee, MD). **B:** Fundus photos of a patient with a left hypertropia due to lateral medullary infarct, showing greater of excyclotorsion of hypotropic **(right)** eye, and mild incyclotorsion of higher **(left)** eye.

EXCYCLOTORSION of lower eye

INCYCLOTORSION of higher eye

B

subjective sensations of tilt or inversion of the world probably also reflect involvement of central projections from the gravireceptors, the utricle and saccule.

Syndrome of the Anterior Inferior Cerebellar Artery

The anterior inferior cerebellar artery (AICA) supplies portions of the vestibular nuclei, adjacent dorsolateral brainstem, and inferior lateral cerebellum. In addition, the AICA is the origin of the labyrinthine artery in most persons and also sends a twig to the cerebellar flocculus in the cerebellopontine angle. Consequently, ischemia in the distribution of the AICA may cause vertigo, vomiting, hearing loss, facial palsy, and ipsilateral limb ataxia, along with gaze holding and pursuit deficits as well as vestibular nystagmus. The ocular motor signs reflect a combination of

involvement of the labyrinth, vestibular nuclei, and the flocculus.

Syndrome of the Superior Cerebellar Artery

Infarction in the territory of the SCA causes ataxia of gait and limbs and vertigo (Fig. 17.6). A characteristic abnormality is **saccadic contrapulsion**. This consists of an overshooting of contralateral saccades and an undershooting of ipsilateral saccades. Attempted vertical saccades are oblique, with a horizontal component away from the side of the lesion. Thus, this saccadic disorder is the opposite of the saccadic ipsipulsion seen in Wallenberg syndrome and probably reflects interruption of outputs from the fastigial nucleus running in the uncinate fasciculus next to the superior cerebellar peduncle. Infarction restricted to

Figure 17.6 Neuroimaging of infarct in the territory of the superior cerebellar artery (SCA) in a 69-year-old man with hypertension. Computed tomographic scan shows a large hypodense area in the left cerebellar hemisphere corresponding to the distribution of the left SCA. The patient had a left horizontal gaze palsy from compression of the left side of the brainstem.

the posterior-inferior vermis can selectively impair pursuit and optokinetic eye movements.

Skew Deviation and the Ocular Tilt Reaction

Skew deviation is a vertical misalignment of the visual axes caused by a disturbance of prenuclear inputs—there is an imbalance in otolithic inputs (i.e., otolith–ocular pathways). Torsional and horizontal deviations may be associated findings. The hypertropia may be the same in all positions of gaze (comitant), or it may vary and may even alternate (e.g., right hypertropia on right gaze, left hypertropia on left gaze) (incomitant or noncomitant). When skew deviation is incomitant—and especially in the pattern of an individual muscle palsy—it can be differentiated from a vertical extraocular muscle palsy by the coexistence of signs of central neurologic dysfunction, and attention to the direction of cyclotorsion (see Fig. 17.7). The utricular–ocular imbalance can often be overridden by altered patterns of otolith stimulation (upright-supine test) affirming the supranuclear origin of the misalignment. Recent studies have shown that in patients with a purely supranuclear deficit (no associated cranial nerve involvement), that the amplitude of vertical and torsional misalignment measured when upright, reduces

by at least one-half when the patient is placed in the supine position.

Skew deviation occurs with a variety of abnormalities in the vestibular periphery, brainstem, or cerebellum and rarely as a reversible finding with raised intracranial pressure (ICP) from supratentorial tumors or pseudotumor cerebri. In infants, a skew deviation may be the harbinger of a subsequent horizontal strabismus.

Utricular projections from the vestibular nuclei probably cross the midline and ascend in the medial longitudinal fasciculus (MLF). Therefore, unilateral **internuclear ophthalmoplegia** (INO) is often associated with a skew deviation. The INO usually is on the side of the hypertropic eye, possibly because lesions of one MLF cause an imbalance of ascending otolithic inputs (Fig. 17.5).

In the **midbrain**, otolith projections contact the oculomotor and trochlear nerve nuclei, as well as the INC. Mesencephalic lesions in or around the INC thus may cause skew deviation and the OTR. When the head tilt is sustained (tonic), it is contralateral to the side of the lesion; in addition, there is usually a hypertropia that is ipsilateral to the lesion and a conjugate cyclotorsion that is characterized by intorsion of the ipsilateral eye. (Fig. 17.5). Associated defects of vertical eye movements and oculomotor or trochlear nerve function are common, including seesaw, pendular, or upbeat nystagmus.

Rarely, skew deviation slowly alternates or varies in magnitude over the course of a few minutes. The periodicity of the phenomenon is reminiscent of periodic alternating nystagmus (PAN), and the two phenomena can, in fact, coexist. Patients with this condition usually have midbrain lesions, while patients with PAN typically have lesions of the cerebellar nodulus.

Ocular Motor Syndromes Caused by Lesions of the Cerebellum

Clinicians are appropriately cautious in attributing eye movement abnormalities specifically to cerebellar dysfunction, because the brainstem is so frequently damaged in patients with lesions of the cerebellum. Nevertheless, most clinical and experimental studies provide convincing evidence that cerebellar lesions alone can cause specific ocular motor abnormalities (Figs. 17.8 and 17.9). In essence, three principal syndromes can be identified: the syndrome of the dorsal vermis and underlying posterior fastigial nuclei, the syndrome of the flocculus and paraflocculus, and the syndrome of the nodulus and ventral uvula. The main features of each of these syndromes are summarized in Fig. 17.10.

SKEW (OTR, ocular tilt reaction)   IV (SUPERIOR OBLIQUE PALSY)

A and B
Observer View

A **SKEW**
Higher eye intorted, lower eye extorted
Usually no or little torsional diplopia

B **SUPERIOR OBLIQUE PALSY**
Higher eye extorted
Torsional diplopia (images point to paretic eye)
Slant (top of object appears closer)

C and D (Patient View)

Figure 17.7 Differentiation between a skew deviation and fourth nerve palsy is often possible on the basis of observing the direction of torsion of the higher eye, on funduscopy as well double Maddox rod testing. In skew **(left)**, the eyes exhibit conjugate cyclotorsion, with the higher eye incyclotorted, and fourth nerve palsy **(right)** exhibits excyclotorsion of the higher eye only, without change in torsion of the contralateral eye. (Modified from Leigh, Zee. *Neurology of Eye Movements.* 5th ed. Figure 10.05, with permission.)

Location of Lesions and Their Manifestations

Experimental lesions of the **dorsal vermis** (lobules VI and VII) and of the underlying fastigial nuclei (called the fastigial oculomotor region or FOR) cause saccadic dysmetria, typically hypometria, when the vermis alone is involved, and hypermetria when the deep nuclei are affected (see Figs. 17.8 to 17.10). Bilateral lesions of the deep nuclei may sometimes lead to macrosaccadic oscillations, as a result of an extreme degree of hypermetria.

Experimental lesions of the **flocculus and paraflocculus** cause gaze-evoked nystagmus, rebound nystagmus, and downbeat nystagmus (see Fig. 17.8). Unilateral lesions produce ipsilateral deficits in pursuit and gaze holding. The flocculus sends climbing fibers via the inferior cerebellar peduncle to support the horizontal and vertical neural integrators. Without this input, the integrators' output is not sustained

("leaky") resulting in impaired gaze holding (gaze-evoked nystagmus and postsaccadic drift).

Experimental lesions of the **nodulus** lead to unwanted perseveration of vestibular responses resulting from a dysregulation of the "velocity storage mechanism." This predisposes the animal to the development of periodic alternating nystagmus, failure of tilt suppression of postrotatory nystagmus, and loss of habituation. Positional nystagmus usually occurs with lesions of the nodulus.

Another ocular motor sign attributable to a focal cerebellar lesion is torsional nystagmus during vertical pursuit. Patients with lesions in the middle cerebellar peduncle show this phenomenon. The direction of the torsional nystagmus changes with the direction of the pursuit, with the eye velocity of the slow phase of the torsional nystagmus being directly proportional to the eye velocity of the slow phase of pursuit.

The cerebellum is also important in long-term **adaptive functions** that keep eye movements

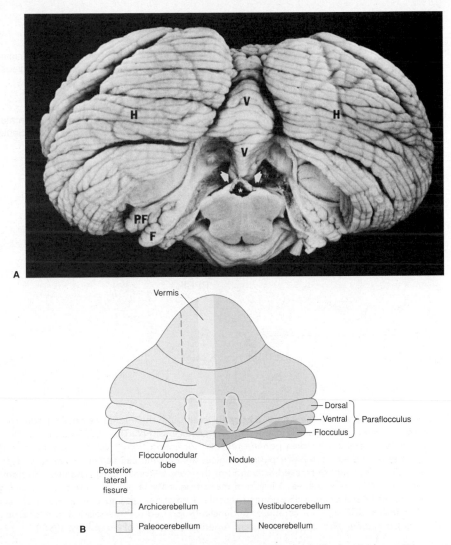

Figure 17.8 The human cerebellum. **A:** Anterior-inferior view shows the cerebellar hemispheres (*H*), vermis (*V*), flocculus (*F*), and paraflocculus (*PF*). *White arrowheads*, nodulus; *asterisk*, fourth ventricle. (Reprinted with permission from Ghuhbegovic N, Williams TH. *The Human Brain: A Photographic Guide.* Hagerstown, MD: Harper & Row; 1980.) **B:** Schematic drawing of the subdivisions of the human cerebellum. The left half of the drawing shows the three main subdivisions: the archicerebellum—the flocculonodular lobe; the paleocerebellum—the anterior vermis, the pyramids, the uvula, and the paraflocculus; and the neocerebellum. The right half of the diagram shows the structures of the vestibulocerebellum—the flocculonodular lobe and the dorsal and ventral paraflocculi. (After Brodal A. *Neurological Anatomy in Relation to Clinical Medicine.* 3rd ed. New York: Oxford University Press; 1981.)

appropriate to the visual stimulus. For example, adaptation of the gain of the VOR is impaired in patients with cerebellar lesions. This adaptive or "repair shop" function of the cerebellum probably accounts for both the enduring nature of the ocular motor deficits that accompany diffuse cerebellar lesions and, perhaps, the somewhat variable effects of cerebellar lesions. Thus, inherent, idiosyncratic abnormalities in brainstem or peripheral ocular motor mechanisms that are normally "repaired" by the cerebellum may reappear after cerebellar lesions.

Etiologies

Developmental Anomalies
The **Arnold-Chiari malformation** is an anomaly of the hindbrain involving the caudal cerebellum (including the vestibulocerebellum, flocculus, paraflocculus [tonsils], uvula, and nodulus) and the caudal medulla. In the type 1 malformation, the cerebellar tonsils are displaced caudally into the foramen magnum, and the medulla is elongated. A meningomyelocele usually is not present. Such patients often present with symptoms

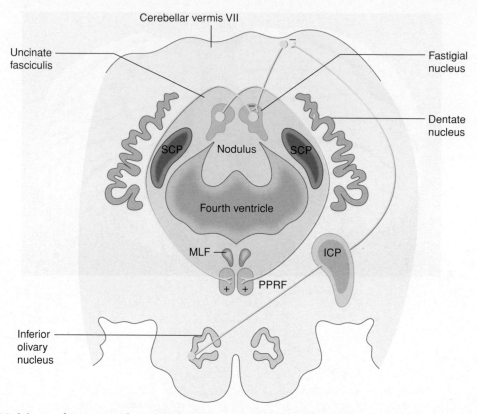

Figure 17.9 Schema of projections from the inferior olivary nuclei through the inferior cerebellar peduncle (*ICP*) to lobule VII of cerebellar cortex, where Purkinje cells inhibit the fastigial nucleus (*FN*). The caudal part of the fastigial nucleus probably excites the contralateral paramedian pontine reticular formation (*PPRF*) via its projections in the uncinate fasciculus. A lesion in the left inferior cerebellar peduncle increases Purkinje cell activity, leading to decreased firing of the ipsilateral fastigial nucleus and decreased activation of the contralateral **(right)** paramedian—pontine reticular formation. This causes ipsipulsion of saccades. A lesion of the left uncinate fasciculus (from the right fastigial nucleus) decreases activity in the ipsilateral paramedian pontine reticular formation, causing contrapulsion of saccades. *MLF*, medial longitudinal fasciculus; *SCP*, superior cerebellar peduncle. (Reprinted with permission from Sharpe JA, Morrow MJ, Newman NJ, et al. *Continuum, Neuro-ophthalmology*. American Academy of Neurology, 1995.)

in adult life. In the type 2 malformation, both the fourth ventricle and the inferior vermis extend below the foramen magnum, the brainstem and spinal cord are thin, and a lumbar meningomyelocele is usually present. Patients with a type 2 malformation usually present in childhood, but in milder cases, the onset of symptoms is delayed until adulthood. Presenting symptoms include oscillopsia that is brought on or exacerbated by head movements, and Valsalva-induced dizziness, vertigo, cervical pain, and headaches. A variety of ocular motor abnormalities, especially downbeat nystagmus (both spontaneous and positional), occur in patients with the Chiari malformation (Table 17.1). Diagnosis is by MRI, with sagittal views of the craniocervical junction being most useful (Fig. 17.11). Patients often improve after suboccipital decompression, although it may take months for the eye movement abnormalities to diminish. A similar ocular motor syndrome may be observed in patients with other lesions located at the craniocervical junction.

The **Dandy–Walker syndrome** consists of a malformation of the cerebellar vermis, a membranous cyst of the fourth ventricle, and malformations of the cerebellar cortex and deep cerebellar nuclei. Patients with this condition often show a mild saccadic dysmetria, although some patients have normal eye movements. Ocular motor abnormalities, including nystagmus and strabismus, also occur in patients with agenesis of the vermis or hypoplasia of the entire cerebellum.

Degenerative Diseases

Many degenerative processes can affect the cerebellum or its connections and produce cerebellar eye signs. These disorders include the cerebellar cortical degenerations, ataxia telangiectasia, and various spinocerebellar and olivopontocerebellar degenerations

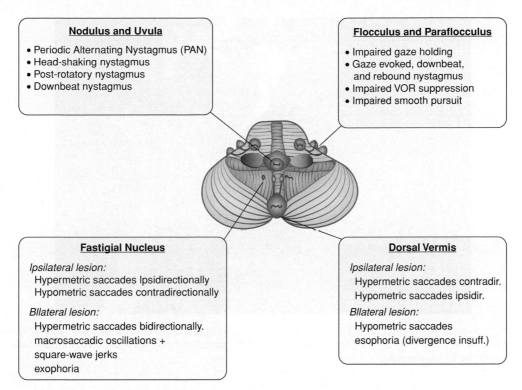

Nodulus and Uvula

- Periodic Alternating Nystagmus (PAN)
- Head-shaking nystagmus
- Post-rotatory nystagmus
- Downbeat nystagmus

Flocculus and Paraflocculus

- Impaired gaze holding
- Gaze evoked, downbeat, and rebound nystagmus
- Impaired VOR suppression
- Impaired smooth pursuit

Fastigial Nucleus

Ipsilateral lesion:
  Hypermetric saccades Ipsidirectionally
  Hypometric saccades contradirectionally

Bilateral lesion:
  Hypermetric saccades bidirectionally.
  macrosaccadic oscillations +
  square-wave jerks
  exophoria

Dorsal Vermis

Ipsilateral lesion:
  Hypermetric saccades contradir.
  Hypometric saccades ipsidir.

Bilateral lesion:
  Hypometric saccades
  esophoria (divergence insuff.)

Figure 17.10 Key clinical signs of damage to various cerebellar structures. (Original courtesy of David S. Zee, MD; modified and adapted to current format.)

(OPCDs). Moreover, many of these conditions also affect brainstem structures. Thus, other, presumably noncerebellar, ocular motor signs may be present (e.g., slow saccades, prolonged saccadic latencies, decreased

Table 17.1 Eye Signs in the Chiari Malformation

1. Downbeat nystagmus (occasionally with a torsional component), worse on lateral gaze
2. Sidebeat nystagmus (primary position, unidirectional, horizontal nystagmus)
3. Periodic alternating nystagmus
4. Divergent nystagmus
5. Esotropia
6. Gaze-evoked nystagmus
7. Rebound nystagmus including torsional rebound
8. Impaired pursuit (and VOR cancelation)
9. Impaired OKN with slow buildup of eye velocity in response to a constant-velocity stimulus
10. Convergence nystagmus
11. Divergence paralysis
12. Skew deviation accentuated or alternating on lateral gaze
13. Saccadic dysmetria
14. Internuclear ophthalmoplegia
15. Increased VOR gain
16. Shortened VOR time constant
17. Positional nystagmus

or absent vestibulo-ocular responses, and ophthalmoplegia).

Paraneoplastic cerebellar degeneration is a rare remote effect of cancer, usually occurring with breast, ovarian, or small-cell lung cancer, and typically associated with serum and cerebrospinal fluid anti-Yo antibodies. The onset of symptoms is usually acute or subacute, with the development of severe midline and appendicular ataxia, dysarthria, and downbeat nystagmus. Pathologic studies indicate total loss of Purkinje cells in patients with this condition. Such patients have lost all output from the cerebellar cortex, and the common finding of primary position downbeat nystagmus thus tends to confirm that asymmetric, inhibitory projections of the cerebellum to the central connections of the semicircular canals can be the cause of this nystagmus. A cerebellar syndrome may also complicate treatment of cancer or leukemia with cytosine arabinoside.

Mass Lesions

Cerebellar hemorrhage, tumors, infarcts, abscesses, cysts, and extra-axial hematomas may all cause cerebellar eye signs by direct damage to the cerebellar parenchyma. Cerebellar lesions, however, may also compress the brainstem and produce additional signs. Vertical or horizontal gaze disorders can occur, depending on whether

Figure 17.11 Neuroimaging of an Arnold-Chiari malformation. T2-weighted sagittal MRI shows herniation of cerebellar tonsils below the foramen magnum with relative hypoplasia of the posterior fossa, enlarged supravermian cistern, and obliteration of the fourth ventricle.

the direction of compression is rostral or forward, respectively. The oculomotor, trochlear, and abducens nerves may also be affected. Ocular motor dysfunction may also be caused by secondary obstructive hydrocephalus and increased ICP.

Vestibular schwannomas (acoustic neuromas) may compress the cerebellar flocculus (which lies in the cerebellopontine angle) and produce eye signs of vestibulocerebellar lesions, including Bruns nystagmus in which there is a coarse (high amplitude) nystagmus beating to the side of the lesion (reflecting a gaze-holding deficit) and a fine (high frequency) nystagmus beating away from the side of the lesion (reflecting a vestibular imbalance). Acute cerebellar hemorrhage frequently causes nystagmus, gaze palsy (usually toward the side of the lesion), abducens nerve palsy, and skew deviation.

Ocular Motor Syndromes Caused by Lesions of the Pons

Lesions of the Internuclear System: Internuclear Ophthalmoplegia

Among the fibers that comprise the MLF, many carry a conjugate horizontal eye movement command from abducens internuclear neurons in the pons to the medial rectus subdivision of the **contralateral** oculomotor nuclear complex in the midbrain. Other fibers in the MLF carry signals for holding vertical and

torsional eye position, for vertical smooth pursuit, and for the vertical VOR.

Manifestations

Lesions of the MLF produce **INO** (Fig. 17.12). When the lesion is unilateral, the INO is characterized by weakness of adduction ipsilateral to the side of the lesion (Fig. 17.13). This weakness can vary from a complete loss of adduction beyond the midline to a mild decrease in the velocity of adduction without any limitation in range of motion. The fibers subserving horizontal gaze in the MLF each carry commands for all types of conjugate eye movements. Thus, vestibular slow phases, pursuit and optokinetic following movements, and saccades and quick phases of nystagmus are all affected by the MLF lesion.

When patients with INO are able to converge, despite absence of voluntary adduction, a caudal lesion with preservation of the medial rectus subdivision of the oculomotor nuclear complex can be assumed. Patients with INO and intact convergence were said to have a **posterior internuclear ophthalmoplegia** by Cogan. Although the presence of intact convergence is important in such cases, the absence of convergence in the setting of an INO (the "anterior" INO of Cogan) does not necessarily imply a rostral lesion involving the medial rectus nuclear subdivision. Some patients simply are not able to produce a strong convergence effort, and the vertical disparity that occurs when a unilateral INO is associated with

Figure 17.12 Neuroimaging in two multiple sclerosis patients presenting with internuclear ophthalmoplegia. On left, T2-weighted MRI, axial view, shows a hyperintense lesion in the paramedian area of the rostal midbrain involving the right medial longitudinal fasciculus (*orange arrow*), just dorsal to the red nucleus. On right, T2-FLAIR MRI, sagittal view, showing a plaque involving the MLF at the level of the pontomesencephalic junction (*orange arrow*). (Courtesy of Carlos Torres, MD.)

a skew deviation (see below) also may interfere with convergence effort.

The second cardinal sign of an INO is **nystagmus on abduction in the contralateral eye**. This nystagmus consists of a centripetal (inward) drift, followed by a corrective saccade that may be hypermetric, hypometric, or orthometric. It is present in nearly all patients with INO. The cause of abduction nystagmus must relate either to lesions outside the MLF or to an adaptive response to the initial adduction weakness. In

Figure 17.13 Unilateral, right internuclear ophthalmoplegia in a 32-year-old man with multiple sclerosis. Note complete lack of adduction in the right eye on attempted left horizontal gaze.

patients with "pseudo-INO" due to disorders of the neuromuscular junction, abducting nystagmus typically does not accompany the deficit of adduction.

Lesions that damage the MLF may also damage the abducens nucleus, fascicle, or both on either side of the brainstem (see Fig. 17.14). Lesions that damage the MLF on one side and the ipsilateral abducens nucleus produce the one-and-a-half syndrome (see below), whereas lesions that damage the ipsilateral abducens fascicle produce horizontal ophthalmoplegia in the ipsilateral eye from the combination of an INO and an abducens nerve palsy. Damage to the MLF on one side and to the contralateral abducens nerve fascicle will produce abduction weakness of the contralateral eye combined with adduction weakness of the ipsilateral eye. In this setting, there will be a "pseudo-horizontal gaze palsy" on attempted horizontal gaze away from the side of the MLF lesion. The diagnosis may be suspected in a patient who appears to have a horizontal gaze palsy that is asymmetric, with one eye (usually the adducting eye) being much more limited than the other.

Etiologies

Table 17.2 summarizes some etiologies of INO. In general, a unilateral INO is most commonly caused by ischemia, although even in these cases there is often subtle involvement of the other side. Bilateral INO is commonly caused by demyelination. Although MRI frequently shows a lesion in the MLF in patients with INO (see Fig. 17.12), there are many exceptions where

A   **B**

Figure 17.14 Drawing of the pons at the level of the abducens nuclei. **A:** Drawing illustrates the important structures involved in the production of horizontal gaze. *MLF,* medial longitudinal fasciculus; *PPRF,* paramedian pontine reticular formation. Note that neurons project from the PPRF to the abducens nucleus and that neurons in the abducens nucleus are both motoneurons whose axons represent the abducens nerve and internuclear neurons whose axons ascend in the *contralateral* MLF. **B:** The areas that may be involved when a one-and-a-half syndrome is present. Note that involvement of either the abducens nucleus or the PPRF can cause the horizontal gaze palsy. Damage to the ipsilateral medial longitudinal fasciculus produces the internuclear ophthalmoplegia. (Modified from Sharpe JA, Rosenberg MA, Hoyt WF, et al. Paralytic pontine exotropia. A sign of acute unilateral pontine gaze palsy and internuclear ophthalmoplegia. *Neurology.* 1974;24:1076–1081.)

Table 17.2 Etiology of Internuclear Ophthalmoplegia
1. Multiple sclerosis (commonly bilateral); postirradiation demyelination
2. Brainstem infarction (commonly unilateral), including complication of arteriography; hemorrhage
3. Brainstem and fourth ventricular tumors and mesencephalic clefts
4. Chiari malformation, and associated hydrocephalus and syringobulbia
5. Infection: bacterial, viral, and other forms of meningoencephalitis; in association with AIDS
6. Hydrocephalus, subdural hematoma, supratentorial arteriovenous malformation
7. Nutritional disorders: Wernicke encephalopathy and pernicious anemia
8. Metabolic disorders: hepatic encephalopathy, maple syrup urine disease, abetalipoproteinemia, Fabry disease
9. Drug intoxications: phenothiazines, tricyclic antidepressants, narcotics, propranolol, lithium, barbiturates, D-penicillamine, toluene
10. Cancer: either due to carcinomatous infiltration or remote effect
11. Head trauma, including cervical hyperextension or manipulation
12. Degenerative conditions: progressive supranuclear palsy
13. Syphilis
14. Pseudointernuclear ophthalmoplegia of myasthenia gravis and Fisher syndrome

the diagnosis is suspected and confirmed by clinical examination alone.

Lesions of the Abducens Nucleus

Lesions of the abducens nucleus cause an ipsilateral palsy of horizontal conjugate gaze because the abducens nucleus contains two groups of neurons: abducens motoneurons that innervate the ipsilateral lateral rectus muscle and abducens internuclear neurons that innervate the contralateral medial rectus motor neurons via the MLF (Fig. 17.15). Vergence movements of the eyes are spared, however, so adduction is possible with a near stimulus. Most often, the abducens nucleus is affected in association with adjacent tegmental structures, particularly the genu of the facial nerve, the MLF, and the PPRF—the so-called eight-and-a-half syndrome (Fig. 17.16). Lesions restricted to the abducens nucleus can often be distinguished from those in the adjacent caudal PPRF, because only in the latter may pursuit and vestibular movements be spared. Gaze-evoked nystagmus on contralateral gaze also occurs in patients with presumed abducens nucleus lesions. Possible mechanisms for the gaze-evoked nystagmus include damage to adjacent vestibular or NPH pathways that are involved in neural integration for gaze holding, or damage to the paramedian cells and tracts that lie in part in the rostral abducens nucleus and have reciprocal connections with the cerebellar flocculus, a structure that supports the brainstem gaze-holding centers.

Figure 17.15 Summary of saccadic and vestibular eye movement control. The center figure shows the supranuclear connections from the frontal eye field (*FEF*) and the parietal eye field (*PEF*) to the superior colliculus (*SC*), rostral interstitial nucleus of the medial longitudinal fasciculus (*riMLF*), and the paramedian pontine reticular formation (*PPRF*). The FEF, PEF, and SC are involved in the production of saccades. The schematic drawing on the left shows the brainstem pathways for horizontal gaze. Axons from the cell bodies located in the PPRF travel to the ipsilateral abducens nucleus (*VI*), where they synapse with abducens motoneurons whose axons travel to the ipsilateral lateral rectus (*LR*) muscle and with abducens internuclear neurons whose axons cross the midline and travel in the medial longitudinal fasciculus (*MLF*) to the portions of the oculomotor nucleus (*III*) concerned with medial rectus (*MR*) function (in the contralateral eye). The schematic drawing on the right shows the brainstem pathways for vertical gaze. Important structures include the riMLF, PPRF, the interstitial nucleus of Cajal (*INC*), and the posterior commissure (*PC*). Note that axons from cell bodies located in the vestibular nuclei (*VN*) travel directly to the abducens nuclei and, most via the MLF, to the oculomotor nuclei. (*IV*), trochlear nucleus.

Lesions of the Paramedian Pontine Reticular Formation

The PPRF is a collection of neurons in the caudal pons that contain burst neurons required for the generation of saccades. The paramedian nucleus raphe interpositus contains pause neurons that inhibit burst neurons at all times except during saccades.

Destructive lesions of the PPRF, such as infarction and hemorrhage, tend to affect all cell groups, along with fibers of passage that convey pursuit and vestibular signals to the ipsilateral abducens nucleus. **Unilateral** destructive lesions cause an ipsilateral, conjugate, horizontal gaze palsy. With acute lesions, the eyes may be deviated contralaterally. Ipsilaterally directed saccades and quick phases are small and slow and do not carry the eye past the midline. Vertical saccades may be slightly slow, and an inappropriate horizontal component, directed away from the side of the lesion, may occur during attempted vertical saccades.

Bilateral pontine lesions may impair vertical eye movements. It is well established that signals for vertical vestibular and smooth pursuit eye movements ascend in the MLF and other pathways through the pons, and it also seems likely that pontine lesions can cause impairment of vertical saccades, likely due to the contributions of the PPRF to vertical eye movement control.

Combined Unilateral Conjugate Gaze Palsy and Internuclear Ophthalmoplegia (One-and-a-Half Syndrome)

Combined lesions of the abducens nucleus or PPRF and adjacent MLF on one side of the brainstem cause an ipsilateral horizontal gaze palsy and an INO. The only preserved horizontal eye movement is abduction of the contralateral eye, hence the name **one-and-a-half syndrome**. Patients with this condition may have

Figure 17.16 A patient with an eight-and-a-half syndrome. **A:** Looking straight ahead, eyes are grossly aligned, with left facial weakness. **B:** Attempted gaze to right, note left INO. **C:** Attempted gaze to the left, note complete left gaze palsy.

an exotropia when attempting to look straight ahead; the eye opposite the side of the lesion deviates outward. This strabismus is thought to be caused by the unopposed drives of the intact pontine gaze center. Thus, the condition is often called **paralytic pontine exotropia**.

Occasionally, the ipsilateral horizontal vestibular responses are preserved when voluntary gaze is abolished, suggesting that the pontine lesion is more rostral in the PPRF or more discrete (less widespread) in the caudal PPRF, thus sparing the vestibular projections to the abducens nucleus. Although attempts at conjugate (version) movements elicit no adduction, vergence movements may be preserved in such cases. The one-and-a-half syndrome may result from brainstem ischemia, hemorrhage, tumor infiltration, trauma, or demyelination.

Slow Saccades from Pontine Lesions

Certain metabolic, toxic, and degenerative conditions can cause selective deficits of ocular motility suggestive of predominant loss of one population of brainstem neurons concerned with eye movements. Such a process may explain both slow saccades and saccadic oscillations in patients with lesions in the pons.

Slow saccades are characteristic of many degenerative and metabolic diseases (Table 17.3). Horizontal saccades may be slowed in patients with spinocerebellar or OPCDs; vertical saccades are often relatively less

Table 17.3 Etiology of Slow Saccades

1. Olivopontocerebellar atrophy and related spinocerebellar degenerations
2. Huntington disease
3. Progressive supranuclear palsy
4. Whipple disease
5. Lipid storage diseases
6. Wilson disease
7. Drug intoxications: anticonvulsants, benzodiazepines
8. Tetanus
9. Dementia: Alzheimer disease (stimulus dependent) and AIDS associated
10. Lesions of the paramedian pontine reticular formation
11. Internuclear ophthalmoplegia
12. Peripheral nerve palsy; diseases affecting the neuromuscular junction and extraocular muscle (chronic progressive external ophthalmoplegia)
13. Paraneoplastic syndromes

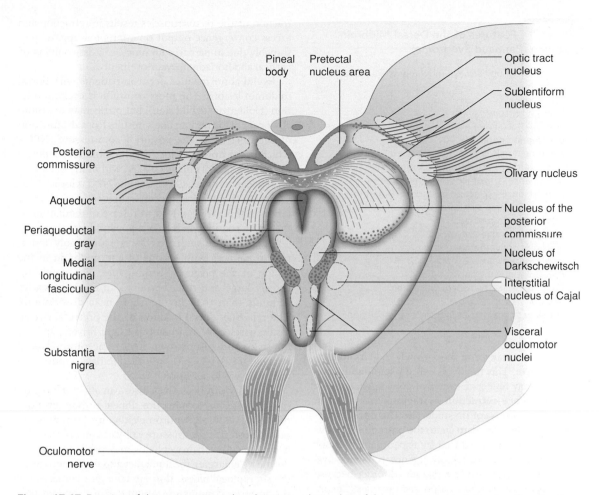

Figure 17.17 Drawing of the major pretectal nuclei. Note relationship of the posterior commissure to other structures. (Reprinted with permission from Carpenter MB, Pierson RJ. Pretectal region and the pupillary light reflex: An anatomical analysis in the monkey. *J Comp Neurol.* 1973;149:271–300.)

affected in such patients. In diseases that principally affect the midbrain, such as progressive supranuclear palsy (PSP), vertical saccades are the first to become slow. Patients with spinocerebellar degenerations usually make saccades that have normal amplitudes despite their low velocity. PSP, however, causes both slow and small horizontal saccades. Patients with slow saccades may use a variety of strategies of eye–head coordination to move their eyes more quickly to the target.

Ocular Motor Syndromes Caused by Lesions of the Mesencephalon

Sites and Manifestations of Lesions

Disturbances of vertical eye movements from midbrain lesions usually are caused by damage to one or more of three main structures: the posterior commissure, the

rostral interstitial nucleus of the medial longitudinal fasciculus (riMLF), and the INC (see Fig. 17.17).

Posterior Commissure

Lesions of the **posterior commissure** cause a syndrome characterized by loss of upward gaze and a number of other associated findings (Table 17.4; Figs. 17.17 and 17.18 and **Video 17.2**. The condition is known by a variety of names: Parinaud syndrome, pretectal syndrome, dorsal midbrain syndrome, and the sylvian aqueduct syndrome. Unilateral midbrain lesions can also create the same ocular motor syndrome, but probably by interrupting the afferent and efferent connections of the posterior commissure.

The dorsal midbrain syndrome is also characterized by disturbances of horizontal eye movements, especially vergence. In some patients, convergence is paralyzed, whereas in others it is excessive, resulting in **convergence spasm**. During horizontal saccades, the

Table 17.4 Features of the Dorsal Midbrain Syndrome (Parinaud Syndrome)

1. Limitation of upward eye movements (Parinaud syndrome)
   Saccades
   Smooth pursuit
   Vestibulo-ocular reflex
   Bell phenomenon
2. Lid retraction (Collier sign); occasionally ptosis
3. Downward gaze preference ("setting sun" sign)
4. Disturbances of vergence eye movements
   Convergence–retraction nystagmus (Koerber–Salus–Elschnig syndrome) on attempted upgaze (saccades in particular)
   Paralysis of convergence
   Spasm of convergence
   Paralysis of divergence
   Pseudo-abducens palsy
5. Fixation instability (square-wave jerks)
6. Skew deviation
7. Pupillary abnormalities (light-near dissociation)

abducting eye may move more slowly than its adducting fellow eye. This finding is called **pseudoabducens palsy** and may reflect an excess of convergence tone.

Convergence–retraction nystagmus may occur in patients with disease of the midbrain. This disorder presumably results from damage to the posterior commissure, and has been produced by experimental lesions restricted to this structure. Convergence–retraction nystagmus is best regarded as a saccadic disorder because it consists of asynchronous, opposed saccades. Cocon-

Figure 17.18 Appearance of a patient with Parinaud dorsal midbrain syndrome. In primary position, the patient has marked upper lid retraction (Collier sign), middilated pupils, and a skew deviation producing a left hypertropia. (Reprinted with permission from Bajandas FJ, Aptman M, Stevens S. The sylvian aqueduct syndrome as a sign of thalamic vascular malformation. In: Smith JL, ed. *Neuro Ophthalmology Focus 1980*. New York: Masson; 1979; 401–406.)

traction of the rectus muscles results in retraction and excess convergence output on attempted upgaze, presumably due in part to supranuclear cross-coupling of vertical and horizontal eye movements.

Eyelid abnormalities occur in patients with dorsal midbrain lesions. The most common is eyelid retraction (Collier tucked lid sign), but ptosis may occasionally occur. This finding likely results from dysfunction of the nucleus of the posterior commissure (NPC), which in the normal state provides inhibitory input to the central caudal nucleus (CCN) within the oculomotor nuclear complex. Given that the NPC is located just ventral to the posterior commissure (see Fig. 17.17), a lesion in this area can lead to release in regulation of the CCN, resulting in bilateral upper lid retraction.

Pupillary size and reactivity are commonly abnormal in patients with lesions of the midbrain in the region of the posterior commissure. The pupils are usually large and react better to an accommodative stimulus than to light (i.e., light-near dissociation). The relatively dorsal location of the pretectal nuclei, results in selective dysfunction of light-driven pupillary miosis in comparison to convergence/accommodation-related miosis, which is presumed to have a more ventral midbrain localization.

A variety of disease processes can affect the region of the posterior commissure. Pineal tumors produce the dorsal midbrain syndrome either by direct pressure on the posterior commissure or by causing obstructive hydrocephalus. Hydrocephalus may produce this syndrome by enlarging the aqueduct and third ventricle or the suprapineal recess, thus stretching or compressing the posterior commissure. Shunt dysfunction may produce Parinaud syndrome before dilation of the ventricles is apparent on neuroimaging or measures of ICP are consistently high. A demyelinating plaque affecting the region of the dorsal midbrain is a common cause of Parinaud syndrome in young adults (see Fig. 17.19).

Rostral Interstitial Nucleus of the Medial Longitudinal Fasciculus

The **riMLF**, which lies in the prerubral fields of the mesencephalon, contains the burst neurons that provide supranuclear input for the generation of vertical and torsional saccades (see Fig. 17.15). The riMLF lies dorsomedial to the rostral half of the red nucleus and immediately rostral to the INC. The right and left riMLF are connected via the posterior commissure dorsally and perhaps also by a commissure that lies ventral to the aqueduct. Bilateral experimental lesions of the riMLF abolish all vertical and torsional saccadic movements. It is postulated that the lateral aspect of each riMLF contain cells involved in upgaze, while the medial subpopulations are devoted to downgaze. Given that upgaze requires input from both riMLF (each riMLF contributes fibers that cross in the posterior

Figure 17.19 A 47-year-old man presented with subacute onset of features consistent with Parinaud syndrome including limitation of upgaze, convergence–retraction nystagmus on attempted upgaze, light-near dissociation, skew deviation, and mild eyelid retraction. On left, a blue circle demarcates the region of acute demyelination on T1-weighted MRI, sagittal view. On right, T2-FLAIR MRI, axial view better demonstrates the plaque at the dorsal thalamomesencephalic junction.

commissure), a unilateral lesion can produce a bilateral upgaze deficit; whereas a unilateral riMLF lesion (likely the medial portion) produces an ipsilateral depression deficit only.

Unilateral lesions of the riMLF produce slowed or abolished saccades in the vertical plane. Unilateral lesions also cause a contralaterally beating torsional nystagmus, a tonic torsional (slow phase) deviation to the contralateral side, and a deficit in generating ipsilateral-directed torsional quick phases (top pole beating to the side of the lesion).

Bilateral lesions of the riMLF are more common than unilateral lesions. They cause either loss of downward saccades or loss of all vertical saccades. Although vertical smooth pursuit and the VOR may be affected with lesions in this area, this probably reflects damage to nearby INC, in addition to the riMLF.

Lesions of the riMLF are usually infarcts in the distribution of a small perforating vessel (the posterior thalamosubthalamic paramedian artery) that arises between the bifurcation of the basilar artery and the origin of the posterior communicating artery. This vessel may be paired or single. It supplies structures that include the riMLF, rostromedial red nucleus, adjacent subthalamus, the posterior-inferior portion of the dorsomedial nucleus, and the parafascicular nucleus of the thalamus.

The vertical one-and-a-half syndrome consists of loss of all downward movements and selective loss of upward movements in one eye or more commonly, impairment of all upward eye movements and a selective deficit of downward saccades in the eye on the side of the lesion (see Fig. 17.20). Unilateral lesions of the midbrain can produce combined upgaze and downgaze palsies, isolated upgaze palsies, or a monocular elevator palsy, as well as the vertical one-and-a-half syndrome. Lesions of the adjacent **periaqueductal gray matter** of the midbrain may cause an imbalance of the vertical gaze-holding mechanism.

Interstitial Nucleus of Cajal

Lesions restricted to the **INC** may produce two distinct deficits: an OTR and a defect in vertical pursuit and vertical/torsional gaze holding. In the OTR, there is a contralesional tonic torsional deviation and an ipsilesional beating torsional nystagmus. If the riMLF is also damaged on the same side then the ipsilesional quick phases will also be abolished, resulting in a tonic torsional rotation of the eyes to the contralesional side. This explains why a lesion of the right INC can result in a right hypertropia and right eye incyclotorsion, and left eye excyclotorsion (skew deviation). A jerk seesaw nystagmus may occur in patients with lesions that damage the INC, usually due to demyelinating disease.

Neurologic Disorders that Primarily Affect the Mesencephalon

Progressive Supranuclear Palsy

PSP is a degenerative disease of later life characterized by disturbances of tone and posture leading to falls, difficulties with swallowing and speech, and mental slowing. The disturbance of eye movements is usually present early in the course of the disease, but it occasionally is noted late or not at all. The condition is usually fatal within 6 years of onset, death commonly being caused by aspiration pneumonia. The disease is usually sporadic.

Figure 17.20 Four days after transsphenoidal surgery to remove a craniopharyngioma, a 43-year-old woman developed sudden-onset binocular vertical diplopia. No saccades or smooth pursuit were present on attempted upgaze; on attempted downgaze, only the right eye depressed **(A).** Bell phenomenon and oculocephalic movements were preserved. In addition, she had a right head tilt, left hypertropia, and bilateral cycloversion (left eye incyclotorsion, right eye excyclotorsion **(B))** consistent with an ocular tilt reaction (OTR). Her findings were characteristic of a vertical one-and-a-half syndrome due to infarction of the left rostral interstitial nucleus of the medial longitudinal fasciculus (riMLF) (*blue circle*), and an OTR due to left interstitial nucleus of Cajal (INC) ischemia (*red circle*) **(C).** (Courtesy of Dr. Josh Beh.)

A variety of eyelid abnormalities occur in patients with PSP. These include typical blepharospasm, apraxia of eyelid closing or opening, lid retraction, and lid lag. More than one of these abnormalities may coexist in a single patient.

The initial ocular motor deficit of PSP consists of **impairment of vertical saccades and quick phases**. Downward saccades are usually affected first and are usually more severely impaired than upward saccades, at least in the early stages of the disease. Impaired saccades are at first slow and later also small, with eventual complete loss of voluntary vertical refixations. Vertical smooth pursuit is usually relatively preserved, and the VOR is intact until later in the disease, although a characteristic nuchal rigidity may make the vertical doll's head maneuver difficult.

Many patients with PSP first complain of visual difficulties related to the disturbance of vertical, and particularly downward, saccades. These complaints include problems with near tasks, particularly reading and eating. Such patients can be helped by providing them with a separate set of reading glasses so that they do not have to use bifocal or progressive lens glasses, which require them to look downward through a small lower area of the spectacle lens for near viewing. They can also be helped by conjugate base down prisms (6 to 8 prism diopters) allowing visualization objects below the direction of gaze.

Horizontal eye movements also show characteristic disturbances in patients with PSP. Typical abnormalities include impaired fixation with square-wave jerks, impaired pursuit, impaired vestibular cancelation, and saccades and quick phases that are small and eventually slow. Late in the disease, the ocular motor deficit may progress to a complete ophthalmoplegia.

PSP is a diffuse brainstem disorder, although cortical involvement may also be important. Histologically, neuronal loss, neurofibrillary tangles, and gliosis principally affect the brainstem reticular formation and the ocular motor nuclei. The midbrain may bear the brunt of the early pathology, accounting for the relative vulnerability of vertical saccades.

Whipple disease is a rare, multisystem infectious disorder characterized by weight loss, diarrhea, arthritis, lymphadenopathy, and fever that may involve and even be confined to the central nervous system (CNS). This disease can cause a defect of ocular motility that may mimic PSP. Initially, vertical saccades and quick phases are abnormal; eventually, however, all eye movements may be lost. A highly characteristic finding is pendular vergence oscillations and concurrent contractions of the masticatory muscles, **oculomasticatory myorhythmia**. The pendular vergence oscillations are always associated with a vertical saccade palsy. Ophthalmoplegia may occur in association with

myorhythmia of the leg, but not of the eyes or jaw. Whipple disease can be diagnosed using molecular analysis and can be treated with antibiotics.

Ocular Motor Abnormalities and Disease of the Basal Ganglia

A number of diseases characterized by damage to the basal ganglia are associated with specific disturbances of ocular motility and alignment.

Parkinson Disease

Patients with Parkinson disease may show a number of ocular findings. Steady fixation is often disrupted by square-wave jerks, and upward gaze is often moderately restricted, although this abnormality frequently is observed in normal, elderly persons. Convergence insufficiency is a particularly common and often symptomatic disturbance.

Saccades in Parkinson disease are characteristically hypometric, particularly when patients are asked to perform rapid, self-paced refixations between two stationary targets. Saccades made in anticipation of the appearance of a target light or to a remembered target location are also hypometric, and patients with Parkinson disease have difficulty in generating sequences of memory-guided saccades to all types of stimuli. In contrast, saccades made **reflexively** to novel visual stimuli are of normal amplitude and usually promptly initiated. Patients with mild Parkinson disease perform normally on the antisaccade task, but with advanced disease, errors increase, especially when patients are also taking anticholinergic drugs. In contrast to PSP, patients with Parkinson disease do not exhibit marked slowing of saccades.

Oculogyric crises, once encountered mainly in patients with postencephalitic Parkinsonism, now occur primarily as an extrapyramidal side effect of drugs, especially neuroleptic agents. A typical attack begins with feelings of fear or depression, which gives rise to an obsessive fixation of a thought. The eyes typically deviate upward and sometimes laterally (Fig. 17.21); they rarely deviate downward. Anticholinergic drugs promptly terminate both the thought disorder and the ocular deviation.

Oculogyric crises are distinct from the brief upward ocular deviations that occur in Tourette syndrome, Rett syndrome, and in most patients with tardive dyskinesia. In some patients with tardive dyskinesias, however, the upward eye deviations are longer lasting and also have the characteristic neuropsychologic features of oculogyric crises, thus making the differentiation between the two entities difficult, if not impossible.

A   B

Figure 17.21 Oculogyric crisis in patients with postencephalitic Parkinsonism. **A:** In a young man. Note hyperextension of neck, opening of the mouth, and conjugate deviation of the eyes up and to the right. **B:** In a middle-aged man. Again, the eyes are conjugately deviated up and to the right. (Reprinted with permission from Kyrieleis W. Die Augenveränderungen bei entzündlichen Erkrankungen des Zentralnervensystems. III. Die nichteitrigen entzündlichen Erkrankungen des Zentralnervensystems. A. Die nichteitrige epidemische Encephalitis (Encephalitis epidemica, lethargica). In: Schieck F, Brückner A, eds. *Kurzes Handbuch der Ophthalmologie.* Vol 6. Berlin: Julius Springer; 1931; 712–738.)

In general, treatment of Parkinson disease with dopaminergic drugs such as L-dopa does not seem to improve the ocular motor deficits, except for saccadic accuracy (i.e., saccades become larger). Occasionally, reversal of saccadic slowing occurs with treatment, and newly diagnosed patients with idiopathic Parkinson disease may experience improved smooth pursuit after institution of dopaminergic therapy. Education regarding ocular surface lubrication, encouraging forced blinking, and base in prisms (for convergence insufficiency) can be helpful for patients having difficulty with reading.

Huntington Disease

Huntington disease produces disturbances of voluntary gaze, particularly **saccades**. Initiation of saccades in patients with Huntington disease may be difficult. Such patients show prolonged latencies, especially when the saccade is to be made on command or in anticipation of a target moving in a predictable fashion. An obligatory blink or head turn may be used to start the eye moving. Saccades may be slow in the horizontal or vertical plane. Patients often have difficulty suppressing reflexive saccades as evidenced by poor performance on the antisaccade task (the patient is instructed to look in the opposite direction to the target).

Smooth pursuit may be impaired with decreased gain in patients with Huntington disease, but it often is relatively spared compared with saccades. By contrast, gaze holding and the VOR are preserved. Late in the disease, rotational stimulation causes the eyes to deviate tonically with few or no quick phases. **Fixation** is abnormal in some patients with Huntington disease because of saccadic intrusions. Thus, these patients have difficulty initiating voluntary saccades but show an excess of extraneous saccades during attempted fixation.

Ocular Motor Syndromes Caused by Lesions in the Cerebral Hemispheres

Acute Unilateral Lesions

Following an acute destructive lesion of one cerebral hemisphere, the eyes usually deviate conjugately

A   B

Figure 17.22 Neuroimaging of an acute infarct in the territory of the left anterior cerebral and middle cerebral arteries. **A:** T2-weighted axial MRI shows diffuse hyperintensity in the distribution of the left anterior cerebral artery (*large arrowheads*). Note also small area of hyperintensity in the right frontal region, consistent with an old infarct (*small arrowhead*). **B:** T2-weighted MRI at a lower plane reveals an area of hyperintensity in the region of the left middle cerebral artery (*arrowhead*). The patient had a supranuclear conjugate gaze paresis to the left side and right hemineglect. He also had difficulty generating rightward saccades. The ocular motor signs were transient as expected from a left-sided cerebral lesion.

toward the side of the lesion (Prevost or Vulpian sign). Gaze deviations are more common after large strokes involving predominantly the right post-Rolandic (parietal) cortex (Fig. 17.22). Visual hemineglect often accompanies such gaze deviations. Gaze deviation that occurs after a stroke usually resolves within a few days to a week. In general, for comparably sized lesions, ocular motor defects—both pursuit and saccades—are more profound when the lesion is in the nondominant hemisphere.

In the acute phase, patients may not be able to voluntarily direct their eyes toward the side of the intact hemisphere, in part because of neglect. Shortly thereafter, however, vestibular stimulation usually produces a full range of horizontal movement (with the slow phase), in contrast to most gaze palsies associated with pontine lesions (see above).

When acute right cerebral hemisphere lesions cause conjugate deviation of the eyes, the lesions are located predominantly in the subcortical frontoparietal region and the internal capsule. In the left hemisphere, the lesions are usually larger, covering the entire frontotemporoparietal area. The larger the lesion, the more persistent the conjugate deviation.

Conjugate eye deviation is occasionally "wrong way"—contralateral to the side of the lesion. The lesions are almost always hemorrhagic, most commonly in the thalamus. Affected patients usually have signs of rostral brainstem dysfunction and a shift of midline structures. Epileptic phenomena, impairment of ipsilateral pursuit pathways, and more caudal damage to descending pathways near the brainstem are evoked as explanations. Acute hemisphere lesions may cause epileptic seizures ("irritative" to the cortex) with contralateral deviation of the eyes or nystagmus, often with an associated head turn.

Persistent Deficits Caused by Large Unilateral Lesions

Persistent ocular motor deficits caused by lesions such as hemidecortication for intractable seizures are summarized in Table 17.5. Although there may be no resting deviation of the eyes, forced eyelid closure may cause a contralateral **spastic** conjugate eye movement, the mechanism of which is not understood. This tonic deviation (Cogan sign) differs from the tonic deviation associated with Wallenberg syndrome; in the former, active or attempted eyelid closure is necessary to cause the eyes to deviate, whereas in the latter, the deviation occurs even with eyes open in darkness. Cogan sign occurs most frequently in patients with parietotemporal lesions.

Table 17.5	Persistent Effects of Large Unilateral Lesions of the Cerebral Hemispheres upon Ocular Motor Function
Fixation	In darkness, eyes usually drift away from the side of the lesion. This may also be evident during fixation (on ophthalmoscopic examination[a]) as nystagmus with quick phases toward the side of the lesion; square-wave jerks.
Saccades	Slower saccades to both sides, especially contralaterally; latency longer for small saccades directed contralateral to the side of the lesion; inaccurate (hypometric and hypermetric) saccades into the "blind" hemifield.
Smooth pursuit	Reduced pursuit gain toward the side of the lesion; smooth pursuit gain away from the side of the lesion may be increased for low-velocity targets.
Optokinetic	Reduced gain for stimuli directed toward the side of the lesion; impaired optokinetic after nystagmus; may be relatively preserved compared with pursuit, with prolonged buildup of slow-phase velocity.[b]
Vestibular	During sinusoidal rotation, VOR gain in darkness may be slightly asymmetric (greater for eye movements away from the side of the lesion); with attempted fixation of an imagined or real stationary target, the asymmetry is increased.
Forced eyelid closure	Eyes usually deviate conjugately away from the side of the lesion ("spasticity of conjugate gaze").

[a]Remember that the direction of eye movements appears inverted during ophthalmoscopy.
[b]Recorded in patients with parietal lobe lesions.

In primary position, a small-amplitude nystagmus may be present that is best seen during ophthalmoscopy. It is characterized by slow phases directed toward the side of the intact hemisphere and may represent an imbalance in smooth pursuit tone. Horizontal pursuit gain (eye velocity/target velocity) is low for tracking of targets moving toward the side of the lesion for all stimulus velocities. For targets moving slowly toward the intact hemisphere, the eye movements may be too fast (pursuit gain >1); for higher target velocities, pursuit gain toward the intact side is normal. This disturbance of smooth pursuit probably reflects loss of both posterior (occipital–parietal–temporal) and frontal influences.

A convenient way to demonstrate the asymmetry of smooth pursuit that occurs with large hemisphere lesions is with a hand-held "optokinetic" tape or drum. The response is decreased when the stripes are moved or the drum is rotated toward the side of the lesion.

Focal Lesions

Ocular motor disturbances that occur from focal lesions of the cerebral hemispheres depend on a variety of factors, including the location and size of the lesion and whether the lesion is unilateral or bilateral.

Occipital Lobe Lesions

A small, unilateral lesion of either occipital lobe causes a contralateral homonymous visual field defect without any significant disturbance of ocular motor function; however, a large, unilateral lesion of either occipital lobe usually causes a contralateral homonymous hemianopia and an ocular motor deficit (saccadic dysmetria) that is related primarily to the field defect. Saccades into the hemianopic visual field are usually hypometric.

Parietal Lobe Lesions

Unilateral lesions of the parietal lobes, especially those involving the inferior parietal lobule and underlying deep white matter, cause abnormalities of visual tracking of moving targets, including an asymmetry of smooth pursuit and of optokinetic response as tested at the bedside with hand-held drums or tapes. Lesions at the temporoparietooccipital junction probably affect secondary visual areas that are important for motion processing and for programming of smooth pursuit eye movements. One such area is likely to be the human homolog of what in monkeys is called the middle temporal (MT) visual area (see Fig. 17.23).

Lesions of MT in monkeys impair the ability to estimate the speed of a moving target that is within the affected visual field, although stationary objects can be seen and accurately localized. The ocular motor consequences of this **scotoma for motion** are that saccades made to targets moving in the affected, contralateral hemifield are inaccurate and that the initiation of smooth pursuit is impaired. Such a behavior deficit occurs in patients with lesions affecting the temporoparietooccipital cortex.

Lesions of adjacent cortex, corresponding to the medial superior temporal (MST) visual area and underlying white matter, lead to a **directional defect** in smooth pursuit that is characterized by impaired tracking (reduced gain) for targets moving toward the

Saccades (FEF and PEF) and Pursuit (MST)

Figure 17.23 Illustration of the cortical regions involved in various supranuclear eye movement systems. Note the frontal eye fields within the inferior frontal lobe, parietal eye fields shaded in gray, motion processing regions MST and MT. *MT*, middle temporal; *MST*, middle superior temporal. (From Leigh RI, Zee DS (2006). *The Neurology of Eye Movements*. 4th ed. New York: Oxford University Press, with permission.)

side of the lesion, irrespective of the visual hemifield in which the target lies.

In some patients, pursuit gain away from the side of the parietal lobe lesion is also somewhat reduced, especially when the eyes move into the contralateral field of gaze. This phenomenon probably results from contralateral neglect. In other patients, contralateral pursuit gain is increased. Subcortical, thalamic, and brainstem lesions may cause an ipsilateral defect from damage to the descending pathway for smooth pursuit.

Unilateral lesions of the parietal lobe may affect saccadic initiation, causing an increase in saccadic latencies, either bilaterally or only for saccades to contralateral targets. These changes are independent of any visual field defect. The latency defects are enhanced when the fixation target remains on and a new target appears in the periphery (the "overlap" task) and are diminished when the fixation target is extinguished before the presentation of the new target in the periphery (the "gap" task). These phenomena likely represent perseveration in processing.

Temporal Lobe Lesions

In patients with posterior temporal lesions, fixation–suppression of caloric-induced nystagmus is impaired when slow phases are directed away from the side of the lesion. This abnormality may reflect impairment of visual motion or smooth pursuit pathways rather than any effect on vestibular nystagmus per se. Patients with homonymous hemianopia and lesions affecting the temporal lobes may lack the sensation of self-rotation (circular vection) that normally occurs during full-field optokinetic stimulation, compared with patients who have a homonymous hemianopia

from occipital lesions and who do experience circular vection. These findings support the localization of the vestibular cortex to the superior temporal gyrus and, perhaps, the adjacent parietal cortex. Patients with parieto-insular lesions may have tilts of the subjective visual vertical, usually contraversive. This is not associated with a skew deviation, although occasionally there is some monocular torsion. Patients with lesions in the same area may also have a defect in generating memory-guided saccades after a vestibular (rotational) stimulus. Finally, patients with lesions in the medial temporal lobe—the hippocampus—show marked impairment of generating sequences of saccades, whereas their spatial memory is intact.

Frontal Lobe Lesions

Lesions of the frontal lobe may produce an ipsilateral conjugate deviation of the eyes that resolves with time. Rarely, contralateral deviation occurs with acute frontal lesions or frontoparietal lesions. Enduring deficits after frontal lobe lesions include abnormalities of saccades and smooth pursuit. Three areas within the frontal lobes that play an important role in the control of eye movements are: (1) the frontal eye fields, (2) the supplementary eye fields (SEF) in the supplementary motor area, and (3) the prefrontal cortex (PFC) (see Fig. 17.23).

Unilateral frontal eye field (FEF) lesions lead to a slight increase in saccade latency to reflexively triggered saccades with a predominantly contralateral hypometria. Latencies are greatest in the overlap task (when the initial fixation target remains on, even after the peripheral target appears), suggesting a role for the FEF in disengagement from central fixation. Saccades may show a prolonged latency to predictable target jumps, particularly in patients with right-sided frontal lesions. Patients with this condition show a bilateral deficit in latency and accuracy for saccades to a remembered visual target but not for remembered saccades after a vestibular (rotation) input. With attempted vertical saccades, a horizontal deflection toward the side of the lesion can occur, resulting in an oblique movement. Mild slowing of contralateral saccades occurs in some patients. Deep, unilateral frontal lobe lesions cause increased latency for contralateral saccades. This deficit is probably caused by damage of efferent and afferent connections of the FEF.

Patients with unilateral frontal lobe lesions also show pursuit deficits. The FEF, SEF, and perhaps the PFC play a role in this abnormality. The defects are in both initiation and maintenance (more so at higher target speeds and frequencies). If lesions are in the SEF, defects are ipsilateral; if lesions are in the FEF, defects are bilateral but usually are greater for ipsilateral tracking. Patients with SEF lesions may have delayed reversal with periodic constant velocity stimuli, implying

Generation of Leftward Saccades

Figure 17.24 Simplified schematic demonstrating ipsilateral cortical (*FEF* and *PEF*) excitatory input to the superior colliculus (*SC*), which then projects to the contralateral *PPRF*. The result of right FEF or PEF stimulation is leftward conjugate gaze. (Courtesy of Dr. David S. Zee.)

impaired anticipation of the target trajectory. Saccades to moving targets are also inaccurate in some of these patients.

Acute bilateral frontal or frontoparietal lesions may produce a striking disturbance of ocular motility that is called **acquired ocular motor apraxia**. It is characterized by loss of voluntary control of eye movements, both saccades and pursuit, with preservation of reflex movements, including the VOR and quick phases of nystagmus. There is also relative preservation of saccades made to visual targets compared with internally guided saccades made on command and with blinking or head movements. Voluntary movements of the eyes are limited in the horizontal and usually also in the vertical plane. The defect of voluntary eye movements probably reflects disruption of descending pathways both from the FEF and the parietal cortex so that the superior colliculus and brainstem reticular formation are bereft of their supranuclear inputs (see Fig. 17.24).

Ocular motor apraxia is characterized by an impaired ability to generate saccades on command. In congenital ocular motor apraxia (COMA), an abnormality in eye movements may be recognized shortly after birth, when the child does not appear to fixate upon objects normally and may be thought to be blind. Between ages 4 to 6 months, characteristic thrusting horizontal head movements develop, sometimes with prominent blinking or even rubbing the eyelids, when the child attempts to change fixation. In children with poor head control, development of head thrusting may be delayed or absent. Almost all patients show a defect in generating quick phases of nystagmus, which can

usually be appreciated at the bedside by manual spinning of the patient, either when holding the child out at arm's length or by rotating the child on a swivel chair (if necessary sitting in an adult's lap). Despite difficulties in shifting horizontal gaze, vertical voluntary eye movements are normal, an important differential diagnostic point because **most acquired cases of ocular motor apraxia cause defects in both the horizontal and vertical planes**.

The head thrusts made by patients with COMA probably reflect one of several adaptive strategies to facilitate changes in gaze. Younger patients appear to use their intact VOR, which drives their eyes into an extreme contraversive position in the orbit. As the head continues to move past the target, the eyes are dragged along in space until they become aligned with the target. The head then rotates back to align with the target, and the eyes maintain fixation as they are brought back to the primary position in the orbit by the VOR. In contrast, older patients appear to use the head movement alone to trigger the generation of a saccadic eye movement that cannot normally be made with the head still. This strategy may reflect the use of a vestigial linkage between head and saccadic eye movements that occurs reflexively in afoveate animals when they desire to redirect their center of visual attention.

A variety of disorders that directly damage the brainstem mechanisms for generating saccades—including structural or degenerative processes within the pontine and mesencephalic reticular formations—are characterized by the development of a strategy of head thrusting or blinking to shift the gaze that superficially resembles COMA. These disorders usually can be differentiated from COMA because all types of saccades and quick phases (both horizontal and vertical) are typically affected, and because saccades may be slow. In the early stages of these diseases, however, the ocular motor apraxia may be indistinguishable from COMA.

Bilateral posterior parietal lesions (Fig. 17.25) can produce a constellation known as Balint syndrome, characterized by acquired ocular motor apraxia, simultagnosia (inability to recognize more than one object at a time within a complex visual scene; see Fig. 17.26), and optic ataxia (difficulty with accurately reaching for a visual target). The deficits are due to damage to cortical visuospatial processing regions.

Abnormal Eye Movements and Dementia

Patients with various dementing processes have abnormal eye movements, reflecting either disturbances in cerebral cortical structures or in other subcortical structures that may also be affected by that

Figure 17.25 A 73-year-old man presented with features of Balint syndrome following cardiac bypass surgery. DWI-weighted MRI, axial view, demonstrates acute bilateral posterior parietal lobe ischemia.

Figure 17.26 A: Classic "cookie theft" picture aimed to simulate a complex visual scene. Patients with simultagnosia will have difficulty perceiving more than one aspect of the scene at a time. **B:** Navon figure. Patients with simultagnosia will notice the series of "s" but not realize that together they comprise a large "H," or less commonly, vice versa.

particular disease. Excessive errors on the antisaccade test, particularly when associated with a "visual grasp reflex," are a useful indicator of an organic process when pseudodementia is a diagnostic consideration in a patient with a possible cognitive decline.

Patients with Alzheimer disease (AD) have excessive numbers of square-wave jerks and defects in saccade latency and, occasionally, accuracy and velocity. AD patients show longer mean fixation durations and a reduced number of exploring saccades when viewing simple but not complex scenes, perhaps reflecting a motivation deficit. Impairment of spatially directed attention may also be reflected in eye movement abnormalities, and a Balint-like syndrome may develop. Pursuit abnormalities also occur in patients with AD. Benson disease (posterior cortical atrophy) is a variant of AD, which may present with visual field changes, simultagnosia and higher order processing issues in the absence of significant cognitive or memory abnormalities.

Patients with Creutzfeldt–Jakob disease may show limitation of vertical gaze and slow vertical saccades as well as two rare forms of nystagmus, PAN and centripetal nystagmus. Cerebellar eye signs are typically found in another prion disorder, Gerstmann–Sträussler–Scheinker disease.

Ocular Motor Manifestations of Seizures

Abnormal eye and head movements are common manifestations of epileptic seizures. A variety of eye movements can occur in this setting, including horizontal or vertical gaze deviation and conjugate, retractory, or monocular nystagmus. Epileptic convergence nystagmus also occurs with periodic lateralizing epileptiform discharges and with burst-suppression patterns. The seizure focus may arise from any lobe, although the lesions usually are more posterior. Epileptic nystagmus occurs with typical absence seizures and with infantile spasms.

Patients with epileptic foci affecting the temporoparietooccipital cortex may show either ipsiversive or contraversive eye deviation and nystagmus. Overall, contraversive deviation of the eyes is more common than ipsiversive deviation during seizures. In cases with posterior foci (temporal, parietal, or occipital lobes), experimental studies suggest that eye movements may be mediated by projections via either the superior colliculus or the FEF. Thus, saccades may be generated by more than one of the descending parallel pathways. Frontal lobe foci are also reported to cause contraversive deviations unless they are bilateral, in which case vertical deviations also may occur. Ipsiversive deviations may reflect abnormal activity within the cortical pursuit pathways.

Eye Movements in Stupor and Coma

The ocular motor examination is especially useful for evaluating the unconscious patient, because both arousal and eye movements are controlled by neurons in the brainstem reticular formation. Comatose patients do not make eye movements that depend upon cortical visual processing. Voluntary saccades and smooth pursuit are in abeyance, and quick phases of nystagmus also may be absent. The ocular motor examination of the unconscious patient therefore consists of observing the resting position of the eyes, looking for any spontaneous movements, and reflexively inducing eye movements.

Gaze Deviations

Conjugate, horizontal deviation of the eyes is common in coma. When the coma is caused by a lesion above the brainstem ocular motor decussation between the midbrain and pons, the eyes are usually directed toward the side of the lesion and away from the hemiparesis that typically is present. A vestibular stimulus, however, can usually drive the eyes across the midline. If the conjugate deviation is caused by a lesion below the ocular motor decussation, the eyes will be directed away from the side of the lesion and toward the hemiparesis. The latter is typically seen with pontine lesions, but also in some patients with thalamic and, rarely, hemispheric disease above the thalamus (so-called wrong-way deviations).

Intermittent deviation of the eyes and head is usually caused by seizure activity. At the onset of each attack, gaze is usually deviated contralateral to the side of the seizure focus and may be followed by nystagmus with contralaterally directed quick phases. Toward the end of the seizure, gaze drifts to an ipsilateral (paretic) position.

Tonic downward deviation of the eyes, often accompanied by convergence, occurs in patients with thalamic hemorrhage and with lesions affecting the dorsal midbrain. It may be induced by unilateral caloric stimulation, after the initial horizontal deviation subsides, in patients with coma induced by sedative drugs.

Forced downward deviation of the eyes can also be seen in patients with nonorganic (feigned) coma or seizures.

Tonic upward deviation of the eyes is uncommon in coma, but it may occur following a hypoxic–ischemic insult, even when no pathologic lesions are found in the midbrain. Patients who survive after manifesting this ocular motor disturbance typically develop downbeating nystagmus, the upward drift of which is thought to be caused by loss of inhibition on the upward vertical VOR (mediated by the anterior semicircular canal). Upward deviation of the eyes also occurs as a component of oculogyric crisis, which usually occurs as a side effect of certain drugs, especially neuroleptic agents. Tonic uninhibited elevation of the lids (**eyes-open coma**) may also occur in unconscious patients and may be related to pontomesencephalic dysfunction.

Spontaneous Eye Movements

Spontaneous eye movements that occur in unconscious patients may help establish the etiology of the coma. **Slow conjugate or disconjugate roving eye movements** are similar to the eye movements of light sleep but slower than the rapid eye movements (REMs) of paradoxic or REM sleep. Their presence indicates that brainstem gaze mechanisms are intact.

Other types of spontaneous eye movements consist of various forms of vertical to-and-fro movements, often called "bobbing." Typical **ocular bobbing** consists of intermittent, usually conjugate, rapid downward movement of the eyes followed by a slower return to the primary position. Reflex horizontal eye movements are usually absent. Ocular bobbing is a classic sign of intrinsic bilateral pontine lesions, usually hemorrhage, but it also occurs in patients with cerebellar lesions that compress the pons and in some cases of metabolic or toxic encephalopathy. **Inverse bobbing** also occurs in this setting. This eye movement abnormality, which is also called **ocular dipping,** is characterized by a slow downward movement, followed by a rapid return to midposition. **Reverse bobbing** consists of rapid deviation of the eyes upward and a slow return to the horizontal, whereas **converse bobbing** (also called **reverse dipping**) is characterized by a slow upward drift of the eyes that is followed by a rapid return to primary position. These variants of ocular bobbing are less reliable for localization than typical ocular bobbing. Nevertheless, the occurrence in some patients of several different types of ocular bobbing during the course of their illness suggests a common underlying pathophysiology. Because the pathways that mediate upward and downward eye movements differ anatomically, it seems likely that these movements represent a varying imbalance of mechanisms for vertical gaze in the setting of bilateral horizontal gaze paralysis due to pontine pathology.

Monocular bobbing movements may occur as a synkinesis with jaw movement. Such movements are similar to those seen in the congenital condition called the Marcus Gunn jaw-winking phenomenon and primarily involve the neural pathways to the inferior rectus muscle.

Ping-pong gaze consists of slow, horizontal, conjugate deviations of the eyes that alternate every few seconds. Although ping-pong gaze can occur in patients with posterior fossa hemorrhage, it is usually a sign of bilateral infarction of the cerebral hemispheres. Sometimes, oscillations with a periodicity similar to that of ping-pong gaze can be induced transiently by a rapid head rotation in patients with bilateral hemisphere disease.

Identification of patients who are conscious but quadriplegic—the **locked-in syndrome** or de-efferented state—depends on identifying preserved voluntary vertical eye movements. The syndrome is typically caused by pontine infarction and is characterized in part by a variable loss of voluntary and reflex horizontal movements, such that eyelid or vertical eye movements may be the only means of communication during the acute illness. The locked-in syndrome also occurs with midbrain lesions, in which case ptosis and ophthalmoplegia may be present.

Reflex Eye Movements

Reflex eye movements may be elicited in unconscious patients either by head rotation (the oculocephalic or doll's head maneuver) or by caloric stimulation. Head rotation, with the patient supine, stimulates the labyrinthine semicircular canals and neck muscle proprioceptors. However, eye rotations induced by head rotation in unconscious individuals principally result from the effects of the semicircular canals and their central connections (Fig. 17.27). Head rotations should not be used in unconscious patients unless it is certain that no neck injury or abnormality is present.

Caloric irrigation of the external auditory meatus causes convection currents of the vestibular endolymph that displace the cupula of a semicircular canal; thus, this procedure also tests the VOR. The canal stimulated depends on the orientation of the head; for example, with the head elevated 30 degrees from the supine position, the horizontal canals are principally stimulated. Before caloric stimulation, the physician should always check that the tympanic membrane is intact. Usually only about 5 mL of ice water need be introduced into the external auditory meatus, but large quantities (100 mL or more) may be necessary to induce a response in some comatose patients.

In testing reflex eye movements in unresponsive patients, it is important to note: (1) the magnitude of the response, (2) whether the ocular deviation is conjugate, (3) the dynamic response to position-step head

rotations, and (4) the occurrence of any quick phases of nystagmus, particularly during caloric stimulation. Impaired abduction suggests an abducens nerve palsy. Impaired adduction usually indicates either an INO or an oculomotor nerve palsy, although occasionally impaired adduction to vestibular stimulation may be observed in patients with metabolic coma or drug intoxication. Vertical responses may be impaired with disease of the midbrain or bilateral lesions of the MLF. Pontine lesions may abolish the reflex eye movements in the horizontal plane but spare the vertical responses. When reflex eye movements are present in an unresponsive patient, the brainstem is likely to be structurally intact. When reflex eye movements are abnormal or absent, the cause may be structural brainstem disease, profound metabolic coma, or drug intoxication.

If reflex eye movements are intact in an unconscious patient, the eyes are carried into a corner of the orbit when the head is rapidly rotated horizontally to a new position (velocity step stimulus). If the head is held stationary in its new position, the eyes may slowly drift back to the midline. This implies that the gaze-holding mechanism (neural integrator) is not functioning normally. Patients with more rapid centripetal drift may have more severe brain injury.

Quick phases of nystagmus are usually absent in acutely unconscious patients. Their presence, without a tonic deviation of the eyes, should raise the possibility of nonorganic (i.e., feigned) coma. In patients who are stuporous but uncooperative, caloric nystagmus may be a useful way of inducing eye movements that cannot be initiated voluntarily. Patients who survive coma but who are left in a persistent vegetative state, with severe damage of the cerebral hemispheres but preservation of the brainstem, regain nystagmus with caloric or rotational stimulation.

Ocular Motor Manifestations of Some Metabolic Disorders

Some babies who ultimately develop normally show transient ocular motor disturbances, including upward or downward deviation of the eyes (but with a full range of reflex vertical movement), intermittent opsoclonus, and skew deviation. However, abnormal eye movements also occur in many metabolic diseases that affect the nervous system, particularly inborn errors of metabolism, in infants, children, and adults.

The **lipid storage diseases** are often characterized by gaze palsies. Tay–Sachs disease impairs vertical and, subsequently, horizontal eye movements. Adult-onset hexosaminidase deficiency also preferentially affects vertical gaze. Variants of Niemann–Pick disease that begin after the first year of life (e.g., the sea-blue histiocyte

Figure 17.27 Direct vertical vestibulo- ocular projections from the vertical semicircular canals. **A** and **B:** Excitatory connections. **C** and **D:** Inhibitory connections. **A:** Excitatory afferents from the anterior semicircular canals (*AC*) synapse in the superior vestibular nucleus (*S*), and their signals are relayed via the brachium conjunctivum (*BC*) to ocular motor subnuclei that drive the ipsilateral superior rectus (*SR*) and contralateral inferior oblique (*IO*) muscles. **B:** Excitatory afferents from the posterior semicircular canals (*PC*) synapse in the medial vestibular nucleus (*M*), and their signals are relayed via the contralateral medial longitudinal fasciculus (*MLF*) to the ocular motor subnuclei that drive the ipsilateral superior oblique (*SO*) and contralateral inferior rectus (*IR*) muscles. **C:** Inhibitory afferents from the anterior semicircular canals. **D:** Inhibitory afferents from the posterior semicircular canals. (Redrawn from Ghelarducci B, Highstein SM, Ito M. In: Baker R, Berthoz A, eds. *Control of Gaze by Brain Stem Neurons.* New York: Elsevier/North Holland Biomedical Press; 1977; 167–175.)

syndrome or juvenile dystonic lipidosis) are characterized by deficits of voluntary vertical eye movements, particularly saccades and smooth pursuit; vertical vestibular and horizontal eye movements are relatively preserved. Gaucher disease is associated with a prominent deficit of horizontal gaze, and slow saccades may be a prominent finding in adults with this condition.

Pelizaeus–Merzbacher disease is an X-linked recessive leukodystrophy with severe cerebellar signs, including saccadic dysmetria. Some patients with this condition also show difficulty initiating saccades and pendular nystagmus.

Wernicke encephalopathy is characterized by the triad of ophthalmoplegia, mental confusion, and gait ataxia. It is caused by thiamine deficiency and is most commonly encountered in alcoholics. The ocular motor findings include weakness of abduction, gaze-evoked nystagmus, primary position vertical nystagmus (which reverses direction upon convergence), impaired vestibular responses to caloric and rotational stimulation, INO, the one-and-a-half syndrome, and horizontal and vertical gaze palsies that may progress to total ophthalmoplegia. The ophthalmoplegia is almost always bilateral but may be asymmetric. Lesions are found in the ocular motor and vestibular nuclei, as well as in the paraventricular regions of the thalamus, the hypothalamus, periaqueductal gray matter, superior vermis of the cerebellum, and dorsal motor nucleus of the vagus.

Most likely, affected areas of the brain contain neurons that use high amounts of glucose and, therefore, are particularly dependent upon thiamine, an important coenzyme in glucose metabolism. Administration of thiamine usually causes rapid improvement of the ocular motor signs, although complete recovery may take several weeks. Coexistent magnesium deficiency should also be treated. In patients with Wernicke disease who go on to develop Korsakoff syndrome, which is primarily characterized by a severe and enduring memory loss, ocular motor abnormalities may persist. The ocular motor abnormalities include slow and inaccurate saccades, impaired smooth pursuit, and gaze-evoked nystagmus. In acute Wernicke syndrome the mammillary bodies may be swollen on neuroimaging, and exhibit atrophy in more chronic cases.

Leigh syndrome is a subacute necrotizing encephalopathy of infancy or childhood characterized by psychomotor retardation, seizures, and brainstem abnormalities, including eye movements. It is invariably fatal. It is an inherited disorder of mitochondrial function and can be caused either by abnormalities of mitochondrial DNA or by chromosomal disease. Both the disturbances of ocular motility and the pathologic findings resemble those caused by experimental thiamine deficiency or Wernicke encephalopathy.

Deficiency of vitamin E may cause a progressive neurologic condition characterized by areflexia, cerebellar ataxia, and loss of joint position sense. Ocular motor involvement includes progressive gaze restriction, sometimes with strabismus. There usually is a dissociated ophthalmoplegia and nystagmus in which adduction is fast but with a limited range and abduction is slow but with a full range (the posterior INO of Lutz). The combination of ocular motor findings in patients with vitamin E deficiency probably reflects a mixture of central and peripheral pathology. Vitamin E deficiency is more common in children, in whom it may be caused by abetalipoproteinemia (Bassen–Kornzweig disease). It is also reported in adults who have bowel or liver diseases that interfere with fat absorption or as part of an inherited ataxia caused by a defect of chromosome 8q13, the site of the α-tocopherol transfer protein gene.

Hepatolenticular degeneration, also called Wilson disease, is an inherited disorder of copper metabolism that is transmitted in an autosomal-recessive fashion. The defect is in a copper-transporting ATPase gene at q14.3 on chromosome 14. The classic clinical picture is a movement disorder with psychiatric symptoms and associated liver disease. Ocular motor disorders in hepatolenticular degeneration include a distractibility of gaze, with inability to voluntarily fix upon an object unless other competing visual stimuli are removed. Slow saccades and apraxia of eyelid opening can also occur.

Amyotrophic lateral sclerosis is associated with various eye movement disorders, including nystagmus, saccade disturbances that suggest a frontal lobe disturbance, and pursuit impairment. However, the existence of multisystem diseases in which motor neuron degeneration is just one neurologic feature makes specific clinical diagnoses difficult.

Effects of Drugs on Eye Movements

Many substances affect eye movements (Table 17.6). In some cases, the drug induces abnormalities of eye movements at therapeutic concentrations (e.g., anticonvulsants). In other cases, abnormalities of eye movements develop only when concentrations of the drug in the CNS are inappropriately elevated. In still other cases, the eye movement abnormalities are caused by substances not meant for internal use.

Patients with drug-induced abnormalities of eye movements most often complain of diplopia, caused by ocular misalignment, or oscillopsia, caused by spontaneous nystagmus or an inappropriate VOR. Many drugs have their effect on central vestibular and cerebellar connections, and they cause ataxia and gaze-evoked nystagmus. Chronic use of alcohol and benzodiazepines can produce a number of cerebellar eye movement control abnormalities including gaze-evoked or downbeat nytagmus, impaired pursuit, and saccadic dysmetria.

Although all classes of eye movements may be affected by **therapeutic doses** of various drugs, smooth pursuit, eccentric gaze holding, and convergence are particularly susceptible. For example, diazepam, methadone, phenytoin, barbiturates, chloral hydrate, and alcohol all impair smooth pursuit tracking.

Table 17.6 Potential Effects of Drugs on Eye Movements

Drug—Reported Effects

Amphetamines
  Reduced saccadic latency
  Increased AC/A ratio
Baclofen
  Reduced VOR time constant
  Complete paralysis of gaze
Benzodiazepines
  Reduced velocity and increased duration of saccades
  Impaired smooth pursuit
  Decreased gain and increased time constant of VOR
  Divergence paralysis
β-Adrenergic blocking agents
  Internuclear ophthalmoplegia
  Exacerbation of myasthenia gravis–related
  ophthalmoplegia
Carbamazepine
  Decreased velocity of saccades
  Impaired smooth pursuit
  Gaze-evoked nystagmus
  Oculogyric crisis
  Downbeat nystagmus
Chloral hydrate
  Impaired smooth pursuit
  Ethyl alcohol
  Reduced peak velocity of saccades
  Increased latency of saccades
  Hypometric saccades
  Impaired smooth pursuit and VOR suppression
  Gaze-evoked nystagmus
Lithium carbonate
  Saccadic dysmetria
  Impaired smooth pursuit
  Gaze-evoked nystagmus

  Downbeat nystagmus
  Oculogyric crises
  Internuclear ophthalmoplegia
  Opsoclonus
Methadone
  Hypometric saccades
  Impaired smooth pursuit
Phenobarbital and other barbiturates
  Reduced peak saccadic velocity
  Gaze-evoked or upbeat nystagmus
  Impaired vergence
  Decreased VOR gain
Phenothiazines
  Oculogyric crises
  Internuclear ophthalmoplegia
Phenytoin
  Impaired smooth pursuit and VOR suppression
  Gaze-evoked nystagmus
  Downbeat nystagmus
  Periodic alternating nystagmus
  Complete paralysis of gaze
  Convergence spasm
Tobacco
  Upbeat nystagmus in darkness (cigarettes)
  Square-wave jerks (nicotine)
  Impaired pursuit (nicotine)
Toluene
  Pendular nystagmus
  Internuclear ophthalmoplegia
Tricyclic antidepressants
  Internuclear ophthalmoplegia
  Opsoclonus

At **toxic levels**, neuroactive drugs can impair all eye movements, particularly when consciousness is also impaired. Phenytoin may cause a complete ophthalmoplegia in an awake patient, and therapeutic levels may cause ophthalmoplegia in patients in stupor. Phenytoin and diazepam can lead to opsoclonus. The tricyclic antidepressants may cause complete ophthalmoplegia or an INO in stuporous patients. Lithium causes a variety of abnormalities, including fixation instability and downbeat nystagmus.

In addition to drugs, certain **toxins** can cause abnormal eye movements. Some, such as chlordecone and thallium, cause saccadic oscillations. Intoxication with hydrocarbons can cause a vestibulopathy, and exposure to trichloroethylene and other solvents may affect pursuit, suppression of the VOR, and saccades. Prolonged exposure to toluene, especially in glue-sniffing addiction, may lead to a variety of ocular motor disturbances, including pendular and downbeat nystagmus, saccadic oscillations, and INO. Tobacco

has a number of ocular motor effects. It can cause upbeat nystagmus, impaired pursuit, decreased saccade latency, and increased square-wave jerks during pursuit, although performance is normal on the antisaccade test. Cocaine can affect eye movements, with opsoclonus being the most dramatic abnormality.

Ototoxicity, especially that associated with administration of aminogylcosides, is an important cause of loss of the VOR. Intravenous gentamycin is most often responsible. Its toxicity may be insidious, occurring without hearing symptoms and even with normal blood levels and relatively short periods of administration. Some patients who develop ototoxicity may be genetically predisposed to its toxic side effects. Topical (intratympanic) gentamicin is used to purposefully ablate labyrinthine function as part of the treatment of intractable Ménière syndrome or Tullio phenomenon, but it may occasionally lead to unwanted labyrinthine loss when used to treat external ear infections.

Nuclear and Infranuclear Ocular Motility Disorders*

Oculomotor (Third) Nerve Palsies
 Congenital
 Acquired

Trochlear (Fourth) Nerve Palsies
 Congenital
 Acquired
 Evaluation and Management of Trochlear
  Nerve Palsy

Abducens (Sixth) Nerve Palsies and Nuclear
Horizontal Gaze Paralysis
 Congenital
 Acquired
 Evaluation and Management of Abducens
  Nerve Palsy

Hyperactivity of the Ocular Motor Nerves
 Ocular Neuromyotonia
 Superior Oblique Myokymia (Superior Oblique
  Microtremor)

Synkineses Involving the Ocular Motor and
Other Cranial Nerves

The ocular motor system is separated anatomically and physiologically into infranuclear (peripheral), nuclear, internuclear, and supranuclear components. In this chapter, we consider ocular motor disturbances caused by congenital and acquired lesions of the nuclear and infranuclear neural structures—the lesions of the ocular motor nuclei and nerves.

Disorders that produce dysfunction of the oculomotor, trochlear, and abducens nerves may be located anywhere from the ocular motor nuclei to the termination of the nerves in the extraocular muscles within the orbit. Ocular motor nerve palsies may present in one of four ways:

1 As isolated partial or complete nerve palsy without any other neurologic signs and without symptoms except those related to the palsy itself.

2 In association with symptoms other than those related to the palsy (e.g., pain, dysesthesia, paresthesias) but without any signs of neurologic or systemic disease.
3 In association with other ocular motor nerve palsies (e.g., the simultaneous onset of an oculomotor palsy and an abducens palsy) but without any other neurologic signs.
4 In association with neurologic signs other than the ocular motor nerve palsy.

Oculomotor (Third) Nerve Palsies

Congenital

Congenital oculomotor nerve palsies constitute nearly half of the oculomotor nerve pareses seen in children (Fig. 18.1). Most cases are unilateral. As a general rule, patients with congenital oculomotor nerve palsies have no other neurologic or systemic abnormalities. Usually, these patients have some degree of amblyopia.

All patients with congenital oculomotor nerve palsy have some degree of ptosis, ophthalmoparesis, and pupillary involvement. In most of these cases, the pupil is miotic rather than dilated, presumably because of misdirected (aberrant) oculomotor nerve regeneration. Abnormalities of the oculomotor nerve that are present at birth may be caused by absent or incomplete development of the nucleus, nerve, or both. Injury to the oculomotor nerve during gestation or at the time of delivery may produce a congenital oculomotor nerve palsy. Such patients may or may not have other physical signs of trauma or other neurologic signs.

In addition to simple congenital oculomotor nerve palsy, several congenital syndromes implicate oculomotor maldevelopment with anomalous or paradoxic innervation of the extraocular muscles. These syndromes include (1) congenital adduction palsy with synergistic divergence, (2) atypical vertical retraction syndrome, and (3) cyclic oculomotor nerve paresis with cyclic spasm.

Congenital Adduction Palsy with Synergistic Divergence
Patients with this syndrome have congenital unilateral paralysis of adduction associated with simultaneous

*The authors acknowledge the past contributions of Jane C. Sargent to this chapter.

Figure 18.1 Congenital left oculomotor nerve palsy with aberrant regeneration in a child with a history of birth trauma. **A:** In primary position, there is a left hypotropia. Note the miotic left pupil. **B:** On attempted downward gaze, there is retraction of the left upper eyelid (pseudo-Graefe sign).

bilateral abduction on attempted gaze into the field of action of the paretic medial rectus muscle (Fig. 18.2). Most patients with congenital adduction palsy with synergistic divergence have no other neurologic abnormalities.

Electromyographic studies in patients with this condition suggest that it is caused by absent oculomotor nerve innervation of the affected medial rectus muscle, combined with absent or minimal innervation of the lateral rectus muscle by the abducens nerve but with a branch of the oculomotor nerve innervating the lateral rectus muscle (Fig. 18.3).

Vertical Retraction Syndrome

The main clinical feature of the vertical retraction syndrome is limitation of movement of the affected eye on elevation or depression, associated with a retraction of the globe and narrowing of the palpebral fissure. There may be an associated esotropia or exotropia on attempted vertical gaze, more marked in the direction of the restricted vertical field of action. The condition is usually unilateral. The results of both electro-oculography and electromyography in patients with this condition are consistent with anomalous oculomotor innervation of the vertical rectus muscles of the affected eye.

Oculomotor Paresis with Cyclic Spasms (Cyclic Oculomotor Paresis, COPS)

Cyclic oculomotor paresis is usually unilateral and is, in the majority of cases, present from birth. The typical patient with this condition has an oculomotor nerve paresis with ptosis, mydriasis, reduced accommodation, and ophthalmoparesis. About every 2 minutes, the ptotic eyelid elevates, the globe begins to adduct, the pupil constricts, and accommodation increases. These spasms last 10 to 30 seconds and then give way to the paretic phase. Cyclic oculomotor palsy usually continues throughout life.

Most patients with unilateral cyclic oculomotor paresis have reduced visual acuity in the affected eye

Figure 18.2 Congenital right adduction palsy and synergistic divergence. Extraocular movements in nine fields of gaze. The right eye abducts somewhat on attempted right lateral gaze, but also abducts on left lateral gaze. (Reprinted with permission from Wilcox LM Jr, Gittinger JW Jr, Breinin GM. Congenital adduction palsy and synergistic divergence. *Am J Ophthalmol.* 1981;91:1–7.)

Synergistic divergence

Figure 18.3 Anomaly of peripheral innervation that may explain synergistic divergence with congenital limitation of adduction. The oculomotor nerve provides major innervation of the lateral rectus muscle (which may or may not also be innervated by the abducens nerve). The thickness of the line representing the nerve represents quantitative innervation. Dashed lines indicate hypoplasia or aplasia of the abducens nucleus and/or nerve. *OD*, right eye; *LR*, lateral rectus muscle; *MR*, medial rectus muscle; *III*, oculomotor nucleus; *VI*, abducens nucleus. (Redrawn from Wilcox LM Jr, Gittinger JW Jr, Breinin GM. Congenital adduction palsy and synergistic divergence. *Am J Ophthalmol.* 1981;91:1–7.)

because of amblyopia. The syndrome is occasionally associated with other pathologic conditions, including birth trauma and congenital infections. Rarely, cases occur after an acquired oculomotor nerve palsy, such as from a posterior fossa tumor. However, patients with true congenital oculomotor nerve paresis with cyclic spasms do not require any workup unless they have other evidence of neurologic disease, or they give a history of progressive neurologic dysfunction. Carbamazepine has been shown to be helpful for some patients. COPS and ocular neuromyotonia (ONM) (discussed later in this chapter) likely share a similar pathogenetic mechanism; however, they differ in that COPS patients typically lack a history of previous radiation treatment and have pre-existing paresis of the oculomotor nerve, unlike ONM patients.

Acquired

Acquired dysfunction of the oculomotor nerve is far more common than its congenital counterpart, being caused by nearly every pathologic process.

Lesions of the Oculomotor Nucleus

Lesions that damage the oculomotor nucleus are relatively uncommon. When they occur, they often produce bilateral defects in ocular motility, eyelid position, or both. The bilaterality of involvement is explained by the anatomy of the nucleus and its fibers. Both levator palpebrae superioris muscles are innervated by a single, midline subnucleus located at the caudal end of the oculomotor nerve complex (central caudal nucleus) (Fig. 18.4). A lesion that damages this region thus produces a bilateral, symmetric ptosis. In some cases, the ptosis is isolated, whereas in others, there is associated ophthalmoplegia.

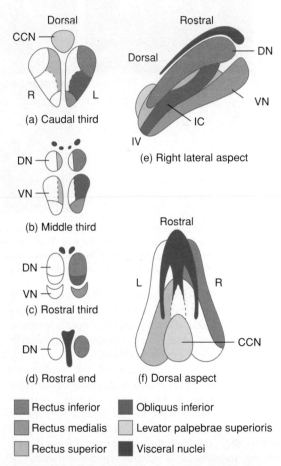

Figure 18.4 Warwick schema of topographic organization within the oculomotor nucleus. Note the caudal dorsal midline position of caudal central nucleus (CCN), the motor pool for the levator palpebrae superioris. The motor pool of the superior rectus (*hashed area*) is **contralateral** to the extraocular muscle it innervates. The visceral (parasympathetic) nuclei are shown in black. *DN*, dorsal nucleus; *IC*, intermediate column; *IV*, region of the trochlear nucleus; *VN*, ventral nucleus. (Reprinted with permission from Warwick R. Representation of the extra-ocular muscles in the oculomotor nuclei of the monkey. *J Comp Neurol.* 1953;98:449–504.)

Figure 18.5 Nuclear oculomotor nerve palsy. There is a complete left oculomotor nerve palsy. In addition, however, there is absence of elevation of the right eye. The right eye also has marked limitation of depression, suggesting that the lesion is not limited to the left oculomotor nerve nucleus but also involves the right nucleus as well. Neither oculocephalic nor caloric stimulation produced any improvement in vertical gaze.

Lesions of the oculomotor nuclear complex may spare the central caudal nucleus. Patients with such lesions have fixed, dilated pupils and ophthalmoparesis affecting one or more of the muscles innervated by the oculomotor nerve but no ptosis.

A second anatomic feature of the oculomotor nuclear complex that results in bilateral ocular damage is the course of the nerve to the superior rectus muscle, which is crossed. The subnucleus for superior rectus function on either side of the brain stem gives rise to fibers that pass through the contralateral superior rectus subnucleus without synapse and innervate the **contralateral** superior rectus muscle. Lesions that affect this region thus cause not only ipsilateral weakness of superior rectus, medial rectus, inferior rectus, inferior oblique, or a combination of these muscles, but also limitation of elevation in the contralateral eye from impairment of superior rectus function on that side. Such patients have bilateral limitation of upward gaze, occasionally worse on the contralateral side (Figs. 18.5 and 18.6; Table 18.1).

Lesions of the oculomotor nucleus are most often caused by ischemia, usually from embolic or thrombotic

Figure 18.6 Computed tomographic scan in the patient whose appearance is seen in Figure 18.5. Note the enhancing lesion in the dorsal mesencephalon (*arrow*).

Table 18.1	Nuclear Oculomotor Nerve Palsy

Obligatory Lesions
Bilateral CN III palsy + spared levator function
Unilateral CN III palsy + contralateral SR paresis
Unilateral CN III palsy + bilateral ptosis

Possible Nuclear Lesions
Bilateral ptosis
Bilateral complete CN III palsies
Isolated weakness of any single muscle except LPS
    or SR

Most Likely Not Nuclear
Unilateral CN III palsy ± pupillary involvement, and
    normal contralateral SR function
Unilateral internal ophthalmoplegia (more likely
    Adie's, trauma, migraine)
Isolated unilateral or bilateral MR weakness (more
    likely INO)
**In any case of motor dysfunction without pupillary
    involvement consider the possibility of myasthenia
    gravis

Modified and adapted from Leigh RI, Zee DS (2006). *Neurology of Eye Movements*, 4th ed. New York: Oxford Publishing, with permission.

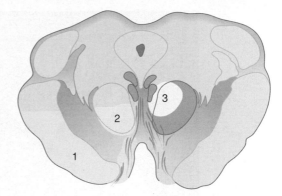

Figure 18.7 Diagram of a section through the mesencephalon showing regions in which the oculomotor nerve fascicle may be injured causing specific neurologic syndromes. (*1*) Weber syndrome. (*2*) Benedikt syndrome. (*3*) Claude syndrome (red nucleus and superior cerebellar peduncle).

occlusion of small, dorsal perforating branches of the mesencephalic portion of the basilar artery or, less often, from occlusion of the distal portion of the basilar artery itself ("top of the basilar syndrome"). Other etiologies include hemorrhage, infiltration by tumor, inflammation, and brain stem compression.

Involvement of the immediate premotor mesencephalic structures located adjacent to the oculomotor nuclei complex may produce difficulties with ocular motility that may initially appear indistinguishable from direct damage to the nucleus itself. Such supranuclear defects can usually be distinguished from their nuclear and infranuclear counterparts by stimulation of the vestibular system using oculocephalic or caloric testing.

Lesions of the Oculomotor Nerve Fascicle

Fascicular lesions of the oculomotor nerves produce both complete and incomplete palsies that cannot be differentiated clinically from palsies caused by lesions outside the brain stem. Although most lesions that affect the fascicle produce an oculomotor nerve palsy with pupillary involvement, occasionally the pupil is spared. A fascicular oculomotor nerve palsy may occur as an isolated finding or in association with other neurologic signs (Fig. 18.7).

Fascicular oculomotor nerve palsies that are associated with other neurologic manifestations produce several characteristic syndromes. Lesions in the area of the brachium conjunctivum (superior cerebellar peduncle) may produce ipsilateral oculomotor nerve palsy and cerebellar ataxia (**Nothnagel syndrome**).

The syndrome of ipsilateral oculomotor nerve palsy combined with contralateral involuntary movements (rubral hemitremor) is known as **Benedikt syndrome** and reflects damage to the red nucleus, especially its dorsocaudal portion, through which the oculomotor fascicle passes (see Fig. 18.7). Mesencephalic lesions ventral to the red nucleus may damage fascicular oculomotor fibers and motor fibers in the cerebral peduncle, producing an oculomotor nerve palsy with contralateral hemiplegia or hemiparesis, including the lower face and tongue (**Weber syndrome**) (Figs. 18.7 to 18.9). Simultaneous damage in the mesencephalon to the red nucleus *and* the brachium conjunctivum produces a syndrome with the features of both Benedikt and Nothnagel syndromes—oculomotor nerve paresis, contralateral asynergia, ataxia, dysmetria, and dysdiadochokinesia—called **Claude syndrome** (see Fig. 18.7). The majority of mesencephalic syndromes are vascular in origin and are caused by occlusion or other injury to the vascular area of the basilar artery or perforating branches of the posterior cerebral artery; however, Claude syndrome can result from thrombosis of the medial interpeduncular branch of the posterior cerebral artery.

Although divisional oculomotor nerve pareses are often caused by lesions in the cavernous sinus or posterior orbit, anatomic separation into superior and inferior divisions begins in the brain stem. Thus, rarely lesions of the oculomotor fascicles can cause isolated dysfunction of either the superior or inferior division of the oculomotor nerve. It is also possible that fascicular lesions can also cause isolated weakness of only one of the muscles innervated by the oculomotor nerve.

As with nuclear oculomotor palsies, fascicular lesions may be ischemic, hemorrhagic, compressive,

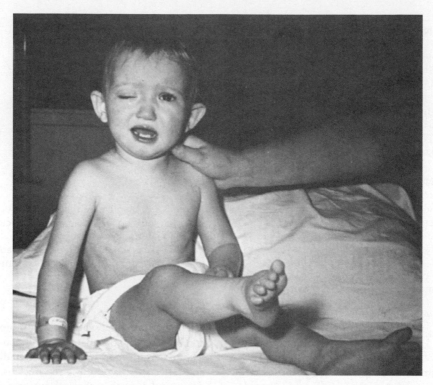

Figure 18.8 Weber syndrome produced by a brain stem glioma infiltrating the mesencephalon. Note the oculomotor nerve palsy on the right, and the hemiplegia on the left.

Figure 18.9 Computed tomogram in a patient with Weber syndrome showing an enhancing lesion in the ventral mesencephalon (*arrow*). The lesion was thought to be a solitary metastasis from a breast carcinoma.

infiltrative, traumatic, or rarely, inflammatory. Because the fascicles are white matter tracts, demyelinating disease may also cause an oculomotor nerve paresis that may occur as an isolated phenomenon or associated with other neurologic manifestations.

Lesions of the Oculomotor Nerve in the Subarachnoid Space

Lesions that damage the oculomotor nerve in the interpeduncular fossa may be located anywhere from the emergence of the nerve at the ventral surface of the mesencephalon to the point at which the nerve penetrates the dura beside the posterior clinoid process to enter the cavernous sinus (Fig. 18.10). Interpeduncular damage to the oculomotor nerve may be partial or complete. In some cases, the palsy is initially incomplete but progresses over hours, days, weeks, or even months. In most cases, there is some degree of accommodative paresis, but pupillary involvement is variable and depends primarily on the nature of the lesion. Oculomotor nerve dysfunction that is produced by damage to its subarachnoid portion may occur as (1) isolated pupillary dilation with a reduced or absent light reaction, (2) ophthalmoplegia with

Figure 18.10 The relationship of the oculomotor nerve to the intracranial arteries in the subarachnoid space. **A:** The oculomotor nerves (III) are viewed from above. On the left, the posterior communicating artery has been retracted to show the groove that it may produce through its contact with the oculomotor nerve. *RN*, red nucleus. **B:** Lateral view of the left oculomotor nerve (III) showing its arterial relationships. **C:** Schematic showing the emergence of the oculomotor nerves from brain stem, accessing the cisternal region from in between the posterior cerebral and superior cerebellar arteries, traveling anterolaterally. **D:** T2-FLAIR MRI, axial view, *arrow* pointing to the right oculomotor nerve (cisternal portion); note proximity to overlying hippocampal gyrus (uncus), denoted by the asterisk.

pupillary involvement, or (3) ophthalmoplegia with normal pupillary size and reactivity.

Isolated Fixed, Dilated Pupil as the Sole Manifestation of Subarachnoid Oculomotor Nerve Palsy

Many different lesions that compress the oculomotor nerve from above and medially rarely may produce isolated pupillary dilation, given that the Edinger–Westphal nuclei are draped over the superomedial aspect of each oculomotor nerve. Intracranial aneurysms, particularly those at the junction of the internal carotid artery and the posterior communication artery, are capable of producing a fixed dilated pupil in the early stages of oculomotor nerve involvement, but **other signs of oculomotor nerve palsy usually develop within a few hours.** Basilar artery aneurysms or basal meningitis can produce an isolated middilated nonreactive or poorly reactive pupil that may be the only sign of an oculomotor nerve palsy for days or even weeks. Hence, close follow-up (daily pupil checks within the first week) is recommended for patients that present with this isolated finding. Nonetheless, truly isolated pupil-

lary dilation from involvement of the interpeduncular portion of the oculomotor nerve is **exceptionally rare.** The occurrence of a widely dilated, nonreactive pupil in an otherwise healthy patient, even a patient complaining of headache, is far more likely to be caused by either ciliary ganglion involvement (i.e., a tonic pupil) or direct pharmacologic blockade, both of which can be diagnosed easily by pharmacologic testing.

Subarachnoid Oculomotor Nerve Palsy with Pupillary Involvement

Intracranial aneurysms are the most common cause of isolated oculomotor nerve palsy with pupillary involvement, particularly when the patient has a history of sudden severe pain in or around the eye (Figs. 18.11 and 18.12). The aneurysms usually arise from the junction of the internal carotid and posterior communicating arteries; however, aneurysms located at the top of the basilar artery and aneurysms located at the junction of the basilar artery and superior cerebellar artery may produce a similar clinical picture. Such aneurysms may injure the oculomotor nerve by direct compression, from a small hemorrhage, or at

Figure 18.11 Complete right oculomotor nerve palsy with involvement of the pupil. The patient also complained of severe right-sided retro-orbital pain.

A   **B**

Figure 18.12 A: Top panels show selective left internal carotid arteriogram showing large aneurysm at the junction of the left internal carotid and left posterior communicating arteries and bottom left panel shows 3D MRA reconstruction of the aneurysm. Bottom left, aneurysm postendovascular coiling. (Courtesy of Dr. Carlos Torres.) **B:** Intraoperative photo shows compression of oculomotor nerve (*red arrow*) from a large posterior communicating artery aneurysm (*blue oval*).

the time of a major rupture. Trauma to the oculomotor nerve may occur during aneurysm surgery.

A painful oculomotor nerve palsy with pupillary involvement may result from a posteriorly draining, low-flow carotid-cavernous sinus fistula. Tumors and other compressive lesions, such as ectatic posterior cerebral or basilar artery vessels, can occasionally stretch or compress the oculomotor nerve in the interpeduncular fossa. Intrinsic lesions of the oculomotor nerve, such as schwannomas or cavernous angiomas, can also produce an acute or progressive oculomotor nerve paresis (Fig. 18.13). The presence of pain in a patient with an oculomotor palsy does not necessarily suggest a compressive lesion since ischemic injury can also produce periorbital pain. However, pain that lasts beyond 1 to 2 weeks should raise suspicion for an alternate process to microvascular ischemia. In the event that the pupil cannot be reliably assessed (surgical distortion, trauma, heavy panretinal photocoagulation), the pupil must be assumed to be involved.

Subarachnoid Oculomotor Nerve Palsy with Pupillary Sparing

Ischemia is the most frequent cause of pupil-sparing oculomotor nerve palsies, particularly those that are unassociated with any other neurologic signs or symptoms (Fig. 18.14). In most instances, the patient has diabetes mellitus, but systemic hypertension, athero-

sclerosis, and migraine can all produce a similar clinical picture. In cases of ischemic oculomotor nerve palsy, the lesion is most often located in the oculomotor nerve fascicle, where the pupillary efferent fibers

Figure 18.13 T1-weighted magnetic resonance image (axial view) in a 31-year-old woman with progressive bilateral pupillary-involved oculomotor pareses and neurofibromatosis. There are bilateral enhancing lesions in the interpeduncular cistern (*arrows*) consistent with schwannomas of the oculomotor nerves.

A

B

Figure 18.14 **A:** Patient with cavernous sinus syndrome from basal meningioma. The patient has right proptosis associated with a complete right oculomotor nerve palsy, a right abducens nerve paresis, and a right Horner syndrome. Note that the right pupil is slightly smaller than the left pupil. **B:** T1-gadolinium–enhanced MRI, coronal view, demonstrates the cranial nerves as they travel within the cavernous sinus. *Red arrow,* oculomotor nerve; *green,* trochlear nerve; *yellow,* ophthalmic division of the trigeminal; *purple,* maxillary division of the trigeminal; and *blue,* abducens nerve.

are anatomically separated from the fibers to the extra-ocular muscles, or in the subarachnoid portion of the nerve, where the pupillary fibers occupy a peripheral (superomedial) location and receive more collateral (pial) blood supply than the main trunk of the nerve.

Patients with oculomotor nerve pareses caused by ischemia often have severe pain regardless of whether or not the pupil is involved. Ischemic oculomotor nerve palsies characteristically resolve within 4 to 16 weeks without treatment. The resolution is almost always complete, and there is almost never evidence of aberrant regeneration. Around 20% of patients with ischemic oculomotor nerve palsies will present with some involvement of the pupil.

Although most pupil-sparing oculomotor nerve palsies (with or without associated pain) are caused by ischemia, such palsies may also be produced by subarachnoid compressive lesions, particularly aneurysms, ipsilateral temporal lobe astrocytomas, and ipsilateral acute subdural hematomas. It is estimated that approximately 5% of compressive oculomotor palsies are pupil sparing. Such palsies are nearly always

incomplete and are often accompanied by persistent ocular or orbital pain. Patients with a painful, incomplete, pupil-sparing oculomotor nerve paresis should undergo MRI as well as either computed tomographic angiography (CTA) or MR angiography (MRA). Depending on the results of these studies, conventional angiography may be appropriate, although very rarely performed at this point for diagnostic purposes given the perpetual advances in imaging resolution and techniques (see Table 18.2).

Subarachnoid Oculomotor Nerve Palsy from Involvement at or near its Entrance to the Cavernous Sinus

The oculomotor nerve is particularly vulnerable to stretch and contusion injuries where it is firmly attached to the dura adjacent to the posterior clinoid process just posterior to the cavernous sinus. Frontal head trauma, aneurysms, and surgery in the parasellar region are the common causes of injury at this site.

Herniation of the hippocampal gyrus (uncus) compresses the oculomotor nerve where it passes over the

Table 18.2	Evaluation of Oculomotor Palsies/Risk of Compressive Lesion		
Internal and External Ophthalmoplegia	**Risk of Compressive Lesion**	**Recommendation**	
Complete internal dysfunction (blown pupil) + complete external dysfunction	Highest	1. MRI/MRA or CTA 2. Angiogram if negative	
+ partial external dysfunction	Highest	1. MRI/MRA or CTA 2. Angiogram if negative	
+ no external dysfunction	Extremely low	No imaging, follow closely for ~1 wk for evolution	
Incomplete internal dysfunction (sluggish pupil) + complete external dysfunction	Low to moderate	1. MRI/MRA or CTA 2. Angio if still suspicious, persistent pain, or evolution	
+ incomplete external dysfunction	Low to minimal	1. MRI/MRA or CTA 2. Angio if still suspicious, persistent pain, or evolution	
+ no external dysfunction	Extremely low	No imaging—likely not an oculomotor nerve palsy	
No internal dysfunction (no pupil involvement) + complete external dysfunction	Very low	1. Observe if ischemic risk factors present 2. Consider GCA 3. MRI/CTA if pain persists or worsens beyond 2 wk	
+ incomplete external dysfunction	Uncertain	1. Consider myasthenia gravis 2. MRI/MRA or CTA 3. Angio if still suspicious, persistent pain, or evolution	

ridge of the dura associated with the attachment of the free edge of the tentorium to the clivus. As the herniating hippocampal gyrus descends into the tentorial incisura, it presses upon the upper surface of the ipsilateral oculomotor nerve that is running beneath it (see Fig. 18.10D) and pulls the oculomotor nerve more firmly into contact with the posterior clinoid process. The herniating cerebral mass ultimately reaches and impinges on the dorsal surface of the pons on the same side. The posterior cerebral arteries are also drawn tightly down across the dorsal surface of the oculomotor nerves, producing even more compression (see Fig. 18.10A). Pupillary dilation is often the first sign of increasing cerebral edema or of an ipsilateral, expanding, supratentorial mass. This initial pupillary sign is caused by pressure on the peripheral portion of the nerve. With increasing compression, additional signs of impaired oculomotor nerve function appear.

Lesions of the Oculomotor Nerve within the Cavernous Sinus and Superior Orbital Fissure

Lesions within the cavernous sinus or superior orbital fissure may produce isolated oculomotor nerve dysfunction but more often cause a cranial polyneuropathy. Because the cavernous sinus contains structures that continue through the superior orbital fissure, it is often impossible to determine with certainty if the lesion is confined to the sinus, is in the fissure, or involves both structures. It is reasonable to consider damage in this region as a single entity, the **sphenocavernous syndrome**. This syndrome is characterized by paralysis or paresis of the oculomotor, trochlear, and abducens nerves, usually associated with the involvement of the ophthalmic division (and in the cavernous sinus, the maxillary division) of the trigeminal nerve (Fig. 18.14). Involvement of the optic nerve either within the orbit or intracranially often causes visual loss. Because of the frequent involvement of the trigeminal nerve by lesions of the cavernous sinus and superior orbital fissure, patients with such lesions often complain of severe pain when they develop ophthalmoplegia. In many cases, there is oculosympathetic paresis, and there may be proptosis, edema of the eyelids, and chemosis of the conjunctiva. In patients with combined oculomotor paresis and sympathetic denervation, the pupil may be small or midposition and poorly reactive. This appearance is almost pathognomonic of a cavernous sinus lesion. Pain with associated hypesthesia (anesthesia dolorosa) suggests a compressive or infiltrative lesion of the trigeminal ganglion or nerve(s) itself; whereas periorbital/hemi-cranial pain without anesthesia in this context may be due to the involvement of the adjacent dura.

The sphenocavernous syndrome may be produced by primary or secondary lesions within the cavernous sinus or superior orbital fissure or by lesions within the orbit or intracranial cavity that compress the cranial nerves that pass through these structures. Common lesions capable of producing the sphenocavernous syndrome include aneurysms, meningiomas, pituitary tumors, craniopharyngiomas, nasopharyngeal tumors, metastatic tumors, lymphoma, and infectious and inflammatory processes.

Idiopathic granulomatous inflammation may produce a painful ophthalmoplegia from involvement of the cranial nerves within the cavernous sinus and superior orbital fissure: the **Tolosa–Hunt syndrome (THS)**. Patients with this syndrome typically improve rapidly and dramatically when treated with systemic corticosteroids; however, both spontaneous and steroid-induced remissions of symptoms and signs, sometimes of prolonged duration, occur in cases of painful ophthalmoplegia caused by tumors, infiltrative conditions, lymphoproliferative conditions, and aneurysms. Thus, because of the similarity of the symptoms, signs, and response to therapy of both inflammatory and noninflammatory lesions of the cavernous sinus (including ischemic lesions), patients with the syndrome of painful ophthalmoplegia require a complete assessment, including neuroimaging, a systemic evaluation for an underlying vascular or inflammatory disorder, and, in most cases, a lumbar puncture (Fig. 18.15A and B), followed by biopsy of the apical lesion if a dramatic resolution is not noted with steroid treatment. Near resolution of the pain is expected in THS within 72 hours of treatment—however, the ocular motor deficits may

Figure 18.15 Neuroimaging in a patient with painful ophthalmoplegia. The patient was a 49-year-old man with right retrobulbar pain and generalized limitation of movement of the right eye. The patient was thought to have the Tolosa–Hunt syndrome and was treated with oral corticosteroids without improvement. The ophthalmoparesis progressed to a complete ophthalmoplegia associated with loss of vision in the eye. **A:** T1-weighted, coronal magnetic resonance image (MRI) after intravenous injection of paramagnetic contrast material reveals enlargement of the right cavernous sinus. **B:** CT scan of the abdomen reveals a left renal mass. The patient was found to have a metastatic renal cell carcinoma. (Reprinted with permission from Mehelas TJ, Kosmorsky GS. Painful ophthalmoplegia syndrome secondary to metastatic renal cell carcinoma. *J Neuroophthalmol.* 1996;16:289–290). **C:** T1-enhanced MRI, axial view, of a patient presenting with bilateral frontal pain, mild proptosis, and right > left chemosis. Note pachymeningeal thickening along left temporo-parietal convexity and bilateral orbital inflammatory infiltrate. Biopsy revealed IgG4 infiltrative disease. (*continued*)

D

Figure 18.15 (*continued*) **D:** T1-enhanced MRI, coronal (**left**) and axial (**right**) views demonstrating avidly enhancing tissue in orbital apex, extending anteriorly. This patient presented with right-sided orbital pain, right upper lid fullness, 3-mm proptosis, and a mild right superior division oculomotor nerve palsy. She responded exquisitely to steroids, suggesting idiopathic orbital inflammation with apical involvement.

persist for weeks or longer. IgG4 infiltrative disease is being increasingly recognized as a potential etiology in many presumed "idiopathic" cases of orbital inflammation. This condition carries systemic implications, including thyroiditis, retroperitoneal fibrosis, para-aortitis, and pachymeningitis (Fig. 18.15C).

Vascular processes can produce a painful ophthalmoplegia from damage to structures in the cavernous sinus and superior orbital fissure. Cavernous sinus thrombosis and carotid-cavernous sinus fistulas can produce typical cavernous sinus syndromes. Painful ophthalmoplegia also occurs in patients with syphilis, giant cell (temporal) arteritis, diabetes mellitus, rheumatoid arthritis, and systemic lupus erythematosus.

The ischemia that produces oculomotor nerve dysfunction in patients with diabetes mellitus is, at least in some instances, caused by a lesion in the intracavernous portion of the nerve. Similar lesions may be responsible for the isolated oculomotor nerve palsies that develop in patients with systemic hypertension, ophthalmoplegic migraine, herpes zoster ophthalmicus, and giant cell arteritis.

Trauma to the cavernous sinus and superior orbital fissure may produce an isolated oculomotor nerve palsy. Such palsies are usually associated with skull fracture and are caused by intraneural and perineural hemorrhage in the cavernous sinus or superior orbital fissure.

Lesions of the Oculomotor Nerve within the Orbit

The sphenocavernous syndrome is characterized by a painful ophthalmoplegia and is generally unassociated with visual loss from an optic neuropathy. Conversely, lesions in the apex of the orbit produce ophthalmople-

gia that may or may not be painful but that are usually associated with loss of vision from optic neuropathy and variable proptosis. The distinction between these two entities—the sphenocavernous syndrome and the orbital apex syndrome—can thus often be made both on clinical grounds and by neuroimaging.

The oculomotor nerve enters the orbit as two separate divisions: the superior division, which innervates the levator palpebrae superioris and the superior rectus muscle; and the inferior division, which innervates the medial and inferior rectus muscle, the inferior oblique muscle, and the motor root of the ciliary ganglion. Thus, an incomplete oculomotor nerve paresis in the distribution of either division is often caused by a lesion of either the sphenocavernous region or the orbital apex (Fig. 18.15D). However, as noted above, the oculomotor nerve has a divisional topographic arrangement beginning in the brain stem. Thus, divisional oculomotor nerve pareses may result from lesions not only in the cavernous sinus and orbital apex, but also from lesions in the brain stem or subarachnoid space, although the latter is quite rare. Further clinical localization is thus based on eliciting additional signs and symptoms, while being cognizant of the relevant relational anatomy. Although neuroimaging is certainly helpful in increasing the precision of localization, discrete lesions are often beyond the resolution of even the most sophisticated imaging techniques.

Recovery from Acquired Oculomotor Nerve Palsy

Oculomotor nerve paralysis, whether complete or incomplete, may have several outcomes. First, complete recovery may occur. In such cases, recovery may be complete within 1 to 2 weeks after the onset of symptoms. In other instances, notably those associated with diabetes mellitus and systemic hypertension, recovery does not begin for a month or more but is usually complete within 3 months. In still other cases, recovery can take much longer, sometimes as long as 3 years. Prolonged recovery occurs especially after damage to the fascicular portion of the nerve.

In some cases of oculomotor nerve palsy, the paralysis persists completely unchanged. In such cases, the nerve has usually been transected by trauma or chronic compression or has been infiltrated by tumor.

Acquired Oculomotor Synkinesis: Misdirection of Regenerating Fibers in the Oculomotor Nerve

Some patients with oculomotor nerve pareses experience partial recovery of oculomotor nerve function. Peripheral motor and sensory nerves, including the autonomic nerves, can regenerate. The regenerative process produces more axons than were present before the nerve was interrupted. Axons sprout from the proximal end of the severed nerve and from collateral nerves that have not been severely damaged. Cords of Schwann cells form in the peripheral segment of the nerve so that the new nerve fibers are conducted to the end organ. The newly formed neurons reach the empty tubes (Schwann tubes) that contained functioning neurons before degeneration. Regenerating axons have the capacity to bridge long gaps in damaged nerves.

In peripheral nerves that innervate more than one muscle, misdirection of regenerating nerve fibers may occur. Thus, regenerating sprouts from axons that previously innervated one muscle group may ultimately innervate a different muscle group with a different function.

Following injury to the oculomotor nerve at any point along its pathway from the brain stem to the orbit, a syndrome of oculomotor nerve synkinesis may occur. In adults, evidence of synkinesis first appears about 9 weeks after injury, whereas in infants with oculomotor nerve palsy from birth trauma, such signs may be observed from 1 to 6 weeks following birth. Oculomotor nerve synkinesis is thought to occur from misdirection of regenerated axons in the nerve. Thus, the levator palpebrae superioris may receive fibers that were originally destined for the medial rectus muscle, or fibers originally intended for the superior rectus muscle may reach the inferior oblique, inferior rectus, or medial rectus muscles. The active elevation of the eyelid during attempted downward eye movement is called the **pseudo-Graefe sign** to distinguish it from the lid lag on downward gaze that occurs in patients with thyroid eye disease (Graefe sign) (Fig. 18.16).

Fibers originally destined for any of the muscles innervated by the oculomotor nerve may reach the ciliary ganglion to synapse with the postganglionic parasympathetic fibers that innervate the iris sphincter muscle, the ciliary body muscle, or both. Often, this anomalous reinnervation of the pupil is easily observed because the pupil constricts only when the patient is asked to look in a direction requiring oculomotor nerve function. In other cases, the pupil may appear to be permanently paralyzed in the middilated position, but slit lamp biomicroscopy will enable the examiner to observe subtle abnormalities of pupillary movement that reflect misregeneration of the iris sphincter (Figs. 18.17 and 18.18).

The signs of aberrant regeneration of the oculomotor nerve may be summarized as follows:

1 **Muscle to Muscle:** Adduction of the involved eye on attempted elevation or depression (SR or IR to MR). Conversely, elevation of the eye on attempted adduction (MR to SR or IO)
2 **Muscle to Eyelid:** *Pseudo-Graefe sign*—retraction and elevation of the eyelid on attempted downward gaze. Elevation of the eyelid on attempted adduction can also occur.
3 **Muscle to Pupil:** *Pseudo-Argyll Robertson pupil*—the involved pupil does not react or reacts poorly and irregularly to light stimulation but does constrict on adduction during conjugate gaze.
4 Limitation of elevation and depression of the eye with occasional retraction of the globe on attempted vertical movement

The phenomenon of **secondary oculomotor nerve synkinesis** occurs in nearly all patients with congenital oculomotor nerve palsy; however, the majority of patients with this syndrome have experienced a primary, acute event that has produced a complete oculomotor nerve palsy. Secondary oculomotor nerve synkinesis occurs commonly following oculomotor nerve palsy from intracranial aneurysms, trauma (including surgical trauma), syphilis, and basal meningitis. As a general rule, synkinetic movements *do not occur* after ischemic insults to the nerve. The release of neurotrophic factors guiding collateral sprouting of axons generally occurs in response to a degree of crush injury. Thus, in a patient suspected of having an ischemic oculomotor nerve palsy, particularly if there have been no previous episodes, the development of oculomotor synkinesis should suggest an alternative etiology, such as compression or aggressive inflammation.

Although the syndrome of acquired oculomotor nerve synkinesis occurs most frequently after acute oculomotor nerve palsy, it also occurs as a "primary" phenomenon; that is, without a pre-existing acute oculomotor nerve paresis. Patients with **primary**

Figure 18.16 Misdirected regeneration of the right oculomotor nerve following trauma (secondary aberrant regeneration). Note elevation of the right upper eyelid in particular on attempted downward gaze (pseudo-Graefe sign) and subtly on attempted adduction of the right eye. Although the right pupil poorly reactive to light and mildly dilated on upgaze, it constricted slightly in the primary position and on attempted adduction of the eye.

oculomotor nerve synkinesis usually harbor slowly growing lesions of the cavernous sinus, usually meningiomas or aneurysms, but also trigeminal schwannomas. Slowly growing lesions in the subarachnoid space, including unruptured aneurysms, can also produce primary oculomotor nerve synkinesis. Lesions that cause primary aberrant regeneration grow so slowly that the mild oculomotor nerve damage that results does not produce major visual difficulties and, in addition, allows regeneration to occur concurrently with damage to the native oculomotor axons.

In patients with partial recovery following a period of observation of at least 6 months, various strabismus procedures may be of benefit in providing binocular single vision, at least in primary position, and ptosis surgery may also be used to improve the position of the affected eyelid. Many patients experience some resolution of their ptosis via aberrantly regenerating fibers (muscle to eyelid), hence begin to notice diplopia over time. Hence, ptosis surgery, if contemplated, should also be delayed until such time that no further

improvement is seen on serial observation. Botulinum toxin injections of the lateral rectus can realign the eyes for better fusion in patients with mild oculomotor nerve palsy who are awaiting improvement. Other patients seem content to simply patch the affected eye or are able to ignore the double image. An opaque contact lens provides a cosmetically acceptable means to alleviate subjective diplopia in these patients.

Trochlear (Fourth) Nerve Palsies

Trochlear nerve palsy is the most common cause of acquired vertical strabismus in the general population, other causes being ocular myopathies (e.g., dysthyroid eye disease), disorders of the neuromuscular junction (e.g., myasthenia gravis), incomplete oculomotor nerve paresis, and skew deviation. Trochlear nerve palsy causes partial or complete paralysis of the superior oblique muscle, usually associated over time with overaction of its antagonist, the ipsilateral inferior

Figure 18.17 Diagram of aberrant regeneration of the oculomotor nerve as it affects pupillary function. **Above:** Before injury, preganglionic fibers serving the pupillary light reaction synapse in the ciliary ganglion with axons that then proceed along short ciliary nerves to supply specific sectors of the iris sphincter. Thus preganglionic fiber *1* synapses with postganglionic fiber *A* to supply sector *A'* of the iris sphincter. **Below:** After injury to the preganglionic pathway, several phenomena may occur. A fiber may be undamaged (fiber *1*). A fiber may be completely destroyed and may never grow (fibers *3* and *4*), or it may be damaged, and regeneration may occur (fibers *2* and *2b*). In such a scenario, a collateral sprout could grow from a preganglionic fiber other than that originally intended for the iris sphincter. If fiber *4a* grew from a nerve originally destined for the inferior rectus muscle, then segment *D'* of the iris sphincter would constrict whenever the patient attempted to look downward. (Redrawn from Czarnecki JSC, Thompson HS. The iris sphincter in aberrant regeneration of the third nerve. *Arch Ophthalmol.* 1978;96:1606–1610.)

oblique muscle (Figs. 18.19 and 18.20). Patients with this disorder complain of vertical diplopia that is greatest in downgaze and to the opposite side. Such patients also have excyclotorsion when tested with double Maddox rods or Lancaster red green glasses. This feature helps to distinguish trochlear nerve palsy from skew deviation, in which the higher eye is invari-ably intorted (see Fig. 18.21). The ability of the superior oblique muscle to intort the eye is particularly important when assessing superior oblique function in patients with an oculomotor nerve palsy. In such cases, the absence of intorsion when the patient attempts to depress the eye while it is abducted indicates lack of superior oblique function as well.

Figure 18.18 Aberrant regeneration of the right oculomotor nerve with involvement of the pupil. **A:** During attempted elevation of the eyes, the right pupil remains middilated. **B:** During depression of the eyes, the right pupil constricts.

Figure 18.19 Bilateral trochlear nerve palsies in a 28-year-old man following a motorcycle accident. The patient suffered a severe blow to the vertex of his head. Note the patient's inability to depress either eye fully in adduction. There is bilateral overaction of both inferior oblique muscles. (Courtesy of Jacqueline Morris, C.O.)

Most patients with trochlear nerve palsy have torticollis. Such patients typically tilt the head to the side opposite the paralyzed superior oblique muscle. This spontaneous ocular torticollis is absent in patients with poor vision in either eye and in patients with large vertical fusional amplitudes that allow them to fuse in all positions of gaze. On occasion, some patients with trochlear nerve palsy tilt their heads to the side of the palsy. This results in greater separation of images, thus allowing one of the images to be ignored.

Figure 18.20 A 39-year-old man with vertical diplopia worse when he looks to the left, with evidence of right inferior oblique overaction. Double Maddox rod testing reveals roughly 10 degrees of excyclotorsion of the right eye. Note that the excyclotorted and hypertrophic right eye sees the lower image, which appears incyclotorted to the patient. Hence he excyclotorts the image by twisting the right lens within the trial frame until the images appear parallel. The degree of excylotorsion can be read from the markings on the trial frame. The above is consistent with a right trochlear nerve palsy.

SKEW (OTR, ocular tilt reaction)   IV (SUPERIOR OBLIQUE PALSY)

A and B
Observer View

A

B

SKEW
Higher eye intorted, lower eye extorted
Usually no or little torsional diplopia

SUPERIOR OBLIQUE PALSY
Higher eye extorted
Torsional diplopia (images point to paretic eye)
Slant (top of object appears closer)

C and D (Patient View)

C

D

Figure 18.21 Differentiation between a skew deviation and fourth nerve palsy is often possible on the basis of observing the direction of torsion of the higher eye, on funduscopy as well double Maddox rod testing. In skew (**left**), the eyes exhibit conjugate cyclotorsion, with the higher eye incyclotorted, and fourth nerve palsy (**right**) exhibits excyclotorsion of the higher eye only, without change in torsion of the contralateral eye. (Modified from Leigh RI, Zee DS (2015). *The Neurology of Eye Movements.* 5th, ed. New York: Oxford University Press, with permission.)

Congenital

Congenital trochlear nerve palsy is common. The etiology of congenital trochlear palsy is unknown; however, aplasia of the trochlear nerve nucleus appears to be responsible in some cases, and hypoplasia in others. Most congenital trochlear nerve palsies are sporadic. Most patients with congenital trochlear nerve palsy are neurologically normal, and many have some degree of facial asymmetry.

Patients with congenital trochlear nerve palsy usually develop large vertical fusion amplitudes that, in association with a head tilt, allow them to compensate for their muscle weakness. Such patients may, however, develop diplopia from decompensation of the palsy after a minor head injury. When these patients are evaluated, a review of old photographs often reveals a pre-existing head tilt. In addition, direct measurement of vertical fusion amplitudes may also establish the diagnosis. Normal persons have a vertical fusion range of only 2 to 4 prism diopters, whereas patients with congenital superior oblique paresis may have 8 to 25 prism diopters of vertical fusion amplitude.

Congenital superior oblique palsy may be bilateral. In some instances, the patients appear to have a unilateral palsy until they undergo surgical correction, at which time the contralateral palsy becomes apparent. In most cases, however, careful measurements of both vertical and torsional deviation permit differentiation between unilateral and bilateral palsies.

Acquired

When an etiology can be determined, blunt head trauma, usually a direct orbital, frontal, basal, or oblique cranial blow, is the most common cause of isolated, acquired, unilateral, and bilateral trochlear nerve palsy in both adults and children. As with other ocular motor nerve palsies, almost any pathologic process can damage the trochlear nerve at any point from its nucleus to its termination in the orbit where it innervates the superior oblique muscle.

Lesions of the Trochlear Nerve Nucleus

Lesions of the brain stem that damage the trochlear nerve nucleus cannot be localized with certainty on clinical grounds unless there are other neurologic signs suggesting intrinsic mesencephalic damage. Even when such signs are present, distinguishing nuclear from fascicular involvement is almost impossible. In addition, extrinsic lesions that compress the dorsal mesencephalon may damage the trochlear nerves as they emerge from the brain stem and at the same time produce damage to intrinsic brain stem structures. Cells of the trochlear nucleus are often damaged by lesions that involve the tegmentum at the junction of the pons and mesencephalon, particularly contusion and hemorrhage caused by impact against the tentorial margin. Other lesions that can produce intrinsic damage to the trochlear nerve nuclei include ischemia, primary and metastatic tumors, and vascular malformations. Paresis of the superior oblique muscle with such lesions can, however, be obscured by associated conjugate or internuclear gaze defects. In such patients, the recognition of a trochlear nerve palsy becomes possible only after the supranuclear difficulties resolve.

Both unilateral and bilateral superior oblique paresis can be associated with Parinaud dorsal midbrain syndrome from pineal tumors, aqueductal stenosis, and hydrocephalus; vertical diplopia in this setting is far more commonly caused by trochlear nerve dysfunction than previously recognized. Trochlear nerve palsy also can follow neurosurgical procedures in the posterior fossa.

Lesions of the Trochlear Nerve Fascicle

Fascicular involvement of the trochlear nerves can be caused by the same processes that cause damage to the trochlear nuclei. These processes include compression, infiltration, ischemia, hemorrhage, trauma, and inflammation, particularly multiple sclerosis.

Because of the dorsal location of the trochlear fascicles, associated neurologic signs are of less help in the topographic diagnosis of such lesions than are neuroimaging studies. Nevertheless, two important associated signs that suggest that the site of a trochlear

nerve paresis is the trochlear nucleus or fascicle are a central Horner syndrome and a relative afferent pupillary defect (RAPD) unassociated with evidence of an optic neuropathy or optic tract syndrome.

The Horner syndrome is caused by damage to descending sympathetic fibers (in the dorsal brain stem), which are usually adjacent to the trochlear nerve nucleus. Thus, the Horner syndrome is usually on the side opposite the trochlear nerve paresis (because the trochlear nerves are crossed). The only exception is if the lesion affects the postdecussation portion of the trochlear nerve fascicle, in which case both the trochlear nerve paresis and the Horner syndrome are on the same side. The latter scenario is indistinguishable from a cavernous sinus localization, unless other signs are seen to shed more light.

The RAPD is caused by damage to afferent pupillary fibers in the brachium of the superior colliculus. If the trochlear nerve paresis is caused by a lesion of the predecussation portion of the fascicle (or the trochlear nerve nucleus), the RAPD is on the same side as the trochlear nerve paresis, whereas if the paresis is caused by damage to the postdecussation portion of the fascicle, the RAPD is on the side opposite the trochlear nerve paresis (Fig. 18.22A).

Lesions of the Trochlear Nerve in the Subarachnoid Space

The trochlear nerve is particularly susceptible to injury or compression as it emerges from the dorsal surface

A   **B**

Figure 18.22 A: Presumed site of damage in a young woman who developed a left trochlear nerve paresis and was found to have a left relative afferent pupillary defect (greater number of nasal retinal fibers decussate than temporal) unassociated with any visual sensory deficit. The shaded portion of the illustration indicates a lesion involving the brachium of the right superior colliculus and the right dorsal mesencephalon, including the right trochlear nucleus or the predecussation portion of the right trochlear nerve fascicle. The patient was found to have an anaplastic astrocytoma of the brain stem. (Reprinted with permission from Eliott D, Cunningham ET Jr, Miller NR. Fourth nerve paresis and ipsilateral relative afferent pupillary defect without visual sensory disturbance: A sign of contralateral dorsal midbrain disease. *J Clin Neuroophthalmol.* 1991;11:169–171.) **B:** Arrow points to the superior (anterior) medullary velum, which forms the roof of the fourth ventricle and is the site of decussation of the trochlear fascicles, and often the site of shearing injury in cases of closed trauma causing bilateral trochlear nerve palsies.

of the brain stem (Fig. 18.22B). Injuries in this location may avulse the rootlets of the emerging nerve, or there may be stretching or contusion injury from hemorrhage within the nerve.

When damage occurs to the trochlear nerves at their exit from the brain stem, both nerves are often involved. The presence of bilateral palsies may first become apparent after the patient undergoes surgical correction of the apparent unilateral palsy. Trauma that is insufficient to produce a skull fracture or loss of consciousness may cause a trochlear nerve palsy because of the extremely fragile nature of the nerve and its long subarachnoid course. The subarachnoid portion of the trochlear nerve can occasionally be damaged by posterior fossa aneurysms. In most cases, the aneurysm arises from the junction of the basilar and superior cerebellar arteries.

The subarachnoid portion of the trochlear nerve may also become affected in patients with basal meningitis. Syphilis, tuberculosis, sarcoidosis, and Lyme disease are the most common causes.

Schwannomas of the trochlear nerve may produce diplopia from trochlear nerve palsy by involvement of the nerve in the subarachnoid space. Other intrinsic lesions of the subarachnoid portion of the trochlear nerve include cavernous angiomas and arteriovenous malformations.

The association of trochlear nerve palsy and elevated ICP is well documented. Some of these patients have pseudotumor cerebri, whereas others have hydrocephalus related to a variety of different processes, including blocked ventriculoperitoneal shunts. Indeed, bilateral trochlear nerve paresis may be a localizing sign of involvement of the superior medullary velum by a dilated sylvian aqueduct or downward pressure from an enlarged third ventricle.

Lesions of the Trochlear Nerve within the Cavernous Sinus and Superior Orbital Fissure

Lesions that produce a cavernous sinus syndrome are discussed above. When such lesions produce combined ocular motor nerve palsies, the trochlear nerve is often involved. However, it is unusual, for isolated trochlear nerve palsy to occur from cavernous sinus disease, although ischemic conditions (e.g., diabetes mellitus) may conceivably affect the trochlear nerve in this location as they do the oculomotor nerve. In this respect, it is also possible that the isolated trochlear nerve palsy that occurs in some patients with herpes zoster may be produced by a local granulomatous angiitis that originates in the ophthalmic division of the trigeminal nerve and spreads to the sphenocavernous portion of the trochlear nerve. This cannot be the only mechanism, however, because trochlear nerve palsy can also occur in patients with geniculate herpes zoster (i.e., the Ramsay Hunt syndrome).

Lesions of the Trochlear Nerve within the Orbit

Trauma (including surgical injury) may damage the trochlear nerve within the orbit; however, in many cases, it is impossible to ascertain if the damage has occurred to the nerve, the trochlea, the superior oblique muscle or tendon, or several of these structures. A similar problem arises in assessing patients with orbital inflammation, ischemia, or vascular malformations that are associated with superior oblique dysfunction. The superior oblique paralysis that occurs in patients with Paget disease of the orbit and with hypertrophic arthritis may also be caused by mechanical disruption of the superior oblique tendon within the trochlea and not by damage to the trochlear nerve itself.

Recovery from an acquired fourth nerve palsy is highly variable. Those resulting from ischemia or demyelination tend to improve over several weeks, often with complete resolution. Fourth nerve palsies due to trauma (surgical or otherwise) should be observed for several months before one considers performing surgical realignment as partial or complete recovery occurs spontaneously in many cases. Patients presenting with decompensated congenital fourth nerve palsies can occasionally regain fusion and improve clinically, but generally maintain some degree of misalignment once they have decompensated.

Evaluation and Management of Trochlear Nerve Palsy

The diagnosis of a trochlear nerve palsy is made primarily by performing the "three-step test". It must be emphasized that this test is only useful if the paresis is of a single cyclovertical muscle. Furthermore, although we believe the three-step test is extremely useful in patients with presumed trochlear nerve palsies, its reliability in the diagnosis of pareses of other vertical muscles is questionable. In addition, restrictive ophthalmoplegia, myasthenia gravis, and skew deviation can mimic a trochlear nerve palsy when they are evaluated using the three-step test (Fig. 18.23).

Treating the vertical or torsional diplopia experienced by patients awaiting resolution of an acquired or a decompensated congenital trochlear nerve palsy can be challenging, particularly for those with significant torsional misalignment or bilateral fourth nerve palsies. In other cases, particularly those with mild vertical displacement, the use of a vertical press-on (Fresnel), or ground-in prism may be of benefit, although some degree of diplopia in extremes of gaze is almost always present given the usual incomitancy of the deviation. Patients with long-standing trochlear nerve lesions often exhibit "spread of comitance" making optical realignment strategies much more effective. In cases of acquired trochlear nerve palsy, no attempt at surgical

Figure 18.23 Orthoptic measurements taken for a patient with a right trochlear nerve palsy. Application of the three- step test demonstrates (1) right hypertropia in primary gaze; (2) worsening of RHT in contralateral gaze; and (3) worsening with ipsilateral head tilt. Note the mild right inferior oblique overaction and superior oblique underaction. Often a fourth step is included, demonstrating increase in hypertropia in downgaze.

correction should be considered until at least 6 months have elapsed without change in orthoptic measurements, unless the physician knows with certainty that the trochlear nerve has been severed.

When a trochlear nerve palsy has been stable over an appropriate period of time, one may attempt to correct persistent diplopia using any one of the several operative procedures. These procedures are designed to (1) strengthen all or a portion of the superior oblique muscle, (2) weaken its antagonist, the ipsilateral inferior oblique muscle, or (3) weaken its yoke muscle, the contralateral inferior rectus muscle. Many surgeons prefer to use adjustable suture technique in such cases given the narrow vertical range of fusion and variability in surgical dosing among individuals. The decision to use one or another of these procedures or to use several in combination depends on the results of a careful orthoptic examination. Similar considerations apply for the treatment of bilateral trochlear nerve palsies. Given the large amount of excyclotorsion in bilateral cases, a Harada–Ito procedure is usually needed. Although the results of surgery for both congenital and acquired trochlear nerve palsies are usually excellent, patients should be counseled at the outset that they may need several surgeries to achieve appropriate alignment, especially in bilateral cases.

Abducens (Sixth) Nerve Palsies and Nuclear Horizontal Gaze Paralysis

The abducens nerve is unique in that damage to its nucleus results not in a sixth nerve palsy but, rather, in a horizontal **gaze** paralysis toward the side of the lesion. In addition, the precise anatomic location of the nerve produces syndromes that are different from those seen with damage to either the oculomotor or trochlear nerves.

Congenital

Congenital absence of abduction as an isolated phenomenon is exceedingly rare but may occur from injury to the abducens nerve shortly before or during birth. That birth trauma is a significant factor indicated by an incidence of congenital abduction weakness in infants that increases progressively from 0% for deliveries by caesarean section, to 0.1% for spontaneous vaginal delivery, to 2.4% for forceps delivery, and to 3.2% for vacuum extraction.

Congenital paralysis of conjugate horizontal eye movements occurs more frequently than does unilateral or bilateral abduction weakness. Congenital horizontal gaze palsy may occur as an isolated sporadic finding, or it may be familial. Histologic findings in patients with isolated bilateral horizontal gaze palsy include absent or hypoplastic abducens nuclei and absent abducens nerves.

Far more common are congenital disturbances of horizontal gaze associated with two conditions: Möbius syndrome and Duane retraction syndrome (DRS).

Möbius Syndrome (Congenital Bulbar Paralysis)

Characteristically, this defect involves the face and horizontal gaze mechanisms bilaterally. Affected patients have a mask-like facies, with the mouth constantly held open. The eyelids often cannot be completely closed. Some patients have only an esotropia associated with unilateral or bilateral limitation of abduction, and some may even be able to converge. In most cases, however, the eyes are straight and do not move horizontally in either direction (Fig. 18.24).

Other congenital defects that are found in patients with this syndrome include deafness, webbed fingers or toes, supernumerary digits, atrophy of the muscles of the chest, neck, and particularly the tongue, and absence of the hands, feet, fingers, or toes. Nearly all patients with Möbius syndrome have some degree of mental retardation.

The diversity of brain stem pathologic findings in patients with Möbius syndrome suggests that the syndrome actually is a heterogeneous group of congenital disorders that in some cases are caused by developmental defects, and in others, by acquired hypoxic or other insults. Most cases of Möbius syndrome are sporadic.

Duane Retraction Syndrome (Stilling–Turk–Duane Syndrome)

DRS is a predominantly congenital eye movement disorder characterized by marked limitation or absence

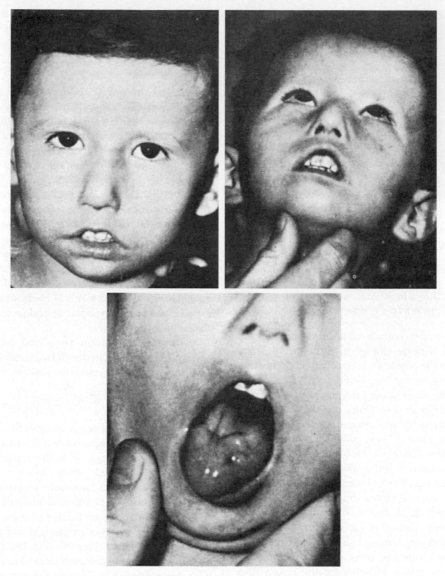

Figure 18.24 Möbius syndrome in a 3-year-old boy. The boy had spontaneous vertical eye movements but no horizontal eye movements. Note bilateral facial palsy and atrophy of the tongue.

of abduction, variable limitation of adduction, and palpebral fissure narrowing and globe retraction on attempted adduction. Vertical ocular movements are often noted on adduction (upshoot), most frequently in an upward direction.

A disorder of horizontal eye movements is common to all patients with DRS. In most cases, the abnormalities are unilateral, but bilateral Duane syndrome occurs in 15% to 20% of affected patients. In most patients, gaze is directed toward the side of the unaffected eye, and in some instances, the face is turned toward the affected side to allow binocular single vision. Vision is almost always normal. Thus, in the majority of cases, no treatment is necessary unless the patient has a marked head turn.

Electromyographic studies show that DRS is a neurogenic disorder in which branches of the oculomotor nerve innervate the lateral rectus muscle. Retraction of the globe is produced by a cocontraction of horizontal rectus muscles. Autopsy studies have confirmed anomalous innervation of the extraocular muscles. Abducens nuclei and nerves are absent and the lateral rectus muscle is innervated by branches from the oculomotor nerve. Interestingly, in the region of the abducens nuclei, cell bodies representing internuclear neurons typically remain intact.

There are three types of DRS: Duane I type consists of limited or absent abduction with relatively normal adduction; Duane II consists of limited or absent adduction with relatively normal abduction; and Duane III is characterized by limited abduction and adduction. In all cases, an anomaly of ocular motor innervation involving the oculomotor and abducens nerves is thought to be responsible.

Although some cases may be caused by birth trauma, 30% to 50% of patients with DRS have associated congenital defects involving ocular, skeletal, and neural structures. The differentiation of these frequently affected structures occurs between the fourth and eighth weeks of gestation, coincident with the development of the ocular motor nerves. Thus, a teratogenic event during the second month of gestation may cause DRS in some cases. Most cases of DRS are sporadic, but familial unilateral and bilateral cases occur and constitute about 10% of observed cases.

Acquired

Lesions of the Abducens Nerve Nucleus

The abducens nucleus contains not only motoneurons that innervate the ipsilateral lateral rectus, but also cell bodies of internuclear neurons that cross the midline and ascend in the contralateral medial longitudinal fasciculus (MLF) to synapse in the medial rectus subnucleus on that side (Fig. 18.25). Thus, lesions that damage the abducens nucleus produce a **conjugate gaze palsy** to the ipsilateral side, and lesions of both abducens nuclei completely eliminate conjugate horizontal gaze. Given that the abducens nucleus provides the final motor command to the respective extraocular muscles, the horizontal gaze palsy that ensues is not overcome using oculocephalic (vestibulo-ocular) reflexes, in contrast to ipsilateral PPRF or contralateral cortical lesions (see Chapter 17). **Neither unilateral nor bilateral isolated abduction weakness ever occurs from a lesion of the abducens nucleus.** In most but not all cases in which the abducens nucleus is damaged, an ipsilateral, peripheral, facial nerve palsy is also present. This palsy occurs because the facial nerve fascicle loops around the abducens nucleus before exiting from the brain stem.

The horizontal gaze palsy that occurs from damage to the abducens nucleus is not always symmetric, perhaps because the cell bodies of the abducens motoneurons are more vulnerable than those of the internuclear neurons to certain insults, thus producing an asymmetric horizontal gaze paralysis that is worse in the abducting eye. Lesions of the abducens nucleus sometimes damage the ipsilateral MLF, producing the **one-and-a-half syndrome**. This syndrome consists of a horizontal gaze palsy combined with an internuclear ophthalmoplegia (INO).

Lesions that produce intrinsic brain stem damage and cause acquired unilateral or bilateral paralysis of horizontal gaze from damage to the abducens nuclei include ischemia, infiltration, trauma, inflammation, and compression (Fig. 18.26).

Patients with the Wernicke–Korsakoff syndrome often develop paralysis of conjugate gaze, presumably from a metabolic insult to the abducens nuclei. Neuronal loss and gliosis can occur in the abducens nuclei of patients with ALS.

Lesions of the Abducens Nerve Fascicle

When an abducens nerve palsy coexists with a gaze palsy to the same side from damage to both the abducens nucleus and the ipsilateral abducens nerve fascicle, identification of the peripheral nerve element in the gaze palsy cannot be assessed unless there is a marked asymmetry between the two eyes, with the abducting eye being more limited in movement than the adducting eye. In other instances, fascicular involvement of the abducens nerve produces an isolated abduction weakness that cannot be differentiated clinically from involvement outside the brain stem. However, most lesions that damage the abducens fascicle produce distinctive clinical syndromes from damage to the surrounding neurologic tissue.

A lesion in the pontine tegmentum may damage the abducens and facial nerve fascicles, the nucleus of the tractus solitarius, the central tegmental tract, the spinal tract of the trigeminal nerve (and its nucleus), the superior olivary nucleus, or a combination of these structures. Such a lesion may produce ipsilateral paralysis of abduction, ipsilateral facial palsy (flaccid), loss of taste from the anterior two-thirds of the tongue, ipsilateral central Horner syndrome, ipsilateral analgesia of the face, ipsilateral peripheral deafness, and contralateral weakness. Together, these signs comprise the syndrome of the anterior-inferior cerebellar artery—**Foville syndrome (medial inferior pontine syndrome)**. The clinical expression of this syndrome is rarely complete, and many of its features may occur in association with ipsilateral paralysis of horizontal gaze rather than ipsilateral paralysis of abduction, indicating nuclear, rather than fascicular involvement.

A lesion located ventrally within the paramedian pons may damage the ventral portion of abducens and facial nerve fascicles, as well as the corticospinal tract. Such a lesion produces an ipsilateral abducens palsy and a contralateral hemiplegia, with (**Millard–Gubler syndrome**) or without (**Raymond Céstan syndrome**) ipsilateral peripheral facial paralysis (Fig. 18.27).

Fascicular lesions of the abducens nerve may be produced by ischemia, tumor compression or infiltration, infection, and inflammation. Demyelination is

Figure 18.25 Diagram on the left shows that the abducens nucleus (VI) contains not only motoneurons that innervate the ipsilateral lateral rectus (LR), but also cell bodies of internuclear neurons that cross the midline and ascend in the contralateral medial longitudinal fasciculus (MLF) to synapse in the medial rectus subnucleus on that side (III). *MR*, medial rectus muscle; *PPRF*, paramedian pontine reticular formation; *VN*, vestibular nucleus; *IV*, trochlear nerve nucleus.

Figure 18.26 MRI of a 62-year-old woman with a slowly progressive right horizontal gaze paresis and ipsilateral facial weakness. Axial proton density (**left**) and T2-weighted (**right**) images demonstrate a lesion in the region of the right abducens nerve nucleus and adjacent facial colliculus (*arrow*, facial nerve fascicles). Evaluation revealed breast carcinoma with evidence of systemic metastases—the brain stem lesion was thought to be a metastasis.

the most common inflammatory etiology for fascicular abducens nerve paresis, and generally improves over several weeks. MS plaques involving the abducens fascicle or nucleus often also implicate the adjacent facial nerve fascicles, resulting in hyperactivity of the seventh nerve (similar to hemifacial spasm), rather than facial weakness. Hence, the workup of a patient presenting with facial muscle hyperactivity, suspected to have microvascular compression of the

seventh nerve root entry zone, should include an MRI of the brain for parenchymal views, in addition to an MRA.

Lesions of the Abducens Nerve in the Subarachnoid Space

Causes of abducens nerve damage in the subarachnoid space are many and varied. The long course of the nerve is usually cited as an explanation for its frequent

Figure 18.27 Millard–Gubler syndrome in a 23-year-old man with an intrapontine hemorrhage. The patient has a right abducens nerve paresis, a right peripheral facial nerve paresis, and a left (contralateral) hemiparesis.

involvement; however, the course of the trochlear nerve is longer and yet trochlear nerve pareses occur less frequently than do abducens nerve pareses. In fact, the location and course of the abducens nerve, rather than its length, are the major factors that lead to an abducens nerve paresis. The abducens nerve lies along the ventral surface of the pons and is bound to that structure by the anterior-inferior cerebellar artery. The nerve may, therefore, be compressed by this vessel, the posterior-inferior cerebellar artery, or the basilar artery, particularly when the vessel is atherosclerotic or dolichoectatic. Aneurysms of these vessels may also cause abducens paralysis. In most of these cases, there are no other cranial nerve findings, but there may be severe headache.

After its exit from the pons, the abducens nerve passes almost vertically through the subarachnoid space to pierce the dura overlying the clivus (Fig. 18.28). During its course, it is vulnerable to damage from a variety of processes in the posterior fossa, including descent of the brain stem associated with vertex blows, space-occupying masses above the tentorium

Figure 18.28 A: Sagittal oblique CISS without contrast demonstrates VI (*black arrow*) emerging from the pontomedullary junction and extending superiorly and anteriorly toward the dorsal clivus. The nerve is shallow in this case, without significant evagination of CSF (*white arrow*). **B:** Axial CISS demonstrates both CN VI segments at the midcisternal component (*arrows*). **C:** Postcontrast sagittal oblique CISS demonstrates CN VI (*black upward arrow*) extending to pierce the inner layer of dura without a significant dural segment (*white upward arrow*). CN VI extends through the petroclival (*white downward arrow*) into the cavernous segment (*black downward arrow*), passing adjacent to the cavernous internal carotid artery (*asterisk*) to enter the superior orbital fissure (*arrowhead*). (Courtesy of Dr. Ari Blitz.)

(transtentorial herniation), posterior fossa masses, and structural abnormalities (e.g., Chiari malformations). In these settings, the abducens nerve may be stretched and injured at its attachment at either the pons or the clivus. Trauma may be direct, including neurosurgical, or indirect from blunt, closed head injury. Both unilateral and bilateral abducens paralysis, usually associated with other neurologic signs and symptoms, have been reported in patients placed in halo-pelvic traction.

Meningitis may produce abducens nerve paralysis. As with other ocular motor nerve palsies produced by meningitis, abducens nerve palsies are often bilateral. Meningitis can result in elevation of ICP, which in and of itself can produce unilateral or bilateral abducens palsies, such as in patients with pseudotumor cerebri, dural venous sinus thrombosis, or acute hydrocephalus. In such instances, the palsies may represent false localizing signs of intracranial tumors. A unilateral (and occasionally bilateral) abducens palsy may develop after a lumbar puncture, whether or not there is increased ICP. Indeed stretch (and resulting paresis) of the abducens nerves as they travel along the clivus, can occur with elevated ICP as well as cerebral hypotension, given the downward pressure exerted by the brain onto the underlying abducens nerves in both scenarios.

Both unilateral and bilateral abducens nerve paresis can also occur in patients with idiopathic hypertrophic cranial pachymeningitis, a condition characterized by chronic, nongranulomatous inflammation of the meninges (Fig. 18.29).

Lesions of the Extradural Portion of the Abducens Nerve at the Petrous Apex

After the abducens nerve penetrates the dura overlying the clivus, it passes beneath the petroclinoid (Gruber) ligament. In this region, it is adjacent to the mastoid air cells. In patients with severe mastoiditis, the inflammatory process may extend to the tip of the petrous bone, producing localized inflammation of the meninges in the epidural space and a classic condition called **Gradenigo syndrome**. The adjacent abducens nerve becomes inflamed and paretic. In addition, because the gasserian ganglion and facial nerve are also nearby, such patients have severe pain on the ipsilateral side of the face and around the eye and may also develop facial paralysis. Abducens paresis may not occur until 2 to 3 days following the onset of pain. Photophobia and lacrimation are often present, and corneal sensation may be diminished. In some patients, meningitis develops, whereas in others, only a localized inflammation occurs. Because of the prompt and almost universal use of antibiotics in children with known or presumed acute otitis media, the incidence of Gradenigo syndrome is extremely low.

Lesions other than inflammation can involve the petrous apex and produce symptoms suggesting Gradenigo syndrome. These lesions include tumors and aneurysms of the intrapetrosal segment of the internal carotid artery. Thus, patients presenting with the petrous apex syndrome should be carefully evaluated with appropriate neuroimaging studies before it is concluded that the involvement is inflammatory.

A **B**

Figure 18.29 A: Neuroimaging in a 39-year-old man with a slowly progressive right abduction deficit associated with headache. Axial T1-weighted MRI shows diffuse meningeal enhancement as well as inflammatory changes in the right cavernous sinus. Biopsy of the meninges established a diagnosis of idiopathic hypertrophic cranial pachymeningitis. The disease was arrested with cranial irradiation and immunotherapy. **B:** T1-enhanced MRI, axial view, of a 43-year-old woman with IgG4 infiltrative disease reveals mostly anterior pachymeningeal enhancement and thickening.

When lateral sinus thrombosis or phlebitis extends into the inferior petrosal sinus (IPS), the abducens nerve may become paretic, given that the abducens nerve and IPS share the narrow space within Dorello canal. A similar situation may occur when one jugular vein (particularly the right jugular) is ligated during radical neck dissection, or a posteriorly draining carotid-cavernous fistula. Thrombosis of the IPS may explain the abducens nerve palsy that sometimes occurs in patients with mastoiditis.

Lesions of the Abducens Nerve in the Cavernous Sinus and Superior Orbital Fissure

Abducens nerve paralysis, either isolated or in combination with other cranial neuropathies, may occur from lesions within the cavernous sinus. The location of the abducens nerve within the body of the sinus itself—rather than in the deep layer of the lateral sinus wall where the oculomotor, trochlear, and ophthalmic nerves are located—predisposes it to damage from intracavernous vascular lesions, including aneurysms, direct and dural carotid-cavernous fistulas, and rarely internal carotid artery dissection.

Tumors that infiltrate the cavernous sinus as well as those that compress the structures within it may produce isolated abducens palsy. These include meningioma, metastatic carcinoma, nasopharyngeal carcinoma, Burkitt lymphoma, pituitary adenoma with and without apoplexy, craniopharyngioma, and a variety of other rare lesions in the region of the optic chiasm and cavernous sinus, including suprasellar germinomas, osteogenic sarcomas, teratomas, and multiple myeloma or plasmacytoma. When such lesions are sufficiently large, they may involve both cavernous sinuses and produce bilateral abducens nerve palsies.

Ischemic conditions, such as hypertension, diabetes mellitus, giant cell arteritis, systemic lupus erythematosus, and migraine, may damage the abducens nerve within the cavernous sinus, as may both granulomatous (e.g., tuberculosis, sarcoidosis, or the Tolosa–Hunt syndrome) and nongranulomatous (e.g., sphenoid sinus abscess or idiopathic hypertrophic pachymeningitis) inflammation. Herpes zoster may also produce abducens palsy from involvement of the abducens nerve in the cavernous sinus.

Although isolated involvement of the abducens nerve by cavernous sinus pathology is not rare, it is far more common for such involvement to be associated with other neurologic signs and symptoms, even if there are no other ocular motor nerve palsies. One of the more important of these cavernous sinus syndromes consists of the combination of isolated abducens paralysis and ipsilateral postganglionic Horner syndrome. This syndrome can occur in association with primary and traumatic intracavernous aneurysms and with both benign and malignant tumors that arise in or invade the

cavernous sinus. The occurrence of this syndrome is explained by the anatomic course of the oculosympathetic fibers within the cavernous sinus, which leave the internal carotid artery and join briefly with the abducens nerve before separating and fusing with the ophthalmic division of the trigeminal nerve.

Lesions of the Abducens Nerve within the Orbit

The abducens nerve has a very short course in the orbit, piercing the lateral rectus muscle only a few millimeters from the superior orbital fissure. For this reason, isolated involvement of this nerve within the orbit is rare, although it may occur in patients with a primary orbital schwannoma that originates from the sheath of the orbital portion of the abducens nerve. Abducens nerve paresis can also occur following injection of an anesthetic solution in preparation for mandibular surgery.

Chronic, Isolated Abducens Nerve Paralysis

Most patients who develop abducens nerve pareses either experience spontaneous improvement of the paresis or are found to have an underlying lesion that has caused the paresis. Some patients, however, do not recover and have no obvious lesion despite an extensive evaluation (see below). We follow such patients at regular intervals, obtaining an interval history and performing a complete examination each time the patient is seen. If, during this time, the patient develops other neurologic signs or the paresis worsens, a complete workup, including neuroimaging and an otolaryngologic evaluation, is performed. If no changes occur over a 3-month period, we perform or repeat a complete assessment of the patient. Although many patients with isolated, chronic abducens nerve palsies that last more than 6 months follow a completely benign course, a substantial number of such patients harbor basal tumors that may be amenable to treatment if identified at an early stage.

Spontaneous recovery of an abducens nerve palsy does not eliminate the presence of a neoplastic process. The possible mechanisms for recovery in such cases include remyelination, axon regeneration, relief of transient compression (e.g., resorption of hemorrhage), restoration of impaired blood flow, slippage of a nerve previously stretched over the tumor, or immune responses to the tumor.

Evaluation and Management of Abducens Nerve Palsy

There is a tendency to assume that all patients with an esotropia associated with unilateral or bilateral abduction weakness have an abducens nerve paresis. In fact, the physician encountering such a patient should first consider the possibility that the condition is myopathic (e.g., thyroid eye disease) or neuromuscular (e.g., myasthenia gravis). A careful history and examination directed at these possibilities may be sufficient to eliminate them as etiologies. Alternatively, the physician may need to perform further studies, including orbital ultrasonography, orbital imaging, thyroid function studies, serum assay for antireceptor antibodies, and single-fiber electromyography.

Once the physician is satisfied that an abducens nerve paresis is likely, he or she should initiate an evaluation that, like the evaluation performed in patients with an oculomotor nerve palsy, depends on the associated symptoms and signs and the age of the patient. All patients with a presumed abducens nerve palsy **must** undergo a thorough neurologic assessment, particularly with respect to the first eight cranial nerves and the integrity of the oculosympathetic pathway. If other neurologic signs (e.g., trigeminal sensory neuropathy, facial paresis, hearing loss, Horner syndrome) are present, such patients should undergo neuroimaging, preferably gadolinium-enhanced MRI of the orbits and brain. An MRA or CTA should be added for patients suspected of an aneurysm or present with mild redness, swelling, or proptosis of the affected eye, given the possibility of a spontaneous dural carotid-cavernous sinus fistula or even cavernous sinus thrombosis if the patient appears lethargic or unwell. Patients with septic cavernous sinus thrombosis nearly always have prominent systemic manifestations of sepsis.

If a patient with an apparent abducens nerve paresis has no other findings and has underlying systemic vascular disease or is in the vasculopathic age group (i.e., over age 60), and if the onset of the palsy is sudden, the patient could be followed at regular intervals, with an interval history obtained and a complete examination performed each time the patient is seen. If, during this time, the patient develops other neurologic signs or the paresis worsens, a complete workup, including neuroimaging and an otolaryngologic evaluation, is performed. If no changes occur over a 3-month period, a complete reassessment of the patient should be performed. On the other hand, if the patient is under age 60 and has no risk factors for ischemic or inflammatory disease, we perform MRI with careful attention to the pathway of the abducens nerve from the brain stem to the orbit. A lumbar puncture may be indicated in some patients.

Abducens nerve paralysis may or may not resolve, and the resolution may be complete or incomplete. Ischemic pareses patients almost always recover completely, usually within 2 to 4 months, whereas some degree of spontaneous recovery of traumatic abducens pareses occurs in 30% to 54% of patients and may take more than 1 year. Among patients who do not recover, serious pathology (e.g., tumor, stroke, aneurysm) is often present, emphasizing the importance of performing an evaluation in patients whose abducens nerve palsy does not recover within 3 to 6 months.

Strabismus surgery should not be considered to correct an abducens nerve palsy until at least 6 months have passed without improvement, unless it is known that the abducens nerve is no longer intact. During this period, some patients prefer to occlude one eye, whereas others are able to ignore their diplopia or visual confusion. Although a patch is the simplest manner in which to occlude one eye, an opaque contact lens can also be used. Patients under 8 years old should undergo alternate patching of the eyes to prevent amblyopia. In most patients with unilateral abducens paresis, prisms are not of great benefit, although they are occasionally useful in achieving binocular single vision in primary position, and if the deviation is not particularly large in cases of partial paresis.

Chemodenervation of the antagonist medial rectus muscle with botulinum toxin can be used to treat patients with both acute and chronic abducens nerve palsy. This can be combined with surgery, when required. Strategies include either weakening of the ipsilateral medial rectus muscle combined with strengthening of the ipsilateral lateral rectus muscle (when partial tone is present in the paretic muscle) or some type of vertical muscle transposition procedure (Knapp full tendon, Hummelsheim, or Jensen) with or without adjustable sutures. For patients with complete palsies, if surgery is contemplated, a tendon transposition procedure is required, and can improve ductions to the paretic field to some degree; however, the primary goal is to improve alignment in primary position. Provided these goals and limitations are clearly understood by the surgeon and the patient, the results are usually very gratifying.

Hyperactivity of the Ocular Motor Nerves

Several ocular motor syndromes are characterized by hyperactivity, rather than hypoactivity, of one or more of the ocular motor nerves. The most common of these are ocular neuromyotonia and superior oblique myokymia (SOM).

Ocular Neuromyotonia

Ocular neuromyotonia is characterized by brief, episodic contractions of muscles supplied by the oculomotor, trochlear, or abducens nerves. The condition is usually unilateral, but bilateral cases occur. In most cases, the extraocular muscles corresponding to only one of the ocular motor nerves are affected; however, some patients have involvement of muscles innervated by more than one of the ocular motor nerves on one side (Fig. 18.30). In most patients, ocular neuromyotonia is permanent; however, it resolves spontaneously in some patients and disappears with treatment in others.

Most patients who develop ocular neuromyotonia have previously received radiation therapy to the base of the skull. This is not always the case, however. For example, some patients have received radiation indirectly, as occurred in a patient who develop ocular neuromyotonia many years after he underwent myelography with iophendylate (Pantopaque, Thorotrast), a substance that is weakly radioactive. Other patients have developed the condition in the setting of dysthyroid orbitopathy.

The evaluation of patients with ocular neuromyotonia, particularly those without a history of prior radiation therapy, should include MRI of the brain, with particular attention to the suprasellar region and posterior fossa. Carbamazepine can be effective in treating this condition, and should be differentiated from cyclic oculomotor paresis (see earlier in this chapter).

Superior Oblique Myokymia (Superior Oblique Microtremor)

SOM is characterized by typical symptoms of monocular blurring of vision or tremulous sensations in the eye. Patients typically experience brief episodes of vertical or torsional diplopia, vertical or torsional oscillopsia, or both. Attacks usually last less than 10 seconds but may occur many times per day. The attacks may be brought on by looking downward, by tilting the head toward the side of the affected eye, or by blinking. The eye movements of SOM are often difficult to appreciate on gross examination, although they are usually apparent during examination with the ophthalmoscope or slit lamp biomicroscope. They consist of spasms of cyclotorsional and vertical movements, and typically unilateral.

The majority of patients with SOM have no underlying disease, although cases have been reported following trochlear nerve palsy, after mild head trauma, in the setting of multiple sclerosis, after brain stem stroke, in a patient with a dural arteriovenous fistula, and in patients with cerebellar tumor. A growing number of reports have demonstrated microvascular compression of the trochlear nerve at its root entry zone in SOM patients. The etiology of SOM may be neuronal damage and subsequent regeneration, leading to desynchronized contraction of muscle fibers.

SOM spontaneously resolves in some patients. Other patients are not bothered by their symptoms and thus do not need treatment. For patients whose symptoms are particularly distressing, both medical and surgical therapies are available. Individual patients may respond to a number of drugs, including Neurontin (typically first line), carbamazepine, baclofen, and topically or systemically administered β-adrenergic blocking agents. Patients who do not respond to drug therapy, who develop side effects from the drugs, or who do not wish to take drugs for their condition may

Figure 18.30 Ocular neuromyotonia. Appearance of a 62-year-old woman who had been treated with whole brain radiation for a pituitary tumor 15 years prior to her presentation. The patient had paroxysmal spasms of adduction of the right eye, left eye **(A)**, or both eyes **(B)**, lasting several seconds. The pupils remained normal during the spasms, and there was no evidence of accommodation spasm as might be expected if the patient was experiencing spasm of the near response. In addition, there was occasional spasm of elevation of the left eye **(C)**. Between episodes of spasm, the eyes were straight **(D)** and horizontal gaze to the right **(E)** and left **(F)** was normal. The spasms initially responded to quinine (tonic water) but later required carbamazepine.

experience complete relief of symptoms after extraocular muscle surgery, the most successful of which is tenectomy of the affected superior oblique muscle combined with ipsilateral inferior oblique myectomy.

Synkineses Involving the Ocular Motor and Other Cranial Nerves

A **synkinesis** is a simultaneous movement or a coordinated set of movements of muscles supplied by different nerves or different branches of the same nerve. Normally occurring cranial synkineses are exemplified by sucking, chewing, conjugate eye movements, and Bell phenomenon.

Abnormal cranial nerve synkineses occur most commonly in DRS (see above) and in the Marcus Gunn jaw-winking phenomenon (trigemino-ocular motor synkinesis). Similar synkineses involving various facial and neck muscles and the extraocular muscles occur in rare patients. A synkinesis between the superior oblique muscle (innervated by the trochlear nerve) and one of the muscles elevating the tongue and hyoid (innervated by the trigeminal, facial, or hypoglossal nerve) can cause double vision produced by swallowing. Similarly, bobbing movements of the eyes may be associated with jaw movements, suggesting a complex form of trigemino-ocular motor synkinesis similar to the classic Marcus Gunn jaw-winking phenomenon but involving more than just the levator muscle.

Disorders of Neuromuscular Transmission

Normal Neuromuscular Transmission

Myasthenia Gravis
   Epidemiology
   Ocular Versus Generalized MG
   Ocular Signs
   Nonocular Signs
   Diagnostic Testing
   Treatment

Congenital Myasthenic Syndromes

Acquired Disorders of Neuromuscular Transmission Other than Myasthenia Gravis
   Lambert–Eaton Syndrome

Neuromuscular Disorders Caused by Drugs or Toxins
   Drug-Induced Autoimmune Damage to the Neuromuscular Junction
   Toxins that Damage Presynaptic Neuromuscular Transmission
   Toxins that Damage Both Pre- and Postsynaptic Neuromuscular Transmission

Normal Neuromuscular Transmission

Acetylcholine (ACh) is a natural transmitter that is synthesized chiefly in the motor nerve terminals and stored in vesicles for subsequent release. Neurotransmission begins with the release of the contents of the vesicles by exocytosis that occurs at specialized release sites located directly opposite the areas of highest concentration of ACh receptors on postsynaptic membranes (Fig. 19.1), thus minimizing the distance that the transmitter must travel to reach the receptor site. When ACh combines with its receptor, a transient increase of permeability to sodium and potassium ions occurs, resulting in membrane depolarization. When a nerve impulse arrives at the motor nerve terminal, the amplitude of the depolarization normally is sufficient to trigger an action potential that is propagated along the muscle membrane. The muscle action potential, in turn, initiates the sequence of events that leads to muscle contraction. The entire process is rapid, on the order of a millisecond. It is terminated by the removal

of ACh, in part by its diffusion away from the neuromuscular junction (NMJ), but mostly by the action of acetylcholinesterase, which rapidly hydrolyzes ACh.

Myasthenia Gravis

Myasthenia gravis (MG) is a disease characterized clinically by muscle weakness and fatigability. It is caused by a reduction in the number of available ACh receptors at NMJs. Receptor depletion is mediated by one or more antibodies directed against ACh receptors or other NMJ postsynaptic membrane constituents, resulting in impaired neuromuscular transmission. Such antibodies, which either degrade or block the receptors, are found in the serum of 80% to 90% of patients with MG, although some patients with MG who have no antireceptor antibodies have an immunoglobulin (Ig) G antibody that binds to muscle specific kinase (MuSK). Finally, about 9% of MG patients are seronegative for both anti-ACh receptor antibodies and anti-MuSK antibodies. These doubly seronegative patients often have purely ocular disease.

Epidemiology

Autoimmune MG affects all races and ages, with an incidence of 4 to 5 per 100,000. There is a female predominance overall, but the sex predilection is age dependent, with women predominating among younger patients and men among those who are older at diagnosis.

Ocular Versus Generalized MG

In about 60% to 70% of patients, MG first or only affects the extraocular muscles, levator palpebrae superioris, orbicularis oculi, or a combination of these. Patients in whom only the ocular muscles are affected are said to have "ocular" MG. Patients in whom nonocular muscles initially are affected or are affected at the same time as the ocular muscles, or who develop nonocular muscle involvement after initial ocular muscle involvement are said to have "generalized" MG. In fact, the vast majority of patients (>90%) with "ocular" MG will, usually within 18 to 24 months after the onset of ocular signs, develop evidence of "generalized" disease. Thus, patients in whom "ocular" MG has been diagnosed on the basis of isolated ocular manifestations should be

Figure 19.1 Drawing of the normal neuromuscular junction. Note the sites of acetylcholine (ACh) release, the location of acetylcholine receptors, and the location of acetylcholinesterase (AChE).

warned about the tendency for generalization, and the symptoms of generalization (see below) reviewed with them. There is some suggestion that treatment of patients with ocular MG with systemic corticosteroids decreases the likelihood of subsequent development of generalized MG (see below).

Ocular Signs

The clinical hallmark of both ocular and generalized MG is variable weakness of the affected muscles. The weakness varies from day to day and even from hour to hour, but typically increases toward evening. Transient weakness is often associated with physical exertion.

Figure 19.2 Unilateral ptosis in a 73-year-old man with myasthenia gravis.

Affected muscles fatigue if contraction is maintained or repeated. In patients with ocular MG, the most commonly affected muscles being the levator palpebrae superioris, the extraocular muscles, and the orbicularis oculi. Indeed, as noted above, the levator palpebrae superioris and extraocular muscles are affected initially in 60% to 70% of cases, and these muscles eventually are affected in over 90% of patients. When weakness of these muscles is combined with weakness of the orbicularis oculi, the combination is highly suggestive of MG.

Ptosis and Other Signs Involving the Levator Palpebrae Superioris

Ptosis may occur as an isolated sign or in association with extraocular muscle involvement. It is characterized by its fluctuating nature and frequently shifts from one eye to the other. Ptosis often initially is unilateral but eventually almost always becomes bilateral (Fig. 19.2). When ptosis is bilateral, it may be symmetric or asymmetric, with symmetric ptosis being more common in patients who also have severe ophthalmoparesis (Fig. 19.3). The ptosis frequently is absent when the

patient awakens but appears later in the day, becoming most pronounced in the evening. Repeated closure of the eyelids may make ptosis appear or may worsen it when it initially is minimal. Prolonged upward gaze also often will result in gradual lowering of the eyelids (Fig. 19.4), but fatigability of bilateral ptosis does not exclude a nonmyasthenic cause, such as dorsal midbrain compression by a mass lesion.

Patients with MG-related ptosis often have worsening of ptosis on one side when the opposite eyelid is elevated and held in a fixed position (Fig. 19.5). The explanation of this "enhancement of ptosis" phenomenon is Hering law of equal innervation, which relates to the levator muscles as it does to the extraocular muscles. Manual eyelid elevation decreases the effort required for eyelid elevation ipsilaterally and thus results in relaxation of the contralateral levator and consequent worsening ptosis on that side (**Video 19.1**). However, enhancement of ptosis is not pathognomonic for MG. It can be seen in patients with congenital ptosis and in patients with acquired ptosis from causes other than MG. Nevertheless, in a patient with an appropriate history, the observation of enhancement of ptosis with manual elevation of the contralateral eyelid is highly suggestive of MG.

Cogan lid twitch is another important sign that suggests MG. When the patient's eyes are directed downward for 10 to 20 seconds and the patient then is instructed to make a vertical saccade back to primary position, the upper eyelid elevates and either slowly begins to droop or else twitches several times before settling into a stable position (**Video 19.2**). This sign is caused by the rapid recovery and easy fatigability of myasthenic muscle.

Ophthalmoparesis and Other Abnormalities of Eye Movement

Involvement of the extraocular muscles, like ptosis, is extremely common in patients with MG, although the

A   **B**

Figure 19.3 Bilateral ptosis in two patients with myasthenia gravis. **A:** Bilateral symmetric ptosis in a 4-year-old girl. **B:** Bilateral asymmetric ptosis in a 58-year-old man.

Figure 19.4 Eyelid fatigue after prolonged upgaze in a patient with myasthenia gravis. The patient was a 52-year-old man with a history of intermittent ptosis and diplopia. **A:** Before prolonged upgaze, the patient has minimal bilateral ptosis. **B:** After about 1 minute of upgaze, the patient's ptosis is much worse.

reason for this is unknown. In most cases, disturbances of ocular motility and alignment are associated with ptosis; however, cases without clinical involvement of the levator muscles frequently occur. There is no set pattern to the diplopia experienced by such patients or to the nature of extraocular muscle involvement. All degrees of ocular motor dysfunction, from apparent involvement of a single isolated muscle to complete

external ophthalmoplegia, occur. Thus, the abnormalities may mimic such neurologic disturbances as ocular motor nerve palsies, unilateral or bilateral internuclear ophthalmoplegia, or vertical or horizontal gaze palsies (Fig. 19.6). Unlike patients with neurologic ophthalmoparesis in whom saccadic (fast) eye movements have reduced velocities, however, patients with MG-related ophthalmoparesis have saccades with normal velocities

Figure 19.5 Enhancement of ptosis in a 61-year-old woman with myasthenia gravis. **A:** The patient has bilateral ptosis. Note also a right exotropia. **B:** When the left eyelid is manually elevated, the right ptosis increases. **C:** When the right eyelid is manually elevated, the left ptosis increases. (See also **Video 19.1**).

Figure 19.7 Orbicularis oculi weakness in a 78-year-old woman with myasthenia gravis. The patient is trying to close her eyes as tightly as possible; however, the closure can be overcome easily with gentle force. Note that she cannot bury the lashes on left.

Figure 19.6 Bilateral pseudo-internuclear ophthalmoplegia in a 72-year-old man with myasthenia gravis. A: On attempted rightward gaze, the left eye adducts only to the midline. B: On attempted leftward gaze, the right eye adducts only to the midline.

or velocities that are increased relative to the extent of the saccade. Even patients with MG-related complete ophthalmoplegia may show tiny "quiver movements" on attempted eccentric gaze.

Orbicularis Oculi Involvement

Patients with MG often have involvement of the orbicularis oculi muscles that may not be apparent when ptosis or ophthalmoplegia predominates. The combination of ptosis, ocular motility disturbances, and weakness of the orbicularis oculi is found in only a few disorders, including MG, myotonic dystrophy, oculopharyngeal dystrophy, and mitochondrial myopathy. Of these, MG is by far the most common. Patients suspected of having MG therefore should have testing of orbicularis oculi strength by having the patient forcefully shut the eyes while the examiner manually attempts to open the eyelids against the forced lid closure (Fig. 19.7).

Some patients with MG exhibit a "peek" sign caused by orbicularis fatigue. In such patients, upon gentle eyelid closure, the orbicularis oculi muscle contracts, initially achieving eyelid apposition; however, the orbicularis muscle rapidly fatigues and the palpebral fissure widens, hereby exposing the sclera. The patient thus appears to "peek" at the examiner.

Pupillary Function

Patients with MG do not have clinically abnormal pupillary reactions to light or near stimulation, although subclinical involvement can sometimes be detected with

pupillometry. Nevertheless, when ocular motor disturbances occur in the setting of a dilated, poorly reactive or nonreactive pupil, MG should not be considered a likely cause. Conversely, in any patient in whom an ocular motor disturbance, ptosis, or both are associated with normally reactive pupils, MG must be in the differential diagnosis.

Nonocular Signs

In patients with generalized involvement of skeletal muscles, the facies may be characteristic, showing a generalized weakness of expression. Weakness frequently affects the neck extensors and proximal limb muscles. When the muscles of expression, phonation, articulation, swallowing, and chewing are affected, there may be a characteristic facial "snarl," dysarthric speech, nasal regurgitation of liquids, and/or the need to prop the jaw closed. When the muscles of respiration or swallowing are involved, the term "myasthenic crisis" indicates the gravity of the disease. Rarely, MG presents with respiratory insufficiency alone. On physical examination, the findings are limited entirely to the lower motor unit, without loss of reflexes or altered sensation or coordination.

Diagnostic Testing

The tests used to diagnose MG include clinical tests, assays for circulating antibodies to components of the NMJ, pharmacologic tests, repetitive nerve stimulation, and single-fiber electromyography (single-fiber EMG).

Clinical Tests

Two simple office tests are particularly helpful in supporting the clinical diagnosis of MG: the sleep test and the ice test. These tests have generally supplanted pharmacologic testing and are particularly useful in elderly or ill patients for whom pharmacologic testing may be potentially dangerous.

Sleep Test. The sleep test is based on the observation that when many patients with MG awaken in the morning, they have little or no ptosis or diplopia; however, these manifestations appear or worsen during the day. The sleep test is performed as follows: The patient first undergoes a complete ocular examination and external photographs. The patient then is taken to a quiet, darkened room and instructed to close the eyes and try to sleep. Thirty minutes later, the patient is awakened, immediately photographed, and measurements taken of his or her palpebral fissures, ocular alignment, and ocular motility. Most patients with MG show marked improvement in ptosis, ocular motor dysfunction, or both immediately upon awakening from sleep (Fig. 19.8). The improvement lasts 2 to 5 minutes, following which the ptosis and ophthalmoparesis recur. Patients with ptosis and ophthalmoparesis caused by disorders other than MG show no such improvement after sleep. In our opinion, the sleep test is a safe, moderately sensitive, and specific way to confirm a presumptive diagnosis of MG.

Ice Test. The strength of myasthenic muscles often improves when the muscles are cooled, probably because lowering the temperature reduces the effects of acetylcholinesterase. In patients with ptosis in whom the diagnosis of MG is considered, the use of local cooling to eliminate or reduce the ptosis is a rapid, simple, and inexpensive test with a high degree of specificity and sensitivity for MG. The ice test is performed as follows: The sizes of the palpebral fissures are measured, photographed, or both. The patient is instructed to close the eyes for 2 minutes, following which the palpebral fissures are again assessed. A surgical glove containing crushed ice or ice cubes is then applied to the ptotic (if unilateral) or more ptotic (if bilateral) eyelid for 2 minutes. After 2 minutes, the glove is removed, and the size of the palpebral fissure is immediately measured or photographed. The test is considered positive if the size of the palpebral fissure is greater after cooling than after the rest period; this difference usually is greater than 2 mm in patients with MG, with the improvement in ptosis typically lasting about 1 minute (Fig. 19.9). The ice test is about 90% sensitive and 100% specific for the diagnosis of MG, making it one of the most useful tests for the clinician. Interestingly, the test is most likely to give false-negative results in those patients with MG in whom there is complete or nearly complete ptosis. The ice test also can be used in patients with ophthalmoparesis but no ptosis, but the results are much less sensitive.

Specific Autoantibody Assays

A radioimmunoassay to detect ACh receptor antibodies is one of the standard diagnostic tests for MG; however, although this test detects antibodies in about 85% of all patients with MG, such antibodies are detected in no more than 50% of patients with weakness confined to the levator and extraocular muscles. In addition, anti-MuSK antibodies only very rarely are found in patients with ocular myasthenia. Thus, should a patient with a clinical diagnosis of ocular MG show no evidence of either antireceptor or anti-MuSK antibodies, the diagnosis should not necessarily be abandoned.

Pharmacologic Tests

The abnormal fatigability of skeletal muscles may be evaluated by observing or quantifying their strength before and after the injection of anticholinesterase agents. Anticholinesterase pharmacologic testing has a sensitivity of about 50% to 75% in MG. Thus, when MG is strongly suspected, and the ice or sleep tests are negative, these tests may be useful.

Figure 19.8 The sleep test for myasthenia gravis. The patient was an 80-year-old woman with new-onset bilateral ptosis. She had cardiac disease and was not considered a good candidate for pharmacologic testing. **A:** On presentation, the patient has bilateral ptosis. Note the use of her frontalis to open her eyes. The patient was put in a reclining chair and told to close her eyes and go to sleep. **B:** After 45 minutes of rest/sleep, the patient no longer has any significant ptosis.

Edrophonium (Tensilon) Test. Edrophonium chloride (usually supplied as the chloride salt under the trade name Tensilon) is a rapidly acting and quickly hydrolyzed anticholinesterase that competes with ACh for acetylcholinesterase and thus allows prolonged and repetitive action of ACh at the synapse. It commonly

Figure 19.9 Results of an ice test in a 62-year-old woman with myasthenia gravis. **A:** The patient has bilateral ptosis. **B:** A surgical glove filled with ice is placed over the left eye for 2 minutes. **C:** Appearance of the patient after removal of the ice. Note marked improvement in ptosis.

is used because of the rapid onset (≤30 sec) and short duration (about 5 min) of its effects. The edrophonium test is performed as follows: The position of the eyelids is verified as is any ocular misalignment and restriction of movement. A total of 10 mg (1 cc) of edrophonium is drawn up in a 1-cc syringe (if performing the test with an intravenous line in place) or a 3-cc syringe (if a direct venous injection is being performed). A test dose of 2 mg of edrophonium is injected intravenously, and the patient is observed for improvement in ptosis, ocular alignment, range of movement, or a combination of these (Fig. 19.10). If definite improvement occurs, the test is considered positive and is terminated. If no such changes occur within 30 seconds, the remainder of the dose (8 mg) is injected as a single bolus, and the patient is observed for improvement in ptosis, ocular alignment, and/or range of movement. Because patients with diplopia and strabismus may not appreciate changes in their ocular alignment, when performing the edrophonium test on a patient with strabismus but without ptosis, it is helpful to have them hold a red glass over one eye (or use red green glasses), fixate a distant white light, and describe any change in the relative positions of the two lights seen after injection of the edrophonium. Another option is to use the Lancaster red green test or the Hess screen to plot the position of

the two eyes before and after the injection. This technique provides an extremely accurate determination of eye position and is much more reliable than asking the patient if he/she sees any improvement in his/her diplopia. The alternate prism–cover test also can be used to document the effects of edrophonium on ocular motor alignment, but this test may be better suited to assessing the more prolonged effects of neostigmine (see below).

Occasionally, a brief paradoxical reaction (e.g., worsening of ptosis) occurs following administration of edrophonium. This should not be considered a positive response. Similarly, virtually all patients experience transient quivering of the eyelids, lacrimation, and salivation. These responses also do **not** constitute a positive test. A positive response generally lasts at least a few minutes.

Because edrophonium is a peripheral anticholinesterase agent, it allows ACh to accumulate briefly in ganglia, at parasympathetic nerve endings, and at NMJs in all types of muscle: cardiac, smooth, and striated. It is the transient excess of ACh at nicotinic synapses that produces a positive test in patients with MG, but this same excess also may produce muscarinic cholinergic side effects from a brief over stimulation of the parasympathetic nervous system. Major side effects

Figure 19.10 Results of a Tensilon (Edrophonium chloride) test in a 34-year-old man with recent onset of ptosis and diplopia. **A:** The patient has bilateral left ptosis, left more than right. Note also bilateral inferior scleral show from laxity of the lower eyelids. **B:** The patient can adduct the right eye only to the midline when attempting to look to the left (pseudointernuclear ophthalmoplegia). **C:** 1 minute after intravenous injection of 2 mg of Tensilon, the patient's ptosis has markedly improved and the inferior scleral show has resolved. **D:** At the same time, the patient's right eye adduction has become full.

occur in about 1 in 1,000 persons and include brady-cardia, asystole, syncope, and seizures. Less severe side effects include near syncope, dizziness, and involun-tary defecation. Although most side effects associated with the edrophonium test probably can be prevented by pretreating patients with an intramuscular injection of atropine sulfate, such reactions are sufficiently rare that it is not necessary to pretreat with atropine. Nev-ertheless, it is prudent always to have the drug available during the test. In addition, great caution should be used in performing edrophonium (or neostigmine) tests in older patients, particularly those with known cardiac disease. Instead, the clinician may depend on the results of other features of the presentation, or the results of an ice or sleep test (see above) to direct a further diag-nostic evaluation. Should it be necessary to perform an edrophonium test in a patient with cardiac disease, the patient should always have an intravenous line in place and be hooked up to an electrocardiograph machine, in an environment with advanced cardiac life support immediately available.

A positive edrophonium test usually, but not always, is indicative of MG. No reliable quantitative estimates of the specificity of the test are available, but the speci-ficity is believed to be fairly high. Nevertheless, on rare occasions, patients with intracranial lesions producing pupil-sparing oculomotor nerve palsies and other ocular motor disorders may show transient improve-ment of their findings when tested with edropho-nium. Some of these patients may have both MG and an intracranial lesion. In others, however, there is no other evidence of MG, and the response to edropho-nium can be considered to be falsely positive. For this reason, it is advisable to perform neuroimaging in all patients with an isolated, unilateral, and pupil-sparing ophthalmoparesis and in selected patients with other ocular muscle pareses, even when the diagnosis of MG seems certain. Other neuromuscular disorders that have been reported to produce a positive edrophonium test include Lambert–Eaton myasthenic syndrome, botulism, envenomation, Guillain–Barré syndrome, amyotrophic lateral sclerosis, and postpoliomyelitis syndrome.

Just as a positive edrophonium test does not neces-sarily indicate MG, a negative edrophonium test does out eliminate the possibility of MG. The sensitivity of the test in patients with generalized MG ranges from 73% to 96%, whereas its sensitivity in ocular MG ranges from 60% to 95%. Thus, in patients suspected of having MG, a negative edrophonium test should be followed either by a neostigmine test or by other non-ocular diagnostic tests (see below).

Figure 19.11 The Prostigmin (neostigmine bromide) test for myasthenia gravis. **A:** The 10-year-old boy has marked right ptosis. **B:** There is limitation of both abduction of the right eye and adduction of the left eye on attempted right lateral gaze. **C:** 45 minutes after intramuscular injection of 1.5 mg of neostigmine combined with 0.3 mg of atropine, the child's ptosis has resolved. **D:** Horizontal eye movements to the right are now full.

Neostigmine (Prostigmin) Test. Because of the transient nature of the ocular (and systemic) changes in muscle strength that occur following the administration of edrophonium, the neostigmine bromide (Prostigmin) test remains an exceptionally valuable method of diagnosing MG, particularly in patients with diplopia but without ptosis and in children. The longer duration of the effects of this drug is sufficient to permit careful assessment not only of eyelid position and strength, but also of ocular motility and alignment. In adults with obvious ptosis and/or ophthalmoparesis, one mixes 0.6 mg of atropine sulfate with 1.5 mg of neostigmine in a 3-cc syringe and injects the mixture into a deltoid or gluteus muscle. A change in ocular motility and ptosis usually is apparent 30 to 45 minutes following the injection (Fig. 19.11). The sensitivity of this test ranges from 70% to 94%.

As noted above, the neostigmine test is particularly helpful in the diagnosis of MG in children, in whom intravenous injection of edrophonium may be accompanied by crying and lack of cooperation, precluding any meaningful assessment of its effect. In such patients, neostigmine is injected intramuscularly, and by the time the neostigmine takes effect, the child usually has stopped crying and the eyelid position and

ocular alignment and motility can be assessed. In children, the amount of neostigmine given is related to body weight and is 0.025 to 0.04 mg/kg, not exceeding a total dose of 1.5 mg (the adult dose). The dose of atropine in children is adjusted to 0.011 mg/kg, up to a maximum of 0.6 mg.

Adverse effects of neostigmine testing include bradycardia, syncope, near syncope, and paradoxical tachycardia (especially at low doses). The combined muscarinic autonomic effects of neostigmine and atropine often are not balanced completely. If neostigmine predominates, the patient may experience transient increased salivation, tearing, borborygmi, and the urge to defecate or urinate. Atropine predominance produces dry mouth, tachycardia, etc. The relative balance of these competing effects may change over time during the test period. In addition, fasciculations almost always occur in normal subjects as well as myasthenic patients after the administration of neostigmine.

As with edrophonium, a positive neostigmine test usually, but not always, indicates MG. Nevertheless, positive responses have been reported in patients with multiple sclerosis, brain stem tumors, and congenital ptosis. Isolated, nonreproducible positive neostigmine tests thus may occur in nonmyasthenics.

Electrophysiologic Tests

Repetitive nerve stimulation has long been used to diagnose MG. In recent years, however, single-fiber EMG has been shown to be a much more sensitive and specific technique.

Repetitive Nerve Stimulation.

The primary technique used by most clinical electrophysiologists in the diagnosis of MG consists of eliciting a decremental response between the first and fourth or fifth response to repetitive supramaximal motor nerve stimulation. Supramaximal electric stimuli are delivered at a rate of 2 to 3 Hz to the appropriate nerves, and compound muscle action potentials are recorded from muscles. A decrement in amplitude of 10% or more usually is considered abnormal. The sensitivity of repetitive nerve stimulation in diagnosing generalized MG varies considerably from 51% to 100%, depending on the technique used and the severity of myasthenia in sampled patients. The wide range of sensitivity of the test indicates that a normal test does not exclude MG.

Single-Fiber Electromyography.

Endplate potentials in the postsynaptic membrane of the NMJ reach the threshold for triggering an action potential of the muscle fiber with random variability, resulting in a variable latency between a nerve stimulus and the action potential of the responding muscle fiber. The latencies of responses of fibers belonging to the same motor unit therefore are not quite synchronous. The variability between any fiber and a reference fiber from the same unit is called "jitter." When the safety factor for transmission is low, these latency variabilities (jitters) are increased. There also are more response failures ("blocking"), in which an action potential of the muscle fiber is not triggered by arrival of a nerve terminal action potential. Jitter and blocking can be detected in human muscles using suitably selective electrodes, and the latencies can be studied statistically during either voluntary contraction or indirect stimulation in a technique called single-fiber EMG. In patients undergoing evaluation for MG who are antibody negative and in whom repetitive nerve stimulation is negative or equivocal, single-fiber EMG is an extremely useful diagnostic test, being positive in 88% to 99% of all patients with MG. An experienced electrophysiologist is required to perform this test.

Like the edrophonium and neostigmine tests, single-fiber EMG initially may be negative only to be positive several months later. Thus, a negative single-fiber EMG test in a muscle with normal strength is not absolute evidence that the patient does not have MG; however, if a clinically weak muscle has normal jitter at all endplates, the diagnosis of MG can be excluded. Conversely, single-fiber EMG abnormalities frequently are seen in other disorders of neuromuscular transmission, including the Lambert–Eaton myasthenic syndrome, congenital myasthenic syndromes, and botulism. Increased jitter may have causes other than defective neuromuscular transmission, such as denervation from many causes, amyotrophic lateral sclerosis, mitochondrial cytopathy, and oculopharyngeal dystrophy.

Additional Tests

Because a thymic tumor is found in about 10% of patients with MG, the evaluation of a patient with suspected or proven MG should include CT scanning or MR imaging of the anterior mediastinum. Chest radiographs have such a low sensitivity as to make them useless for such screening.

A complete blood count, erythrocyte sedimentation rate, antinuclear antibody test, and thyroid function tests should be performed in all patients diagnosed with MG because of the increased prevalence of other autoimmune diseases in these patients. Any patient who may be a candidate for corticosteroid treatment should be screened for diabetes mellitus, and all patients should undergo a skin test for tuberculosis prior to institution of chronic immunosuppression.

Treatment

Most patients with both ocular and generalized MG can lead full and productive lives with proper therapy. Treatment includes anticholinesterase inhibitors, thymectomy, immunomodulatory drugs, and, for selected patients with ocular manifestations, local therapy. Although anticholinesterase inhibitors tend to be the primary therapy for patients with MG, the ocular manifestations of the disease, particularly the diplopia and strabismus, often are refractory of these drugs, being more responsive to systemic corticosteroids or thymectomy. In addition, there is some evidence that early treatment of "ocular" MG with systemic corticosteroids prevents generalization of the disease. Thus, the choice of therapy for a given patient with "ocular" MG is best left to a specialist in neuromuscular diseases with appropriate input from the ophthalmologist.

Congenital Myasthenic Syndromes

Congenital MG comprises a heterogeneous group of genetic neuromuscular transmission disorders. These conditions can be differentiated from acquired autoimmune MG by clinical, electromyographic, electrophysiologic, cytochemical, structural, and molecular genetic testing. Many but not all cases present neonatally or in infancy with ptosis, fluctuating ophthalmoparesis, poor feeding, and respiratory difficulty. Symptoms may be episodic or may demonstrate fatigability that is worsened by crying, activity, or fever. Persistence of symptoms, rather than a transient monophasic course, distinguishes a congenital myasthenic syndrome from neonatal MG. Some syndromes may not even present until adolescence or adulthood. Serum ACh receptor antibodies are absent. In many cases, siblings or parents are affected, but a negative family history does not exclude autosomal-recessive inheritance. The edrophonium test, which relies on intact acetylcholinesterase and normal channel open times for its effect, is negative in many congenital myasthenic syndromes. Thus, a negative test does not exclude the diagnosis, and a positive test cannot distinguish any of the congenital myasthenic syndromes from autoimmune myasthenia. The diagnosis instead rests on the results of electrophysiologic testing and other key features.

Congenital myasthenic syndromes may be separated into those in which the defect is primarily presynaptic and those in which the defect is primarily postsynaptic. The major syndromes in which the defect is presynaptic are related to defects in ACh synthesis, mobilization, or release. Postsynaptic syndromes are mainly those caused by endplate acetylcholinesterase deficiency and ACh receptor deficiency, as well as disorders of the ACh receptor kinetics, including the fast- and slow-channel syndromes. Nevertheless, almost any gene or process involved in neuromuscular transmission is a potential target for these rare genetic mutations.

Acquired Disorders of Neuromuscular Transmission Other than Myasthenia Gravis

As with congenital "myasthenic" syndromes, acquired disorders of neuromuscular transmission other than MG may be caused by presynaptic or postsynaptic abnormalities. In addition, some syndromes are characterized by both pre- and postsynaptic abnormalities. Most of the acquired disorders of neuromuscular transmission other than MG are caused by the effects of exogenous agents on the NMJ.

Lambert–Eaton Syndrome

Lambert–Eaton syndrome is characterized primarily by weakness, but also by fatigability, hyporeflexia, and autonomic dysfunction. Weakness is proximal and more prominent in legs and truncal muscles than in arms. Ocular and bulbar muscles sometimes are affected but mildly so, in contrast to their prominent involvement in MG. Lambert–Eaton syndrome usually occurs as a paraneoplastic syndrome associated with small-cell lung cancer and occasionally with non-

Hodgkin lymphoma, leukemia, and other malignancies. Paraneoplastic Lambert–Eaton syndrome presents before the discovery of the neoplasm in over 80% of patients, with the vast majority of patients being found to have a tumor within 2 years of onset of neurologic symptoms. Although most affected patients are adults, the disorder can also occur in children. The Lambert–Eaton syndrome also may develop in patients with other autoimmune disorders including pernicious anemia, thyroid disease, systemic lupus erythematosus, celiac disease, type I diabetes mellitus, ulcerative colitis, Addison disease, rheumatoid arthritis, and Sjögren syndrome.

Pathophysiology
The neuromuscular transmission defect in Lambert–Eaton syndrome is presynaptic. It is caused by impaired release of ACh at motor nerve terminals because of antibodies directed against voltage-gated calcium channels in the motor nerve terminal and cholinergic autonomic nerve terminals. These antibodies reduce the number of calcium channels and thus the probability of synaptosomal release of ACh at active zones. Small-cell lung carcinomas enriched with voltage-gated calcium channels provide the shared antigenic stimulus in paraneoplastic Lambert–Eaton syndrome. Thus, almost all patients with the syndrome associated with small-cell lung carcinoma have antibodies to voltage-gated calcium channels. In patients with the Lambert–Eaton syndrome without underlying cancer, 85% to90% have voltage-gated calcium channel antibodies.

ACh synthesis and mobilization are unimpaired in Lambert–Eaton syndrome, and the amount of depolarization produced by single quanta is normal. The impaired ACh release results in compound endplate potentials that may be too small to trigger muscle action potentials. As a result, muscles fatigue and evoked compound muscle action potentials are low in amplitude. The normally increased mobilization of calcium that occurs in the nerve terminal immediately following exercise or electric activation of motor nerves at rates above 10 Hz transiently increases the release of ACh, producing an increased endplate potential amplitude. This "facilitation" is the basis for the electrophysiologic diagnosis.

Ocular Manifestations
Ocular symptoms and signs are much less common in Lambert–Eaton syndrome than in MG, but ptosis and both clinical and subclinical ocular motor involvement do occur. Nevertheless, a patient with obvious ptosis and ocular motor dysfunction without pupillary involvement is much more likely to have MG or chronic progressive external ophthalmoplegia (see Chapter 20) than Lambert–Eaton syndrome.

Therapy

In general, the Lambert–Eaton syndrome responds to therapy somewhat less well than MG. An individualized, combined approach to therapy includes treatment of any underlying cancer, pharmacotherapy of the neuromuscular transmission defect, and immunomodulation. Because the syndrome may precede the discovery of a tumor by several years, the evaluation should include not only an initial extensive search for underlying malignancy, including chest CT or MRI, but also frequent surveillance if the initial evaluation is negative. Partial and event complete remission may be achieved by removal or control of the underlying small-cell cancer with surgery, radiation therapy, or chemotherapy.

Neuromuscular Disorders Caused by Drugs or Toxins

Substances that cause neuromuscular disturbances do so by affecting presynaptic mechanisms, postsynaptic mechanisms, or both. These substances are primarily drugs and toxins.

The common settings in which the effects of drugs appear are as follows: (a) in a patient at increased risk because of abnormally increased drug concentration; (b) as part of a drug–induced generalized immunologic disorder; (c) with delayed recovery of strength following general anesthesia during which neuromuscular blocking agents may have been used; and (d) unmasking or worsening of MG or the myasthenic syndrome. Drug-induced disturbances of neuromuscular transmission usually resemble naturally occurring MG, causing prominent ptosis and ophthalmoparesis as well as variable degrees of facial, bulbar, and extremity muscle weakness. Respiratory difficulties may occur early and are often severe. Treatment consists of discontinuing the offending agent and reversing the block with various agents, including calcium gluconate, potassium, and anticholinesterases.

Toxins that disturb neuromuscular transmission may be acquired from many sources, including bacteria, arthropods, and snakes. Treatment depends on the recognition of the specific toxin, the availability of antitoxin, and supportive therapy.

Drug-Induced Autoimmune Damage to the Neuromuscular Junction

A myasthenic syndrome may develop in patients receiving D-penicillamine for rheumatoid arthritis or Wilson disease. The syndrome may consist of ocular symptoms and signs alone or may be associated with generalized muscle involvement. It mimics true MG not only in its clinical features but also in that affected patients have the same histocompatibility antigens and ACh receptor antibodies that either block or increase the degradation of ACh receptors, just as they do in true MG. D-penicillamine thus has no direct neuromuscular blocking effect but produces a myasthenic syndrome in much the same way that MG occurs naturally. The onset averages 8 months after the onset of therapy, and the syndrome is unrelated to D-penicillamine dosage or cumulative dosage.

Drugs that Affect Neuromuscular Transmission Through Presynaptic or Postsynaptic Effects

A variety of drugs act at both pre- and postsynaptic sites of the NMJ to disturb neuromuscular transmission in humans. Such drugs can "unmask" subclinical MG or worsen known MG. Table 19.1 lists some of the drugs that interfere with the function of the NMJ.

Toxins that Damage Presynaptic Neuromuscular Transmission

Arthropod Envenomation

Envenomation by a variety of arthropods, including the female black widow spider (*Latrodectus mactans*), the brown widow spider (*Latrodectus geometricus*), several species of scorpions, and a variety of ticks such as Dermacentor, Amblyomma, *and Ixodes holocyclus* species cause a variety of systemic and ocular disturbances related to the effects of the venom on the presynaptic portion of the NMJ. Treatment of this type of envenomation is generally supportive.

Botulism

Botulism occurs in three forms: food borne, wound, and infantile. The disease is produced by a polypeptide toxin elaborated by the organism *Clostridium botulinum*. In food-borne botulism, symptoms begin 8 to 36 hours after food containing the preformed toxin is eaten. The toxin is intact because proper cooking that normally would denature the toxin has not been performed. In wound botulism, organisms contaminating wounds produce toxin that is absorbed systemically. Nearly all cases develop either from extremity wounds that occur outside the home or intravenous drug abuse. Symptoms begin 4 to 17 days after the injury, with an average incubation time of 7 days. Wounds that cause botulism may appear clinically uninfected; however, when the wound is carefully explored and cultured, the organism is usually found. In infantile botulism, organisms in the gastrointestinal tract produce toxin that is systemically absorbed.

At least eight types of botulinum toxin are characterized (A, B, Cα, Cβ, D, E, F, and G). Types A and B are the most common causes of botulism in the United States, although type E should be suspected when seafood is eaten. All of these toxins impair neuromuscular

Table 19.1 Drugs that Interfere with Function of the Neuromuscular Junction

Drug	Site of Action
Neuromuscular blocking agents (pancuronium, vecuronium, alcuronium)	Postsynaptic
Acetylcholinesterase inhibitors Medications—pyridostigmine, neostigmine Pesticides—organophosphates, carbamates Biowarfare agents—Sarin, VX	Postsynaptic
Phenothiazines	Postsynaptic
Trimethaphan	Postsynaptic
D,L-Carnitine	Postsynaptic
Inhalational anesthetics (ether, ketamine, halothane)	Postsynaptic
Amphetamine	Presynaptic
Corticosteroids	Pre- and postsynaptic
Antiarrhythmics (procainamide, quinidine)	Pre- and postsynaptic
Antibiotics Aminoglycosides (e.g., gentamicin) Polymyxins (e.g., polymyxin B) Penicillins (e.g., ampicillin) Macrolides (e.g., erythromycin) Tetracyclines (e.g., minocycline) Quinolones (e.g., ciprofloxacin) Monobasic amino acids (e.g., clindamycin)	Pre- and postsynaptic
Anticonvulsants (e.g., phenytoin)	Pre- and postsynaptic
Beta-adrenergic blocking agents	Pre- and postsynaptic
Chloroquine	Pre- and postsynaptic
Cis-platinum	Unknown
Lithium	Pre- and postsynaptic
Magnesium	Pre- and postsynaptic
Iodinated radiographic contrast agents	Unknown

The diagnosis of botulism depends on clinical, epidemiologic, and electrophysiologic findings and may be confirmed by the discovery of the toxin or the organism in food, stool, or a wound. Signs of infantile botulism are constipation, listlessness, poor suck, regurgitation, and generalized weakness. In children and adults, the symptoms of botulism include nausea, vomiting, blurred vision, dysphagia, and pooling of secretions in the mouth and pharynx, followed by generalized weakness mostly proximal in the upper extremities and diplopia. Examination of affected patients reveals facial, pharyngeal, and generalized proximal weakness but normal sensation.

Ophthalmologic findings in patients with botulism include bilateral ptosis associated with ophthalmoparesis or ophthalmoplegia (**Video 19.3**). In this respect, the condition superficially mimics MG; however, such patients invariably also have dilated pupils with little or no pupillary light reaction, accommodation weakness or paralysis, and decreased lacrimation.

The diagnosis of botulism should be suspected by the history and the clinical findings. When needed, electromyography can be performed that shows findings consistent with a presynaptic disorder analogous to the Lambert–Eaton syndrome.

Botulism is treated with bivalent (A and B) or trivalent (A, B, and E) antitoxin in addition to removal of stomach and intestinal contents if ingestion is thought to be the likely route of entry. In patients with wound botulism, the most important treatment is to open and extensively debride the wound. Penicillin or another antibiotic should be given, with the choice of the antibiotic being based on sensitivities from wound culture. Regardless of the apparent severity of the disease when the patient is first seen, full respiratory and nutritional support may be required. With appropriate and timely therapy, most patients recover completely (**Video 19.4**). Patients with botulism normally do not respond to treatment with anticholinesterase agents.

Tetanus
Like *Clostridium botulinum*, *Clostridium tetani* produces a neurotoxin that blocks the calcium-dependent release of ACh at NMJs, but these effects—including bilateral ptosis, ophthalmoplegia, and dilated nonreactive pupils—are overshadowed by its effects on the CNS. The diagnosis usually is obvious from the history and clinical findings. Treatment is antitoxin and supportive care, with the prognosis depending on rapid diagnosis and treatment.

Toxins that Damage Both Pre- and Postsynaptic Neuromuscular Transmission

Envenomation by poisonous snakes is an important problem around the world. Of the four largest families

transmission presynaptically by interfering with the exocytotic release of ACh vesicles after the stimulus-induced influx of calcium into the nerve terminal. Recovery eventually occurs when nerve fibers sprout, and new NMJs are established, but the process may take months or even years.

of poisonous snakes (Elapidae, cobras, coral snakes, mambas, kraits; Hydrophiidae, sea snakes; Viperidae, Old World vipers; and Crotalidae, rattlesnakes and related species), only the first two have venom with potent neuromuscular blocking properties. In most cases of Elapidae envenomation, neuromuscular blocking activity of the venoms is a major cause of death and disability. Envenomation is followed in minutes to hours by signs of neuromuscular blockade resembling that caused by competitive neuromuscular blocking drugs. Patients initially develop bilateral ptosis, ophthalmoparesis, and dysphagia, followed by tongue, laryngeal, and pharyngeal weakness. Respiratory paralysis eventually occurs, leading to death if patients are not treated. Ophthalmoparesis and ptosis are frequent components, related to both pre- and postsynaptic effects on neuromuscular transmission. Sea snakes, members of Hydrophiidae, produce a neurotoxic venom that can also produce ptosis and ophthalmoplegia. Many of the symptoms show improvement with anticholinesterase agents, although antivenom administration and ventilatory and cardiocirculatory support are the mainstays of treatment.

Myopathies of Neuro-Ophthalmologic Significance

Developmental Disorders of Extraocular Muscle
    Agenesis of the Extraocular Muscles
    Anomalies of Extraocular Muscle Origin, Insertion, and Structure
    Congenital Adherence and Fibrosis Syndromes
Congenital Myopathies
Muscular Dystrophies
    Congenital Muscular Dystrophies
    Myotonic Muscular Dystrophies
    Oculopharyngeal Muscular Dystrophy
    Ion Channel Disorders (Myotonia)
Mitochondrial Myopathies
    Chronic Progressive External Ophthalmoplegia
    CPEO Plus Syndromes
    Genetics
    Diagnosis
Encephalomyopathy with Ophthalmoplegia from Vitamin E Deficiency
Other Acquired Myopathies

In this chapter, we consider disorders that produce ocular motor dysfunction from involvement of the extraocular muscles. Some of these disorders affect only the extraocular muscles, whereas others are multisystem disorders in which various organ systems are also affected.

Developmental Disorders of Extraocular Muscle

Anomalous development of extraocular muscles probably is more common than the literature would indicate. Many of these anomalies are recognized only during surgical procedures or at autopsy. The most common congenital anomalies of the extraocular muscles are agenesis, anomalous insertions or origins, and the adherence and fibrosis syndromes.

Agenesis of the Extraocular Muscles

Most cases of agenesis of the extraocular muscles involve only a single muscle. Isolated agenesis of the lateral rectus muscle, medial rectus muscle, inferior rectus muscle, superior rectus muscle, and superior oblique muscle are all well described, particularly in children with craniostenosis.

Anomalies of Extraocular Muscle Origin, Insertion, and Structure

Abnormal origins of extraocular muscles are rare. Somewhat more commonly responsible for ocular motor dysfunction is an abnormal insertion of an extraocular muscle. Abnormal insertions of extraocular muscles, like agenesis of the muscles, often occur in children with craniostenosis.

Occasionally, an extraocular muscle shows underaction because of an abnormally increased length. In other instances, an anomalous muscle slip or fibrous band may be present. This phenomenon appears to be responsible for most of the congenital cases of superior oblique tendon dysfunction called Brown syndrome. Patients with this syndrome show absence of elevation in adduction, improvement of elevation in the primary position, and normal or near-normal elevation in abduction (Fig. 20.1). Forced duction testing (see Chapter 16) reveals mechanical limitation of motion upward and inward in the involved eye, but upward saccadic velocities are normal.

Congenital Adherence and Fibrosis Syndromes

Congenital fibrosis of the extraocular muscles (CFEOM) is the term used to describe several hereditary disorders characterized by (a) ophthalmoplegia, (b) ptosis, (c) fibrosis of all the extraocular muscles, (d) fibrosis of Tenon capsule, (e) adhesions between muscles, Tenon capsule, and globe, and (f) inelasticity and fragility of the conjunctiva (Fig. 20.2). CFEOM is associated with mutations at three distinct loci, FEOM1, FEOM2, and FEOM3, located on chromosomes 12, 11, and 16, respectively. FEOM1 and FEOM3 mutations produce autosomal-dominant CFEOM, whereas the FEOM2 mutation produces autosomal-recessive CFEOM. Most patients with these disorders have only ocular motor dysfunction, but some patients have facial diparesis, and individual patients have been described who also have inguinal hernias and cryptorchidism or a cleft palate.

Figure 20.1 Congenital Brown syndrome in an 8-year-old girl. Note the patient's inability to elevate the right eye in adduction. (Courtesy of Dr. Michael X. Repka.)

Although histopathologic findings in some patients with CFEOM include replacement of muscle tissue with fibrous tissue and degenerative changes in the muscles, these findings are secondary to maldevelopment of the oculomotor (III) nerve, trochlear (IV) nerve, or both. Thus, CFEOM is actually a disorder similar in origin to Duane and Möbius syndromes.

Congenital Myopathies

Two types of congenital, primarily nonprogressive myopathies can affect the extraocular and eyelid muscles, producing bilateral ptosis, ophthalmoparesis, and facial weakness (Fig. 20.3). One group consists of disorders that are similar to one another clinically but have distinctive histopathologic features. They are called collectively **structurally defined congenital myopathies** and include: (1) central core myopathy, (2) nemaline myopathy, (3) centronuclear (or myotubular) myopathy, (4) multicore disease, and (5) congenital fiber-type disproportion.

A second group of congenital myopathies remains to be characterized fully. These disorders generally present with congenital hypotonia or with early-onset generalized weakness that does not progress. Some have ocular features; others do not. Skeletal deformities, such as high-arched palate, scoliosis, and a slender body habitus may be present.

Most congenital myopathies are mild and nonprogressive or slowly progressive. Some cases, however, are severe, relentlessly progressive, or both, resulting in substantial debilitation.

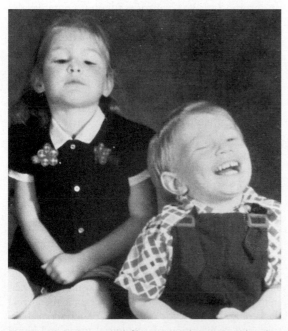

Figure 20.2 Congenital fibrosis syndrome in a brother and sister. Because of the bilateral ptosis and ophthalmoplegia, both children have adopted a head posture with the chin elevated. (Courtesy of Dr. Stewart M. Wolff.)

Figure 20.3 Appearance of a 14-year-old girl with severe congenital fiber-type disproportion. Note bilateral asymmetric ptosis, inferior scleral show due to laxity of lower lids, and flaccid facies. The patient also has orbital dystopia. (Courtesy of Dr. Thomas Crawford.)

Congenital myopathies must be differentiated from other causes of congenital hypotonic weakness such as various forms of spinal muscular atrophy. This distinction usually is fairly simple, however, as most of these latter conditions are not associated with either ptosis or ophthalmoparesis/plegia. Thus, an infant with congenital hypotonia associated with ptosis, external ophthalmoplegia, or both almost always has a myopathy. Nevertheless, conditions other than congenital myopathies, including neonatal myasthenia gravis and infant botulism, also can cause hypotonia, weakness, facial paresis, and ophthalmoparesis.

Muscular Dystrophies

The term "muscular dystrophy" covers a group of genetically determined disorders that cause **progressive** weakness and wasting of the skeletal muscles and that are assumed to affect the muscle cell directly. Some forms cause death after 15 to 20 years, whereas others are compatible with a normal life expectancy. The distinction between the terms "myopathy" and "dystrophy" breaks down, however, when it is realized that some glycogenolytic myopathies, like acid maltase deficiency, can progress inexorably like dystrophies, and some dystrophies, like Becker dystrophy, may hardly progress at all. Nevertheless, the diagnostic category is a tradition. Although the diagnosis of this group of disorders cannot be established by morphology alone, histologic examination of an affected muscle can exclude other myopathies (e.g., the congenital myopathies and the mitochondrial myopathies). In others, molecular genetic testing can provide the correct diagnosis.

Muscular dystrophies are historically subdivided on the basis of age of onset, mode of inheritance, and clinical features as follows:

1 The dystrophin-deficient dystrophies, including the severe X-linked pseudohypertrophic muscular dystrophy of Duchenne and its more benign "Becker" variant
2 The dystrophin-associated glycoprotein disorders that may resemble Duchenne or Becker dystrophy, including mutations of merosin and the α-, β-, γ-, or δ-sarcoglycans
3 Various limb-girdle dystrophies, including severe childhood-onset autosomal-recessive (chromosome 13) muscular dystrophy, juvenile scapulohumeral dystrophy of Erb, pelvifemoral dystrophy of Leyden and Möbius, and adult-onset autosomal-dominant limb-girdle dystrophy
4 The facioscapulohumeral dystrophy of Landouzy and Déjérine
5 Distal dystrophies (myopathies) of Welander, Miyoshi, and others

6 Congenital muscular dystrophies (CMDs), including Fukuyama dystrophy, muscle–eye–brain disease, and Walker–Warburg syndrome
7 Myotonic muscular dystrophy
8 Proximal myotonic myopathy (PROMM)
9 Oculopharyngeal muscular dystrophy (OPMD)

Only the last four of these disorders are of neuroophthalmologic importance and are discussed below.

Congenital Muscular Dystrophies

Patients with dystrophic muscle pathology associated with symptoms present at birth and a variable clinical course are said to have CMD. These individuals have generalized muscle atrophy and weakness that is symmetric and predominates in proximal muscles. In addition, nonmuscular ocular involvement is common in three congenital dystrophy syndromes that are really multisystemic disorders of eye, brain, and skeletal muscle. These three—the Fukuyama type of CMD, so-called muscle–eye–brain disease, and the Walker–Warburg syndrome—are associated with mutations that result in protein glycosylation defects.

Fukuyama Congenital Muscular Dystrophy
The Fukuyama type of CMD is transmitted as an autosomal-recessive trait with no gender predilection, a high incidence of consanguinity, and a high frequency of affected siblings. The mutant gene, located on chromosome 9q31, encodes fukutin, a putative glycosyltransferase.

Patients with Fukuyama dystrophy have CMD associated with central nervous system (CNS) involvement, including mental retardation and convulsions. Children are severely weak from birth, and only a few children can walk without assistance. Most survive beyond infancy to remain relatively stable, but the average life span is 8 to 10 years. Serum levels of creatinine kinase (CK) are elevated, and the muscle biopsy shows myopathic and fibrotic changes. Ventricular enlargement and hypoplasia of the cerebellar vermis are seen with computed tomographic (CT) scanning, and magnetic resonance (MR) imaging shows severe signal abnormalities in white matter.

The neuropathologic findings in Fukuyama dystrophy include polymicrogyria of the cerebrum and cerebellum, loss of cerebral cytoarchitecture with demyelination and proliferation of interstitial tissue, occasionally absent or hypoplastic corpus callosum, and brain stem pyramidal tract abnormalities. Chronic meningeal thickening, lymphocytic infiltration of intracranial tissues, and proliferation of meningeal tissue and blood vessels are less common.

Ocular involvement in Fukuyama CMD is inconsistent, but it is milder than that in muscle–eye–brain disease and Walker–Warburg syndrome (see below). Reported findings include occasional optic nerve hypoplasia and optic atrophy, as well as high myopia, cataracts, weakness of the orbicularis oculi muscles, and retinal abnormalities that may be mild or severe, including mottling of the retinal pigment epithelium, abnormal retinal vessels, incomplete retinal vascularization with temporally displaced foveae, and dysplasia.

Muscle–Eye–Brain Disease

This autosomal-recessive disorder is associated with homozygous mutations in O-mannose beta-1,2–N-acetylglucosaminyltransferase (POMGnT1), an enzyme that participates in O-mannosyl glycan synthesis. It is characterized by severe congenital hypotonic weakness from both progressive CNS disease and CMD. Although the cerebral and visual abnormalities are severe, most patients reach adulthood (average age of death, 18 years). As in Fukuyama dystrophy, levels of serum CK are elevated, and muscle biopsy shows mild myopathy with fibrosis.

Ocular abnormalities are more consistent and severe in muscle–eye–brain disease than in Fukuyama dystrophy, but they are less uniform than in Walker–Warburg syndrome. High myopia is common. Other ocular findings include severe generalized loss of retinal ganglion cells, retinochoroidal scars, a pronounced preretinal membrane and gliosis, mottled retinal pigment epithelium, and mild optic nerve and chiasm atrophy with reactive gliosis. The microscopic and macroscopic features of the cortex in these cases tend to be highly abnormal, showing argyric areas, coarse and nodular gyri, or total disorganization. The cerebellar vermis and brainstem may be hypoplastic.

Walker–Warburg Syndrome

The Walker–Warburg syndrome is an autosomal-recessive disorder with more severe findings than either Fukuyama dystrophy or muscle–eye–brain disease. It is caused by homozygous mutations in the gene encoding O-mannosyltransferase 1 (POMT1) that, like POMGnT1 (the mutant protein in muscle–eye–brain disease), participates in O-mannosyl glycan synthesis. The neuropathologic features of Walker–Warburg syndrome are the same as those of muscle–eye–brain disease, but they are more extensive and include the macroscopic features of arrhinencephaly: cephalocele, hemispheric fusion, agenesis of the corpus callosum, or a combination of these manifestations.

The ocular malformations in Walker–Warburg syndrome, like the neuropathologic features, are more severe than in muscle–eye–brain disease. Typical ocular features include retinal dysplasia and nonattachment, persistent hyperplastic primary vitreous, optic nerve atrophy, microphthalmia, corneal opacities, congenital cataract, and congenital glaucoma.

The skeletal muscle biopsy changes in Walker–Warburg syndrome are similar to those of muscle–eye–brain disease and less severe than those in Fukuyama dystrophy. Levels of serum CK are elevated in this disorder as it is in the other two.

Myotonic Muscular Dystrophies

Myotonic dystrophy (dystrophia myotonica 1 [DM1]) and the less severe PROMM (DM2) are autosomal-dominant disorders associated with nucleotide repeat expansions in untranslated regions of the respective target genes. The genetic defect in DM1 is amplification of an unstable trinucleotide CTG repeat located in the $3'$ untranslated region of the gene that encodes dystrophia myotonica protein kinase (DMPK) on chromosome 19. DM1 is highly variable in severity and age of onset, and it exhibits "anticipation," the phenomenon of increasing severity of inherited disease in successive generations of an affected family. The number of CTG repeats ranges from about 50 in patients who are mildly affected to thousands in severely affected patients. Amplification of the CTG repeat is the molecular basis for genetic anticipation. Although the mutation does not alter the protein-coding region of the DMPK gene, the CTG repeats can disrupt RNA splicing and cellular metabolism by interacting with RNA-binding proteins.

PROMM/DM2 is caused by a CCTG expansion (approximately 5,000 repeats) in intron 1 of the gene encoding zinc finger protein 9 (ZNF9). Like the CTG expansion of the DMPK gene in DM1, the CCTG expansion does not alter the protein-coding region of the ZNF9 gene. However, the CCTG repeats can disrupt RNA splicing and cellular metabolism by interacting with RNA-binding proteins.

Myotonic Dystrophy

Myotonic dystrophy (DM1) is the most common inherited myopathy in adults, with a prevalence of approximately 5 per 100,000 and men and women being equally affected. It is a multisystem disorder characterized by progressive wasting and weakness of distal muscles and myotonia.

Systemic and Ocular Manifestations. Many patients can be recognized instantly by their characteristic frontal balding, long face, ptosis, hollowing of the masseter and temporalis muscles, slackened mouth, facial weakness, and thin neck and limbs (Fig. 20.4). Other features include intellectual impairment, testicular atrophy, excessive daytime somnolence, insulin resistance, and cardiac conduction defects. The most important finding on physical examination is myotonia—involuntary delayed relaxation following a contraction, such as after sustained handgrip; however, most patients with DM1 complain of weakness, not myotonia.

Figure 20.4 Clinical appearance of a 56-year-old man with myotonic dystrophy (DM1). Note bilateral ptosis, exotropia, myopathic facies, and frontal baldness typical of this disorder.

Cataract is the most common ocular abnormality in patients with DM1, occurring in nearly 100% of patients with the disease. The severity of the cataract is not related to the severity of the disease. Myotonic cataracts may be of two types. The first consists of tiny opaque, white, or—most often—iridescent, colored (usually red, green, or blue) crystals that are located in a thin band of anterior and posterior cortex just beneath the lens capsule (Fig. 20.5A). The second type is a stellate grouping of opacities at the posterior pole along the posterior suture lines, producing a spoke-like appearance (Fig. 20.5B).

In addition to cataracts, ptosis frequently is present in patients with DM1 and may be mild (Fig. 20.4) or profound (Fig. 20.6A). In addition, there may be weakness of the orbicularis oculi muscles (Fig. 20.6B), producing infrequent blinking and difficulty closing the eyes. When the orbicularis is affected, there may be bilateral lower lid retraction or delayed opening of the eyes after forceful closure.

Abnormal eye movements are present in many patients with DM1. In its mildest form, the ocular motor involvement consists of slowed saccades in patients who have a full range of eye movements and no visual complaints. In other patients, however, there are varying degrees of ophthalmoparesis (Fig. 20.7). The ophthalmoparesis, particularly when combined with ptosis and orbicularis weakness, may suggest a diagnosis of myasthenia gravis or chronic progressive external ophthalmoplegia (CPEO), the two disorders with which DM1 most often is confused.

The pupils in patients with DM1 tend to be miotic, react sluggishly and incompletely to both light and near stimuli, react normally to psychosensory stimuli, and do not tend to fatigue on repeated stimuli any more than normal pupils. Despite these abnormalities, most patients with DM1 appear clinically to have normally reactive pupils.

Vascular abnormalities of the iris occur in many patients with DM1. These iris neovascular tufts usually

A   B

Figure 20.5 Typical appearance of cataracts in myotonic dystrophy (DM1). **A:** Numerous dot opacities, each having a different color, located primarily in the posterior subcortical region of the lens. **B:** Spoke-like opacities of the posterior subcortical region of the lens.

Figure 20.6 Severe ptosis and orbicularis weakness in a 65-year-old man with myotonic dystrophy (DM1). **A:** The patient has marked bilateral ptosis. **B:** On attempted forced lid closure, the patient has mild right-sided lagophthalmos and cannot bury the lashes on either side.

can be identified by slit-lamp biomicroscopy. In most cases, they are of no consequence, but they can bleed spontaneously or after mild ocular trauma, resulting in a hyphema.

The ciliary processes may be short and depigmented in patients with DM1. These abnormalities may explain the finding of ocular hypotony in many patients with this disorder.

Retinal abnormalities occur in patients with DM1. The involvement ranges from abnormalities of dark adaptation and electroretinography in patients with no visual complaints and normal-appearing fundi to decreased vision with pigmentary retinopathy involving the macula, peripheral retina, or both (Fig. 20.8). Regardless of the degree of retinopathy, it is never as severe as retinitis pigmentosa and does not cause

Figure 20.7 Asymmetric ophthalmoparesis in the patient with myotonic dystrophy (DM1) seen in Figure 20.6. Note bilateral pseudointernuclear ophthalmoplegia, right more than left, as well as moderate bilateral limitation of depression.

Figure 20.8 Chorioretinopathy involving the posterior pole in myotonic dystrophy (DM1).

blindness. Indeed, the retinopathy observed in patients with DM1 is similar in appearance, electrophysiologic dysfunction, and visual prognosis to that in patients with the Kearns–Sayre variant of CPEO (see below).

Abnormal visual evoked potentials may be detected in patients with DM1 who have no visible retinal abnormalities and a normal electroretinogram (ERG), suggesting that at least some patients with DM1 have dysfunction in the visual sensory conducting system other than at the retinal level.

Pathology. The characteristic features in the muscles of patients with DM1 are a marked variation in the caliber of the fibers, myofiber degeneration and regeneration, ringed fibers ("ringbinden") or myofibrils with an aberrant course, sarcoplasmic masses of tightly packed disordered myofilaments, focal areas of myofibrillar disruption and Z-band streaming, and associated secondary changes in mitochondria or the sarcotubular system. In the advanced stages of the disease, a large proportion of the fiber population is replaced by connective tissue and fat cells. This pathologic end stage is indistinguishable from the advanced stage of other muscular dystrophies.

In patients with DM1 who have ophthalmoparesis, the extraocular muscles may undergo changes similar to those of striated muscle. In addition, some patients show a proliferation of mitochondria in the extraocular muscles.

The iridescent crystals that comprise some myotonic cataracts are not crystals at all but represent whorls of lens fiber plasma membrane.

Pathologic changes in the iris and ciliary body in patients with DM1 are nonspecific and consist of hyalinization, vacuole degeneration, and interstitial proliferation. Whether these changes are responsible for the pupillary abnormalities observed in patients with DM1 is unclear.

The retinal lesions observed in patients with DM1 are many and varied. Atrophy of the inner retinal layers with preservation of photoreceptors occurs, particularly in the peripheral retina. In the macula, increased pigmentation with a granular, striate, or stellate pattern may occur. Foci of pigmented cells in the outer plexiform layer and macular edema over subretinal fluid also are observed.

Diagnosis. The diagnosis of DM1 may be suspected by a combination of the patient's external appearance, ptosis that may be associated with an external ophthalmoparesis, multihued subcortical iridescent crystals and/or spoke-like posterior cataracts, hypotony, and retinal changes. The diagnosis can be confirmed by findings of myotonia on EMG. Genetic testing for the CTG repeat can be performed when the diagnosis is not clinically obvious, thus eliminating the need for a muscle biopsy.

Treatment. When troublesome, myotonia can be treated medically, but few patients require such therapy. Distal weakness causing foot drop is treated with ankle-foot orthoses. Patients with cardiac conduction defects may require pacemakers.

Treatment of the ophthalmoparesis associated with DM1 usually is unnecessary because the limitation of eye movement usually is symmetric. Thus, such patients do not commonly report diplopia. Prisms can be used to treat patients with diplopia in primary position. Extraocular muscle surgery usually is unwarranted but may be appropriate in rare instances.

Treatment of ptosis is somewhat problematic in patients with DM1 because of the commonly associated orbicularis weakness. If the eyelids are raised to a "normal" level, such patients may develop severe tearing and irritation from exposure keratopathy, and some may even develop corneal ulceration, leading to blindness. Thus, the eyelids should be raised only when ptosis is interfering with function and only as high as needed to improve vision.

Proximal Myotonic Myopathy (PROMM/DM2)
Proximal myotonic myopathy (PROMM/DM2) has certain features in common with DM1 but a very different clinical presentation. The clinical features of PROMM/DM2 are muscle stiffness, myotonia, weakness, muscle pain, and cataracts. These problems can occur singly or in various combinations. Initial symptoms usually develop between 20 and 60 years of age. Many patients first complain of intermittent stiffness in the thigh muscles of one or both legs and of intermittent grip myotonia. In other patients, cataracts are the first manifestation of the disorder. These may appear in late childhood or early adolescence and are indistinguishable from those in DM1, being posterior

subcapsular, iridescent, multicolored opacities. Cardiac arrhythmias occur in some patients.

EMG usually reveals myotonic discharges in affected patients, including those without obvious clinical myotonia; however, these discharges are scarce and difficult to detect. Muscle biopsy usually reveals a nonspecific myopathy. In contrast to DM1, there are no ringbinden or subsarcolemmal masses, and there is no evidence of selective type 1 fiber atrophy.

The prognosis of PROMM/DM2 is more favorable than that of DM1. Most patients do not show any deterioration of mental status, dysarthria, dysphagia, or respiratory failure. Nonsteroidal anti-inflammatory drugs and muscle relaxants can be used to treat the muscle pain experienced by these patients, and antimyotonia therapy can be used in patients with severe myotonic stiffness and grip myotonia. Cataract surgery is warranted in some patients.

Oculopharyngeal Muscular Dystrophy

OPMD is a hereditary disorder usually transmitted in an autosomal-dominant fashion, although rare autosomal-recessive cases have been reported. The mutation is located on chromosome 14q11 and increases the length of a polyalanine sequence located at the N terminus of the polyadenylate-binding protein nuclear 1 (PABPN1).

The two essential clinical characteristics of OPMD are ptosis and dysphagia (Fig. 20.9). Neither manifestation usually presents until late in life, but mild ptosis usually precedes any significant dysphagia, often by several years. The ptosis eventually becomes bilateral but rarely is complete. It usually is symmetric, although one lid may become ptotic weeks or months before the other. External ophthalmoplegia is present in most but not all patients. The pupils are never clinically abnormal.

Figure 20.9 Bilateral ptosis and mild ophthalmoparesis in a 78-year-old man with oculopharyngeal muscular dystrophy (OPMD).

Dysphagia may be disabling in patients with OPMD. At first there is difficulty only in swallowing solid foods, but eventually swallowing liquids also becomes difficult, and several attempts at swallowing may be necessary to empty the upper pharynx. Examination of the swallowing mechanisms in affected patients usually reveals weak movements in the pharynx and larynx. The pharyngeal musculature cannot propel the bolus of food into the upper esophagus, partly because of dysfunction of the pharyngeal musculature and partly because of the absence of reflex relaxation of the cricopharyngeal muscle. Degeneration of the pharyngeal striated musculature evidently results in uncoordinated activity, with material pooling in the pyriform sinuses and regurgitating into the nasopharynx rather than passing into the esophagus. Ingested material thus may be aspirated. Some patients with severe dysphagia are treated successfully with cricopharyngeal myotomy, but a percutaneous feeding gastrostomy is a more practical treatment and is more commonly used.

The morphologic hallmark of OPMD is intranuclear filamentous inclusions that contain PABPN1, sequestered polyadenylated RNA, and ubiquitin and that are confined to muscle cells, where PABPN1 plays a specific role in differentiation. It is believed that the reduced solubility of mutant PABPN1 and its tendency to form intranuclear aggregates play a direct role in the pathogenesis of OPMD.

As in other dystrophies, biopsies from affected muscles show advanced degenerative changes, fibrosis, abundant central nuclei, altered myofibrils and Z-bands, and other nonspecific changes. "Ragged-red" fibers (RRFs) with mitochondrial proliferation and other mitochondrial abnormalities are sometimes found, but these probably are the result of age-related mitochondrial DNA (mtDNA) mutations and are unrelated to the pathogenesis of OPMD.

Ion Channel Disorders (Myotonia)

Myotonia is a phenomenon in which muscle fibers have a pathologically persistent activity after a strong contraction or are continuously active when they should be relaxed. Myotonia is identified physiologically as a delay in muscle relaxation after percussion or electric stimulation of a muscle, or after a voluntary contraction. The phenomenon is caused by mutations affecting chloride, sodium, and calcium ion channels in surface membranes. It persists after blockage of either the peripheral nerve or the neuromuscular junction. In patients with myotonia, the spontaneous action potentials as recorded in the EMG are high-frequency discharges of single muscle fibers that wax and wane in both amplitude and frequency. When translated into sound, these discharges produce a noise resembling that of a motorcycle engine.

Clinical myotonia is a common feature of a number of different genetically determined primary muscle diseases, including autosomal-dominant and autosomal-recessive myotonia congenita, paramyotonia congenita, the familial periodic paralyses, and chondrodystrophic myotonia.

Myotonia Congenita

Autosomal-dominant and autosomal-recessive myotonia congenita result from allelic mutations of the chloride channel gene encoded on chromosome 7q35. Myotonic symptoms, noted in the first years of life and often worse in males than females, frequently lessen by the 20s or 30s. Myotonia of limb muscles is more likely to occur when strenuous exertion is initiated after a period of rest; myotonia is then followed by transient weakness. Unlike paramyotonia, the myotonia is not aggravated by cooling, and long-lasting paralysis does not occur. This is one of a few myopathies in which prominent hypertrophy can occur, particularly in the masseter, proximal arms, thighs, calves, and extensor digitorum brevis.

Patients with myotonia congenita often have eyelid myotonia. At the very least, lid lag usually is present, and blepharospasm may occur in some patients after forced closure of the eyelids. Strabismus is said to occur in some patients, but not ptosis or generalized ophthalmoplegia. Swallowing and voice are spared, but chewing sometimes is affected.

Needle EMG shows typical myotonic runs. Muscle biopsy is nonspecific. Specific genetic diagnosis is possible.

The pathophysiology of the myotonia is thought to be caused by both low chloride channel conductance and abnormal reopening of sodium channels. Treatment is best undertaken several days before vigorous activity rather than on a regular basis.

Paramyotonia Congenita

Paramyotonia congenital is an autosomal-dominant condition characterized by paradoxic myotonia (i.e., myotonia that worsens with exercise), exacerbation of myotonia by cold, and periodic attacks of weakness. The disorder is caused by mutations in the sodium channel gene and is allelic to hyperkalemic periodic paralysis, accounting for the great overlap between the two syndromes. Neither ptosis nor ophthalmoplegia occurs in patients with this disease; however, some patients show myotonic lid lag similar to that observed in other myotonic disorders, including myotonia congenita.

Familial Periodic Paralysis

Familial periodic paralysis is a rare syndrome characterized by abnormal flux of potassium across muscle membranes and spells of severe flaccid weakness in the limb muscles that last minutes to hours and are provoked by rest following exercise. Bulbar and ocular muscles rarely are affected; thus, patients with this disorder typically do not present to the ophthalmologist.

Respiratory muscles are almost never affected. The syndrome is subdivided into hyper-, hypo-, and normokalemic types, but all three types are characterized by presentation in the third decade of life, greater severity in males, autosomal-dominant inheritance, and oliguria preceding attacks. In rare patients, hypo- or hyperkalemia causes a complicating cardiac arrhythmia. Examination shows normal strength between attacks, but if the attacks are frequent and not treated, mild fixed proximal weakness may develop. Myotonia, especially eyelid myotonia, may be seen, manifesting as intermittent lid lag or staring episodes. During paralytic attacks, muscles are nonexcitable and deep tendon reflexes are hypoactive or absent. The histologic hallmark is a vacuolar myopathy most consistently associated with the permanent myopathy that develops after repeated attacks.

Chondrodystrophic Myotonia (Schwartz–Jampel Syndrome)

This rare syndrome of dwarfism, abnormalities of long bones and the face, blepharospasm, and myotonic symptoms is caused by mutation of a gene that is located on chromosome 1p34–36.1 and that encodes perlecan, a heparan sulfate proteoglycan component of the basement membrane that is responsible for the localization of acetylcholinesterase in the postsynaptic clefts of the neuromuscular junction.

The facial appearance of blepharospasm, puckered lips, myokymic twitching of the chin, low-set ears, receding chin, a high-pitched forced voice, and high-arched palate is distinctive. Frequent ophthalmologic features include myopia, cataract, strabismus, and nystagmus. Serum CK levels are usually normal. Although muscle biopsies show many changes, none are specific. This condition is not a true myotonia, because EMG discharges from affected muscles are abolished by *d*-tubocurarine. Instead, the abnormal activity of affected muscles appears to reflect prolonged activation of postsynaptic receptors resulting from the impaired degradation of acetylcholine at the neuromuscular junction.

Mitochondrial Myopathies

The mitochondrial myopathies are a genetically and biochemically diverse set of disorders caused by mitochondrial dysfunction. The histologic hallmark of these disorders is the abnormal accumulation of increased numbers of enlarged mitochondria beneath the sarcolemma of affected muscle fibers. Because of their irregular appearance and their strikingly dark red color when stained with the modified Gömöri trichrome stain, these abnormal muscle fibers are called **RRFs** (Fig. 20.10). In patients with ophthalmoplegia, RRFs are present not only in skeletal muscles, but also in the orbicularis oculi and in the extraocular muscles.

Figure 20.10 "Ragged-red" muscle fibers in a patient with chronic progressive external ophthalmoplegia. Modified Gömöri trichrome stain.

When viewed with the electron microscope, the mitochondria in affected muscle fibers appear more numerous and more variable in size than in normal muscle fibers. The mitochondria often are enlarged, with distorted or disorganized cristae that sometimes are arranged concentrically. Paracrystalline inclusions are invariably present within the cristae, and similar inclusions also may be observed outside the cristae. Similar mitochondrial inclusions may be seen in liver cells, in sweat glands, and in the granular and Purkinje cells of the cerebellum of affected patients.

The most common mitochondrial myopathy in which ophthalmoplegia is a prominent feature is CPEO and its variants, including the Kearns–Sayre syndrome (KSS) and the mitochondrial neurogastrointestinal encephalomyopathy (MNGIE) syndrome.

Chronic Progressive External Ophthalmoplegia

The syndrome known as CPEO is by far the most common of the mitochondrial myopathies. Most patients with CPEO also have generalized skeletal muscle weakness. Nevertheless, some patients have either no evidence of weakness elsewhere or their weakness is sufficiently mild as to be overlooked by patient and physician alike.

Figure 20.11 Bilateral ptosis in a 26-year-old woman with chronic progressive external ophthalmoplegia.

Ptosis is usually the first evidence of involvement and may precede ophthalmoparesis by months to years (Fig. 20.11). The ptosis is slowly progressive and tends to become complete in most cases. Characteristically, it is bilateral, but unilateral ptosis can be present for years before the opposite side becomes involved or ophthalmoparesis is observed. As ptosis progresses, it eventually interferes with vision, and the patient must tilt the head backward and use the frontalis muscles to elevate the eyelids. The ptosis in patients with CPEO usually is fixed, unlike the variable, fatigable ptosis in myasthenia gravis, but in some patients, the ptosis increases later in the day and/or with extended upgaze.

The clinical hallmark of CPEO is **an external ophthalmoparesis** that progresses slowly over years and that eventually may become a complete external ophthalmoplegia. It can begin simultaneously with ptosis, months to years after onset of ptosis, or even prior to ptosis. Like the ptosis of CPEO, the external ophthalmoparesis/plegia usually is bilateral but it may begin as a unilateral phenomenon and remain unilateral for months to years.

Because limitation of ocular movements is generally symmetric, most patients with CPEO do not report diplopia and are not aware of a problem with ocular motility until it is of such severity that it limits peripheral vision or until someone points it out to them. For this reason, immobility of the eyes is often severe when such patients are first examined (Fig. 20.12).

Figure 20.12 Moderate ptosis and external ophthalmoparesis in a 15-year-old boy with CPEO.

Figure 20.13 CT scanning of extraocular muscles in a patient with CPEO. **A:** Axial view shows marked thinning of left medial rectus muscle (*arrow*). **B:** Coronal view shows similar thinning of left superior rectus muscle (*arrow*). (Reprinted with permission from Wallace DK, Sprunger DT, Helveston EM, et al. Surgical management of strabismus associated with chronic progressive external ophthalmoplegia. *Ophthalmology.* 1997;104:695–700.)

Both ultrasonography and CT scanning in patients with long-standing CPEO show thin, presumably atrophic, extraocular muscles (Fig. 20.13). The thinning usually is symmetric.

Most patients with CPEO have generalized, symmetric limitation of eye movement and have no diplopia. Thus, they do not require surgical realignment of the eyes. In the rare patients who have asymmetric limitation of movement and complain of double vision, prism therapy or surgery may be used to improve ocular alignment. Surgery to raise the eyelids can be performed in patients with severe ptosis that prevents them from functioning normally, but because such patients also may have or eventually develop weakness of the orbicularis oculi muscles, care must be taken to avoid raising the eyelids so much that the patient develops exposure keratopathy from inability to close the eyes.

CPEO Plus Syndromes

Several variants of CPEO warrant a separate discussion. These variants, often referred to as "CPEO Plus," have important nonocular manifestations the recognition of which may have major implications for management.

Kearns–Sayre Syndrome

The KSS is a variant of CPEO characterized by a typical external ophthalmoparesis/plegia associated with a bilateral pigmentary retinopathy and cardiac conduction abnormalities including complete heart block. Most patients develop these manifestations before the age of 20 years.

In contrast to retinitis pigmentosa, which usually initially affects the peripheral and midperipheral retina, the retinopathy of KSS usually occurs initially in the posterior fundus (Fig. 20.14). In advanced cases, a metallic sheen or mottled fluorescent appearance surrounds the optic nerve. "Bone spicule" pigment formation, a common feature of retinitis pigmentosa, rarely occurs. Examination of affected fundi usually shows diffuse depigmentation of the retinal pigment epithelium with a characteristic mottled "salt-and-pepper" pattern of pigment clumping similar to that seen in patients with congenital rubella retinopathy. This appearance may be most marked around the macula. Pallor of the optic disc, attenuation of retinal vessels, and posterior cataracts—all common in patients with retinitis pigmentosa—rarely occur. As might be expected, visual symptoms such as night blindness or diminished visual acuity generally are mild and occur in about 40% to 50% of patients. Thus, the retinopathy of KSS is similar to that in myotonic dystrophy type 1. There are, however, rare cases of KSS with CNS involvement in which bone spicule formation and pigment clumping in the macula are associated with profound loss of visual acuity.

As might be expected, the results of electrophysiologic tests performed on patients with KSS also differ from those in patients with retinitis pigmentosa. Although exceptional cases exist, electroretinography usually is normal or only mildly abnormal.

The cardiac conduction disturbances that occur in patients with KSS typically do so years after the onset of ptosis and ophthalmoplegia. Thus, any patient with CPEO and a pigmentary retinopathy or neurologic dysfunction but with a normal ECG should be warned of the possibility of future cardiac disease, and such patients should be told to undergo cardiac examinations at regular intervals, regardless of their age.

Although the cardiac dysfunction that occurs in patients with KSS can often be managed effectively with an artificial pacemaker, patients may die suddenly even after insertion of a pacemaker because of a decreased ventilatory response to hypoxia and hypercarbia caused

Figure 20.14 Pigmentary retinopathy in Kearns–Sayre syndrome. Note diffuse stippled retinal pigmentary disturbance.

by deficient brain stem respiratory control mechanisms. Cardiac failure in patients with KSS also can be treated with cardiac transplantation.

Cardiac abnormalities other than conduction defects occur uncommonly in patients with KSS but include intraventricular septal hypertrophy of the idiopathic hypertrophic subaortic stenosis type and mitral valve prolapse with mitral regurgitation.

Some patients with KSS have weakness of skeletal muscles in addition to ptosis and ophthalmoplegia. Facial muscles, particularly the orbicularis oculi muscles, may be affected. Patients in whom this occurs may be unable not only to open the eyelids, but also to close them tightly. With involvement of the frontalis muscle, there is inability to wrinkle the forehead and brow ptosis, resulting in an even lower position of the upper eyelids. All muscles of the face eventually may become affected, with the face becoming thin and relatively expressionless. In some patients, the muscles of mastication become involved, and the patients report difficulty chewing.

With progression of the disease, there often is weakness and wasting of the neck and shoulder muscles. Although the muscles of the extremities may be involved, the weakness usually is mild.

Patients with KSS usually have evidence of neurologic dysfunction. Abnormalities include cerebellar ataxia, pendular nystagmus, vestibular dysfunction, hearing loss, impaired intellectual function, and peripheral neuropathy. In addition, in many patients there is elevation of CSF protein content. Spongiform changes in the brain are present in almost every patient in whom an autopsy is performed.

CNS involvement in KSS is reflected in MR imaging abnormalities with high signal intensity for proton density, T2-weighted, and T2-weighted fluid attenuated inversion recovery (FLAIR) sequences. These abnormalities are present in the brain stem, globus pallidus, thalamus, and white matter of the cerebrum and cerebellum. In addition, regional abnormalities of brain metabolism can be demonstrated in patients with KSS using MR spectroscopy (MRS). These changes include an increase in the lactate/creatine resonance intensity ratio (an index of impairment of oxidative metabolism) in resting occipital cortex and a decrease in N-acetylaspartate/creatine (a measure of neuron loss or dysfunction) in cerebral cortex.

Endocrine dysfunction is common in patients with KSS. In addition to short stature, other manifestations include hypoparathyroidism with tetany as a presenting symptom, gonadal dysfunction, and diabetes mellitus.

There is no adequate treatment for KSS, although rare patients appear to respond to controlled carbohydrate intake and coenzyme Q10 therapy. As is the case with CPEO, some patients with diplopia benefit from treatment with prisms or strabismus surgery. Ptosis also may be treated surgically.

Mitochondrial Neurogastrointestinal Encephalomyopathy Syndrome

The MNGIE syndrome is characterized by progressive intestinal dysmotility, external ophthalmoplegia, leukoencephalopathy, and peripheral neuropathy. Most patients develop manifestations around age 18 years, but there is a wide range. Men and women are equally

Figure 20.15 Bilateral ptosis and ophthalmoparesis in a 26-year-old woman with mitochondrial neurogastrointestinal encephalomyopathy (MNGIE) syndrome. The patient had been admitted for management of severe gastrointestinal dysmotility and was noted to have bilateral ptosis. She had no visual concerns and specifically denied diplopia.

affected. Gastrointestinal symptoms and signs (recurrent diarrhea, nausea, vomiting, pseudo-obstruction, weight loss, and cachexia) are the presenting manifestation in about 45% of patients, but they eventually develop in all patients. External ophthalmoparesis is the presenting sign in about 25% of patients but, again, it eventually develops in all patients (Fig. 20.15). About 15% of patients first present with a peripheral neuropathy. Other clinical manifestations include ataxia, hearing loss, and cognitive dysfunction.

The laboratory findings in the MNGIE syndrome include a diffuse cerebral leukoencephalopathy and abnormal electromyographic and nerve conduction responses usually indicating both neurogenic and myogenic dysfunction. Skeletal muscle biopsies in these patients demonstrate neurogenic atrophy and fibers deficient in cytochrome oxidase.

The MGNIE syndrome is an autosomal-recessive disorder. It is associated with mutations in a gene on chromosome 22 (22q13.32-qter) that encodes the enzyme thymidine phosphorylase (TP). The mutations severely reduce enzyme activity, resulting in elevated plasma levels of thymidine. The accumulation

of thymidine alters deoxynucleoside and nucleotide pools and impairs mtDNA replication and/or repair, leading to mtDNA mutations. The mutations, in turn, render the mitochondria incapable of de novo thymidine synthesis.

Without treatment, the MNGIE syndrome is fatal, with most patients dying at around age 40 years from such complications as aspiration pneumonia, electrolyte imbalance, metabolic acidosis, and cardiac arrhythmias. A few patients have been treated with an allogeneic stem cell transplantation and at least one patient has been reported who was treated with erythrocyte-encapsulated recombinant *Escherichia coli* TP. Although these patients experienced improvement in both GI and neurologic manifestations, the long-term effects of such treatments are unknown.

Sensory Ataxic Neuropathy with Dysarthria and Ophthalmoplegia

A sensory ataxic neuropathy with dysarthria and ophthalmoplegia (SANDO) occurs as a sporadic disorder in association with multiple mtDNA deletions.

Genetics

Most cases of CPEO and KSS are sporadic, but some are hereditary, being transmitted in an autosomal-dominant or autosomal-recessive fashion. Most of the sporadic cases of CPEO and KSS are caused by single deletions of mtDNA, with the deleted mtDNAs distributed to a wider variety of tissues in KSS than CPEO. Furthermore, duplications of mtDNA appear to be present in all cases of KSS but are absent in CPEO. Deletions of mtDNA impair mitochondrial protein synthesis, with the severity of dysfunction within an affected cell correlating with the proportion of deleted mtDNA. The close association between deletions of mtDNA and dysfunction of the extraocular muscles may be related to the relatively high metabolic activity of these muscles, which are tonically active while the eyes are maintained in primary position.

Most autosomal dominantly inherited cases of CPEO (as well as some sporadic cases) are caused by mutations in three main nuclear genes: (1) adenine nucleotide translocator-1 (ANT1) located on chromosome 4q35. This gene regulates the adenine nucleotide pool within mitochondria and is a structural element of the mitochondrial permeability pore; (2) chromosome 10 open reading frame 2 (C10*orf2*) gene. This gene produces Twinkle, an adenine nucleotide-dependent mtDNA helicase, alterations in which impair mtDNA replication; and (3) polymerase gamma (POLG), a gene located on chromosome 15q22–26 that produces the α subunit of polymerase γ, an enzyme required for mtDNA replication.

A number of different clinical phenotypes are associated with autosomal-dominant ophthalmoplegia. In one lineage, they included dysphagia, exercise intolerance, lactic acidosis, cataract formation, and early death; in another, affected family members had muscle atrophy, proximal muscle weakness, hearing loss, and ataxia; in another pedigree, affected individuals had cataracts, ataxia, tremor, peripheral neuropathy, mental retardation, or a combination of these manifestations.

As noted above, the MNGIE syndrome is an autosomal-recessive form of CPEO associated with a mutation in the gene on chromosome 22 that encodes the enzyme TP. Another autosomal recessively inherited form—one without ptosis—has been linked to a genetic defect at chromosome 17p13.1-p12, the nature of which has not yet been clarified. By contrast, SANDO occurs as a sporadic disorder in association with multiple mtDNA deletions.

Diagnosis

It is important to distinguish the mitochondrial myopathies from other conditions in which there is ptosis and ophthalmoparesis, such as autosomal-dominant OPMD and myasthenia gravis, because these disorders have distinctly different therapeutic and genetic implications. Muscle biopsy is the single most useful diagnostic tool for evaluating patients with suspected mitochondrial disease. The presence of RRFs on muscle biopsy, in excess of what can be accounted for by age, establishes the diagnosis of mitochondrial myopathy, and mutations of mtDNA (both deletions and point mutations) can be detected in muscle, blood, and other biopsied tissue.

The diagnosis of KSS is aided by the finding of elevated levels of lactic acid in blood or CSF and by low-density lesions in the basal ganglia on MR imaging. MRS is a valuable tool for diagnosing abnormalities of energy metabolism in brain and other tissues, but it is not available for generalized screening of patients with suspected mitochondrial mutations.

All patients with known or presumed CPEO should undergo a careful ophthalmologic assessment, including a dilated ophthalmoscopic examination to determine if a pigmentary retinopathy is present. In addition, patients with CPEO with pigmentary retinopathy or neurologic dysfunction should undergo an immediate assessment of cardiac function, and patients in whom no disturbances are found should nevertheless be monitored with periodic ECGs. Patients with CPEO who also have GI symptoms should be evaluated by a GI specialist as well as genetic testing to determine if they have the MNGIE syndrome.

Encephalomyopathy with Ophthalmoplegia from Vitamin E Deficiency

Abetalipoproteinemia, also called the Bassen–Kornzweig syndrome, is characterized by acanthocytosis, pigmentary retinopathy, progressive ataxia, and neuropathy. The disorder results from the lack of apolipoprotein B, which is essential to the transport of fat-soluble vitamins and is caused by lack of vitamin E because of impaired intestinal absorption of lipids and lipid-soluble vitamins. In fact, the neurologic disorder of abetalipoproteinemia is identical with that observed in other forms of human vitamin E deficiency, whether caused by malabsorption, cholestatic liver disease with impaired secretion of bile salts, bowel resection, or cystic fibrosis. The neurologic signs in patients with vitamin E deficiency include ataxia, areflexia, and loss of vibratory sensation due both to demyelinating neuropathy and neuronal degeneration of the cerebellum. The ocular motor abnormalities in patients with this disorder include abnormally slow voluntary saccades, slow or absent fast components of vestibular and optokinetic nystagmus, strabismus, pseudointernuclear ophthalmoplegia with dissociated nystagmus in the adducting eye on attempted horizontal gaze, moderate to severe progressive external ophthalmoplegia, and internuclear ophthalmoplegia of abduction (e.g., the posterior internuclear ophthalmoplegia of Lutz).

Many patients with vitamin E deficiency syndromes develop pigmentary retinopathy in addition to ocular motor abnormalities. This retinopathy is similar in appearance and visual outcome to the retinopathies observed in patients with mitochondrial cytopathies (see above).

Vitamin E deficiency produces a true multisystem disorder. The disease appeared initially to be a pure myopathy, because biopsy specimens from affected patients showed distinctive autofluorescent inclusions in muscle fibers. However, there is also extensive involvement of peripheral and central nerve tissue, including dystrophic changes in the brain, spinal cord, and dorsal roots.

In patients with the vitamin E deficiency syndrome, the neurologic defects, including the ocular motor disturbances, can be improved if the serum vitamin E level is restored to normal with supplemental vitamin E therapy, administered via either an oral or parenteral route. Other fat-soluble vitamins should also be administered.

Other Acquired Myopathies

The most common acquired myopathies that may have neuro-ophthalmologic significance are infectious and inflammatory myositis and dysthyroid orbitopathy. These conditions can cause diplopia from direct muscle involvement or from ischemic or inflammatory damage to one or more ocular motor nerves. They can also be associated with the development of unilateral or bilateral optic neuropathy. The optic neuropathy that occurs in patients with myositis tends to be an inflammatory or infectious optic neuritis whereas the optic neuropathy associated with dysthyroid orbitopathy results from compression of the nerve by enlarged extraocular muscles at the orbital apex. The diagnosis of these conditions usually is obvious from the clinical picture combined with appropriate imaging. The treatment depends on the manifestations and etiology and includes medical therapy, radiation therapy, strabismus surgery, orbital decompression, or a combination of these modalities.

Nystagmus and Related Ocular Motility Disorders

21

General Concepts and Clinical Approach
Normal Mechanisms for Gaze Stability
Types of Abnormal Eye Movements that Disrupt Steady Fixation: Nystagmus and Saccadic Intrusions
Differences Between Physiologic and Pathologic Nystagmus
Methods of Observing, Eliciting, and Recording Nystagmus
Classification of Nystagmus Based on Pathogenesis

Nystagmus Associated with Disease of the Visual System and Its Projections to Brainstem and Cerebellum
Origin and Nature of Nystagmus Associated with Disease of the Visual Pathways
Clinical Features of Nystagmus with Lesions Affecting the Visual Pathways
Acquired Pendular Nystagmus and Its Relationship to Disease of the Visual Pathways

Nystagmus Caused by Vestibular Imbalance
Nystagmus Caused by Peripheral Vestibular Imbalance
Nystagmus Caused by Central Vestibular Imbalance
Periodic Alternating Nystagmus
Seesaw Nystagmus

Nystagmus due to Abnormalities of the Mechanism for Holding Eccentric Gaze
Gaze-Evoked Nystagmus
Convergence-Retraction Nystagmus
Divergence Nystagmus
Centripetal and Rebound Nystagmus

Congenital Forms of Nystagmus
Congenital Motor Nystagmus
Latent (Fusional Maldevelopment) Nystagmus
Spasmus Nutans

Saccadic Intrusions
Square-Wave Jerks
Macrosquare-Wave Jerks (Square-Wave Pulses)
Macrosaccadic Oscillations
Saccadic Pulses, Ocular Flutter, and Opsoclonus

Voluntary Saccadic Oscillations or Voluntary Nystagmus

Oscillations with Disease Affecting Ocular Motoneurons and Extraocular Muscle
Superior Oblique Myokymia (Superior Oblique Microtremor)
Ocular Neuromyotonia

Spontaneous Eye Movements in Unconscious Patients

Treatments for Nystagmus and Saccadic Intrusions
Pharmacologic Treatments
Optical Treatments
Botulinum Toxin Treatment of Nystagmus
Surgical Procedures for Nystagmus
Other Forms of Treatment

General Concepts and Clinical Approach

This chapter concerns abnormal eye movements that disrupt steady fixation and thereby degrade vision. In the first section, the mechanisms by which gaze is normally held steady to achieve clear and stable vision are discussed. Next are described the pathogenesis and clinical features of each of the disorders that disrupt steady gaze, including the various forms of pathologic nystagmus and saccadic intrusions. Finally, currently available treatments for these abnormal eye movements are summarized.

Normal Mechanisms for Gaze Stability

In order for a person to see an object best, its image must be held steady over the foveal region of the retina. Although the visual system can tolerate some motion of images on the retina, if this motion becomes excessive, vision declines. Furthermore, if the image is moved from the fovea to peripheral retina, it will be seen less clearly.

In healthy persons, three separate mechanisms work together to prevent deviation of the line of sight from the object of regard. The first is fixation, which has two distinct components: (a) the visual system's ability to detect retinal image drift and program corrective eye movements; and (b) the suppression of unwanted saccades that would take the eye off target. The second mechanism is the vestibulo-ocular reflex (VOR), by which eye movements compensate for head perturbations at short latency and thus maintain clear vision during natural activities, especially locomotion. The third mechanism is the ability of the brain to hold the eye at an eccentric position in the orbit against the elastic pull of the suspensory ligaments and extraocular muscles, which tend to return it toward central position. For all three gaze-holding mechanisms to work effectively, their performance must be tuned by adaptive mechanisms that monitor the visual consequences of eye movements.

Types of Abnormal Eye Movements that Disrupt Steady Fixation: Nystagmus and Saccadic Intrusions

The essential difference between nystagmus and saccadic intrusions lies in the **initial** eye movement that takes the line of sight off the object of regard. For nystagmus, it is a slow drift (or "slow phase"), as opposed to an inappropriate saccadic movement that intrudes on steady fixation. After the initial movement, corrective or other abnormal eye movements may follow. Thus, nystagmus may be defined as a repetitive, to-and-fro movement of the eyes that is initiated by a slow phase (drift). Saccadic intrusions, on the other hand, are rapid eye movements that take the eye off target. They include a spectrum of abnormal movements, ranging from single saccades to sustained saccadic oscillations.

Differences Between Physiologic and Pathologic Nystagmus

Not all nystagmus is pathologic. **Physiologic nystagmus** preserves clear vision during self-rotation. Under most circumstances, for example, during locomotion, head movements are small and the VOR is able to generate eye movements that compensate for them. Consequently, the line of sight remains pointed at the object of regard. In response to large head or body rotations, however, the VOR alone cannot preserve clear vision because the eyes are limited in their range of rotation. Thus, during sustained rotations, quick phases occur to reset the eyes into their working range: **Vestibular nystagmus**. If rotation is sustained for several seconds, the vestibular afferents no longer accurately signal head rotation, and visually driven or **optokinetic nystagmus** takes over to stop excessive slip of stationary retinal images. In contrast to vestibular and optokinetic nystagmus, **pathologic nystagmus** causes excessive drift of stationary retinal images

that degrades vision and may produce illusory motion of the seen world: **Oscillopsia**. An exception is congenital nystagmus, which may be associated with normal visual acuity and which seldom causes oscillopsia.

Nystagmus, both physiologic and pathologic, may consist of alternating slow drifts (slow phases) in one direction and corrective, resetting saccades (quick phases) in the other: **Jerk nystagmus** (Fig. 21.1A). Pathologic nystagmus may, however, also consist of smooth to-and-fro oscillations: **Pendular nystagmus** (Fig. 21.1D). Conventionally, jerk nystagmus is described according to the direction of the quick phase. Thus, if the slow movement is drifting up, the nystagmus is called "downbeating"; if the slow movement is to the right, the nystagmus is "left beating." Although it is convenient to describe the frequency, amplitude, and direction of the quick phases of the nystagmus, it is the slow phase that reflects the underlying abnormality.

Nystagmus may occur in any plane, although it is often predominantly horizontal, vertical, or torsional. Physiologic nystagmus is essentially conjugate. Pathologic nystagmus, on the other hand, may have different amplitudes in the two eyes (dissociated nystagmus), may go in different directions leading to different trajectories of nystagmus in the two eyes, or may have different temporal properties; that is, phase shift between the two eyes, leading to movements that are sometimes in opposite directions (disconjugate nystagmus).

Methods of Observing, Eliciting, and Recording Nystagmus

It is often possible to diagnose the cause of nystagmus through careful history and systematic examination of the patient. History should include duration of nystagmus, whether it interferes with vision and causes oscillopsia, and accompanying neurologic symptoms. The physician should also determine if nystagmus and attendant visual symptoms are worse with viewing far or near objects, with patient motion, or with different gaze angles (e.g., worse on right gaze). If the patient habitually tilts or turns the head, the physician should determine if these features are evident in old photographs.

Before assessing eye movements, the physician must examine the visual system to determine if the patient has any congenital or acquired afferent deficits that may indicate the cause of the nystagmus. The stability of fixation should be assessed with the eyes close to central position, viewing near and far targets, and at eccentric gaze angles. It is often useful to record the direction and amplitude of nystagmus for each of the cardinal gaze positions. If the patient has a head turn or tilt, the eyes should be observed in various

EYE POSITION

TIME

Figure 21.1 Four common slow-phase waveforms of nystagmus. **A:** Constant-velocity drift of the eyes. This occurs in nystagmus caused by peripheral or central vestibular disease and also with lesions of the cerebral hemisphere. The added quick phases give a "saw-toothed" appearance. **B:** Drift of the eyes back from an eccentric orbital position toward the midline (gaze-evoked nystagmus). The drift shows a negative exponential time course, with decreasing velocity. This waveform reflects an unsustained eye position signal caused by a "leaky" neural integrator. **C:** Drift of the eyes away from the central position with a positive exponential time course (increasing velocity). This waveform suggests an unstable neural integrator and is usually encountered in congenital nystagmus. **D:** Pendular nystagmus, which is encountered as a type of congenital nystagmus and with acquired brainstem disease. (Reprinted with permission from Leigh RJ, Zee DS. *The Neurology of Eye Movements.* 3rd ed. New York: Oxford University Press; 1999.)

directions of gaze when the head is in that position as well as when the head is held straight. During fixation, each eye should be occluded, in turn, to check for latent nystagmus. The presence of pseudo-nystagmus and oscillopsia in patients with head tremor who have lost their VOR must be differentiated from true nystagmus.

Subtle forms of nystagmus, due to low amplitude or inconstant presence, require prolonged observation over 2 to 3 minutes. Low-amplitude nystagmus may be detected only by viewing the patient's retina with an ophthalmoscope. Note, however, that the direction of horizontal or vertical nystagmus is reversed when viewed through the ophthalmoscope. The effect of **removal of fixation** should always be determined. Nystagmus caused by peripheral vestibular imbalance may be apparent **only** under these circumstances. Lid closure will, of course, remove fixation, but lid closure itself may affect nystagmus. Thus, it is better to evaluate the effects of removing fixation with the eyelids open. Several clinical methods are available, such as Frenzel goggles: 10- to 20-diopter spherical convex lenses placed in a frame that has its own light source. The goggles defocus the patient's vision, thus preventing fixation of objects, and also provide the examiner with a magnified, illuminated view of the patient's eyes. An alternative is to use two high-plus spherical lenses from a trial case, or to determine the effect of transiently covering the viewing eye during ophthalmoscopy in an otherwise dark room.

Evaluation of nystagmus is incomplete without a systematic examination of each functional class of eye movements (vestibular, optokinetic, smooth pursuit, saccades, vergence) and their effect on the nystagmus because different forms of nystagmus can be directly attributed to abnormalities of some of these movements. For example, the vestibular system can be assessed with the oculocephalic maneuver or by rotating the patient in a swivel chair for 30 seconds, then stopping the rotation and observing the eyes for the development of postrotational nystagmus. The optokinetic system can be assessed by rotating a small drum or moving a tape on which a repetitive pattern is printed. The slow phases generated with this technique represent visual tracking, including smooth pursuit, whereas the resetting quick phases are saccadic in origin.

It is often helpful to **determine the nystagmus waveform** because the shape of the slow phase often provides a pathophysiologic signature of the underlying disorder. To properly characterize nystagmus, it is important to measure eye position and velocity, as well as target position, during attempted fixation at different gaze angles, in darkness, and during vestibular, optokinetic, saccadic, pursuit, and vergence movements. Common slow-phase waveforms of nystagmus are shown in Figure 21.1.

Conventionally, nystagmus is measured in terms of its amplitude, frequency, and their product: intensity; however, visual symptoms caused by nystagmus usually correlate best with the speed of the slow phase and displacement of the image of the object of regard from the fovea.

There are many different methods now available for recording eye movements. Because many patients with nystagmus cannot accurately point their eyes at visual targets, precise measurement is best achieved with the magnetic search coil technique. This is the only technique that permits precise measurement of horizontal, vertical, and torsional oscillations over an extended range of amplitudes and frequencies. Although originally introduced as a research tool, the technique is now widely used to evaluate clinical disorders of eye movements and is well tolerated.

Classification of Nystagmus Based on Pathogenesis

The classification of nystagmus starts by relating the various forms of nystagmus to disorders of visual fixation, the VOR, or the mechanism for eccentric gaze holding.

Nystagmus Associated with Disease of the Visual System and Its Projections to Brainstem and Cerebellum

Origin and Nature of Nystagmus Associated with Disease of the Visual Pathways

Disorders of the visual pathways are often associated with nystagmus. The most obvious example is the nystagmus that accompanies blindness. At least two separate mechanisms are responsible: dysfunction of the visual fixation mechanism itself and dysfunction of the visually mediated calibration mechanism that optimizes its action. The smooth visual fixation mechanism normally stops the eyes from drifting away from a stationary object of regard. This fixation mechanism depends upon the motion detection portion of the visual system that is inherently slow, with a response time of about 100 msec that encumbers all visually mediated eye movements, including fixation, smooth pursuit, and optokinetic responses. If the response time is delayed further by disease of the visual system, the attempts by the brain to correct eye drifts may actually add to the retinal error rather than reduce it, thus leading to ocular oscillations.

Vision is also needed for recalibrating and optimizing all types of eye movements. These functions depend on visual projections to the cerebellum. Lesions at any part of this recalibration pathway can deprive the brain of signals that hold each of the eyes on the object of regard, the result being drifts of the eyes off target, leading to nystagmus.

Clinical Features of Nystagmus with Lesions Affecting the Visual Pathways

Disease of the Retina
Congenital or acquired retinal disorders causing blindness, such as Leber congenital amaurosis, lead to continuous jerk nystagmus with components in all three planes and that changes direction over the course of seconds or minutes. This nystagmus is associated with a drifting "null point"—the eye position at which nystagmus changes direction—that probably reflects inability to calibrate the ocular motor system. This type of nystagmus often shows an increasing-velocity waveform (Fig. 21.1C). Recent developments in gene therapy for retinal disorders suggest that if vision can be restored, this type of nystagmus will be suppressed.

Disease Affecting the Optic Nerves
Optic nerve disease is commonly associated with pendular nystagmus. With unilateral disease of the optic nerve, nystagmus largely affects the abnormal eye, resulting in monocular or markedly asymmetric nystagmus. When both optic nerves are affected, the amplitude of nystagmus is often greater in the eye with poorer vision (the Heimann–Bielschowsky phenomenon). This phenomenon also occurs in patients with profound amblyopia, dense cataract, and high myopia (**Video 21.1**). Oscillations may disappear when vision is restored, supporting the contention that in such cases, the ocular oscillations are caused by loss of vision rather than by any primary disorder of the ocular motor system.

Disease Affecting the Optic Chiasm
Parasellar lesions such as pituitary tumors have traditionally, albeit rarely, been associated with **seesaw nystagmus** (see below). Seesaw nystagmus also occurs in persons whose optic nerve axons do not cross in the optic chiasm, such as some patients with severe albinism. Thus, it is possible that visual inputs, especially crossed inputs, are important for optimizing vertical–torsional eye movements and if interrupted, lead to seesaw oscillations.

Disease Affecting the Postchiasmal Visual Pathway
Horizontal nystagmus is a documented finding in patients with unilateral disease of the cerebral hemispheres, especially when the lesion is large and posterior. Such patients show a constant-velocity drift of the eyes toward the intact hemisphere (i.e., quick phases directed toward the side of the lesion, which is often low amplitude) and also usually show asymmetry of horizontal smooth pursuit that can be brought out using an optokinetic tape or drum. The response is reduced when the stripes move, or the drum is rotated, toward the side of the lesion. Whether this asymmetry occurs primarily

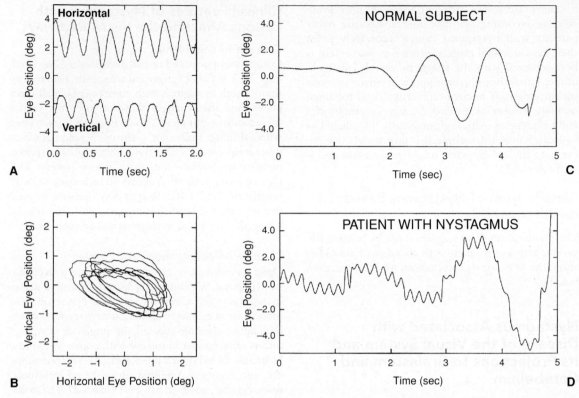

Figure 21.2 Acquired pendular nystagmus. Note both horizontal and vertical pendular waveforms. Represented as a function of time **(A)** or with coincident horizontal and vertical components at any given timepoint **(B)**. Normal subject shows volitional, slow, smooth side-to-side movements **(C)** whereas a nystagmus patient has a much faster, smaller amplitude to-and-fro movement **(D)**.

from impairment of parietal cortex necessary for directing visual attention or from disruption of cortical areas important for processing motion vision is unclear.

Acquired Pendular Nystagmus and Its Relationship to Disease of the Visual Pathways

Acquired pendular nystagmus (Fig. 21.2) is one of the more common types of nystagmus and is associated with the most distressing visual symptoms. Its pathogenesis is undefined, and more than one mechanism may be responsible. It is encountered in a variety of conditions (Table 21.1).

Acquired pendular nystagmus usually has horizontal, vertical, and torsional components with the same frequency, although one component may predominate. The temporal waveform usually approximates a sine wave, but more complex oscillations have been noted. The frequency of oscillations ranges from 1 to 8 Hz, with a typical value of 3.5 Hz. For any particular patient, the frequency tends to remain fairly constant; only rarely is the frequency of oscillations different in the two eyes. In some patients, the nystagmus stops momentarily after a saccade (**Video 21.2**). This phenomenon is called

postsaccadic suppression. Acquired pendular nystagmus may be suppressed or brought out by eyelid closure or evoked by convergence.

Acquired Pendular Nystagmus with Demyelinating Disease

Acquired pendular nystagmus is a common feature of acquired and congenital disorders of central

Table 21.1	Etiology of Pendular Nystagmus
Visual loss (including unilateral disease of the optic nerve)

Disorders of central myelin
  Multiple sclerosis
  Pelizaeus–Merzbacher disease
  Peroxisomal assembly disorders
  Cockayne syndrome
  Toluene abuse

Oculopalatal myoclonus
Acute brainstem stroke
Whipple disease
Spinocerebellar degenerations
Congenital nystagmus

myelin, such as multiple sclerosis (MS), toluene abuse, Pelizaeus–Merzbacher disease, and peroxisomal disorders. Because optic neuritis often coexists in patients with MS who have pendular nystagmus, prolonged response time of the visual processing might be responsible for the ocular oscillations. However, the nystagmus often remains unchanged in darkness, when visual inputs should have no influence on eye movements. A more likely possibility is that visual projections to the cerebellum are impaired, leading to instability in the reciprocal connections between brainstem nuclei and cerebellum that are important for recalibration.

Oculopalatal Myoclonus (Oculopalatal Tremor)

Acquired pendular nystagmus may be one component of the syndrome of oculopalatal (pharyngo-laryngo-diaphragmatic) myoclonus. This condition usually develops several months after brainstem or cerebellar infarction, although it may not be recognized until years later. Oculopalatal myoclonus also occurs with degenerative conditions. The term "myoclonus" is misleading because the movements of affected muscles are to-and-fro and are approximately synchronized, typically at a rate of about 2 cycles per second. The palatal movements thus may be termed "tremor" rather than myoclonus, and the eye movements are really a form of pendular nystagmus. Although the

palate is most often affected, movements of the eyes, facial muscles, pharynx, tongue, larynx, diaphragm, mouth of the eustachian tube, neck, trunk, and extremities may occur.

The ocular movements typically consist of to-and-fro oscillations. They often have a large vertical component, although they may also have small horizontal or torsional components. The movements may be somewhat disconjugate (both horizontally and vertically), with some orbital position dependency, and some patients show cyclovergence (torsional vergence) oscillations. Occasionally, patients develop the eye oscillations without movements of the palate, especially following brainstem infarction. Eyelid closure may bring out the vertical ocular oscillations. The nystagmus sometimes disappears with sleep, but the palatal movements usually persist. The condition is usually intractable, and spontaneous remission is uncommon.

The main pathologic finding with palatal myoclonus is hypertrophy of the inferior olivary nucleus (Fig. 21.3A), which may be seen using magnetic resonance (MR) imaging (Fig. 21.3B and C). There may also be destruction of the contralateral dentate nucleus. Histologically, the olivary nucleus has enlarged, vacuolated neurons with enlarged astrocytes. It has been postulated that the nystagmus of oculopalatal tremor results from instability in the projection from the inferior olive

A

B

C

Figure 21.3 Pathology of oculopalatal myoclonus. **A:** Section through the cerebellum and medulla shows marked demyelination of the right dentate nucleus and restiform body. The left inferior olive is hypertrophic and shows mild demyelination (*arrow*). (Reprinted with permission from Nathanson M. Palatal myoclonus; further clinical and pathophysiological observations. *Arch Neurol Psychiatr.* 1956;75:285–296.) **B:** FLAIR and **(C)** T2-weighted imaging in a patient with oculopalatal myoclonus after resection of a pontine cavernous malformation, showing left hypertrophic olivary degeneration (*arrows*).

to the cerebellar flocculus, a structure thought to be important in the adaptive control of the VOR.

Convergent-Divergent Pendular Oscillations

Vergence pendular oscillations occur in patients with MS, brainstem stroke, and cerebral Whipple disease. In Whipple disease, the oscillations typically have a frequency of about 1.0 Hz and are accompanied by concurrent contractions of the masticatory muscles, a phenomenon called oculomasticatory myorhythmia (**Video 21.3**). Supranuclear paralysis of vertical gaze also occurs in this setting and is similar to that encountered in progressive supranuclear palsy.

At least two possible explanations have been offered to account for the convergent-divergent nature of vergence pendular oscillations: A phase shift between the eyes, produced by dysfunction in the normal yoking mechanisms, or an oscillation affecting the vergence system itself. The latter explanation is more likely because patients who have been studied show no phase shift (i.e., are conjugate) vertically, and because the relationship between the horizontal and torsional components is similar to that occurring during normal vergence movements (excyclovergence with horizontal convergence).

Nystagmus Caused by Vestibular Imbalance

Nystagmus related to imbalance in the vestibular pathway can be caused by damage to peripheral or central structures. Because the nystagmus varies, it usually is possible to distinguish nystagmus caused by peripheral vestibular imbalance from nystagmus caused by central vestibular imbalance.

Nystagmus Caused by Peripheral Vestibular Imbalance

Clinical Features of Peripheral Vestibular Nystagmus

Disease affecting the peripheral vestibular pathway (i.e., the labyrinth, vestibular nerve, and its root entry zone) causes nystagmus with linear slow phases (Fig. 21.1A). Such unidirectional slow-phase drifts reflect an imbalance in the level of tonic neural activity in the vestibular nuclei. If disease leads to reduced activity, for example, in the vestibular nuclei on the left side, then the vestibular nuclei on the right side will drive the eyes in a slow phase to the left. In this example, quick phases will be directed to the right—away from the side of the lesion. Two features of the nystagmus itself are useful in identifying the vestibular periphery as the culprit: Its trajectory (direction) and whether it is suppressed by visual fixation.

The trajectory of nystagmus can often be related to the geometric relationships of the semicircular canals and to the finding that experimental stimulation of an individual canal produces nystagmus in the plane of that canal. Thus, complete unilateral labyrinthine destruction leads to a mixed horizontal–torsional nystagmus (the sum of canal directions from one ear), whereas in benign paroxysmal positional vertigo (BPPV), a mixed upbeat–torsional nystagmus reflects posterior semicircular canal stimulation. Pure vertical or pure torsional nystagmus almost never occurs with peripheral vestibular disease because this would require selective lesions of individual canals from one or both ears, an unlikely event.

Nystagmus caused by disease of the vestibular periphery often is more prominent, or may only become apparent, when visual fixation is prevented. The reason for this is that when visually generated eye movements are working normally, as they usually are in patients with peripheral vestibular disease, they will slow or stop the eyes from drifting.

Another common, but not specific, feature of nystagmus caused by peripheral vestibular disease is that its intensity increases when the eyes are turned in the direction of the quick phase—**Alexander's law**. This probably reflects an adaptive strategy developed to counteract the drift of the vestibular nystagmus and so establish an orbital position (i.e., in the direction of the slow phases) in which the eyes are quiet and vision is clear. This phenomenon forms the basis for a common classification of unidirectional nystagmus. Nystagmus is called "first degree" if it is present only on looking in the direction of the quick phases, "second degree" if it is also present in the central position, and "third degree" if it is present on looking in all directions of gaze.

Although these clinical features help make the diagnosis of peripheral vestibular disease, it is important to realize that brainstem and cerebellar disorders may sometimes mimic peripheral disease and, especially in elderly patients or those with risk factors for vascular disease, careful observation is the prudent course.

Peripheral Vestibular Nystagmus Induced by Change of Head Position

Vestibular nystagmus is often influenced by changes in head position. This feature can be used to aid in diagnosis, especially of **BPPV**. Patients with BPPV complain of brief episodes of vertigo precipitated by change of head position, such as when they turn over in bed or look up to a high shelf. The condition may follow head injury or viral neurolabyrinthitis.

To test for nystagmus and vertigo in a patient with possible BPPV, the examiner should place the patient supine and turn the head toward one shoulder and then quickly move the head and neck together into a head-hanging (down 30 to 45 degrees) position. About 2 to 5 seconds after the affected ear is moved to this dependent position, a patient with BPPV will report the onset of vertigo, and a mixed upbeat–torsional nystagmus, best viewed with Frenzel goggles, will develop. The direction of the nystagmus changes with the direction of gaze. Upon looking toward the dependent ear, it becomes more torsional; on looking toward the higher ear, it becomes more vertical. This pattern of nystagmus corresponds closely to stimulation of the posterior semicircular canal of the dependent ear (which causes slow phases mainly by activating the ipsilateral superior oblique and contralateral inferior rectus muscles). The nystagmus increases for up to 10 seconds, but it then fatigues and is usually gone by 40 seconds. When the patient sits back up, a similar but milder recurrence of these symptoms occurs, with the nystagmus being directed opposite to the initial nystagmus. Repeating this procedure several times will decrease the symptoms and make the signs more difficult to elicit. This habituation of the response is of diagnostic value because a clinical picture similar to that of BPPV can be caused by cerebellar tumors, MS, or posterior circulation infarction. With such central processes, however, there is no latency to onset of nystagmus and no habituation of the response with repetitive testing.

Otolithic debris in the respective canals (canalolithiasis) interferes with the flow of endolymph or movement of the cupula and is probably responsible for BPPV. Neck movement causing vertebrobasilar kinking and vertigo as an isolated manifestation of transient brainstem ischemia is an uncommon mechanism; in such cases, associated neurologic symptoms are usually present.

Peripheral Vestibular Nystagmus Induced by Proprioceptive and Auditory Stimuli

The perception of passive body motion relies primarily on vestibular and visual information. However, an illusion of body rotation accompanied by a conjugate, horizontal, jerk nystagmus—**arthrokinetic nystagmus**—can be induced when the horizontally extended arm of a normal, stationary subject is passively rotated about a vertical axis in the shoulder joint. The slow phase of the nystagmus is in a direction opposite to that of the arm movement. The mean slow-phase velocity increases with increasing arm velocity, and the nystagmus continues for a short time following cessation of arm movement (arthrokinetic after-nystagmus). The existence of arthrokinetic circularvection and nystagmus suggests that there exists in normal humans a functionally significant somatosensory–vestibular interaction within the vestibular system, at least for afferent pathways carrying position and kinesthetic information from the joints.

Normal stationary subjects in darkness may experience illusory self-rotation when exposed to a rotating sound field. This illusion is generally accompanied by **audiokinetic nystagmus**, which is conjugate and horizontal, with the slow phase in the direction opposite to that of the experienced self-rotation. This nystagmus indicates that apparent, as well as actual, body orientation can influence ocular motor control. Neither the illusory self-rotation nor the nystagmus occurs when the subject is exposed to a rotating sound field in the light, suggesting that visual information must dominate auditory information in determining apparent body orientation and sensory localization. Patients who develop vestibular symptoms and nystagmus when exposed to certain sounds—**Tullio phenomenon**—often have dehiscence of the superior semicircular canal or pathologic stimulation of otolithic organs.

Peripheral Vestibular Nystagmus Induced by Caloric Stimulation

Nystagmus induced by caloric stimulation of one ear has all the features of that caused by unilateral or asymmetric peripheral vestibular disease. During caloric stimulation, a temperature gradient across the temporal bone induces a convection current in the endolymph of a semicircular canal if it is orientated vertical to the earth. Before attempting to induce caloric nystagmus, the physician must first check that the tympanic membrane is visible and intact. The subject is then placed supine and the neck is flexed 30 degrees. A cold stimulus (30°C) induces horizontal slow-phase components directed toward the stimulated ear (quick phases in the opposite direction). With a warm stimulus (44°C) and the same head orientation, quick phases are toward the stimulated ear (hence the mnemonic, **COWS:** Cold-opposite, warm-same).

Caloric stimulation is an important way to test each peripheral labyrinth. Testing with ice-cold water is especially useful in the evaluation of the unconscious patient. In this setting, tonic eye deviation indicates preservation of pontine function. Induction of caloric nystagmus is also a useful way to confirm preservation of consciousness in patients feigning coma.

Nystagmus Caused by Central Vestibular Imbalance

Clinical Features of Central Vestibular Nystagmus

In this section, we describe the clinical features of three common forms of nystagmus thought to be caused by imbalance of central vestibular connections: Downbeat, upbeat, and torsional nystagmus. We also discuss the less common phenomenon of horizontal nystagmus caused by central vestibular imbalance. Finally, we offer a pathophysiologic scheme to account for these forms of central vestibular nystagmus.

Table 21.2 Etiology of Downbeat Nystagmus

Cerebellar degeneration, including familial episodic ataxia, and paraneoplastic degeneration

Craniocervical anomalies, including Chiari I malformation

Infarction of brainstem or cerebellum

Dolichoectasia of the vertebrobasilar artery

Multiple sclerosis

Cerebellar tumor, including hemangioblastoma

Syringobulbia

Encephalitis

Head trauma

Toxic–metabolic

Anticonvulsant medication

Lithium intoxication

Alcohol

Wernicke encephalopathy

Magnesium depletion

Vitamin B_{12} deficiency

Toluene abuse

Congenital

Transient finding in otherwise normal infants

Figure 21.4 One cause of downbeat nystagmus. Sagittal MRI shows Chiari I malformation with characteristic cerebellar tonsillar descent through the foramen magnum. Decompression of the malformation resulted in resolution of the nystagmus.

Downbeat nystagmus occurs in a variety of disorders (Table 21.2), but it is most commonly associated with disease affecting the vestibulocerebellum—the flocculus, paraflocculus, nodulus, and uvula—and the underlying medulla. These include intrinsic brainstem and cerebellar lesions, such as MS and the Chiari I malformation (Fig. 21.4), and extrinsic lesions of the craniocervical junction such as meningioma. It may also be a manifestation of drug intoxication, notably by lithium. Downbeat nystagmus is usually present with the eyes in central position, but its amplitude may be so small that it can only be detected by viewing the ocular fundus with an ophthalmoscope. Generally, Alexander's law is obeyed in that the nystagmus intensity is greatest in downgaze and least in upgaze. Most often, it is enhanced by having the patient look down and to one side (**Video 21.4**). Unlike patients with peripheral vestibular nystagmus, downbeat nystagmus does not change substantially with removal of fixation (e.g., with Frenzel goggles).

A variety of ocular motor abnormalities often accompany downbeat nystagmus and reflect coincident cerebellar involvement. These include abnormal vertical smooth pursuit and vertical VOR, skew deviation, and impairment of eccentric horizontal gaze holding, smooth pursuit, and combined eye-head tracking.

Upbeat nystagmus that is present with the eyes close to central position occurs in many clinical conditions (Table 21.3). It is most commonly reported in patients with medullary lesions that affect the perihypoglossal nuclei and adjacent medial vestibular nucleus (structures important for gaze holding) and the ventral tegmentum, which contains projections

Table 21.3 Etiology of Upbeat Nystagmus

Cerebellar degenerations, including familial episodic ataxia

Multiple sclerosis

Infarction of medulla, midbrain, or cerebellum

Tumors of the medulla, midbrain, or cerebellum

Wernicke encephalopathy

Brainstem encephalitis

Behçet syndrome

Meningitis

Leber congenital amaurosis or other congenital disorder of the anterior visual pathways

Thalamic arteriovenous malformation

Organophosphate poisoning

Tobacco

Associated with middle ear disease

Congenital

Transient finding in otherwise normal infants

Figure 21.5 One cause of upbeat nystagmus. Axial MRI shows hyperintense signal in the medulla of a patient with upbeat nystagmus and multiple sclerosis.

Table 21.4	Etiology of Torsional Nystagmus
Syringobulbia, with or without syringomyelia and Chiari I malformation	
Brainstem stroke (Wallenberg syndrome)	
Brainstem arteriovenous malformation	
Brainstem tumor	
Multiple sclerosis	
Oculopalatal myoclonus	
Head trauma	
Congenital	
Associated with the ocular tilt reaction	

from the vestibular nuclei that receive inputs from the anterior semicircular canals (Fig. 21.5). It also occurs in patients with lesions affecting the caudal medulla, anterior vermis of the cerebellum, or the adjacent brachium conjunctivum and midbrain. Regardless of the location or nature of the lesion, nystagmus intensity is usually greatest in upgaze (e.g., it obeys Alexander's law), it usually does not increase on right or left gaze, and removal of visual fixation has little or no effect on its waveform (**Video 21.5**). Convergence may enhance or suppress upbeat nystagmus and may even convert it to downbeat nystagmus. As is the case with downbeat nystagmus, patients with upbeat nystagmus often show asymmetries of vertical vestibular and smooth pursuit eye movements, as well as associated cerebellar eye movement findings.

Torsional nystagmus is a much less common form of central vestibular nystagmus than downbeat or upbeat nystagmus. It is often difficult to detect except by careful observation of conjunctival vessels or by noting the direction of retinal movement on either side of the fovea, using an ophthalmoscope or contact lens (**Video 21.6**). Although both peripheral vestibular and congenital nystagmus may have torsional components, purely torsional nystagmus, like purely vertical nystagmus, indicates disease affecting central vestibular connections (see Table 21.4). Torsional nystagmus shares many of the features of downbeat and upbeat nystagmus, including modulation by head rotations, variable slow-phase waveforms, and suppression by convergence.

Horizontal nystagmus in central position from central vestibular imbalance is an uncommon but well-documented phenomenon. The underlying disorder usually is a Chiari malformation. The slow-phase waveform in this form of nystagmus may be of the increasing-velocity type, making distinction from congenital nystagmus potentially difficult. However, patients with acquired central vestibular horizontal nystagmus typically report recent onset of visual symptoms, such as oscillopsia, and measurements usually demonstrate an associated vertical component that is absent in congenital nystagmus. Patients with horizontal nystagmus that is present in the central position always should be observed continuously for 2 to 3 minutes to exclude the possibility that the nystagmus is actually periodic alternating nystagmus (see below).

Periodic Alternating Nystagmus

Periodic alternating nystagmus (PAN) is a spontaneous horizontal nystagmus, present in central gaze that reverses direction approximately every 90 to 120 seconds (**Video 21.7**). Because the period of oscillation is about 4 minutes, the disorder may be missed unless the examiner observes the nystagmus for several minutes. As the nystagmus finishes one half-cycle (e.g., of right-beating nystagmus), a brief transition period occurs during which there may be upbeating or downbeating nystagmus or saccadic movements before the next half-cycle (e.g., of left-beating nystagmus) starts. A congenital form of PAN also exists, but this is usually much less regular in the timing of reversal of direction and shows slow-phase waveforms typical of congenital nystagmus. PAN must be differentiated from "ping-pong gaze," an ocular deviation that reverses direction not over several minutes but every few seconds and that is encountered in unconscious patients with large bihemispheric lesions.

Acquired PAN occurs in association with a number of conditions (Table 21.5), many of which affect the

Table 21.5 Etiology of Periodic Alternating Nystagmus

Chiari malformations and other hindbrain anomalies

Multiple sclerosis

Cerebellar degenerations

Cerebellar tumor, abscess, cyst, and other mass lesion

Creutzfeldt–Jakob disease

Ataxia telangiectasia

Brainstem infarction

Anticonvulsant medications

Lithium intoxication

Infections affecting cerebellum, including syphilis

Hepatic encephalopathy

Trauma

Following visual loss (from vitreous hemorrhage or cataract)

Congenital nystagmus

Table 21.6 Etiology of Seesaw Nystagmus

Mesodiencephalic disease[a]

Parasellar masses

Brainstem stroke

Septo-optic dysplasia

Chiari I malformation

Syringobulbia

Retinitis pigmentosa

Head trauma

Congenital form, including agenesis of optic chiasm, and as a transient finding in albinism

[a]Includes hemi-seesaw nystagmus.

nodulus and uvula of the cerebellum. Baclofen abolishes this nystagmus.

Seesaw Nystagmus

In seesaw and hemi-seesaw nystagmus, one half-cycle consists of elevation and intorsion of one eye and synchronous depression and extorsion of the other eye; during the next half-cycle, the vertical and torsional movements reverse (Fig. 21.6, **Video 21.8**). Seesaw nystagmus may be congenital or acquired (Table 21.6), and the waveform may be pendular or jerk.

Jerk seesaw nystagmus is often referred to as "hemi-seesaw" nystagmus and often occurs in patients with lesions in the region of the interstitial nucleus of Cajal (INC). Such patients also often have a contralateral **ocular tilt reaction**. With a right INC lesion, the reaction consists of a left head tilt, a skew deviation with a right hypertopia, tonic intorsion of the right eye and extorsion of the left eye, and misperception that earth-vertical is tilted to the left.

Pendular seesaw nystagmus occurs most often in patients with large tumors in the region of the optic chiasm and diencephalons. Although these oscillations have been attributed to either compression of the diencephalon or to the effects of chiasmal visual field defects, both the jerk and pendular forms probably arise from imbalance or miscalibration of vestibular responses that normally function to optimize gaze during head rotations in roll.

Nystagmus due to Abnormalities of the Mechanism for Holding Eccentric Gaze

Gaze-Evoked Nystagmus

Nystagmus that is induced by turning the eye to an eccentric position in the orbit is called **gaze-evoked nystagmus**. It is the most common form of nystagmus encountered in clinical practice. Although the terms gaze-evoked nystagmus, end-point nystagmus, and gaze-paretic nystagmus are often used synonymously, gaze-evoked nystagmus is a general term that includes both physiologic and pathologic nystagmus. When gaze-evoked nystagmus is physiologic, the term **end-point nystagmus** is appropriate (see below). When gaze-evoked nystagmus is associated with a paresis of gaze, as in patients with ocular motor nerve palsies or weakness of the extraocular muscles, the term **gaze-paretic nystagmus** is appropriate.

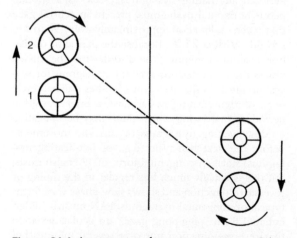

Figure 21.6 Appearance of seesaw nystagmus. Schematic drawing showing that as the right eye elevates, it also intorts. At the same time, the left eye depresses and extorts. The right eye then depresses and extorts, while the left eye elevates and intorts.

Gaze-evoked nystagmus usually occurs on lateral or upward gaze, seldom on looking down. If fixation is impaired or prevented (e.g., in darkness), the slow phases consist of centripetal drifts that may have an exponentially decaying waveform (Fig. 21.1B). If visual fixation is possible, however, the slow phases have a more linear profile.

Gaze-evoked nystagmus is caused by a deficient step of innervation, such that the eyes cannot be maintained at an eccentric orbital position and are pulled back toward the central position by the elastic forces of the orbital fascia. Corrective quick phases then move the eyes back toward the desired position in the orbit.

Gaze-evoked nystagmus may be caused by a variety of medications, including alcohol, anticonvulsants, and sedatives. It may also be caused by structural lesions that damage the gaze-holding neural network, particularly lesions of the nucleus prepositus hypoglossi/medial vestibular nucleus region.

Another cause of gaze-evoked nystagmus is familial episodic ataxia type 2 (EA-2), which is characterized by attacks of ataxia and vertigo lasting hours, with interictal nystagmus. The nystagmus is typically gaze-evoked, with a vertical component that can be downbeat or upbeat.

Differences Between Physiologic End-Point Nystagmus and Pathologic Gaze-Evoked Nystagmus

Gaze-evoked nystagmus is commonly encountered in normal subjects, in which case, as noted above, it should be referred to as end-point nystagmus. End-point nystagmus typically occurs on looking far to the right or left and is poorly sustained. It usually is horizontal and symmetric, but it may be asymmetric, being more prominent on looking to one side than to the other. Most importantly, however, end-point nystagmus is not accompanied by any other ocular motor abnormalities, whereas pathologic gaze-evoked nystagmus tends to be accompanied by other defects of eye movements, such as impaired smooth pursuit.

Dissociated Nystagmus

A special type of pathologic gaze-evoked nystagmus is dissociated or "ataxic" nystagmus. This type of nystagmus is most commonly encountered in patients with an **internuclear ophthalmoplegia** (INO). In such cases, the nystagmus is present only in the abducting eye, not the adducting eye (**Video 21.9**). Several explanations have been offered to account for dissociated nystagmus in INO, with the most plausible suggestion being that it represents an attempt by the brain to adaptively correct hypometric saccades due to the weak medial rectus muscle.

Dissociated nystagmus is, in fact, a series of saccades followed by postsaccadic drift that occurs when the patient attempts to look laterally away from the side of the lesion. Because the oscillations are initiated by saccades, this ocular motor abnormality is not a true nystagmus, but rather a series of saccadic pulses.

In addition to previous extraocular muscle surgery, both myasthenia gravis and the Miller Fisher variant of Guillain–Barré syndrome may produce a dissociated nystagmus similar to that seen in an INO.

Dissociated nystagmus characterized by larger movements in the **adducting** eye occurs when some patients with abducens nerve palsy look into the paretic field (9). Indeed, whenever a patient habitually prefers to fixate with a paretic eye, the normal eye will show a dissociated nystagmus while looking in the direction of action of the paretic muscle, regardless of the pathogenesis of the weakness.

Bruns Nystagmus

Tumors in the cerebellopontine angle, such as meningiomas or schwannomas of the vestibulocochlear nerve, may produce a low-frequency, large-amplitude nystagmus when the patient looks toward the side of the lesion, and a high-frequency, small-amplitude nystagmus when the patient looks toward the side opposite the lesion. The nystagmus that occurs on gaze toward the side of the lesion is gaze-evoked nystagmus caused by defective gaze holding, whereas the nystagmus that occurs during gaze toward the side opposite the lesion is caused by vestibular imbalance. This special nystagmus is called **Bruns nystagmus**.

Convergence-Retraction Nystagmus

The so-called convergence-retraction nystagmus is characterized by quick phases that converge or retract the eyes on attempts to look up. It is elicited either by asking the patient to make an upward saccade or by using a handheld optokinetic drum or tape and moving the stripes or figures down. This maneuver produces slow, downward, pursuit eye movements, but upward quick phases are replaced by rapid convergent movements, retractory movements, or both. Affected patients usually have impaired or absent upward gaze for both pursuit and saccadic eye movements; however, in some cases there is pursuit-saccadic dissociation: Upward pursuit appears normal, whereas upward saccades are obviously slow or absent.

Convergence-retraction nystagmus is commonly produced by lesions of the mesencephalon that damage the posterior commissure, such as pineal tumors (Fig. 21.7, **Video 21.10**). It may also occur with a Chiari malformation or during epileptic seizures.

Convergence-retraction nystagmus is usually intermittent, being determined by saccadic activity, and it thus can be differentiated from other more continuous forms of disjunctive nystagmus, such as

Figure 21.7 Lesion causing convergence-retraction nystagmus. Pineal gland involvement in a 22-year-old man with germinoma resulted in partial dorsal mibrain syndrome with an inability to elevate the eyes above the horizontal midline.

convergent-divergent pendular nystagmus and the oculomasticatory myorhythmia characteristic of Whipple disease (**Video 21.3**).

Divergence Nystagmus

Jerk-waveform **divergence nystagmus** is rare, but it may occur in patients with chronic cerebellar dysfunction, such as that which occurs in the Chiari malformation or MS. In such cases, slow phases are directed inward and fast phases outward.

Centripetal and Rebound Nystagmus

If a patient with gaze-evoked nystagmus attempts to look eccentrically for a sustained period, the nystagmus may begin to decrease in amplitude and may even reverse direction, so that the eye begins to drift centrifugally ("centripetal nystagmus"). If the eyes are then returned to the central position, a short-lived nystagmus with slow drifts in the direction of the prior eccentric gaze occurs. This is called **rebound nystagmus**. Rebound nystagmus typically occurs in patients with chronic cerebellar disease, most often MS.

Congenital Forms of Nystagmus

In this section, we review those forms of nystagmus that develop during infancy. Three distinct syndromes are currently recognized: congenital motor nystagmus, latent (fusional maldevelopment) nystagmus, and spasmus nutans.

Congenital Motor Nystagmus

Clinical Features

Congenital nystagmus is usually diagnosed during infancy, but occasionally presents during adult life when it may create a diagnostic problem, especially if the patient has other symptoms, such as headaches or dizziness. Certain clinical features usually differentiate congenital nystagmus from other ocular oscillations. It is almost always conjugate and horizontal, even on up or down gaze. A small torsional component to the nystagmus is common but difficult to identify clinically. Only rarely is congenital nystagmus purely vertical. Congenital nystagmus is usually accentuated by the attempt to visually fixate a distant object, whereas eyelid closure and convergence usually suppress it. Congenital nystagmus often decreases when the eyes are moved into a particular position in the orbit, called the "null" region.

Congenital nystagmus has one of three waveforms: jerk, pendular, or mixed. Frequently superimposed on these waveforms are **foveation periods**—the hallmark of congenital nystagmus. During each cycle, usually after a quick phase, there is a brief period when the eye is still and is pointed at the object of regard. Such periods probably are one reason (along with elevated thresholds for motion detection) that most patients with congenital nystagmus do not complain of oscillopsia, despite otherwise nearly continuous movement of their eyes, and why many have normal visual acuity. Foveation periods are not invariably present in congenital nystagmus, however, and when they are absent or poorly developed, vision is usually impaired. Patients with acquired nystagmus almost never have foveation periods.

A commonly described finding in patients with congenital nystagmus is "inverted pursuit" or "reversed optokinetic nystagmus." With a handheld optokinetic drum or tape, quick phases are directed in the same direction as the drum rotates or the tape moves. This is different from normal persons who make pursuit movements in the direction of drum rotation or tape movement and quick phases in the opposite direction.

Head turns are common in patients with congenital nystagmus and are an adaptive strategy to bring the eyes close to the null position in the orbit, where nystagmus is reduced. The observation of such a head turn in childhood photographs is often helpful in diagnosing congenital nystagmus. Another strategy used by patients with either congenital or latent nystagmus is to purposely induce an esotropia to suppress the nystagmus. Such an esotropia requires a head turn to direct the viewing eye at the object of interest. This phenomenon is called the nystagmus blockage syndrome.

Some patients with congenital nystagmus also show head oscillations. Such head movements cannot act as an adaptive strategy to improve vision, however, unless the VOR is negated. Because most patients with congenital nystagmus have a normal VOR, their head movements are not compensatory but rather represent a pathologic process.

Pathogenesis of Congenital Nystagmus

Congenital motor nystagmus may arise when abnormal tendon end organs of the extraocular muscles fail to provide adequate proprioceptive feedback to the ocular motor system. By contrast, afferent visual pathway disorders may produce a clinical similar but pathologically distinct early-onset nystagmus. Disorders associated with this "sensory" congenital nystagmus include ocular and oculocutaneous albinism, achromatopsia, retinal cone dystrophy, optic nerve hypoplasia, Leber congenital amaurosis, retinal coloboma, aniridia, corectopia, congenital stationary night blindness, Chédiak–Higashi syndrome, Joubert syndrome, and peroxisomal disorders. Clinical distinction of the two forms is essential because successful treatment of motor nystagmus is associated with improvement in visual sensory function, whereas elimination of sensory nystagmus does not result in improved vision. Because of the many diagnostic possibilities, a complete ophthalmologic evaluation and an electroretinogram should be performed in patients with congenital nystagmus associated with decreased visual acuity or visual dysfunction.

Congenital nystagmus, both with and without associated visual system abnormalities, may be familial. Several modes of inheritance have been reported, including autosomal-recessive, autosomal dominant, and X linked.

Latent (Fusional Maldevelopment) Nystagmus

Latent nystagmus is a horizontal jerk nystagmus that is absent when both eyes are viewing but appears when one eye is covered. This conjugate nystagmus is characterized by quick phases of both eyes that beat toward the side of the fixating eye; this phenomenon is not seen in other types of nystagmus. In many patients, a low-amplitude nystagmus is also present when both eyes are viewing, and is called "manifest latent nystagmus." Latent nystagmus usually reverses direction upon covering of either eye.

Latent nystagmus is usually associated with strabismus, typically esotropia. Amblyopia is frequent, whereas binocular vision with normal stereopsis is rare. Latent nystagmus usually follows Alexander's law, with the nystagmus being greatest on looking in the direction of the quick phases, away from the covered eye. Thus, some patients turn the head to keep the viewing eye in an adducted position, where nystagmus is minimal. In addition to strabismus, patients with latent nystagmus frequently show an upward deviation of the covered eye (dissociated vertical deviation). In such patients, the nystagmus often has a torsional component.

Latent nystagmus may be caused by a defect in cortical motion processing that results from lack of development of binocular vision. A related theory is that latent nystagmus is caused by an imbalance in the subcortical optokinetic system, perhaps secondary to a loss of cortical motion detectors. Another theory is that latent nystagmus is caused by a defect in the influence of the internal representation of egocentric coordinates upon the direction of gaze. These proposed mechanisms are not mutually exclusive.

Latent nystagmus is quite common, and its recognition and accurate diagnosis are important to avoid inappropriate investigations.

Spasmus Nutans

Spasmus nutans is characterized by the triad of nystagmus, head nodding, and an anomalous head position, such as torticollis. It usually begins in the first year of life, although it may not be detected until the child is 3 or 4 years old. Neurologic abnormalities are absent, although strabismus or amblyopia may coexist. The syndrome is sometimes familial and has been reported in monozygotic twins. Spasmus nutans spontaneously remits, usually within 1 to 2 years after onset, although it may last for over 8 years.

The most consistent feature of spasmus nutans is the nystagmus, although head nodding may be the first abnormality to be noticed (**Video 21.11**). Because the nystagmus is usually intermittent and has a small-amplitude, high-frequency (3 to 11 Hz) pendular waveform, it can easily be overlooked. When recognized, however, it has a "shimmering" quality.

The nystagmus of spasmus nutans almost always differs in the two eyes, and it may even be monocular. Other features that differentiate it from simple congenital nystagmus are the variability of the amplitude of nystagmus in each eye and the difference in the phase relationship between the two eyes. Even over the course of a few seconds or minutes, the oscillations may variably be conjugate, disconjugate, dissociated, or purely monocular. The plane of the nystagmus is predominantly horizontal, but it may have vertical or torsional components. It may be brought out by evoking the near response.

The head nodding of spasmus nutans is irregular, with horizontal or vertical components. It is usually more prominent when the child attempts to inspect something of interest. About two-thirds of patients have an additional head tilt or turn. In some patients, the head nodding appears to turn off the nystagmus; however, it is unclear if head nodding, turning, or tilting are always adaptive strategies adopted to reduce the nystagmus or are simply another manifestation of the underlying abnormality in the central nervous system.

Spasmus nutans is a benign, self-limited disorder. However, retinal and optic pathway disease, including chiasmal glioma, may cause a clinically indistinguishable syndrome (**Video 21.12**). Thus, a careful ophthalmologic evaluation must be performed in all children, and neuroimaging studies should be obtained unless serious contraindications are present.

Saccadic Intrusions

Several types of inappropriate saccadic eye movements may intrude upon steady fixation. These **saccadic intrusions** must be differentiated from nystagmus, in which a drift of the eyes from the desired position of gaze is the primary abnormality, and from saccadic dysmetria (Fig. 21.8A), in which the eye over- or under-shoots a target, sometimes several times, before achieving stable fixation. In this section, we first describe the characteristics of each type of saccadic intrusion and then review possible mechanisms of pathogenesis.

Square-Wave Jerks

Square-wave jerks, also called Gegenrücke, are a common finding in healthy persons, particularly the elderly. They are best seen when the patient attempts to fixate a distant or near target and consist of small, conjugate saccades, ranging from 0.5 to 5.0 degrees in size that take the eye away from fixation and return it after about 200 msec (Fig. 21.8C, **Video 21.13**). Their profile on ocular motor recordings (the eyes move rapidly away from fixation, stay in a stable position for about 200 msec, and then return to fixation, thus producing a "square-wave" pattern) is the source of their name.

Square-wave jerks with an increased frequency (up to 2 Hz) occur in certain cerebellar syndromes, in progressive supranuclear palsy, and in cerebral hemispheric disease. When very frequent, they are called square-wave oscillations, and such movements may be mistaken for nystagmus. Cigarette smoking increases the frequency of square-wave jerks.

Macrosquare-Wave Jerks (Square-Wave Pulses)

Macrosquare-wave jerks are large eye movements, typically greater than 5 degrees that occur at a frequency

Figure 21.8 Schematic drawings of various saccadic oscillations. **A:** Saccadic dysmetria: Saccades with inappropriate amplitudes that occur in response to target jumps. **B:** Macrosaccadic oscillations: Hypermetric saccades about the position of the target. **C:** Square-wave jerks: Small, inappropriately occurring saccades away from and back to the position of the target. **D:** Macrosquare-wave jerks: Large, uncalled-for saccades away from and back to the position of the target. **E:** Ocular flutter: To-and-fro back-to-back saccades without an intersaccadic interval. (Reprinted with permission from Leigh RJ, Zee DS. *The Neurology of Eye Movements*. 3rd ed. Philadelphia, PA: FA Davis; 1991.)

of about 2 to 3 Hz. After taking the eye off the target, they return it after a latency of about 80 msec (Fig. 21.8D). Macrosquare-wave jerks are present in both light and darkness, occur in bursts, and vary in amplitude. They are encountered in disease states that disrupt cerebellar outflow, such as MS.

Macrosaccadic Oscillations

Macrosaccadic oscillations consist of horizontal saccades that occur in bursts, initially building up and then decreasing in amplitude, with intersaccadic intervals of about 200 msec (Fig. 21.8B). Described originally in patients with cerebellar disease, macrosaccadic oscillations are thought to be an extreme form of saccadic dysmetria, in which the patient's saccades are so hypermetric that they overshoot the target continuously in both directions and thus oscillate around the fixation point. They usually are induced by a gaze shift, but they may also occur during attempted fixation and thus are often visually disabling. They may have vertical or torsional components and, occasionally, the former may be quite prominent clinically. Macrosaccadic oscillations are occasionally encountered in patients with myasthenia gravis after administration of edrophonium.

Saccadic Pulses, Ocular Flutter, and Opsoclonus

Saccadic pulses are brief intrusions upon steady fixation. They are produced when a saccadic pulse is unaccompanied by a step command. The eye movement thus consists of a saccade away from the fixation position, with a rapid drift back. Saccadic pulses may occur in series or as doublets. They are encountered in some normal subjects and in patients with MS.

Normally, there is a period of inactivity after a voluntary saccade. This intersaccadic interval usually lasts about 150 msec. Some saccadic pulses occur back-to-back without an intersaccadic interval. When these pulses occur in only one plane, usually the horizontal, they are called **ocular flutter** (Fig. 21.8E and **Video 21.14**); when they are multivectorial, they are termed **opsoclonus** or **saccadomania** (**Video 21.15**). The frequency of the oscillations of ocular flutter and opsoclonus is usually high, typically 10 to 15 cycles per second.

Sustained opsoclonus is a striking finding, in which multidirectional conjugate saccades, usually of large amplitude, interfere with steady fixation, smooth pursuit, or convergence. These movements may persist during sleep. Opsoclonus is often accompanied by myoclonus—brief jerky involuntary limb movements—hence the term "opsoclonus-myoclonus." In children, this syndrome is called "dancing eyes and dancing feet." Ataxia and encephalopathy may also accompany opsoclonus.

The causes of ocular flutter and opsoclonus are summarized in Table 21.7. In children, about 50% of cases of opsoclonus are a paraneoplastic phenomenon, resulting from the distant effect of tumors of neural crest origin, such as neuroblastoma. The remaining cases occur after a known or presumed viral infection or are of unclear origin. In adults, opsoclonus is most often a paraneoplastic condition that is associated with small-cell lung carcinoma, breast carcinoma, or other malignancies, but it also may follow a viral infection or occur spontaneously. Both children and adults with paraneoplastic opsoclonus have a variety of autoantibodies in their serum, CSF, or both, including anti-Ri, anti-Hu, and an antibody to neurofilaments.

The prognosis of idiopathic opsoclonus (including patients with manifestations of brainstem encephalitis) is generally good, although many children have

Table 21.7 Etiology of Ocular Flutter and Opsoclonus[a]
Viral encephalitis
As a component of the syndrome of myoclonic encephalopathy of infants ("dancing eyes and dancing feet")
Paraneoplastic (occult tumor, especially small-cell lung and breast cancers)
Neuroblastoma
Other tumors
Trauma (in association with hypoxia and sepsis)
Meningitis
Intracranial tumors
Hydrocephalus
Thalamic hemorrhage
Multiple sclerosis
Hyperosmolar coma
Associated with systemic disease; for example, viral hepatitis, sarcoid, AIDS
Side effects of drugs: Lithium, amitriptyline, phenytoin, and diazepam
Toxins: Chlordecone, thallium, strychnine, toluene, and organophosphates
Transient phenomenon of healthy neonates
Voluntary "nystagmus" or psychogenic flutter

[a]Not all case reports have documented the abnormality with eye movement recordings.

persistent neurologic deficits. Patients with paraneoplastic opsoclonus-myoclonus syndrome may show spontaneous remissions, irrespective of the underlying tumor. In addition, those whose tumor can be identified and treated successfully may recover completely.

Voluntary Saccadic Oscillations or Voluntary Nystagmus

About 5% to 8% of normal persons can voluntarily induce saccadic oscillations, usually by converging, a phenomenon called voluntary nystagmus (**Video 21.16**). The oscillations are conjugate, with frequency and amplitude similar to those of ocular flutter and opsoclonus. Although usually confined to the horizontal plane, voluntary nystagmus can occasionally be vertical or torsional and may be accompanied by a head tremor. Voluntary nystagmus can be produced in the light or dark and with the eyes open or closed. It causes oscillopsia and reduced visual acuity and is often accompanied by eyelid flutter, a strained facial expression, and convergence. The clinical challenge is to distinguish voluntary forms of saccadic oscillations, which have no pathologic significance, from disorders such as ocular flutter and opsoclonus, which require a complete evaluation. Voluntary nystagmus may occur as a familial trait.

Oscillations with Disease Affecting Ocular Motoneurons and Extraocular Muscle

Superior Oblique Myokymia (Superior Oblique Microtremor)

Superior oblique myokymia (SOM) is characterized symptomatically by monocular blurring of vision, tremulous sensations in the eye, brief episodes of vertical or torsional diplopia, and vertical or torsional oscillopsia. The eye movements themselves consist of monocular spasms of cyclotorsional and vertical movements that are often difficult to appreciate on gross examination, but that are usually apparent during ophthalmoscopy or slit-lamp biomicroscopy (**Video 21.17**). The attacks last less than 10 seconds and may occur many times per day. They may be elicited on by looking downward, by tilting the head toward the side of the affected eye, and by blinking.

The majority of patients with SOM have no underlying disease, although cases have been reported following trochlear nerve palsy, after mild head trauma, in the setting of MS, after brainstem stroke, and in patients with cerebellar tumor.

The etiology of SOM is unknown, but many authors believe it is a cranial nerve hyperfunction syndrome similar to trigeminal neuralgia and hemifacial spasm that is caused by vascular compression of the trochlear nerve. Relief has been reported after microvascular decompression of the trochlear nerve.

Although SOM may spontaneously resolve, it usually is a chronic disorder with variable length periods of remission. Many patients do not require treatment, but for those who do, some can be treated successfully with medication or extraocular muscle surgery (see below).

Ocular Neuromyotonia

This rare, usually monocular disorder is characterized by episodes of diplopia that are usually precipitated by holding the affected eye in eccentric gaze. These symptoms are caused by involuntary contraction of the lateral rectus muscle, the superior oblique muscle, or one or more extraocular muscles innervated by the oculomotor nerve. Extraocular muscles innervated by more than one ocular motor nerve may occasionally be affected, and rare patients with bilateral ocular neuromyotonia have been reported.

Most patients with ocular neuromyotonia have undergone previous radiation to the parasellar region, but rare cases have been reported with other pathologies (**Video 21.18**). The mechanism responsible for the condition is unknown, although both ephaptic neural transmission and changes in the pattern of neuronal transmission following denervation have been suggested.

The episodic nature of the diplopia associated with ocular neuromyotonia often suggests myasthenia gravis, but anticholinergic medicines are ineffective in this condition. Other conditions that may mimic ocular neuromyotonia include superior oblique myokymia, thyroid eye disease, and cyclic oculomotor palsy.

Spontaneous Eye Movements in Unconscious Patients

The examination of eye movements often provides important diagnostic information in unconscious patients. For example, slow conjugate or disconjugate roving eye movements similar to the eye movements of light sleep but slower than the rapid movements of paradoxic or rapid eye movement (REM) sleep indicate that brainstem gaze mechanisms are intact.

Ocular bobbing consists of intermittent, usually conjugate, rapid downward movement of the eyes followed by a slower return to central position. Reflex-induced horizontal eye movements are usually absent. Classic ocular bobbing is a sign of intrinsic pontine lesions, usually hemorrhage (Fig. 21.9), but it has also been reported in patients with cerebellar lesions that compress the pons and in patients with metabolic and toxic encephalopathies.

An inverse form of ocular bobbing is characterized by a slow downward movement and rapid return to midposition. This condition is called **ocular dipping**.

Reverse ocular bobbing is characterized by a rapid deviation of the eyes upward and a slow return to the horizontal, whereas **reverse ocular dipping** (also called converse bobbing) describes a slow upward drift of the eyes followed by a rapid return to central position. In general, the variants of ocular bobbing are less reliable for localization than is the classic form.

Ping-pong gaze consists of slow, horizontal, conjugate deviations of the eyes alternating every few seconds. Ping-pong gaze usually occurs with bilateral infarction of the cerebral hemispheres or of the cerebral peduncles.

Periodic alternating gaze deviation, in which conjugate gaze deviations change direction every 2 minutes, occurs in some patients with hepatic encephalopathy. This phenomenon is related to PAN (see above).

A

B

Figure 21.9 Pathology of ocular bobbing. **A:** Section through the midpons demonstrating a massive area of hemorrhage and necrosis in a 2-year-old girl with a pontine glioblastoma who developed a left hemiparesis, obtundation, seizures, and ocular bobbing. **B:** Organizing hematoma in the caudal portion of the basis pontis on the right side in a 57-year-old woman who developed a right gaze palsy, right facial palsy, and obtundation. (**A,** Reprinted with permission from Daroff RB, Waldman J. Ocular Bobbing. *J Neurol Neurosurg Psychiatry.* 1965;28:375–377. **B,** Reprinted with permission from Katz B, Hoyt WF, Townsend J. Ocular bobbing and unilateral pontine hemorrhage. Report of a case. *J Clin Neuroophthalmol.* 1982;2:193–195.)

Treatments for Nystagmus and Saccadic Intrusions

Although a number of drugs have been reported to improve nystagmus in individual patients, few have been subjected to controlled clinical trials. When drug treatments fail or effective drugs cannot be tolerated by the patient, certain optical devices may be used to either suppress the nystagmus or negate its visual consequences. Finally, surgery can be performed to either weaken the extraocular muscles or reattach them to the globe in such a way that the resting position of the eyes is at the null position.

Pharmacologic Treatments

Vestibular Nystagmus

Peripheral Vestibular Imbalance. Nystagmus caused by peripheral vestibular lesions usually resolves spontaneously over the course of a few days. Present approaches use vestibular suppressants for 24 to 48 hours, primarily for severe vertigo and nausea. If the nystagmus persists after this time, exercises are used to accelerate the brain's ability to redress the imbalance. In the case of BPPV, maneuvers to displace otolithic debris from the affected semicircular canal and exercises to sustain recovery are usually effective.

Central Vestibular Nystagmus. A number of drugs have been used to treat patients with downbeat nystagmus, and the most effective appears to be 4-aminopyridine, a potassium channel blocking agent. Patients must be monitored for possible seizures when using this medication. The only drug that has been found to be effective in some cases of upbeat nystagmus is baclofen.

Periodic Alternating Nystagmus

Most cases of acquired PAN respond to baclofen. Indeed, this form of nystagmus is that which is most likely to respond to medical therapy.

Acquired Pendular Nystagmus

This type of nystagmus used to be treated with barbiturates, but their efficacy is limited by their sedative side effects. Other drugs that have been found to be useful in selected patients, including those with oculopalatal myoclonus, include trihexyphenidyl, intravenous scopolamine, valproate, isoniazid, gabapentin, and memantine (Fig. 21.10). In addition to these more or less "traditional" treatments, alcohol has been reported to suppress acquired pendular nystagmus as has smoking cannabis.

Seesaw Nystagmus

Improvement in seesaw nystagmus has been reported in some patients treated with alcohol. Clonazepam

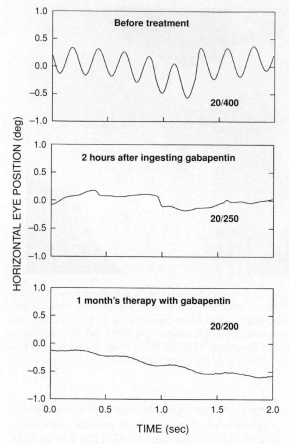

Figure 21.10 Effect of gabapentin on the horizontal component of pendular nystagmus in a 41-year-old woman with multiple sclerosis. After the initial recording (**top**), the patient was given 300 mg of gabapentin, which reduced her oscillations and improved her vision (**middle**). The effect was still present 2 months later, while she was taking a dose of 300 mg three times per day. Visual acuity measurements of the recorded eye are shown at the **right** in each panel.

reduces this type of nystagmus and its associated oscillopsia in occasional patients, as does gabapentin.

Familial Episodic Ataxia with Nystagmus

The attacks of ataxia as well as the nystagmus that occur in patients with episodic ataxia type 2 (EA-2), a calcium channelopathy, respond well to treatment with acetazolamide, as do some cases of EA-1, a potassium channelopathy.

Square-Wave Jerks and Macrosaccadic Oscillations

Several benzodiazepines (diazepam, clonazepam) and the barbiturate phenobarbital may be effective in abolishing high-amplitude square-wave jerks and macrosaccadic oscillations. There is also evidence

that amphetamines can suppress square-wave jerks in some patients.

Ocular Flutter and Opsoclonus

Patients with parainfectious opsoclonus-myoclonus often improve spontaneously, but intravenous immunoglobulin may speed recovery. Similarly, although propranolol, verapamil, clonazepam, gabapentin, and thiamine have all been reported to diminish microsaccadic ocular flutter in such patients, the effect may have been due to spontaneous remission. Opsoclonus associated with neural crest tumors in children usually responds to corticosteroid treatment; however, as noted above, up to 50% of such children have persistent neurologic disabilities, including ataxia, poor speech, and cognitive problems. Similar responses to steroids may occur in children with parainfectious or idiopathic opsoclonus. Treatment with steroids is not uniformly successful in such cases, nor are plasmapheresis, intravenous immunoglobulin, and immunoadsorption therapy.

Superior Oblique Myokymia and Ocular Neuromyotonia

Patients with SOM who request treatment may benefit from carbamazepine, propranolol, baclofen, or gabapentin given systemically or topically. Patients who do not respond to drug therapy, who develop side effects from the drugs, or who do not wish to take drugs for their condition, may experience complete relief of symptoms after extraocular muscle surgery (see below).

Ocular neuromyotonia is usually responsive to carbamazepine.

Optical Treatments

Convergence prisms provide one optical approach for patients with congenital or acquired nystagmus whose nystagmus dampens when they view a near target. In some patients with congenital nystagmus, the resultant improvement of vision is sufficient for them to qualify for a driver's license. Patients whose nystagmus is worse during near viewing may benefit from wearing base-in (divergence) prisms.

Contact lenses sometimes suppress congenital nystagmus. This effect is not from the mass of the lenses but is probably mediated via trigeminal afferents.

The main optical therapy for latent nystagmus consists of measures to improve vision, particularly patching for amblyopia in children.

Botulinum Toxin Treatment of Nystagmus

Paralysis of the extraocular muscles by direct muscular or retrobulbar injection will reduce or eliminate nystagmus in the treated eye. However, ptosis, diplopia, and worsening of nystagmus in the fellow eye frequently occur. Indeed, in one study, nystagmus was abolished or reduced in the treated eye for about 2 to 3 months, but no patient was pleased with the results because of these side effects, and none elected to continue the treatment. Botulinum toxin injection thus is not recommended for treatment of either congenital or acquired nystagmus.

Surgical Procedures for Nystagmus

Patients with congenital motor nystagmus and an eccentric null position may benefit from the Anderson–Kestenbaum operation, which is designed to move the attachments of the extraocular muscles, so that the new central position of the eyes is at the null position. It is performed after first making careful eye movement measurements of nystagmus intensity with the eyes in various positions of gaze and determining the approximate null position. The appropriate extraocular muscles are then weakened or strengthened as necessary to achieve the required shift in the position of the null. The Anderson–Kestenbaum procedure not only shifts and broadens the null region, but also results in decreased nystagmus outside the region. It is of uncertain value in the treatment of acquired forms of nystagmus.

Weakening the medial rectus muscles also may help patients with congenital nystagmus that dampens or is suppressed during near viewing and who have stereopsis. Studies comparing these two methods indicate that the artificial divergence operation generally results in a better visual outcome than the Anderson–Kestenbaum procedure alone.

Several authors have recommended performing large recessions of all of the horizontal rectus muscles

for treatment of patients with congenital nystagmus. Hertle and Dell'Osso subsequently demonstrated in a controlled trial that disinserting and reinserting the horizontal rectus muscles reduces nystagmus and improves fixation in some patients with congenital nystagmus. The mechanism by which this type of procedure suppresses nystagmus is unclear.

The role of surgery in the treatment of acquired nystagmus is not well established, although individual patients may benefit from recession operations; however, it is clear that suboccipital decompression (with opening of the dura) improves downbeat nystagmus in patients with a Chiari malformation and also prevents progression of other neurologic deficits.

As noted above, SOM that does not respond to treatment with medication may respond to extraocular muscle surgery. The procedure used by most surgeons is a superior oblique tenotomy combined with myectomy of the ipsilateral inferior oblique muscle.

Other Forms of Treatment

A variety of methods other than those described above have been used to treat nystagmus, principally the congenital variety. Electrical stimulation or vibration over the forehead may suppress congenital nystagmus. It is thought that the suppressive effect on congenital nystagmus of this treatment, like that associated with contact lenses, may be exerted via the trigeminal system, which receives extraocular proprioception. Acupuncture administered to the neck muscles may suppress congenital nystagmus in some patients via a similar mechanism. Biofeedback has also been reported to help some patients with congenital nystagmus. The role of any of these treatments in clinical practice has yet to be demonstrated.

22

Normal and Abnormal Eyelid Function

Examination of Eyelid Function
Anatomy of the Eyelid System
Anatomy of the Muscles of Eyelid Opening
Anatomy of the Muscles of Eyelid Closure

Abnormalities of Eyelid Opening
Ptosis
Apraxia of Eyelid Opening
Eyelid Retraction

Abnormalities of Eyelid Closure
Insufficiency of Eyelid Closure
Excessive or Anomalous Eyelid Closure

Disorders of neuro-ophthalmologic significance may affect not only visual sensory, ocular motor, and pupil function but also the function of the eyelids. Indeed, the inability of a patient to fully open or close his or her eyelids may be the first sign of a more extensive process, the early diagnosis and treatment of which may be crucial to the ultimate well being of the patient. This chapter describes the elements that make up a complete assessment of eyelid function, the anatomy of the structures that provide normal eyelid function, and the various pathologic processes that impair eyelid opening and closure. We focus on eyelid disorders of neuro-ophthalmologic significance and direct the reader to oculoplastic texts for coverage of other causes of ptosis.

Examination of Eyelid Function

Detailed observation of eyelid position and movement is an important but often neglected part of the neuro-ophthalmologic examination (Table 22.1). In evaluating the eyelids, one should note the resting position of the upper and lower eyelids, assess the ability of the upper eyelid to open and close, and observe the various settings in which eyelid opening and closing occur, including voluntary, reflex, and spontaneous blinking, and lid movements accompanying eye movements.

Patients with eyelid dysfunction often complain of visual problems. Many of these problems are neurologic

in origin. For example, laxity of the eyelids from a facial palsy can cause exposure keratopathy with associated blurring of vision, ocular pain, and tearing. However, the same clinical symptoms can also result from involutional changes in the elastic connective tissue supporting the lids. Ptosis, which also can be neurologic and nonneurologic in origin, can produce visual problems, even when incomplete, if the eyelashes or lid margin cover the pupil. When obtaining a history, it is important to inquire about the onset, duration and progression of the problem, and fluctuations of symptoms at different times of the day, in different seasons, and in different environmental conditions. Systemic diseases often affect eyelid function, but patients may have no reason to associate them with their eye problems. Therefore, a thorough medical history with particular attention to thyroid conditions, diabetes mellitus, systemic hypertension, myopathies, myasthenia gravis, sarcoidosis, and facial paresis should be obtained. In many situations, old photographs are useful in establishing the presence of a pre-existing condition such as ptosis or eyelid retraction, which may have only recently become symptomatic or noticed by the patient.

The detailed examination of the eyelids should proceed as outlined in Table 22.1, with the examiner noting any abnormalities or asymmetries. In addition, because abnormalities of eyelid position, function, or both often are associated with other neuro-ophthalmic signs, a complete eyelid evaluation must be accompanied by an assessment of visual sensory function, ocular motility and alignment, pupil function, function of the trigeminal and facial nerves, and the status of the orbit, particularly for signs of orbital disease such as proptosis or enophthalmos.

All lid movements result from the interaction of four simple forces: (a) an active closing force produced by the orbicularis oculi muscle; (b) an active opening force generated by the levator palpebrae superioris muscle (often called the levator muscle or, simply, "the levator"); (c) an active opening force generated by a smooth muscle—Müller muscle (also called the superior tarsal muscle); and (d) passive lid-closing forces produced by stretching of ligaments and tendons of the eyelid. For example, normal blinks result from a cessation of the tonically active levator followed by a transient burst

Table 22.1	Examination of the Eyelids

1. General observation of contour, shape, and symmetry of eyelids
2. Abnormal movements (involuntary twitches, fasciculations, and synkinesis with other facial muscles)
3. Palpebral fissure (opening) measured in primary position, and upgaze and downgaze, for each eye (contralateral eye occluded if strabismus or apparent eyelid retraction seen)
4. Measurement of the distance between the upper eyelid margin and the corneal light reflex (marginal-reflex distance, or MRD-1)
5. Levator function assessed: excursion of upper eyelid margin from downgaze to upgaze, with brow manually immobilized
6. Eyelid movement during slow pursuit from upgaze to downgaze observed for lid lag
7. Sustained upgaze for at least 1 min to assess fatigability of the levator
8. Observation for a Cogan lid-twitch (upward overshoot of the eyelid on refixation from downgaze to primary position)
9. Inspection for synkinesis between the levator and other muscles (especially the ocular motor muscles, but also occasionally with muscles innervated by cranial nerves V, VII, IX, and XI)
10. Observation of abnormal spontaneous contractions of the orbicularis oculi, procerus, frontalis, and corrugators
11. Assessment of orbicularis oculi strength by attempting to open forcibly closed eyelids

of the normally quiescent orbicularis oculi. The active orbicularis oculi force combined with passive lid-closing forces rapidly lower the lid. When the orbicularis oculi activity terminates, the tonic levator activity resumes. This action slowly raises the eyelid until the passive closing forces match the active opening forces generated by the levator. Moving the lid in conjunction with vertical eye movements involves changes only in the activity of the levator. This muscle receives an eye movement input qualitatively identical with that of its developmental progenitor, the superior rectus muscle. As the eye elevates, the tonic activity on the levator increases and raises the eyelid. With decreases in levator activity, the passive downward forces pull the lid down until the passive closing and active opening forces again match. By understanding these forces, it is possible to determine which element or elements of the lid system are affected by a local, systemic, or neurologic disorder.

Anatomy of the Eyelids

The eyelids contain three main muscles innervated by three different neural networks. The oculomotor

nerve (see Chapter 18) provides innervation to the levator palpebrae superioris muscle that keeps the eyelids open, a function assisted somewhat by Müller muscle, which is innervated by the sympathetic nervous system. Eyelid closure is achieved by contraction of the orbicularis oculi muscle, innervated by the facial nerve (see below).

Anatomy of the Muscles of Eyelid Opening

The principal muscle involved in opening the upper eyelid and in maintaining normal lid posture is the levator palpebrae superioris. Two accessory muscles of lid opening, Müller muscle and the frontalis muscle, play only minor roles.

Levator Palpebrae Superioris

The levator palpebrae superioris muscle originates at the annulus of Zinn and courses anteriorly along the superior aspect of the orbit, passing through a suspensory structure, Whitnall ligament (also called the superior transverse ligament), to which it is attached by bands of connective tissue (Fig. 22.1). The levator does not extend all the way from its origin to the superior tarsus. Instead, it begins to gradually transition from muscle to tendon just posterior to Whitnall ligament. Anterior to Whitnall ligament, it exists only as a tendinous aponeurosis. It is this aponeurosis that fuses with the orbital septum and attaches to the superior tarsus. The levator palpebrae superioris is innervated by branches of the superior division of the oculomotor nerve.

Müller Muscle

Müller muscle is a thin band of smooth muscle about 10 mm in width that inserts on the superior border of

Figure 22.1 Anatomy of the levator palpebrae superioris muscle and its aponeurosis.

Figure 22.2 Anatomy of Müller muscle. Anterior view of transected and partially dissected upper and lower eyelids. The lateral portion of the orbital septum and the levator have been excised to demonstrate adjacent relationships. Note that Müller muscle (mm) is located just underneath the levator aponeurosis (la) and inserts directly into the upper aspect of the superior tarsus (st), whereas the levator aponeurosis inserts into the anterior aspect of the tarsus (la-in). *it,* inferior tarsus; *la-lh,* lateral horn of levator aponeurosis; *lct,* lateral canthal tendon; *lg-ol,* orbital lobe of lacrimal gland; *lg-pl,* palpebral lobe of lacrimal gland; *llr,* lower lid retractors; *lof,* lateral orbital fat; *os,* orbital septum (cut edge); *paf,* preaponeurotic fat; *wl,* Whitnall ligament. (Reprinted with permission from Rootman J, Stewart B, Goldberg RA. *Orbital Surgery: A Conceptual Approach.* Philadelphia, PA: Lippincott-Raven, 1995.)

the upper tarsus (Fig. 22.2). The muscle originates 10 to 12 mm above the tarsus from tendons inserted near the origin of the levator aponeurosis. Müller's muscle is innervated by fibers of the oculosympathetic pathway.

Although Müller muscle is located in the upper eyelid, there is a similar, much smaller, sympathetically innervated muscle located in the lower eyelid. Hypofunction of this muscle (such as occurs in Horner syndrome) results in slight elevation of the lower eyelid ("upside-down" ptosis).

Frontalis and Associated Muscles

The muscles controlling the eyebrow contribute to the eyelid appearance and, to a lesser extent, its elevation. Control of the eyebrow involves three sets of muscles: frontalis, procerus, and corrugator superciliaris (Fig. 22.3). The frontalis has cutaneous insertions at the level of the eyebrow, and frontalis fibers also intermingle with peripheral orbicularis oculi muscle fibers. Contraction of the frontalis raises the entire eyebrow and the upper eyelid through its cutaneous and orbicularis

Figure 22.3 Anatomy of the orbicularis oculi, frontalis, procerus, and corrugator muscles.

oculi connections. The procerus muscle originates from the medial portion of the lower region of the frontalis muscle and inserts on the nasal bone. Contraction of this muscle pulls the medial portion of the eyebrow downward. The corrugator supraciliaris originates from the frontal bone and lies beneath the frontalis and orbicularis oculi. It extends 2 to 3 cm laterally, where it blends with the frontalis and orbicularis oculi fibers. Contraction of the corrugator supraciliaris pulls the eyebrow medially and downward.

Anatomy of the Muscles of Eyelid Closure

The primary muscle responsible for eyelid closure, the **orbicularis oculi**, is a typical striated muscle. It completely covers the orbital opening, forming concentric rings around the palpebral fissure and surrounding bone (Fig. 22.3). It is responsible not only for active eyelid closure, but also for much of the facial expression around the eyes. It can be divided into three parts: orbital, preseptal, and pretarsal.

Abnormalities of Eyelid Opening

Abnormalities of eyelid opening include **ptosis**—insufficient opening of the eyelid—which can be caused by a variety of congenital and acquired disorders, many of which are of neuro-ophthalmologic importance, **apraxia of eyelid opening (AEO)** caused by supranuclear inhibition of levator function, and eyelid **retraction**, the only pathognomonic sign of thyroid eye disease and an important sign of other neuropathic, neuromuscular, myopathic, and mechanical disorders.

Ptosis

A deficiency of levator tonus produces the clinical sign called blepharoptosis or ptosis. Ptosis may be produced by damage to the motor system controlling eyelid elevation and position at any point along the pathway, from the cerebral cortex to the levator muscle itself. Topical diagnosis of ptosis depends on the character of the deficiency and on evidence of neuropathic, neuromuscular, aponeurotic, developmental, mechanical, or myopathic disease. In this chapter, only a subset of these topics will be considered.

The degree of ptosis can be quantified clinically by measuring the height of the palpebral fissure—about 9 mm in normal subjects—assuming the lower eyelid is normally positioned. A more useful measure is the distance between the upper lid margin and the mid-corneal reflex when the globe is in primary position. This is called the MRD-1. Ptosis can be defined as an MRD-1 less than 2 mm or an asymmetry of more than 2 mm between eyes. Using this definition, most patients with ptosis exhibit a contraction of the superior visual field to 30 degrees or less.

Neurogenic Ptosis

Neurogenic ptosis may be caused by supranuclear, nuclear, or infranuclear dysfunction. In some cases, associated symptoms and signs make the distinctions among these causes obvious; in other cases, however, neither the location nor the nature of the lesion is clear.

Supranuclear Ptosis. Unilateral ptosis is a rare manifestation of hemisphere dysfunction. This manifestation, called **cortical ptosis**, usually, although not invariably, is contralateral to the lesion. Unilateral ptosis has been described contralateral to lesions of the angular gyrus, to seizure foci in the temporal lobe, to hemispheric stroke, and to frontal lobe arteriovenous malformations (AVMs). It also has been described ipsilateral to ischemic hemispheric strokes (Fig. 22.4).

Bilateral cortical ptosis can also occur. It is associated most frequently with extensive nondominant hemisphere lesions. In most instances, the ptosis is accompanied by midline shift, gaze deviation to the right, and other signs of right hemisphere dysfunction, including left hemiparesis. The ptosis is often asymmetric. In the setting of cerebral infarction, the ptosis is transient, lasting from several days to 5 months or more.

Ptosis may develop in certain eccentric positions of gaze from congenital supranuclear inhibition of the levator; that is, **supranuclear oculopalpebral synkinesia**. In such cases, lid position in primary gaze may be normal, or the lid may be slightly ptotic. When the patient adducts (or occasionally abducts) the eye on the affected

Figure 22.4 Unilateral supranuclear (cortical) ptosis. The patient developed a left ptosis associated with a left hemiparesis from a right hemisphere stroke. The patient also has a pre-existing right ptosis from dehiscence of the levator tendon. (Reprinted with permission from Caplan LR. Cerebral ptosis. *J Neurol Neurosurg Psychiatry.* 1974;37:1–7.)

Figure 22.7 The inverse Marcus Gunn phenomenon. A: When the patient looks straight ahead, she has a mild left ptosis. B: When the patient opens her mouth, the ptosis increases from inhibition of the left levator muscle.

Figure 22.5 Congenital unilateral supranuclear oculopalpebral synkinesia. A: This young child has moderate right ptosis when looking straight ahead. B: When the patient looks to the right, the position of both upper eyelids is normal. C: On left gaze, there is almost complete right ptosis from inhibition of the levator muscle. Note that the left upper eyelid remains in a normal position in all positions of gaze. (Courtesy of Dr. C. Hedges.)

which the ipsilateral eyelid closes when the external pterygoid muscle moves the jaw to the opposite side (Fig. 22.7). Patients with this condition have mild ptosis of the affected eyelid when the eyes are in primary position and the mouth is closed. The associated ptosis is consequent to levator inhibition without contraction of the orbicularis oculi. This syndrome is an inverse of the Marcus Gunn jaw-winking phenomenon (see below) and probably represents a supranuclear synkinesis affecting the oculomotor and trigeminal nerves.

side, however, the eyelid drops abruptly because of a loss of levator muscle tone. When the eye returns toward center, or toward the opposite side, the levator contracts and the eyelid returns to a normal position. The synkinesia may be unilateral (Fig. 22.5) or bilateral (Fig. 22.6). It may occur as an isolated phenomenon or in association with other congenital syndromes, such as the Duane retraction syndrome. The causes of supranuclear paradoxical levator inhibition are unclear. They may involve a variety of mechanisms, including ephaptic transmission or disturbances in the supranuclear pathways responsible for levator tonus, excitation, and inhibition.

Ptosis associated with mouth opening—**the inverse Marcus Gunn phenomenon**—is a rare condition in

Ptosis from Lesions of the Oculomotor Nucleus, Fascicle, or Nerve

By far, the most common causes of acquired neurogenic ptosis are related to dysfunction of the oculomotor nucleus, fascicle, or nerve. Because the central caudal subnucleus of the oculomotor nucleus supplies bilateral equal innervation to the levator muscles, ptosis resulting from a nuclear midbrain lesion is always bilateral and symmetric as well as usually complete or at least very severe (Fig. 22.8). This **midbrain ptosis** is commonly associated with other signs of mesencephalic dysfunction. However, in some cases, only the central caudal subnucleus of the oculomotor nuclear complex is affected or is much more severely affected than the other oculomotor subnuclei, and bilateral, severe, symmetric ptosis is the predominant or only manifestation of the nuclear lesion.

Midbrain ptosis may be congenital, occurring as a consequence of dysplasia or aplasia of the oculomotor nucleus, or acquired. Acquired causes include ischemia, inflammation, infiltration, compression, and metabolic and toxic processes.

Lesions of the **fascicle of the oculomotor nerve** produce unilateral oculomotor nerve dysfunction that may be mild or severe (see Chapter 18). When ptosis occurs in patients with a lesion of the oculomotor fascicle, it is always unilateral, of variable severity, and,

Figure 22.6 Congenital bilateral supranuclear oculopalpebral synkinesia. **Center:** In primary position, the patient has a moderate right ptosis. On right gaze **(right)**, the patient develops a marked left ptosis, whereas on left gaze **(left)**, the patient develops a marked right ptosis. (Courtesy of Dr. H. Rose.)

Figure 22.8 Midbrain ptosis. Isolated, bilateral ptosis in a patient with a mass lesion infiltrating the posterior and caudal midbrain. **A:** Severe bilateral ptosis. **B:** T1-weighted axial MRI with gadolinium shows a nonenhancing lesion involving the central aspect of midbrain. Ocular motility was completely normal.

in our experience, associated with weakness of one or more of the extraocular muscles innervated by the oculomotor nerve (Fig. 22.9). Pupillary involvement is commonly but not invariably present.

The ptosis that accompanies a lesion of the **peripheral oculomotor nerve** is, like that caused by a fascicular lesion, unilateral and usually accompanied by ophthalmoparesis, pupillary involvement, or both (Fig. 22.10). Rarely, however, ptosis precedes the other signs of oculomotor nerve dysfunction by days, weeks, or even months, depending on the location and nature of the lesion. Isolated ptosis caused by peripheral oculomotor nerve dysfunction has been reported in patients with aneurysms, pituitary adenomas, meningiomas, and meningitis. Some of these cases are examples of truly isolated ptosis. In others, there are other symptoms, for example, headache, or subtle signs of oculomotor dysfunction, a mildly dilated but reactive pupil, an incomitant phoria, or asymptomatic underaction of the superior rectus that is only evident on extreme upgaze. Recurrent, isolated ptosis lasting 6 to 8 weeks has been described with ophthalmoplegic migraine. Isolated, complete, neurogenic ptosis can also occur from orbital trauma that generates forceful anterior displacement of the upper eyelid with denervation of the levator muscle. This form of ptosis usually resolves spontaneously within weeks.

Ptosis from Lesions of the Oculosympathetic Pathways. Lesions of the oculosympathetic pathway produce **Horner syndrome**, a condition that is characterized in part by a partial, unilateral ptosis from hypofunction of Müller muscle. The ptosis of Horner syndrome is often mild, variable, and always associated with ipsilateral miosis (Fig. 22.11), in contrast to the more severe ptosis with mydriasis in an oculomotor nerve lesion. Horner syndrome is discussed in detail in Chapter 15 of this text.

The ptosis occasionally observed after conjunctival instillation of timolol maleate, a β-adrenergic–blocking agent, may be caused by Müller muscle blockade. Similarly, thymoxamine, an α-adrenergic–blocking agent, may cause ptosis when given topically or parenterally.

Myopathic Ptosis

Ptosis that occurs from damage to the levator palpebrae superioris muscle itself (as opposed to its tendon) may be either congenital (i.e., developmental) or acquired; the latter is discussed below.

Acquired Myopathic Ptosis. Acquired myopathic ptosis occurs in a number of the mitochondrial cytopathies characterized by chronic progressive external ophthalmoplegia (CPEO) (see Chapter 20). In some

Figure 22.9 Unilateral ptosis associated with other evidence of a right third nerve paresis caused by damage to the fascicle of the third nerve from a cryptococcal abscess. **A and B:** Appearance of patient; **(C)** axial and **(D)** sagittal MRI showing a ring-enhancing lesion along the path of the right oculomotor nerve fascicle (*arrows*).

Figure 22.10 Unilateral ptosis associated with other evidence of a right third nerve paresis caused by damage to the subarachnoid portion of the third nerve from an intracranial aneurysm. **A:** Appearance of patient; in primary gaze and **(B)** in different gaze positions. **C:** Angiogram in a different patient showing aneurysm (*arrow*) at the junction of the left internal carotid artery and left posterior communicating artery.

distinguish the condition from other causes of ptosis except myasthenia gravis and myotonic dystrophy.

Because the manifestations of the disease are so slowly progressive and in part because they tend to be symmetric, patients with ptosis associated with CPEO are remarkably tolerant of their symptoms, and thus generally present relatively late in their course.

Bilateral partial ptosis contributes to the characteristic appearance of patients with myotonic dystrophy.

The levator palpebrae superioris muscle may be damaged by a variety of inflammatory, ischemic, or infiltrative processes affecting the orbit. Occasionally, ptosis is the most prominent manifestation. For example, lymphoid infiltration, sarcoidosis, amyloidosis, and idiopathic inflammatory disease of the orbit can sometimes selectively affect the levator and spare the extraocular muscles. Patients with diabetes mellitus also may develop unilateral or bilateral ptosis in association with other evidence of microangiopathic changes elsewhere in the body. Although most of these patients probably have a localized infarction in the midbrain, which affects either the oculomotor nerve nucleus or fascicle, or in the peripheral oculomotor nerve, chronic hypoxia of the levator muscle is responsible for this form of ptosis in some diabetic patients.

Neuromuscular Ptosis

Recognition of neuromuscular ptosis depends in part on the absence of clinical signs of an oculomotor or sympathetic lesion and the presence of clinical signs of neuromuscular disease. Ptosis in myasthenia gravis may occur in isolation, but it is more often associated with diplopia, varying degrees of ophthalmoparesis, weakness of the orbicularis oculi, and normal pupillary function by clinical testing (see Chapter 19). Ultimately, ptosis occurs in the majority of patients with myasthenia gravis. Regardless of when it develops, the ptosis of myasthenia gravis may be unilateral or bilateral, and when it is bilateral, it may also be symmetric or asymmetric (Fig. 22.13).

The hallmark of myasthenic ptosis is its fatigability and tendency to fluctuate in severity, although this feature is by no means pathognomonic. A similar tendency to fatigue (although not to the same degree) occurs in patients with aponeurotic defects and oculomotor nerve palsies. Patients with ptosis from myasthenia gravis, myasthenic syndromes, botulism, or drugs affecting neuromuscular transmission usually have sufficient signs and symptoms to allow the correct diagnosis to be made, such as the Cogan lid-twitch sign (**Video 22.1**), enhancement of ptosis with manual elevation of the contralateral eyelid (**Video 22.2**), and the orbicularis "peek" sign (Fig. 22.14). In addition, unless it is complete, myasthenic ptosis often improves when ice is held to the affected eyelid for 2 minutes (Fig. 22.15; see Chapter 19).

Figure 22.11 Horner syndrome. Note mild unilateral ptosis, anisocoria with smaller pupil on side of ptosis, and redness from associated cluster headache. The usual "upside-down" ptosis (i.e., elevation) of the lower lid is masked by coexisting eyelid laxity and blepharitis, which can be confounding factors in older adults.

patients, the ptosis is the presenting sign and may persist in isolation for months to years before the development of ophthalmoplegia. Ptosis of this type usually is bilateral, relatively symmetric, and very slowly progressive. The superior palpebral lid fold may be completely absent. Excessive wrinkling of the brow and backward head tilting are commonly employed to facilitate vision beneath the drooping lids (Fig. 22.12). Orbicularis oculi function, tested by forced lid closure, is frequently weak, and this combination of weakness of both eyelid opening and eyelid closure serves to

Figure 22.12 Ptosis in a patient with CPEO. Note also flat, expressionless facial features associated with continuous frontalis effort to lift the brows. (Pupil dilation is pharmacologic.)

Figure 22.13 Ptosis in a patient with myasthenia gravis. **A:** Before injection of neostigmine, the patient has bilateral ptosis. **B:** Thirty minutes following an intramuscular injection of 1.5 mg neostigmine and 0.6 mg atropine, the ptosis has disappeared.

Ptosis may be produced by neuromuscular disorders other than myasthenia gravis, including botulism and certain envenomations. In such cases, the history as well as accompanying signs or symptoms—particularly pupillary involvement—allow the correct diagnosis.

Pseudoptosis

Pseudoptosis is an apparent ptosis unrelated to defects in the neural, neuromuscular, or myogenic components of eyelid elevation. Pseudoptosis may be present because the eye on the same side is abnormal in size, shape, or position; for example, in patients with anophthalmos, phthisis bulbi, microphthalmos, or enophthalmos. Conversely, patients who present with isolated unilateral lid

Figure 22.14 The orbicularis "peek" sign in myasthenia gravis. **Left:** The patient has bilateral mild ptosis. **Right:** Within 2 seconds, the lids slip apart, exposing the sclera. (Reprinted with permission from Osher RH, Griggs RC. Orbicularis fatigue: The "peek" sign of myasthenia gravis. *Arch Ophthalmol.* 1979;97:677–679.)

retraction and proptosis from thyroid orbitopathy are sometimes mistakenly thought to have ptosis of the other eye.

Pseudoptosis often occurs in patients with a hypotropia who fixate with the higher eye. The position of the upper eyelid on the side of the hypotropia is appropriate to the position of that eye, but because the patient is fixing with the higher eye, the eyelid on the side of the hypotropic eye appears ptotic. When the hypertropic eye is covered and the patient is forced to fixate with the previously hypotropic eye, the "ptosis" disappears (Fig. 22.16).

Pseudoptosis may occur in patients with downgaze paralysis. When such patients attempt to look downward, their eyes remain in the primary position, but their eyelids lower normally.

Narrowing of the lid fissure from hemifacial contracture, hemifacial spasm (HFS), blepharospasm, or previous facial nerve palsy may mimic ptosis. In such patients, the presence of other evidence of abnormal facial movement usually suggests the correct diagnosis.

Apparent ptosis can be caused by voluntary stimulation of one or both orbicularis oculi muscles. Patients with nonorganic overactivity of the orbicularis oculi usually show mild or pronounced wrinkling of the eyelids proportional to the amount of narrowing of the fissure and depression of the brow (although occasionally the brow is elevated). Indicative of levator tone, the upper eyelid crease is present in primary gaze and may deepen in upgaze. In addition, one can often see—and always feel—fine tremors of the affected eyelid as the patient attempts to maintain the "ptotic" lid position. Patients with organic ptosis do not show a delay in returning to their baseline lid position after manual elevation of the eyelid. In contrast, patients with nonorganic ptosis may sometimes exhibit a slight lag before the orbicularis oculi is factitiously reactivated. Nonorganic ptosis may occur in isolation or in association with other somatic complaints.

Apraxia of Eyelid Opening

A more common supranuclear insufficiency of eyelid opening than cortical ptosis is AEO. The main clinical features of AEO include a transient inability to initiate lid opening, the absence of any significant evidence of orbicularis oculi contraction, such as lowering of the brow beneath the orbital rim (Charcot sign), frontalis contraction during attempts to open the eyelids, and the absence of any other signs of neural or myopathic dysfunction. Most patients with AEO show a paucity of blinking interrupted by gentle closure of both eyelids that may last up to 30 seconds or longer. AEO occurs most commonly in patients with progressive

Figure 22.15 The ice test for myasthenia gravis. **A:** Before placement of ice, patient has severe bilateral ptosis. **B:** Placement of ice over both eyelids. **C:** After 2 minutes of ice application, the ptosis has resolved.

supranuclear palsy, Parkinson disease, and atypical parkinsonism including that induced by methyl-phe-nyl-tetrahydropyridine (MPTP). Other associations are listed in Table 22.2.

Treatment of involuntary eyelid closure caused by supranuclear inhibition of levator activity is not particularly successful. Individual case reports suggest that several drugs may be useful, including desipramine and L-dopa. Injection of the orbicularis oculi and frontalis muscles with botulinum toxin produces variable results, depending on the degree of orbicularis contraction that often accompanies the levator inhibition, and we believe this treatment is worth trying in patients with AEO, even though the results are less than satisfactory.

Eyelid Retraction

Inappropriate and excessive elevation of the eyelids—eyelid retraction—makes a patient appear to be staring and also produces an illusion of exophthalmos. Mild degrees of lid retraction are frequently difficult to evaluate. The resting position of the upper lid is influenced by many factors, including age, alertness, and direction of gaze. Normal variations in resting lid position, or upper lid posture, are exemplified by the striking

difference between infants and adults. The infant's eyelid, which barely touches the upper corneal limbus, may appear normal, whereas a similar lid position in an adult is abnormal and represents excessive lid elevation. In general, upper lid position is abnormal if it exposes sclera between the lid margin and the upper

Table 22.2   Disorders Associated with Apraxia of Eyelid Opening
Progressive supranuclear palsy
Parkinson disease
Parkinsonism (including parksinsonism–dementia complex)
Shy–Drager syndrome
Adult-onset Hallervorden–Spatz disease
Huntington chorea
Frontotemporal gunshot injury
Right hemisphere stroke
Wilson disease
Amyotrophic lateral sclerosis
Idiopathic

Figure 22.16 Pseudoptosis caused by ipsilateral hypotropia and limitation of upward gaze in a patient who is fixing with the contralateral (hypertropic) eye. **A:** When the patient looks straight ahead and fixes with the left eye, she has a right hypotropia and appears to have a moderate right ptosis. **B:** When the patient fixes with the hypotropic right eye, however, the apparent ptosis disappears. (Courtesy of Dr. Nicholas T. Iliff.)

corneal limbus when the patient's head is straight and both of the patient's eyes are directed straight ahead.

Eyelid retraction may be unilateral or bilateral. The levator muscle is unique in being subjected to the influence of **two** yoke muscles—the contralateral levator and the ipsilateral superior rectus. Thus, eyelid retraction can result from inappropriate excitation or hyperactivity of ipsilateral levator neurons directly or indirectly via its yoke muscles, from oculosympathetic excitation or inappropriate hyperactivity, and from contracture or shortening of the levator muscle or its tendon, Müller muscle, or the superior rectus muscle. Causes of eyelid retraction may be classified as neuropathic, neuromuscular, myopathic, and mechanical.

Neuropathic Eyelid Retraction

Neuropathic eyelid retraction may be caused by supranuclear, nuclear, or infranuclear mechanisms. In some cases, the pathophysiology is clear; in others, it is either unknown or multifactorial.

Supranuclear Eyelid Retraction. Although true retraction of the eyelids does not usually occur from lesions in the cerebral hemisphere, intermittent or prolonged inappropriate eyelid opening sometimes develops in patients with unilateral nondominant or bilateral cerebral hemisphere disease. Such patients may be unable to close their eyelids on command (i.e., compulsive eye opening), or they may close their eyes only briefly before opening them again (i.e., motor impersistence). These patients have a supranuclear disturbance of orbicularis control and have normal levator relaxation.

Supranuclear bilateral eyelid retraction—**Collier sign**—most commonly occurs with lesions of the dorsal mesencephalon. This type of lid retraction is almost invariably associated with other evidence of dorsal

Figure 22.17 Bilateral eyelid retraction in a patient with a dorsal mesencephalic syndrome (Collier sign). Composite figure shows eyelid retraction in primary position and with attempted upgaze, and normal eyelid position on downgaze.

mesencephalic dysfunction, most often a deficiency of upward gaze, but also convergence-retraction nystagmus and pupillary light-near dissociation. The dorsal mesencephalic syndrome, also called Parinaud syndrome, is discussed in Chapter 17 of this text. It suffices here to emphasize that the eyelid retraction that occurs with lesions of the dorsal mesencephalon is usually symmetric and sustained as long as the patient directs the eyes straight ahead or slightly upward, increases as the patient looks up, and follows the eyes in a normal fashion when the patient looks down (Fig. 22.17). These features distinguish eyelid retraction from lesions of the dorsal mesencephalon from the more common form of lid retraction seen in thyroid orbitopathy, in which lid lag is invariably present.

The nucleus of the posterior commissure (nPC) appears to be the premotor structure responsible for mesencephalic lid retraction. As noted above, lesions that damage this structure in the dorsal mesencephalon generally produce bilateral lid retraction; however, in addition, they may damage the oculomotor nerve fascicle on one side, producing a ptosis on the side of the fascicular damage. This results in a condition characterized by ptosis on one side and primary eyelid retraction (i.e., not secondary to the contralateral ptosis) on the other. This condition is called the "plus-minus syndrome" (Fig. 22.18). Imaging studies

in patients with this syndrome show unilateral paramedian lesions, usually infarctions, dorsal and rostral to the red nucleus in the area of the nPC, extending ventrocaudally to the fascicle of the oculomotor nerve on the ptotic side. Thus, damage to the nPC apparently causes bilateral supranuclear lid retraction that may be masked on one side by an associated fascicular oculomotor nerve palsy.

Sustained eyelid retraction may be observed with any of the disorders known to produce a dorsal mesencephalic syndrome. Some common causes include hydrocephalus, stroke, MS, shunt malfunction, and both intrinsic and extrinsic tumors (Fig. 22.19).

Neurodegenerative conditions that cause supranuclear disturbances in upgaze may cause lid retraction. For example, lid retraction is common among patients with progressive supranuclear palsy, Parkinson disease, and Machado–Joseph disease (spinocerebellar ataxia, type 3), and some patients with severe Guillain–Barré syndrome (GBS) demonstrate marked bilateral limitation of upper lid descent during the acute phase of their illness.

Lid retraction and slight downward gaze of both eyes in response to a sudden decrease in ambient light is a physiologic reflex seen in infants between 1 and 5 months of age. Sometimes called the "eye-popping reflex" or "nonpathologic lid retraction," it is a useful

Figure 22.18 Unilateral ptosis associated with contralateral upper eyelid retraction from a lesion of the dorsal mesencephalon that also damages the fascicle of the oculomotor nerve on one side (plus-minus syndrome). **A:** The patient has marked eyelid retraction on the right and marked ptosis on the left. **B to E:** Show upward gaze paresis, left third nerve palsy, and lid-lag on downgaze. Computed tomographic scanning showed a paramedian midbrain infarct located ventrally and laterally to the aqueduct, extending from the midline to the area of the red nucleus laterally. (Reprinted with permission from Gaymard B, Lafitte C, Gelot A, et al. Plus-minus syndrome. *J Neurol Neurosurg Psychiatry.* 1992; 55:846–848.)

Figure 22.19 Bilateral eyelid retraction in a baby with communicating hydrocephalus. **A:** Eyes deviated slightly downward at rest. **B:** On attempted upgaze, there is no upward movement of the eyes (in fact, the eyes are resting slightly below the horizontal midline), but the eyelids elevate normally. This appearance is often called (the "setting sun" sign).

way of assessing levator function in infants. Transient, clonic, bilateral lid retraction with spastic downward gaze deviation that resolves after several weeks also occurs in otherwise healthy neonates. This may be a variant of the benign, transient, supranuclear disturbances of ocular motility that frequently occur in such infants.

Coma and stupor are commonly associated with eyelid closure caused by an absence of levator tonus. Occasionally, however, levator tonus persists and produces the incongruous picture of intermittently open lids in an unresponsive patient (coma vigil). This sign usually indicates disease of the ventral mesencephalon and pons, but it may occur with diffuse hemisphere disease (persistent vegetative state). Comatose patients with Cheyne–Stokes respiration sometimes open their eyes during the rapid-breathing phase and close them during the slow-breathing phase.

Some patients with extrapyramidal syndromes (e.g., postencephalitic parkinsonism, progressive supranuclear palsy) have defective inhibition of their eyelids during downward gaze. Such patients have normal lid position when they look straight ahead; however, the lids lag behind briefly as the eyes follow an object downward. Patients with a unilateral midbrain lesion dorsal to the red nucleus may also exhibit lid lag without lid retraction. The lesion in these patients is postulated to disrupt the pathways between the rostral interstitial nucleus of the medial longitudinal fasciculus (MLF) and the central caudal subnucleus of the oculomotor nuclear complex while sparing the nPC.

Synkinetic Eyelid Retraction. Elevation of the ipsilateral eyelid may be observed in normal subjects during abduction and, less commonly, on adduction. Lid retraction on attempted abduction in patients with Duane retraction syndrome and in patients with acquired abducens nerve palsies may represent an exaggerated expression of this physiologic synkinesis (**Video 22.3**).

The **Marcus Gunn jaw-winking phenomenon** is a paradoxical elevation of one eyelid that occurs with certain movements of the jaw. It is caused by a synkinesis between the pterygoid muscles and the levator. The condition is usually diagnosed shortly after birth as the infant suckles to feed; the cause of this synkinesis is unknown, and treatment is dependent upon the ophthalmologic and cosmetic status. Amblyopia should always be treated aggressively, and vertical strabismus should be corrected before attempting surgical repair of ptosis. Eyelid surgery should only be contemplated after the patient (when age permits), parents, and surgeon agree that the jaw-winking, ptosis, or both, are objectionable. Surgery usually consists of weakening the levator aponeurotic complex combined with a lid elevation procedure.

Eyelid Retraction Caused by Oculomotor Nerve Dysfunction. The most common cause of this type of retraction is congenital or acquired **aberrant regeneration of the oculomotor nerve.** In this setting, the retraction is not present at all times and, in fact, ptosis may be present when the patient is looking straight ahead; however, the lid retracts or at least "hangs up" during attempted infraduction, adduction, or both.

Lid retraction due to aberrant regeneration of the oculomotor nerve usually develops several months after an acute, nonischemic oculomotor nerve palsy, in which case the condition is known as **secondary aberrant regeneration of the oculomotor nerve.** However, when a slowly progressive compressive process (such as an aneurysm, meningioma, or schwannoma that is usually, but not always, located within the cavernous sinus; see Chapter 18) damages the nerve so slowly that the nerve has time to regenerate, the condition is called **primary aberrant regeneration of the oculomotor nerve.**

Other conditions involving the oculomotor nerve that may cause periodic eyelid retraction are oculomotor palsy with cyclic spasms, a condition that usually is congenital, and ocular neuromyotonia (see Chapter 18). In both conditions, the eyelid retraction usually is unilateral and associated with pupillary constriction and spasms of one or more of the extraocular muscles innervated by the oculomotor nerve.

Unilateral Eyelid Retraction Associated with Contralateral Ptosis. Patients with unilateral ptosis who, for any of a number of reasons (e.g., congenital or acquired strabismus, amblyopia, cataract), fixate with the eye on the side of the ptosis, may develop retraction of the eyelid on the opposite side (Fig. 22.20). This phenomenon can most easily be diagnosed by prolonged (>5 minutes) occlusion of the eye on the side of the ptosis, which will result in the retracted eyelid assuming a more normal position. Conversely, brief occlusion of the eye on the side of the ptosis probably is the least sensitive method because the contralateral retracted eyelid may not reposition immediately.

The explanation for the phenomenon of unilateral cyclic retraction associated with contralateral ptosis is based on equal output to both levator muscles from the central caudal subnucleus of cranial nerve III. Others have invoked Hering law, which states that yoked extraocular muscles receive equal degrees of innervation. In either case, the innervational drive to both lids increases in an effort to elevate the ptotic side. The ptotic lid assumes a more normal position, and the unaffected lid retracts. Secondary retraction of the eyelid in patients with contralateral ptosis is most likely to occur when the ptosis is severe, acquired, and ipsilateral to the dominant eye. The failure to recognize this phenomenon may lead to the erroneous diagnosis of thyroid orbitopathy.

Eyelid Retraction from Sympathetic Hyperfunction. Patients with neck trauma may develop sympathetic irritation or hyperactivity that produces recurrent throbbing headaches and oculosympathetic

A

B

C

Figure 22.20 Unilateral eyelid retraction secondary to contralateral ptosis (secondary eyelid retraction) in a patient with myasthenia gravis. **A:** The patient has moderate right ptosis and marked left upper eyelid retraction. **B:** When the right eye is covered with an occluder, the left eyelid retraction disappears as levator tonus is reduced bilaterally. **C:** After an intravenous injection of edrophonium chloride (Tensilon), the right eyelid elevates, and the left eyelid retraction disappears.

hyperactivity characterized by ipsilateral lid retraction, hyperhidrosis, and mydriasis—the **Pourfour du Petit syndrome.** During the headache-free interval, some of these patients have a Horner syndrome.

Sympathetic hyperactivity is thought to be responsible for some cases of lid retraction observed in patients with thyroid orbitopathy. Indeed, dilute solutions of both direct and indirect adrenergic stimulants (e.g., cocaine, hydroxyamphetamine, phenylephrine, apraclonidine, naphazoline) will widen the palpebral fissure in such patients.

Neuromuscular Eyelid Retraction

Transient, spontaneous eyelid retraction may occur in patients with **myasthenia gravis** without evidence of thyroid dysfunction. This phenomenon, which usually occurs on return of the eyes from upward gaze to primary position, appears to be caused by posttetanic facilitation of the levator muscle. Like the lid retraction of midbrain disease (i.e., Collier sign), neuromuscular lid retraction may be bilateral and symmetric, bilateral but asymmetric, or completely unilateral. Unlike the eyelid retraction of the dorsal mesencephalic syndrome, however, in patients with neuromuscular eyelid retraction, the levator usually fails to "relax" smoothly and completely, and the lid fold fails to smooth out as the eyes move downward. Momentary lid retraction also may be seen in patients with myasthenia after the patient makes an upward saccade from downgaze to primary position (Cogan lid-twitch) (**Video 22.1**). Finally, patients with myasthenia may develop retraction of the eyelid secondary to ptosis of the contralateral eyelid (Fig. 22.20, see above).

Eyelid retraction may result from topical or systemic administration of drugs that affect the neuromuscular junction. The anticholinesterase agents edrophonium chloride (Tensilon) and neostigmine methylsulfate (Prostigmin) produce eyelid retraction in some patients with myasthenia gravis. In addition, subparalytic doses of succinylcholine can produce shortening of the levator muscle fibers associated with the depolarization effect of the drug, resulting in lid retraction.

Myopathic Eyelid Retraction

Congenital myopathic eyelid retraction can be unilateral or bilateral and may be associated with nonspecific strabismus, underaction of the superior rectus on the side of the retraction, or lower lid retraction. The condition also may be associated with other developmental anomalies, including optic disc hypoplasia, craniosynostosis, and Down syndrome. In such cases, levator excursion is normal and there often is lagophthalmos on downgaze, indicating either failure of appropriate inhibition of levator tonus or decreased elasticity of the levator or its suspensory ligaments.

Dysthyroid orbitopathy is the most common cause of acquired unilateral and bilateral sustained lid retraction in both children and adults. The treatment of eyelid retraction in patients with dysthyroid orbitopathy is primarily surgical and consists of various levator-lengthening procedures.

A

B

Figure 22.21 Myotonic eyelid retraction and lid lag (levator myotonia) in a patient with hyperkalemic periodic paralysis. **A:** When the patient looks straight ahead, the eyelids are slightly retracted. **B:** On downward gaze, there is marked eyelid lag. (Reprinted with permission from Layzer RB, Lovelace RE, Rowland LP. Hyperkalemic periodic paralysis. *Arch Neurol.* 1967;16:455–471.)

Eyelid retraction occurs with increased frequency in patients with severe liver disease (Summerskill sign). The appearance is similar to that seen in patients with thyroid orbitopathy.

Myotonic eyelid retraction, lid lag, or both may be observed in patients with familial periodic paralysis (Fig. 22.21). A similar myotonic lid lag may occur in patients with myotonic dystrophy and in patients with congenital myotonia (see Chapter 20).

Abnormalities of Eyelid Closure

As with eyelid opening, abnormalities of eyelid closure may occur from disorders involving any part of the pathway for contracture of the orbicularis oculi, from the cerebral cortex to the muscle itself. Such disorders may be congenital or acquired and may be caused by either hypofunction or hyperfunction of the orbicularis muscle and, to a lesser extent, by the muscles that assist the orbicularis in eyelid closure (i.e., the frontalis, procerus, and corrugator superciliaris).

Insufficiency of Eyelid Closure

As with eyelid opening, insufficient eyelid closure can be neuropathic, neuromuscular, or myopathic in origin. Arriving at the correct diagnosis thus requires a careful history and complete examination, sometimes followed by appropriate ancillary studies.

Figure 22.22 Central volitional (supranuclear) paralysis of the orbicularis oculi after a subcortical hematoma that caused a left hemiplegia and a left facial nerve paresis. **A:** When the patient is told to close her eyes tightly, the left orbicularis oculi, left corrugator muscle, and the other muscles of the left lower side of the face fail to respond. **B:** Volitional control of the forehead is normal. **C:** Left lower facial weakness is evident when the patient attempts to show her teeth. **D:** A spontaneous smile (emotional-extrapyramidal-facial innervation) evokes symmetric contraction of all facial muscles, including the orbicularis oculi, indicating that nuclear and infranuclear pathways are intact.

Neuropathic Insufficiency of Eyelid Closure

Neuropathic causes of insufficient eyelid closure may be supranuclear, nuclear, or infranuclear. In some cases, the cause is clearly neuropathic, but the precise mechanism is unknown or multifactorial.

Supranuclear Insufficiency of Eyelid Closure. Voluntary eyelid closure is mediated by the pyramidal system. Patients with localized subcortical capsular lesions usually can close both eyes, although the force of closure is diminished, and the ability to wink may be lost on the contralateral

paretic side (Revilliod sign). In some cases, paresis is profound and yet spontaneous involuntary or emotional movements of the facial and orbicularis muscles remain undisturbed (automatic voluntary dissociation) (Fig. 22.22).

Bilateral inability to voluntarily close the eyelids may result from a unilateral lesion, usually in the nondominant frontal lobe, but it more commonly develops with bilateral frontal lobe lesions. This phenomenon is called **supranuclear paralysis of voluntary lid closure** or compulsive eye opening. Patients with this syndrome are unable to initiate voluntary

A

B

Figure 22.23 Supranuclear paralysis of voluntary eyelid closure (compulsive eyelid opening) in a patient with Creutzfeldt–Jakob disease. **A:** The patient has no movement of the eyelids when told to close his eyes, even though he understands what he is being told to do and is attempting to do it. **B:** The patient shows some ability to blink to a visual threat. (Reprinted with permission from Russell RW. Supranuclear palsy of eyelid closure. *Brain*. 1980;103:71–82.)

closure of either eyelid, even though they retain their ability to comprehend the task and have intact reflex eyelid closure (Fig. 22.23). Supranuclear paralysis of eyelid closure can occur in patients with unilateral or bilateral infarcts or tumors in the frontal lobe, Creutzfeldt–Jakob disease, progressive supranuclear palsy, and motor neuron disease.

Motor **impersistence** of eyelid closure also occurs in patients with bilateral or unilateral hemispheric lesions. When such patients are instructed to close the eyelids and keep them closed, they are unable to obey. The eyelids close, often develop a fine tremor, and then almost immediately reopen. This phenomenon most frequently is seen in patients with a nondominant hemisphere stroke and is most evident during the first week after the stroke. Occasionally, the condition is unilateral.

Nuclear and Fascicular Insufficiency of Eyelid Closure.

Unilateral weakness of eyelid closure and facial movement may result from unilateral damage to the facial nerve nucleus or fascicle. In such instances, other evidence of brainstem disease is almost always present, including reduction in corneal sensation, ipsilateral abducens nerve paresis or horizontal gaze paralysis, and ipsilateral cerebellar ataxia.

Bilateral weakness of eyelid closure occurs as part of the facial diplegia that is caused by lesions of the pontine tegmentum. Such lesions may be congenital or acquired. Acquired processes include ischemia, inflammation, infiltration, and compression (**Video 22.4**). When insufficiency of eyelid closure results from damage to the facial nerve fascicle within the brainstem, there usually is complete facial paralysis associated with other signs of brainstem dysfunction, such as ipsilateral horizontal gaze palsy from damage to the ipsilateral abducens nucleus or paramedian pontine reticular formation, ipsilateral abduction weakness from damage to the ipsilateral abducens nerve fascicle, and contralateral hemiparesis from damage to the ipsilateral pyramidal tract (Millard–Gubler syndrome).

Insufficiency of Eyelid Closure from Peripheral Facial Nerve Palsy.

Insufficiency or weakness of eyelid closure associated with lesions of the facial nerve is usually combined with weakness of other facial muscles supplied by that nerve. Topographic diagnosis of facial nerve paresis may be facilitated by the relationship of the facial nerve to surrounding structures and by the fact that along its course, the nerve gives off various branches that subserve specific functions. The facial nerve, in addition to innervating the facial musculature, is also responsible for reflex tearing (via the greater superficial petrosal nerve), hearing (via the nerve to the stapedius muscle), taste on the anterior two-thirds of the tongue (via the chorda tympani), and salivation (via nerve branches to the sublingual and submandibular glands) (Fig. 22.24). Thus, by testing reflex tearing, hearing, taste, and ability of an individual with peripheral facial weakness to produce saliva, one often can determine the location of the responsible lesion. In addition, various electrodiagnostic tests, including nerve excitability, electromyography, blink reflex, and electroneurography help determine the extent of dysfunction and prognosis for facial nerve recovery.

Lesions in the cerebellopontine angle (CPA) that produce unilateral facial nerve paresis usually also produce signs and symptoms related to dysfunction of the vestibulocochlear and trigeminal nerves. Common manifestations thus include unilateral sensorineural hearing loss, tinnitus, vertigo, facial pain and numbness, corneal hypoesthesia, and unsteadiness of gait. All of the components of the facial nerve may be affected. Less common manifestations include HFS, nystagmus, evidence of cerebellar dysfunction (e.g., ataxia and tremor), and hydrocephalus. Nevertheless, although most patients with lesions in the CPA present with multiple neurologic findings, facial nerve paralysis may be the only manifestation, particularly in children.

Lesions of the CPA that may cause a facial nerve paresis include vestibular and trigeminal schwannomas,

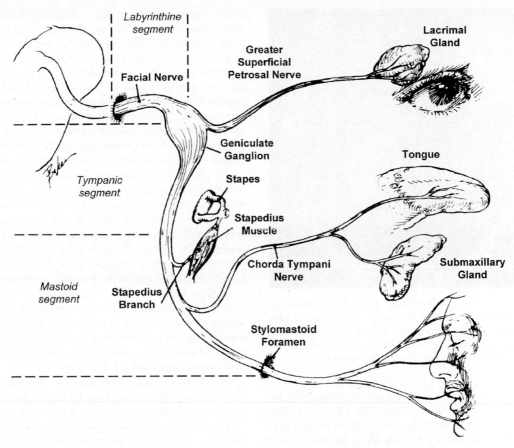

Figure 22.24 Schematic drawing of the branches of the facial nerve showing the different functions of those branches. The branches and their functions include the greater superficial petrosal nerve (reflex tearing), the nerve to the stapedius muscle (stapedius reflex), the chorda tympani nerve (taste on the anterior two-thirds of the tongue and submaxillary gland secretion), and peripheral motor branches to the facial muscles. (Reprinted with permission from Alford BR, Jerger JF, Coats AC, et al. Neurophysiology of facial nerve testing. *Arch Otolaryngol.* 1973;97:214–219.)

meningiomas, epidermoids, lipomas, arachnoid cysts, aneurysms, metastatic lesions, and glomus jugulare tumors (Fig. 22.25). Granulomas associated with tuberculosis, sarcoid, syphilis, or certain fungal infections can also damage the facial nerve in the CPA.

A facial nerve lesion located within the facial canal between the internal auditory meatus and the geniculate ganglion produces many of the same signs as those encountered with lesions in the CPA, except that brainstem signs are absent, and there is no evidence of dysfunction of the trigeminal nerve. Lesions between the geniculate ganglion and the branch to the stapedius muscle produce similar manifestations except that reflex lacrimation is preserved because the lesion is distal to the superficial petrosal nerve. Damage to the facial nerve between the branch to the stapedius muscle and the chorda tympani produces facial paralysis, loss of taste on the

anterior two-thirds of the tongue, and diminution of salivary secretion.

Lesions of the facial nerve distal to the takeoff of the chorda tympani produce only facial motor paralysis. Facial neuropathies that localize to the intratemporal portion of the facial nerve may be caused by fractures of the temporal bone, herpes zoster (Ramsey Hunt syndrome), otitis media, and neoplasms. The condition called "Bell palsy" belongs in this category. Lesions distal to the stylomastoid foramen may affect one or more peripheral branches of the facial nerve and are usually caused by facial trauma, facial surgery, or disease of the parotid gland.

Most isolated facial nerve palsies are idiopathic and are called Bell palsy. The diagnosis of Bell palsy is based on a constellation of findings and the exclusion of other known causes. The condition usually is unilateral. About 60% of patients with Bell palsy have a history of a viral prodrome. The onset of facial motor

Figure 22.25 Large vestibular schwannoma seen on gadolinium-enhanced T1 MR imaging in a patient who had preoperative hearing loss but no facial weakness. She had postop diplopia from a left sixth nerve palsy as well as complete left peripheral facial nerve palsy.

weakness is acute and frequently accompanied by pain or numbness of the face, neck, or tongue. The pain is characteristically located in the retroauricular area. Hypoesthesia or dysesthesia in the distribution of the trigeminal or glossopharyngeal nerve occurs in 25% to 35% of patients. Sensory findings may precede the onset of facial paresis and usually do not persist beyond 7 to 10 days. Dysgeusia and dysacusis are fairly common accompaniments. Both subjective and objective signs of dry eye may be present, and epiphora from exposure or paralytic ectropion is common. Both a direct viral neuropathology (likely from herpes simplex) and swelling of the nerve within the facial canal have been proposed as being causative.

Overall, about 85% of patients with Bell palsy eventually recover completely or are left with only slight residual deficits. The remainder have permanent deficits consisting of residual weakness, tonic contracture, synkinesis, spasms, or gustatory lacrimation (crocodile tears). Clinical factors that adversely affect recovery include advanced age (over 60), diabetes mellitus, complete paralysis, decreased tearing, hyperacusis, and delay in the onset of recovery. Corticosteroid administration during the acute phase of disease significantly increases the likelihood of recovery, while antiviral therapy remains of uncertain benefit.

An isolated facial nerve palsy that may mimic Bell palsy can occur in a number of systemic disorders. These include infections and inflammations (herpes zoster oticus, acquired immune deficiency syndrome, otitis media, mastoiditis, Lyme disease, syphilis, sarcoidosis, tetanus), ischemia (diabetes mellitus, hypertension), and immune-mediated inflammatory diseases (periarteritis, GBS, postvaccination demyelination, MS). Neoplastic causes of isolated peripheral facial palsy include vestibular and facial nerve schwannomas, meningiomas, glomus jugulare tumors, lipomas, dermoids, epidermoids, parotid tumors, carcinomatous meningitis, cholesteatomas, metastatic tumors, and lymphoid lesions. Miscellaneous causes include toxic agents (thalidomide, ethylene glycol, organophosphate poisoning), trauma (temporal bone fractures, facial injuries, barotrauma from scuba diving), iatrogenic injuries (from local anesthetic blocks and facial surgery), amyloidosis, Paget disease, and pseudotumor cerebri.

Because so many conditions can cause an acute, initially isolated, facial nerve paresis, progression of a facial palsy for longer than 3 weeks, lack of recovery after 3 to 6 months, development of HFS, prolonged otalgia or facial pain, or recurrence of paralysis after recovery should prompt closer investigation of a "Bell palsy" to rule out an underlying systemic inflammatory or infectious etiology or a neoplasm.

In patients with congenital or developmental facial nerve paresis, there may be other evidence of incomplete development (i.e., hypoplasia) or agenesis of the facial nerve. Such patients may have Möbius syndrome, congenital unilateral lower lip paralysis (CULLP), hemifacial microsomia, or other associated developmental defects, such as aural atresia and microtia. Acquired prenatal causes include birth trauma and exposure to thalidomide or rubella virus.

Less than 1% of all facial nerve palsies are bilateral and simultaneous. Such cases usually are idiopathic (i.e., Bell palsy) or caused by Lyme disease, sarcoidosis, GBS, Fisher syndrome, brainstem encephalitis, or neoplasia (e.g., carcinomatous meningitis, glioma). Less common causes include meningitis (e.g., from syphilis, tuberculosis, cryptococcus), diabetes mellitus, head trauma, pontine hemorrhage, systemic lupus erythematosus, ethylene glycol ingestion, and Wernicke–Korsakoff syndrome.

The rehabilitation and supportive management of patients with facial nerve palsy depends on the stage and severity of facial weakness. Preventing corneal exposure is the primary treatment goal in the acute phase. This task is best accomplished by copious eye lubrication; use of a moisture barrier also may be needed. More severe exposure requires temporary or permanent tarsorrhaphy and/or eyelid weight placement. If recovery is incomplete, then later surgical intervention may help to restore upper and lower eyelid positions; nerve grafting may improve overall facial function as well

A
B

Figure 22.26 Aberrant regeneration of the left facial nerve after an acute peripheral facial nerve paresis (Bell palsy) producing facial contracture and partial closure of the left eyelid associated with certain movements of the mouth. **A:** The patient has a narrowed left interpalpebral fissure and a deepened left nasolabial groove. **B:** Any spontaneous or voluntary movement of the lower face, such as trying to smile, produces comovements of all muscles on the left side of the face, resulting in eyelid closure.

Abnormal Eyelid Closure Associated with Aberrant Regeneration of the Facial Nerve. Aberrant regeneration of the facial nerve may occur after damage to the facial nerve, particularly after compression, trauma, or Bell palsy. The previously paralyzed side of the face is invariably weak and may appear contracted (Fig. 22.26). Typically, each closure of the eye occurs simultaneously with a twitch at the corner of the mouth that also may be accompanied by dimpling of the chin and contraction of the platysma. During forced lid closure, there is an exaggerated contraction of all facial muscles on the side of the previously paretic facial nerve. Conversely, both voluntary and involuntary movements of the lips or the corner of the mouth precipitate cocontraction of the orbicularis oculi on the affected side that may superficially resemble HFS or the inverse Marcus Gunn jaw-winking phenomenon (see above); however, unlike HFS, which occurs spontaneously (see below), the eyelid and facial spasms that occur in patients with aberrant regeneration of the facial nerve are induced by voluntary or involuntary movements of the eyelid or mouth. Similarly, unlike the inverse Marcus Gunn phenomenon, in which the eyelid closure is caused by levator inhibition, narrowing of the lid fissure in aberrant regeneration of the facial nerve is caused by inappropriate contraction of the orbicularis oculi muscle.

Neuromuscular Insufficiency of Eyelid Closure
The orbicularis oculi often is weak in diseases that affect the neuromuscular junction. **Myasthenia gravis**
characteristically produces weakness of eyelid closure, usually combined with ptosis. This weakness of orbicularis function is responsible for the "peek phenomenon," in which a patient with myasthenia gravis initially is able to close the eyelids, but as closure is maintained, the orbicularis fatigues and the eyelids separate, exposing the globe. Weakness of the orbicularis oculi in patients with neuromuscular disease also may be characterized by retraction of the lower eyelid. Botulism also can cause weakness of the facial muscles, including the eyelids, as can certain envenomations (e.g., snake and spider bites) that affect the neuromuscular junction. The diagnosis of neuromuscular disease, particularly myasthenia gravis, should be considered in any patient with weakness of eyelid closure associated with ptosis, ophthalmoparesis, or both.

Myopathic Insufficiency of Eyelid Closure
The orbicularis oculi muscle is frequently involved in any disease that weakens the facial musculature. Weakness of the orbicularis muscle may be characterized not only by weakness of spontaneous or forced eyelid closure but also by lack of upper facial expression, wasting of eyelid tissue, and fatigue of the eyelids during attempted sustained closure. In addition, there may be retraction of the lower eyelid or paralytic ectropion (Fig. 22.27). Myogenic weakness of the orbicularis oculi is usually bilateral. Because lacrimal drainage depends in part on normal muscle action in the lower eyelid, epiphora may result. The most common causes of myopathic

Figure 22.27 Bilateral, symmetric lower eyelid retraction in a patient with myotonic dystrophy and generalized facial weakness. (Reprinted with permission from Cohen MM, Lessell S. Retraction of the lower eyelid. *Neurology.* 1979;29:386–389.)

insufficiency of eyelid closure are congenital muscular dystrophy, myotonic dystrophy, and the mitochondrial cytopathies associated with CPEO (Fig. 22.28).

Excessive or Anomalous Eyelid Closure

Unlike insufficient eyelid closure, which can be caused by neurologic, neuromuscular, or myopathic causes, excessive or inappropriate eyelid closure usually is neurologic in origin.

Essential Blepharospasm and the Blepharospasm-Oromandibular Dystonia Syndrome (Meige Syndrome; Brueghel Syndrome)

Blepharospasm is an involuntary closure of the eyelids evoked by contraction of the orbicularis oculi. When

Figure 22.28 Bilateral orbicularis oculi weakness in a patient with the Kearns–Sayre syndrome variant of CPEO. The patient is attempting to close her eyelids as tightly as possible. Note lack of folds in the upper eyelids and inability to bury the lashes.

Figure 22.29 Essential blepharospasm. The patient first noted intermittent spasms of lid closure several years earlier. By the time she was examined, she was experiencing almost continuous, bilateral symmetric spasms of the orbicularis oculi muscles.

blepharospasm occurs in isolation without other evidence of neurologic or ocular disease, the condition is called essential blepharospasm (Fig. 22.29 and **Video 22.5**). When these focal dystonic eyelid movements spread to other cranial muscles, the syndrome is called blepharospasm-oromandibular dystonia or Meige syndrome. The disorder occurs most frequently in women over 50 years of age. Initially, there is an increased frequency of blinking, particularly in response to sunlight, wind, noise, movement, or stress. This blinking progresses to involuntary spasms, initially on one side, but inevitably on both. Certain maneuvers like touching the eyelid, coughing, vocalizing, or chewing gum may alleviate the spasms, which increase in frequency and severity as the disease progresses.

Patients with Meige syndrome may experience involuntary chewing movements, lip pursing, trismus, wide opening of the mouth, spasmodic deviations of the jaw, abnormal tongue movements (protrusion, retraction, and writhing), spasmodic dysphonia, and, rarely, difficulty swallowing. In addition to orofacial spasms, such patients may have oculogyric crises, platysmal contractions, torticollis, retrocollis, or other forms of focal dystonia. Generalized dystonia is rare, however.

Many patients with essential blepharospasm and Meige syndrome stop reading, watching television, and driving; some become depressed, occupationally disabled and, in some cases, functionally blind. The disorder may plateau at any point along its progression. Remission occurs in about 11% of patients, almost always within 5 years of the onset of symptoms.

Most cases of essential blepharospasm and Meige syndrome are sporadic, although there are familial occurrences. In addition, patients with essential blepharospasm and Meige syndrome often have a family history of other movement disorders, or they may give a past history of tics or excessive blinking, sometimes dating back to childhood. Thus, familial blepharospasm and craniocervical dystonia may be phenotypically heterogeneous and autosomal dominantly inherited with incomplete penetrance.

Many patients with blepharospasm, whether of the essential variety or part of Meige syndrome, complain of dryness, grittiness, irritation, or photophobia. Some of these patients have evidence of dry eyes or ocular surface disease by slit-lamp biomicroscopy or Schirmer testing, whereas in others, there is no apparent reason for their complaints. The clinician should ensure that the blepharospasm does not occur as a secondary phenomenon (**reflex blepharospasm**); if instillation of topical anesthetic abolishes excessive blinking, then ocular surface dryness should be treated before considering blepharospasm therapy.

The cause of essential blepharospasm and Meige syndrome is unknown, but there is abundant clinical and neurophysiologic evidence that essential blepharospasm and Meige syndrome are **focal dystonias** caused by dysfunction of the basal ganglia or brainstem.

Botulinum toxin type A is the primary form of therapy for patients with blepharospasm. Its effect generally lasts 2 to 4 months. Other drugs, such as clonazepam, trihexiphenidyl, and tetrabenazine, can also be used to treat essential blepharospasm and Meige syndrome, but they are less efficacious. Some patients may benefit from wearing spectacles with a specific (Corning FL-41) tint. Essential blepharospasm also can be treated surgically by removing all or part of the orbicularis oculi muscle; however, complications, variable effectiveness, and frequent recurrence are major limitations of this approach. Thus, surgery should be reserved for patients with disabling blepharospasm that does not respond to botulinum toxin, oral medications, or a combination of these treatments, or for patients who cannot tolerate these treatments.

Patients with essential blepharospasm often have associated dermatochalasis, ptosis, or both. These can be treated with blepharoplasty and ptosis surgery, both of which often reduce the severity of the blepharospasm to some extent. However, these procedures are merely adjuncts to the treatment of blepharospasm and should not be considered as primary treatments for the condition.

Blepharospasm Associated with Lesions of the Brainstem and Basal Ganglia

Blepharospasm may be caused by a variety of lesions and disorders of the basal ganglia and mesodiencephalic region. These include strokes, MS, progressive supranuclear palsy, Parkinson disease, Huntington disease, Wilson disease, Lytico-Bodig syndrome, Hallervorden–Spatz syndrome, olivopontocerebellar atrophy, communicating hydrocephalus, and encephalitis lethargica.

Blepharoclonus

Typical blepharospasm is characterized by repetitive episodes of tonic contractions of the orbicularis oculi, and EMG studies show that the orbicularis contractions in many such patients consist of rhythmic phasic bursts at a rate of 3 to 6 Hz. When such contractions result in visible repetitive upward jerks of the eyelids, the term **blepharoclonus** is used. Blepharoclonus occurs in patients with brainstem syndromes caused by stroke or trauma, hydrocephalus from aqueductal stenosis in the setting of parkinsonism, and MS.

Blepharospasm Associated with Drug-Induced Tardive Dyskinesia

Patients with tardive dyskinesia have blepharospasm and facial tics similar to those seen in patients with Meige syndrome (see above); however, patients with tardive dyskinesia have choreic movements of the extremities as opposed to the more sustained, dystonic movements observed in patients with Meige syndrome. The most important distinguishing feature of tardive dyskinesia, however, is that it is always drug-induced, usually developing 1 to 2 years after starting the medication. In most instances, the responsible agents are antipsychotic or neuroleptic drugs, such as dopamine-blocking or dopamine-stimulating agents. Drug-induced dyskinesia can also occur after the use of antiemetics, anorectics, or nasal decongestants that contain sympathomimetic agents and antihistamines.

The blepharospasm and facial tics of tardive dyskinesia may improve if the drug responsible is identified and discontinued. If the symptoms persist, or if the drug cannot be stopped for medical reasons, botulinum toxin can be used to control the spasms.

Facial Tics and Tourette Syndrome

In contrast to the sustained, dystonic movements typical of blepharospasm, facial tics are usually brief, clonic, and jerk like. They tend to be stereotyped and repetitive. They can vary in frequency, increasing when the patient is bored, tired, or anxious. Eye-winking tics are most commonly observed in childhood, tend to be unilateral, and affect boys more often than girls. They resolve spontaneously after months or years.

When facial tics begin between 2 and 15 years of age, last more than 1 year, fluctuate in severity, and are associated with tics in multiple other bodily locations, vocalizations (e.g., grunting, sniffing, barking, throat clearing, utterance of obscenities), obscene gestures, and other aberrancies of behavior, Tourette syndrome (also called Gilles de la Tourette syndrome) is the likely diagnosis (**Video 22.6**). Ocular manifestations are common in this condition and include increased blinking, blepharospasm, forced staring, and involuntary gaze deviation.

Nonorganic Blepharospasm

Nonorganic blepharospasm generally has a sudden onset and usually is preceded by an emotionally traumatic event. Although quite rare, it is more likely in children and young adults with serious psychologic problems. The blepharospasm is frequently bilateral and may last for hours, weeks, or even months, at which point it may resolve spontaneously. The eyelids are sometimes gently, sometimes forcibly, closed. In some patients, psychotherapy, behavior therapy, hypnosis, or biofeedback are of benefit. In others, a single injection of botulinum toxin is sufficient to eliminate the spasms permanently.

Focal Seizures

Several eyelid phenomena are associated with seizures. An adversive (jacksonian) seizure from an irritative focus in the frontal eye fields can evoke contralateral spasmodic eyelid closure, twitching of the face, and "spastic" lateral gaze. Blinking or fluttering of the eyelids also may be observed in psychomotor or absence seizures. Blinking is usually bilateral and symmetric, although unilateral blinking ipsilateral to the seizure focus has been described.

Lid-Triggered Synkinesias

Eyelid closure occasionally triggers movements of muscles that are not innervated by the facial nerve, presumably from a central or supranuclear disturbance. In some patients with such eyelid-triggered dyskinesias, firm external stimulation of the cornea elicits a brisk anterolateral jaw movement to the side opposite the stimulus associated with eyelid closure: the **corneomandibular reflex.** In other patients, an acquired **palpebromandibular synkinesia** is present that is similar to the corneomandibular reflex except that the jaw movements that regularly accompany spontaneous eye blinks can occur without an external corneal stimulus. The palpebromandibular reflex usually is associated with bihemispheric or upper brainstem pathology.

Facial Myokymia (With and Without Spastic-Paretic Facial Contracture)

The term facial myokymia refers to involuntary, fine, continuous, undulating contractions that spread across facial muscles. The contractions are usually unilateral. Electrophysiologically, affected muscles show brief tetanic bursts of motor-unit potentials that recur in a rhythmic or semirhythmic fashion several times a

second as singlets, doublets, or groups. These bursts recur at a rate of 3 to 8 Hz.

The most common type of facial myokymia occurs in otherwise normal persons and affects only the orbicularis oculi of the lower (or, occasionally, the upper) eyelid on one side. This **eyelid myokymia** often begins at times of excessive fatigue or stress. It usually occurs intermittently for several days, but it may persist for a few weeks and even for several months. Patients with this condition may become alarmed, particularly because they can feel the eyelid fasciculations. They often believe that their eye is "jumping," and some patients actually experience oscillopsia from the effects of the myokymic eyelid against the globe; however, this type of transient eyelid myokymia is almost always benign. Isolated lower eyelid myokymia does not warrant additional workup.

Many disorders characterized by involuntary movements of the facial muscles can begin with eyelid myokymia including essential blepharospasm, Meige syndrome, HFS, and **spastic-paretic facial contracture.** This last disorder is characterized by myokymia that first begins in the orbicularis oculi muscle and gradually spreads to most of the muscles on one side of the face. At the same time, associated tonic contracture of the affected muscles becomes evident. Over a period of weeks or months, the nasolabial groove slowly deepens, the corner of the mouth is drawn laterally, the palpebral fissure narrows, and all the facial muscles become weak. As the contracture becomes more pronounced, voluntary facial movements on the affected side diminish (Fig. 22.30). Spastic-paretic facial contracture is a sign of pontine dysfunction in the region of the facial nerve nucleus. Disorders that may produce it include MS, intrinsic brainstem neoplasms (particularly gliomas but also metastatic tumors), extra-axial neoplasms compressing the brainstem (e.g., chordomas), syringobulbia, brainstem vascular lesions, GBS, obstructive hydrocephalus, subarachnoid hemorrhage, basilar invagination, Machado–Joseph disease, brainstem tuberculoma, cysticercosis, and autosomal-dominant striatonigral degeneration. In most instances, the phenomenon and the pathology that causes it are unilateral, but bilateral facial myokymia from bilateral pontine disease may occur in patients with GBS, following cardiopulmonary arrest, during the course of a lymphocytic meningoradiculitis, and following exposure to a variety of toxins.

The pathophysiology of transient facial myokymia is unknown; however, MR imaging in patients with MS who have continuous facial myokymia often shows changes consistent with demyelination in the postgenu portion of the fascicle of the facial nerve in the dorsolateral pontine tegmentum. In all autopsy cases in which a brainstem tumor is responsible for the condition, the tumor infiltrates the pontine tegmentum, basis pontis,

Figure 22.30 Spastic paretic facial contracture associated with a pontine astrocytoma. **A:** The patient's face is at rest. Note deepened nasolabial groove and narrowed palpebral fissure on the left. **B:** On attempted left gaze, the patient shows a horizontal gaze palsy. **C:** Voluntary forced eyelid closure exposes the paresis of the left orbicularis oculi and the left side of the face. The patient subsequently died and an autopsy was performed. **D:** Serial sections through the brainstem of the patient show a left-sided astrocytoma. (Reprinted with permission from Sogg RL, Hoyt WF, Boldrey E. Spastic paretic facial contracture: A rare sign of brain stem tumor. *Neurology.* 1963;13:607–612.)

A

B

Figure 22.31 T2-weighted MRI in a patient with left hemifacial spasm showing compression of the root exit zones of (A) cranial nerve VII and (B) cranial nerve VIII by a markedly dolichoectatic basilar artery (labeled "B").

or both, sparing the facial nerve nucleus and its neurons. It has therefore been suggested that the lack of direct damage to the ipsilateral facial nerve nucleus in the presence of more rostrally placed lesions produces a functional deafferentation, possibly of local circuit neurons. This, in turn, results in hyperexcitability of facial nerve neurons, thus causing myokymia or spastic-paretic facial contracture. When the facial nerve nucleus itself is damaged by the pathologic process, the facial spasm resolves, leaving only facial paralysis and contracture.

Hemifacial Spasm

HFS is characterized by involuntary paroxysmal bursts of painless, unilateral, tonic or clonic contractions of muscles innervated by the facial nerve (**Video 22.7**). It occurs most commonly in middle-aged adults, but it may develop at any age. The condition is almost always sporadic, but there are familial cases. Bilateral cases occur but are exceptionally rare, and most reported cases probably are examples of essential blepharospasm or Meige syndrome.

HFS usually first appears as spasms of the orbicularis oculi and then spreads slowly to the lower facial muscles over months to years. The spasms may occur spontaneously or be triggered by voluntary facial movements or changes in position, and they may worsen with fatigue, stress, or anxiety. Long-standing HFS almost always is associated with ipsilateral lower facial weakness, although this may be hard to detect, either because it usually is fairly mild or because of the constant spasms. In addition, many patients with HFS have clinical evidence, EMG evidence, or both, of synkinesis between the orbicularis oculi and orbicularis oris muscles.

Most cases of HFS are likely to be caused by pulsatile compression of the proximal region of the facial nerve at the root entry zone (the transitional zone between central and peripheral myelin) by normal vessels in an aberrant location or by dolichoectatic vessels. The blood vessels most commonly responsible for the compression are the anterior-inferior cerebellar artery, the posterior-inferior cerebellar artery, and the vertebral artery. Less commonly, one or more veins accompanying these vessels appear to be responsible. A variety of imaging techniques, including CT scanning, MR imaging, MR angiography, and CT angiography may show ipsilateral displacement, tortuosity, or enlargement of the basilar or vertebral arteries in patients with HFS (Fig. 22.31).

Although HFS appears to be caused by vascular compression from otherwise normal arteries or veins in over 99% of cases, a variety of other structures also can compress the facial nerve at the root entry zone, producing HFS. These lesions include aneurysms, AVMs, infratemporal hemangiomas, and arterial dissections as well as extra-axial tumors located in the CPA such as epidermoids, vestibular schwannomas (acoustic neuromas), meningiomas, cholesteatomas, and lipomas. Occasionally, HFS is produced by intraparenchymal brainstem lesions, including tumors and granulomas. Other rare causes include arachnoid cysts, MS, pontine infarction, hemosiderosis, arachnoiditis, and lesions or structural abnormalities of the bone of the skull base. In some cases, HFS is associated with evidence of hyperactivity of other cranial nerves. The most common association is with trigeminal neuralgia.

The only way to cure most cases of HFS is to decompress the facial nerve at the root entry zone by moving the offending vessel or vessels. Although this procedure has potential mortality and a well-defined morbidity, including permanent ipsilateral hearing loss, facial weakness, or both, the results are generally excellent. When performed by an experienced surgeon, the overall cure rate is 90% or greater. In most patients who are cured, the HFS disappears within 3 to 10 days after surgery, although in a smaller group, resolution can take weeks to months. Among patients whose HFS persists or recurs after apparently successful surgery (i.e., the vessel compressing the nerve is identified and moved), the majority are cured after a second operation.

The results of medical therapy for HFS are generally disappointing. The most commonly used drugs are carbamazepine, diphenylhydantoin, and dimethylaminoethanol. Gabapentin has also been reported to be of value in selected patients.

Intramuscular injections of botulinum toxin can be used to control, but not cure, HFS. In our opinion, this mode of therapy is the best alternative for patients who are unwilling or unable to undergo posterior fossa microvascular decompression of the facial nerve. Other injectable drugs are under investigation.

Excessive Eyelid Closure of Neuromuscular Origin

Neuromuscular hyperexcitability of the orbicularis oculi usually is part of a generalized disorder. The excitability may be latent, spasmodic, or constant. In hypoparathyroidism or during hyperventilation, a tap over the lateral orbital margin produces contraction of the ipsilateral orbicularis muscles and the surrounding facial muscles (latent hyperexcitability). Strychnine poisoning causes spasmodic hyperexcitability and tetanus causes a constant or sustained neuromuscular hyperexcitability manifested in the facial muscles as **risus sardonicus** (Fig. 22.32).

Excessive Eyelid Closure of Myopathic Origin

Myotonia of the orbicularis oculi may occur in association with a number of disorders. For example, patients can develop eyelid myotonia in association with primary hypothyroidism. The myotonia typically disappears after such patients are treated with replacement thyroid medication.

Figure 22.32 Risus sardonicus in a child with tetanus. Increased tone of all facial muscles is evident. Note that the child appears to be smiling. Her apparent bilateral ptosis is caused by myotonia of the orbicularis oculi muscles. (Reprinted with permission from Ford FR. *Diseases of the Nervous System in Infancy, Childhood and Adolescence.* 5th ed 5. Springfield, IL: CC Thomas, 1966:621.)

Patients with both the congenital and adult forms of myotonic dystrophy may show myotonia of the orbicularis oculi. In adults with myotonic dystrophy, EMG studies demonstrate evidence of prolonged contraction in the orbicularis oculi following a blink (see Chapter 20).

Myotonia of the orbicularis oculi may occur in patients with hyperkalemic familial periodic paralysis. Slowness of eyelid opening or temporary narrowing of the palpebral fissure may occur following sustained eyelid closure, application of ice to the lids, or administration of potassium salts. Eyelid myotonia can also occur in patients with chondrodystrophic myotonia (Schwartz–Jampel syndrome) (see Chapter 20).

Neuro-Ophthalmologic Manifestations of Nonorganic Disease

General Considerations

Terminology
    Malingering
    Munchausen Syndrome
    Psychogenic Disturbance

Specific Nonorganic Neuro-Ophthalmologic Disorders
    Nonorganic Disease Affecting the Afferent Visual Pathway
    Nonorganic Disease Affecting Fixation, Ocular Motility, and Alignment
    Nonorganic Disorders of Pupillary Size and Reactivity
    Nonorganic Disturbances of Accommodation
    Nonorganic Disturbances of Eyelid Function
    Nonorganic Disturbances of Ocular and Facial Sensation
    Nonorganic Disturbances of Lacrimation

Patients who have physical signs and symptoms for which no adequate organic cause can be found may receive any one of a large range of diagnostic labels, including functional illness, functional overlay, hysteria, hysterical overlay, conversion reaction, psychophysiologic reaction, somatization reaction, hypochondriasis, invalid reaction, neurasthenia, psychogenic reaction, psychosomatic illness, malingering, and Munchausen syndrome. This plethora of labels highlights the confusion that occurs when one tries to fit patients with nonorganic disease into a formal classification.

General Considerations

The **nature of the symptom** and the manner of its communication are crucial in the understanding of a nonorganic disorder. The patient may be stoic and restrained, or histrionic and dramatizing. The symptom may take the form of a physical dysfunction (e.g., strabismus) that is displayed with a minimum of verbal description, or the symptom may be described verbally during the examination. Thus, one must also determine the **nature of the physical dysfunction** and the degree of disability. It is important to determine why the symptoms have focused in a particular area (e.g., the visual system).

Another consideration is the amount of time a patient spends thinking about his or her symptoms and the precise nature of the thoughts in phenomenologic terms. This concept is called **ideation**.

A patient's **affect** may tell the physician much about the patient's complaints. Some patients clearly are depressed, whereas others are truly indifferent, and still others are anxious. Of particular interest is a patient's **attitude toward those involved in the diagnosis and treatment of his or her condition**. These are persons with whom one would expect the patient to cooperate in an attempt to get well. Is the patient hostile, suspicious, fearful, flirtatious, pleading, aloof, or excessively cooperative and agreeable?

Understanding a patient's **motivation** or incentive for achieving the "sick role" and the degree to which he or she is conscious of it may be the most difficult part of the diagnostic process, but it may be the most crucial. The nature of motivation may range from an unconscious seeking of the dependency-gratifying and guilt-allaying aspects of the "sick role" to the overtly conscious attempt to obtain attention, sympathy, material gain, or a combination of these. Hence, the presentation needs to be contextualized to the patient's overall state and circumstances.

Mere observation of the patient in waiting room or examination room can be very rewarding. For example, individuals with a claim of profound visual loss may be limited in their capacity to navigate, use his/her phone, or perform detailed tasks. However, many patients with nonorganic disease perform well on these types of near-habitual tasks, without realizing the inconsistency. It is also important to remember that "real" disease, at least to some extent, often accompanies a nonorganic component. Hence, the examiner must be thorough and not assume that a patient presenting with nonorganic visual loss must have "normal" vision.

Terminology

Most nonorganic disturbances are categorized by three types: (a) malingering; (b) Munchausen syndrome; and (c) psychogenic.

Malingering

Patients whose symptoms are consciously and voluntarily produced are said to be **malingering**. Malingering can be divided into several different categories, including simulation of nonexistent disease, elaboration of pre-existing disease, and attribution of a disability to a different cause. The most common settings in which malingering occurs are potential compensation after a real or feigned injury, avoidance of a particular task, such as military service or a simple school examination for which the patient is unprepared, or an attempt to seek special attention from family or friends.

Munchausen Syndrome

Malingering must be differentiated from **factitious disorder with physical symptoms**, also called the **Munchausen syndrome**. Patients with this condition intentionally produce physical symptoms and signs, some of which may be ocular. Manifestations might include swelling and redness of the conjunctiva simulating an orbital cellulitis, scarring of the eyelids and conjunctiva, and even chorioretinal scarring, all of which are then presented to members of the medical profession. Patients with Munchausen syndrome are thought to harbor a psychological internal need to adopt the role of a sick person.

Psychogenic Disturbance

Patients whose symptoms seem truly independent of volition are said to have a somatoform disorder or **psychogenic disturbance**. Examples of psychogenic disturbances include body dysmorphic disorder, conversion disorder (hysteria, conversion reaction), hypochondriasis, and somatization disorder.

A **body dysmorphic disorder** is characterized by a patient's perception of a single physical defect, most often in the facial region, including the eye. The patient is preoccupied with this sign, even though it is minimal (e.g., a mild ptosis or anisocoria) or is not present at all.

A **conversion disorder** is diagnosed if alterations or a loss of physical functioning are present that seem to express a psychological conflict or need rather than indicating organic illness. This disorder comprises the clinical syndromes that were previously classified as "hysteria" or "conversion neurosis." Patients in whom such disorders occur may subconsciously obtain both primary gain (e.g., protection from trauma or reduction of stress) and secondary gain (e.g., increased attention).

Hypochondriasis is the fear of, or strong belief in, specific serious physical conditions accompanied by excessive self-observation and the reporting of numerous physical signs and symptoms. It differs from body dysmorphic disorder in that it includes both symptoms and signs from multiple organ systems throughout the body.

A **somatization disorder** features recurrent and multiple somatic complaints. As in hypochondriasis, multiple organ systems may be mentioned, but the patient's descriptions are vague, and anxiety or depression usually is present.

Unfortunately, there remains a large group of patients in whom a clear distinction between malingering, Munchausen syndrome, and psychogenic or somatoform disturbances simply cannot be made. In such cases, the physician must recognize that there is no organic basis for the patient's symptoms and signs and manage the patient accordingly.

Specific Nonorganic Neuro-Ophthalmologic Disorders

From a neuro-ophthalmologic standpoint, there are five areas that may be affected by nonorganic disease.

1 Vision, including visual acuity and visual field
2 Ocular motility and alignment
3 Pupillary size and reactivity
4 Eyelid position and function; and
5 Corneal and facial sensation.

The physician faced with a patient complaining of decreased vision or some other disturbance related to the **afferent** or **efferent** visual systems for which there is no apparent biologic explanation has two responsibilities. First, the physician must ascertain that an organic disorder is not present. Second, the physician must determine if the patient can see or do something that would not be possible if the condition were organic in nature. To best achieve these goals, the physician must adopt an **empathetic** attitude toward the patient regardless of the patient's history, attitude of the patient toward the physician or the disease, or the clinical findings. Keeping an open mind will be helpful for the physician to not miss something important and will likely gain more cooperation from the patient than if a confrontational or dismissive tone is taken.

Nonorganic Disease Affecting the Afferent Visual Pathway

Nonorganic disease that affects the **afferent** visual system is extremely common. It may occur as monocular or binocular decreased visual acuity, abnormal visual fields, or both. Color vision often is abnormal in such patients (depending on the manner in which it is tested), but abnormal color vision is rarely a primary complaint.

Decreased Visual Acuity

Decreased visual acuity is probably the most common nonorganic disturbance in ophthalmology. It occurs most often in children and young adults, but it may be observed in patients 60 years of age and older. It may be psychogenic or caused by malingering. Nonorganic visual loss that is psychogenic seems to be more common in children, with females being affected much more often than males. Malingerers are most often adult males, perhaps because men are more often involved in motor vehicle and work-related accidents than are women.

Patients with nonorganic loss of visual acuity complain of a variable loss of vision in one or both eyes that is not accompanied by a refractive error, a disturbance of the ocular media, or other evidence of retinal or optic nerve dysfunction. Abnormal color perception, an abnormal visual field, or both, may accompany the visual loss.

In many cases, the physician may suspect that the patient's visual loss is nonorganic during the medical history, as noted above, is perhaps the most crucial aspect of the evaluation. In addition, the way the patient acts during the history taking may be helpful. Patients who are truly blind in both eyes tend to look directly at the person with whom they are speaking, whereas patients with nonorganic blindness, particularly patients who are malingering, often look in some other direction. Similarly, patients claiming complete or nearly complete blindness often wear sunglasses, even though they do not have photophobia, and the external appearance of the eyes is perfectly normal. In any event, the physician who suspects a nonorganic

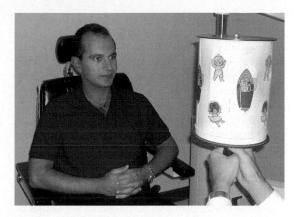

Figure 23.1 Use of the optokinetic drum to detect nonorganic bilateral blindness. The patient is asked to look straight ahead with both eyes open, while the drum is rotated, first in one direction, then in the other.

visual process may be able to orient the examination in a way to bring out the nonorganic nature of the visual disturbance.

If a patient claims no perception of light, light perception only, or perception of hand motions by one or both eyes, one can use a rotating optokinetic drum or horizontally moving tape to produce a horizontal jerk nystagmus that indicates intact vision of at least 20/400 (Fig. 23.1). It is important in this regard that the images on the tape or drum be sufficiently large, so that the patient is not able to look around them. When testing a patient who claims complete loss of vision in one eye only, the test is begun by rotating the drum or moving the tape in front of the patient, who has **both** eyes open. Once good optokinetic nystagmus is elicited, the unaffected eye is suddenly covered with the palm of the examiner's hand or a handheld occluder (Fig. 23.2).

Figure 23.2 Use of optokinetic drum to detect nonorganic unilateral blindness. **A:** In a patient claiming unilateral blindness, the drum is first rotated, while the patient is instructed to look straight ahead with both eyes open. **B:** Once nystagmus is elicited, the examiner continues to rotate the drum and suddenly covers the "normal" eye with the palm of the hand and observes the "blind" eye for continued nystagmus.

Patients with nonorganic loss of vision in one eye will continue to show a jerk nystagmus.

A second test that is helpful in detecting visual function in an eye or eyes that are said to have either no perception of light or light perception only is the "mirror test." A large mirror is held in front of the patient's face, and the patient is asked to look directly ahead. The mirror is then rotated and twisted back and forth, causing the images in the mirror to move. Patients with vision better than light perception will show a nystagmoid movement of the eyes since they cannot avoid following the moving reflection in the mirror.

An excellent way to detect nonorganic visual loss in a patient who claims to be unable to see shapes or objects in one or both eyes is to ask the patient to touch the tips of the first fingers of both hands together. If the patient claims loss of vision in one eye only, the opposite eye is patched before the test is performed. The ability to touch the tips of the fingers of two hands together is based not on vision but on proprioception. Thus, patients with organic blindness can easily bring the tips of the first fingers of both hands together, whereas patients with nonorganic blindness, particularly those who are malingering, will often demonstrate an inability to do so (Fig. 23.3). Similarly, a patient with organic blindness can easily sign his or her name without difficulty, whereas patients with blindness caused by malingering

may produce an extremely bizarre signature that often runs off the page or very large script.

A variety of tests may be performed in patients who claim vision in the range of 20/40 to hand motions in one or both eyes. None of these tests is invariably reliable, but one or more usually is sufficient to provide convincing evidence that visual acuity loss either is nonexistent or not as severe as the patient claims. Visual acuity may be tested not by starting from the largest letters or numbers and moving progressively to smaller ones, but by beginning with the **smallest** line ("bottom-up acuity"). Assuming that the patient cannot see this first line after being allowed to concentrate for several minutes, the physician tells the patient that the size of the print is now going to be "doubled" in size, and the patient is shown the next larger line and given several minutes to read it. This process is continued until the patient is able to read the line. This method of testing often produces visual acuity better than that initially claimed by the patient. In addition, some projector slides have several 20/20 lines, and these lines may be shown to the patient in succession as the examiner tells the patient the size of the letters is increasing. The key is to encourage the patient that each subsequent line presented should be "much easier" to see.

Testing of near vision is also important in patients claiming decreased acuity. A discrepancy in the distance

Figure 23.3 Testing nonorganic visual loss by asking a patient who claims monocular or binocular blindness to touch the tips of the first fingers of each hand together. **A and B:** A person who is truly blind can easily touch the tips of the fingers together, using proprioception, as the person in these photographs is doing despite having both eyes occluded. **C:** A man with nonorganic loss of vision in both eyes is unable to touch the tips of the fingers together, even though he should be able to do so. A person with monocular nonorganic visual loss may touch the tips of the fingers together when viewing with the "normal" eye (**D**), but may claim to be unable to do so when viewing with the "blind" eye (**E**).

and near-visual acuity that is not attributable to a refractive error or a disturbance of the media, such as an oil drop cataract, usually is evidence of a nonorganic disturbance.

Patients claiming decreased vision in one eye only may undergo a "refraction" in which the normal eye is fogged with a high plus lens (e.g., a +5.00 or higher sphere), and a lens with minimal power (e.g., a ±0.50 sphere or cylinder) is placed before the worse eye. The patient is then told to read the chart with "both eyes." A variation of this test is the use of paired cylinders. A plus cylinder and a minus cylinder of the same power (usually 2 to 6 diopters) are placed at parallel axes in front of the "normal" eye in a trial frame. The patient's normal correction is placed in front of the affected eye. The patient is asked to read, with both eyes open, a line that previously had been read with the normal eye but not with the affected eye. As the patient begins to read, the axis of one of the cylinders is rotated about 10 to 15 degrees. The axes of the two cylinders thus will no longer be parallel, blurring vision in the normal eye. If the patient continues to read the line, or can read it again when asked to do so, he or she must be using the affected eye.

Red–green glasses used with a red and green duochrome slide superimposed on the normal vision chart can be used to induce a patient to read with an eye that supposedly cannot see (or cannot see well) by making the patient think that he or she is using both eyes. In this test, the eye behind the red lens will see the letters on both sides of the chart, whereas the eye behind the green lens will see only those letters on the green side of the chart. The lenses are arranged, so that the red lens is over the eye with decreased vision, and the patient is then asked to read the chart with both eyes open. If the patient reads the entire line, it is obvious that the abnormal eye must be functioning better than the patient claims. The fogging refraction and duochrome testing are highly effective methods to "trick" the patient into using the affected eye to see what they admit to seeing with the normal eye. However the physician's performance of these tests needs to be fluid and deliberate. If the patient begins to alternate closing the eyes behind the phoropter or red/green glasses, the physician should be aware that the patient be suspicious of the premise.

A variant of the red–green glasses/duochrome chart test that employs the red–green glasses and Ishihara color plates can be performed in patients with presumed nonorganic monocular visual loss that is worse than 20/400. The patient should first be tested for "congenital" color vision as described below. Once it has been established that color vision is normal, the patient is asked to view the Ishihara color plates while wearing red–green glasses with the red lens over the affected eye. With the exception of plates 1 and 36, the numbers and lines on the Ishihara plates cannot be seen by the eye over which the green filter is placed. Even with visual acuity of 20/400, however, all of the color plates can be seen through a red filter. Thus, a patient who has normal color vision in at least the unaffected eye, who then views the plates through red–green spectacles with the red lens in front of the affected eye, and who correctly identifies the figures on the plates, must have visual acuity of 20/400 or better in the affected eye.

Polarizing lenses can be used in several ways to detect nonorganic visual loss in a patient with decreased vision in one eye only. In the American Optical Polarizing Test, the patient wears polarizing glasses, and the test object, a Project-O-Chart slide, projects letters alternately so that one letter is seen by both eyes, the next by the right eye, the next by the left eye, etc. Another test uses a polarizing lens placed before a projector. The patient is asked to read the chart while wearing polarizing lenses, with one eye or the other being allowed to see the whole projected image at a time.

A prism that is 4 diopters in strength can be used to detect vision in an eye said to have reduced or no vision. The patient is asked to look with both eyes at the vision chart. A 4-prism diopter loose prism is then placed, base-out, over the "affected eye." A patient with normal binocular vision will show a movement of both eyes toward the direction of the apex of the prism followed by a shift of the fellow eye back toward the center. A patient with true decreased or absent vision in the eye over which the prism is placed will show no conjugate movement at all. Similarly, when the prism is placed over the "better eye" of a patient whose other eye truly is blind or has extremely reduced sight, only the first conjugate binocular shift will occur. There will be no compensatory movement of the fellow eye back toward the center.

Several **prism dissociation tests** can be used to detect mild degrees of nonorganic monocular visual loss. In this test, the patient is first asked if he or she has experienced double vision in addition to loss of vision in the affected eye. If the answer is no, the patient is told that the examiner will test the alignment of both eyes and that the test should produce vertical double vision. A 4-prism diopter loose prism is then placed base down in front of the unaffected eye at the same time that a 1/2-prism diopter prism is simultaneously placed with the base in any direction over the eye with decreased vision. In this way, the patient does not become suspicious that the examiner is paying specific attention to one eye or the other. A 20/20 or larger size Snellen letter is then projected in the distance, and the patient is asked if he or she has double vision. When the patient admits to diplopia, he or she is then asked whether the two letters are of equal quality or sharpness, and an assessment of visual acuity can then be made.

Testing of stereopsis may be valuable in detecting nonorganic visual loss. There is a definite correlation

Table 23.1	Relationship of Visual Acuity and Stereopsis

Visual Acuity	Average Stereopsis[a]
20/20	40
20/25	43
20/30	52
20/40	61
20/50	78
20/70	94
20/100	124
20/200	160

[a]Measured in seconds of image disparity.
(Modified from Levy NS, Glick EB. Stereoscopic perception and Snellen visual acuity. *Am J Ophthalmol.* 1974;78:722–724.)

between binocular visual acuity and stereopsis (Table 23.1). For instance, a patient with 20/20 vision in one eye and organic visual loss producing visual acuity of 20/200 in the fellow eye has stereoacuity of only about 180 seconds of arc, whereas a patient with 20/20 visual acuity OU has stereoacuity of 40 seconds of arc. A variety of stereoacuity tests are available, all of which have advantages and disadvantages. The patient can be told that the examiner "just wants to make sure the good eye is seeing well."

Examination of pupillary responses can be helpful in diagnosing nonorganic visual loss. Patients who report complete blindness in both eyes should have pupils that do not react to light stimulation unless the process affects the postgeniculate visual pathways. Thus, the pupils of a patient who cannot perceive light with either eye because of bilateral retinal, optic nerve, or optic tract lesions, or because of damage to the optic chiasm, do not react to light stimulation, whereas the pupils of a patient who is blind from bilateral lesions of the optic radiations or striate cortex will react relatively normally to light. Pupils that react briskly to light stimulation in a patient who claims complete loss of vision in both eyes indicate either that the patient is cerebrally blind (usually from damage to the striate cortex—cortical blindness) or that the patient has nonorganic loss of vision.

Patients with unilateral or asymmetric optic neuropathy invariably have a relative afferent pupillary defect (RAPD) that can easily be detected by performing a swinging flashlight test (see Chapters 14 and 15). The absence of an RAPD in a patient with monocular visual loss indicates either that the patient does not have a unilateral optic neuropathy (and thus may support a diagnosis of nonorganic visual loss) or that the patient has a **bilateral** optic neuropathy that is mildly asymmetric. It must be emphasized that patients with electrophysiologic evidence of bilateral optic neuropathy may

nevertheless have very asymmetric visual acuity in the two eyes unassociated with an RAPD. Thus, if there is no indication of nonorganic disease in a patient with unexplained, unilateral visual loss without an obvious RAPD, such a patient should undergo electrophysiologic testing, particularly full-field and multifocal electroretinography and pattern-reversal and flash-evoked visual-evoked potentials. Deliberate defocusing during VEP studies can often produce a reduction of amplitude, but not prolonged latency. In addition, ERG and mFERG testing generally provides a strong objective measure of retinal sensitivity.

The management of patients who have nonorganic loss of visual acuity is problematic and often depends on whether the patient is a child or an adult and whether the condition is thought to be psychogenic or caused by malingering. Nonorganic visual loss in children usually occurs as a situational phenomenon caused by a wide range of academic, social, or familial difficulties. Once it is certain that the condition is nonorganic, one can first attempt to "cure" the visual loss by informing the child that the only problem is a slight refractive error. A minimal correction is then placed into a trial frame or phoropter, and the patient is told that they "should see normally" with this set of glasses. If this is successful, the patient is told not to worry about the visual process and that the refractive error is sufficiently minimal that it probably is not necessary for glasses to be worn. If this maneuver is unsuccessful, the parents can be privately informed of the findings, so that they will not continue to be concerned about an organic process. The child is then informed that, fortunately, there is **no irreversible damage to the eyes** and that vision should improve spontaneously with time. No particular time frame is indicated during which this will occur, and the child is encouraged to "do as well as you can" in school, at home, etc., until vision improves. This approach usually is sufficient to solve the problem in the vast majority of cases. Nevertheless, dealing with children whose visual loss is associated with complex interpersonal relationships within the family, such as sexual abuse or other social difficulties, is much more difficult and may require the services of a psychotherapist, child psychiatrist, or other specialist. Parents are often reluctant to accept a diagnosis of nonorganic visual disturbance for their child. Such discussion needs to be thoughtful, and often a sensitive matter. Offering the family a second opinion if there is an impasse in communication, is appropriate and potentially supportive for the parents and physician.

The treatment of adults with nonorganic loss of visual acuity is more complicated than the treatment of children, particularly when there is evidence of malingering, and the outcome usually is much less satisfactory. As long as there is a motivation for material secondary gain, it may be impossible to "treat" such a patient for his or her visual loss. In many cases, the physician must be content that the loss of vision is nonorganic and to record this fact in the patient's chart. There is no purpose in confronting the patient with our belief that the visual loss is nonorganic unless one can convince the patient that ultimately it is not in his or her best interest to continue the charade because there is objective evidence that the visual loss is nonorganic and that such evidence will eventually cost the patient time, money, or even freedom.

Visual Field Defects

Nonorganic visual field defects can be of several types. The most common nonorganic visual field defect is a nonspecifically constricted visual field. When the field is tested kinetically, using either a Goldmann perimeter or a tangent screen, the field may have a spiraling nature, becoming smaller and smaller as the test object is moved around the field (Fig. 23.4). Alternatively, the visual field may remain the same size (tunnel field) or nearly the same size regardless of the size or brightness of the test stimulus, or it may be inconsistent when tested repeatedly in one or more meridians. Other

nonorganic visual field defects, however, include unilateral or bilateral central scotomas, unilateral hemianopia, bitemporal hemianopia, binasal hemianopia, and even homonymous hemianopia.

A nonorganically constricted visual field may be diagnosed in a variety of ways. In some cases, the patient can be cajoled into enlarging the field. After completion of perimetry, the patient is told that he or she did fine but that it was clear to the examiner that the patient was responding only when he or she was "absolutely certain" that he or she saw the test object. The examiner then explains that the test is to be repeated and encourages the patient to respond at an earlier stage when he or she just barely detects the stimulus.

Nonorganic visual field constriction can also be detected by testing the field using a tangent screen with the patient at two different distances from the screen (usually 1 and 2 meters). The size of the test object is varied, so that the ratio of the size of the test object and the distance of the patient from the screen remain constant; that is, a 9-mm-diameter white test object is used when the patient is 1 m from the screen, and an

Figure 23.4 In a patient claiming visual difficulties in the right eye, there is a nonorganic spiral field when the eye is tested kinetically using a Goldmann perimeter.

18-mm-diameter white test object is used when the patient is 2 m from the screen, to ensure that the target subtends the same degree of arc on the patient's retina. Patients with an organically constricted visual field (e.g., patients with retinitis pigmentosa) will show an increase in the absolute size of the visual field under these conditions when they are moved from 1 to 2 m away from the screen, whereas patients with nonorganic visual field constriction will maintain the same absolute size of the field constriction. Automated kinetic perimetry can give similar results.

Nonorganic monocular hemianopias and scotomas as well as both binasal and bitemporal hemianopic defects usually can be diagnosed by first performing visual field testing monocularly and then binocularly (Fig. 23.5). If the field defect is present in only one eye when the eyes are tested separately, but is still present when binocular simultaneous field testing is performed, the defect can be assumed to be nonorganic. This method cannot distinguish between organic and nonorganic homonymous hemianopic defects or bilateral central scotomas.

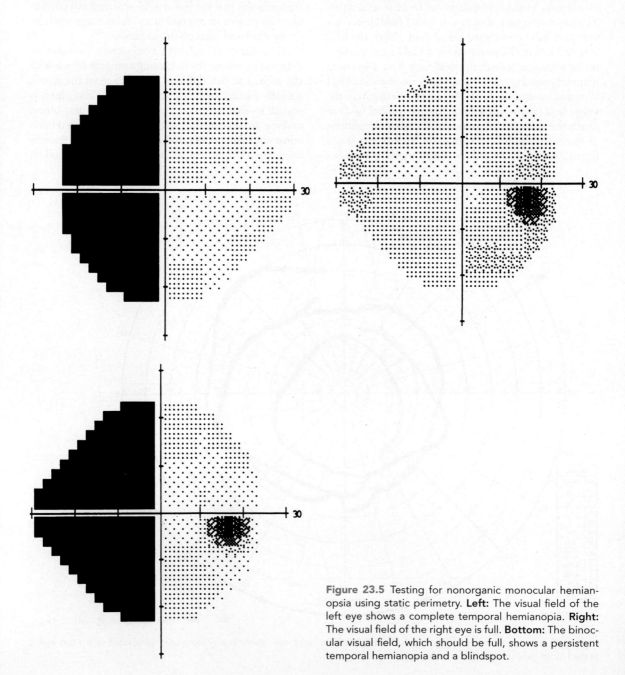

Figure 23.5 Testing for nonorganic monocular hemianopsia using static perimetry. **Left:** The visual field of the left eye shows a complete temporal hemianopia. **Right:** The visual field of the right eye is full. **Bottom:** The binocular visual field, which should be full, shows a persistent temporal hemianopia and a blindspot.

A quick and easy method of detecting nonorganic visual field loss of all types is to test saccadic eye movements into the supposedly absent portion of the field. The patient assumes that the eye movements and not the visual fields are being tested. This assumption is strengthened by first asking the patient if it hurts to move the eyes. Regardless of the patient's answer (which, interestingly, is often affirmative), the patient is told that the examiner is going to test the eye movements, and the patient is asked to pursue an object in various directions. The patient is then asked to look from the straight ahead position to an eccentric location where the examiner holds an object. The object is subsequently moved from one location to another with the patient being asked each time to look from the center to the object. If the patient complains that he or she "cannot see" that far in the periphery, the examiner explains that he or she understands and that is why the patient should look **directly** at the object rather than to try to see it in the peripheral vision.

It should be noted that patients can create reproducible nonorganic visual field defects not only when tested with kinetic perimetry but also when tested using automated static perimetry (Fig. 23.6) with marked respect for the vertical and horizontal meridians. Such patients do not necessarily show an increased number of fixation losses or false-positive or false-negative errors.

The management of patients with nonorganic visual field constriction is similar to that of patients with nonorganic visual loss. Children and adults who do not seem to be malingering are told that they eventually will improve, and this usually is the case. Interestingly, most patients with nonorganic visual field loss deny that their visual field disturbance significantly limits their daily activities or state that despite their visual difficulties they are able to maintain their normal lifestyle. Such patients thus rarely require psychiatric or psychological counseling for these patients.

Monocular Diplopia

Most patients who complain of double vision are suffering from misalignment of the visual axes. In such cases, the diplopia immediately resolves as soon as one eye is covered. Patients in whom diplopia remains despite occlusion of one eye are said to have **monocular diplopia**. This condition is caused most often by a refractive error, particularly by uncorrected or improperly corrected astigmatism; by incorrectly fitted glasses; or by some irregularity of the cornea or lens. Most patients with this type of organic monocular diplopia will recognize a difference in the intensity of the two images that they see. One image will be fairly clear, but the second image will be perceived as "fuzzy" and may be described as a "ghost image" that overlaps the clear image. The "diplopia" in such cases usually

resolves with a pinhole, a better refraction or fitting of spectacles, or a contact lens.

True monocular diplopia (i.e., two separate and equal images of an object seen with one eye only) is almost never caused by organic disease. It is seen it most often in children who have found themselves in stressful academic, social, or family situations. Once both the child and the parents are reassured as to the benign nature of the condition, it usually resolves within a short period of time.

Nonorganic Disease Affecting Fixation, Ocular Motility, and Alignment

Nonorganic disturbances of ocular motor function include disturbances of fixation, ocular motility, and alignment.

Disturbances of Fixation: Voluntary Nystagmus and Voluntary Saccadic Oscillations

Saccadic oscillations in most patients are involuntary eye movements caused by a neurologic disease affecting the brainstem, cerebellum, or both. Nevertheless, some persons can produce saccadic oscillations that resemble nystagmus, ocular flutter, or opsoclonus.

Voluntary nystagmus is characterized by a rapid to-and-fro movement of the eyes that is willfully initiated. It can be produced by 5% to 8% of the population and may occur as a familial trait. Voluntary nystagmus consists of rapidly alternating saccades with frequencies that range from 3 to 42 Hz and amplitudes that range from 0.5 to 35 and that can be sustained for only a few seconds. Voluntary nystagmus usually is horizontal; however, rarely it can be vertical or torsional, and it can be produced in the light or dark and with the eyelids open or closed. It is almost always binocular and conjugate but has been reported as a monocular phenomenon.

Patients with voluntary nystagmus typically complain of oscillopsia and reduced vision. Such patients have fluttering of the eyelids and a strained facial expression during the episodes of nystagmus. In addition, the eyes tend to converge during the nystagmus.

Voluntary nystagmus has no pathologic significance. It may, however, be mistaken for certain pathologic conditions that affect fixation, including acquired nystagmus and saccadic intrusions. Rare patients appear to be able to produce large-amplitude, to-and-fro rapid eye movements. These **voluntary saccadic oscillations** are actually bursts of conjugate saccades in opposing directions, with no intersaccadic interval. Unlike the saccades of voluntary nystagmus, they are multidirectional (horizontal, vertical, or oblique), have amplitudes up to 40, and sometimes have curvilinear trajectories. These characteristics are similar to those of ocular flutter and opsoclonus; however, patients

PIГHT

AGE   36
FIXATION LOSSES   0/20
FALSE POS ERRORS   0/11
FALSE NEG ERRORS   0/10
QUESTIONS ASKED   342
FOVEA: 37 06
TEST TIME 00:10:31

30°

A

60°   60°   60°   60°

B

30°   30°

C

Figure 23.6 Fabricated visual field defects. **A:** Artificially produced quadrantanopsia with the Humphrey field analyzer, using a 24-2 program. Note the excellent reliability. **B:** Fabricated bitemporal hemianopia, using the Humphrey Full Field 120-point screening test **(left and right)**. **C:** Fabricated incongruous right homonymous hemianopia, using Humphrey Central 30-2 threshold test. (*continued*)

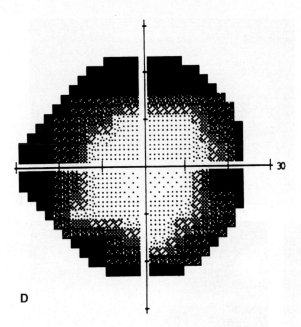

D

Figure 23.6 (*Continued*) **D:** Fabricated constricted visual field in a patient with no clinical or electrophysiologic evidence of retinopathy or optic neuropathy. Note the "squaring" of the field defect, a phenomenon common to nonorganic visual field constriction recorded by automated perimetry. (**A:** Reprinted with permission from Glovinsky Y, Quigley HA, Bissett RA, et al. Artificially produced quadrantanopsia in computed visual field testing. *Am J Ophthalmol.* 1990;110:90–91. **B and C:** Reprinted with permission from MacLeod JDA, Manners RM, Heaven CJ, et al. Visual field defects. *Neuroophthalmology.* 1994;14:185–188.)

with true ocular flutter or opsoclonus generally have other neurologic manifestations. Thus, when saccadic oscillations that appear to be ocular flutter or opsoclonus are found in patients who do not have other neurologic signs or symptoms, the possibility of a nonorganic cause should be considered. True opsoclonus is sustained and relentless, whereas nonorganic eye movements cannot be maintained indefinitely.

Disorders of Ocular Motility and Alignment

Several nonorganic disorders of ocular motility and alignment may be observed in patients both with and without visual complaints. These disorders include insufficiency or paralysis of convergence, spasm of the near reflex, supranuclear horizontal and vertical gaze paresis, and forced downward deviation of the eyes.

Convergence Insufficiency or Paralysis. Convergence insufficiency or paralysis may be nonorganic in nature. We have seen several cases, usually in adolescents, but also in adults. Patients with apparent weakness of convergence may nevertheless show normal convergence when asked to read a paragraph at length during which the eyes are alternately covered. Asking

the patient to perform other near tasks such as telling time by looking at his or her wristwatch or phone, may also be associated with normal convergence.

Spasm of the Near Reflex. The most common nonorganic disturbance of ocular motility and alignment is **spasm of the near reflex** (Fig. 23.7). The syndrome is characterized by episodes of intermittent convergence, increased accommodation, and miosis. The degree of convergence is variable. Some patients exhibit marked convergence of both eyes, resulting in a marked esotropia. Others show a lesser degree of convergence such that one eye remains relatively straight while the other converges. In all cases, however, the patient seems to have unilateral or, more often, bilateral limitation of abduction during testing of versions although not necessarily during testing of ductions. The degree of accommodation spasm also is variable. Some patients produce only a few diopters of myopia, whereas others produce 8 to 10 diopters of myopia. Miosis is invariably significant in patients who exhibit spasm of the near reflex regardless of the degree of accommodation and convergence spasm.

Spasm of the near reflex may be mistaken for unilateral or bilateral abducens nerve paresis, divergence insufficiency, horizontal gaze paresis, or even myasthenia gravis. However, the lack of other neurologic deficits, the variability of the eye movements, and the constant occurrence of miosis associated with the adductive eye movements generally permit the correct diagnosis to be made. In addition, despite apparent unilateral or bilateral abduction weakness during testing of versions (with both eyes open), when ductions are tested directly with one eye occluded or indirectly using oculocephalic testing, both eyes invariably have full abduction and the miosis seen when the eyes are in the esotropic position immediately resolves. Covering one eye during a typical spasm also may cause dramatic reversal of the miosis. Finally, refraction with and without cycloplegia during a period of spasm establishes the presence of pseudomyopia.

Several organic conditions, in addition to abducens nerve paresis and horizontal gaze paresis, may mimic spasm of the near reflex. Pretectal esotropia, also called pseudo-abducens paresis or pseudo-sixth nerve palsy, is a general disordered cocontraction of extraocular muscles and is not related to the near reflex (can be seen in dorsal midbrain syndrome). Convergence-retraction nystagmus jerks are not accompanied by miosis in this condition. Convergence substitution sometimes occurs when patients with supranuclear horizontal gaze paresis use convergence to move the adducting eye into the limited field of gaze. The resulting eye movement may suggest spasm of the near reflex.

True convergence spasm may occasionally be caused by organic lesions, such as intrinsic lesions of

Figure 23.7 Spasm of the near reflex. The patient is a healthy 15-year-old girl. **A:** In primary position, the eyes are eso-tropic, and the pupils are constricted. **B:** On attempted right gaze, the right eye does not abduct, even to the midline, and the pupils become more constricted. **C:** On attempted left gaze, the left eye does not abduct beyond the midline, and the pupils become more constricted. **D:** When the left eye is patched and the patient is asked to pursue a target to the right or is asked to fixate a stationary target while the head is rotated to the left, the right eye abducts fully and the pupil becomes less constricted.

the mesencephalon or extrinsic lesions compressing the dorsal mesencephalon. Thus, the examiner who is unsure whether or not spasm of the near reflex is organic must be prepared to give the patient the benefit of the doubt and perform appropriate neuroimaging studies.

Management of persons with nonorganic spasm of the near reflex may consist only of reassurance. Psy-chiatric counseling may be appropriate in other cases. In some patients, symptomatic relief may be produced using a cycloplegic drug combined with bifocal specta-cles or reading glasses, or even glasses with an opaque inner third of the lens such that they occlude vision when the eyes are esotropic. Spasm of the near reflex should never be treated with strabismus surgery as it will not eliminate the esotropia that is present during the spasms and will produce an exotropia between spasms.

Paralysis of Horizontal and Vertical Gaze.
Patients with nonorganic **paralysis of horizontal and vertical eye movements** will not make voluntary

horizontal or vertical saccades or pursuit movements and will not fixate on a distant object to allow ocu-locephalic testing; however, when such patients are observed through a one-way mirror, they can be seen to make absolutely normal pursuit and saccadic eye movements. In addition, measurements of eye move-ments during chair rotation in light and darkness indicate normal pursuit and saccadic systems.

Forced Downward Deviation of the Eyes in Nonorganic Coma and Seizures

The typical response of a patient with organic coma is either no movement of the eyes, such as occurs in patients with brainstem disease or drug-induced coma, or a smooth movement of the eyes in the direction **opposite** of a head turn. The eyes of a patient feigning a comatose state, however, are often deviated tonically toward the floor as if to avoid looking at the observer. There is often associated convergence to "hold" the eyes in the tonically deviated direction. On moving the head to the opposite side, the eyes will either saccade directly to the side facing the floor (i.e., in the **same** direction as the head turn) or they occasionally will dart from side to side before coming to rest. Although a true seizure focus may certainly produce a deviation of the eyes to one side, turning the head from side to side in such a setting will not affect this deviation.

Nonorganic Disorders of Pupillary Size and Reactivity

A variety of pupillary phenomena have been described in patients with various types of psychiatric and psychogenic diseases. For example, anxious patients occasionally have widely dilated and poorly reacting pupils that fail to dilate further to a psychosensory stimulus as they are already maximally dilated. The pupils of schizophrenic patients are sometimes dilated and unreactive, and some patients develop widely dilated pupils during acute attacks of panic and that are associated with generalized autonomic disturbances consistent with sympathetic hyperfunction, including profuse sweating, trembling, tachycardia, and tachypnea. The pupils of such patients appear normal between attacks, and will constrict to light and/or a near stimulus.

Perhaps the most common induced pupillary disturbance seen in ophthalmologic practice is a unilateral (and occasionally bilateral), fixed, dilated pupil caused by purposeful topical administration of a mydriatic agent (Fig. 23.8A). Pharmacologically dilated pupils are extremely large—larger than the dilated pupils associated with an oculomotor nerve palsy—usually very uniformly dilated and completely nonreactive to light or near stimulation. They are unassociated with ptosis, diplopia, or strabismus unless there is a preexisting disturbance of eyelid function or ocular motility. The diagnosis of a pharmacologically dilated pupil is made by placing 1 to 2 drops of 1% pilocarpine in each lower cul-de-sac. A neurologically dilated pupil (i.e., oculomotor nerve paresis, tonic pupil) will constrict maximally within 30 minutes; however, a pharmacologically dilated pupil either is not affected and remains widely dilated (Fig. 23.8B) or constricts minimally. Unresponsiveness or even partial responsiveness of a dilated, fixed pupil to a solution of pilocarpine that is of sufficient strength to constrict the opposite, normally reacting pupil is absolute evidence of pharmacologic blockade.

Nonorganic Disturbances of Accommodation

The role of accommodative spasm in the condition called spasm of the near reflex is discussed above. In addition, however, nonorganic **weakness or paralysis of accommodation** may occur, primarily in children and young adults. Such patients are unable to read

A

B

Figure 23.8 Diagnosis of unilateral pupillary dilation caused by voluntary use of a topical parasympatholytic drug using 1% pilocarpine. **A:** Before instillation of pilocarpine, the right pupil is markedly dilated and very uniform (much more so than in a third nerve palsy or Adie tonic pupil). The size of the left pupil is normal. The right pupil was nonreactive to both direct and consensual light stimulation. **B:** Forty-five minutes after instillation of 1% pilocarpine in both lower cul-de-sacs, the right pupil is still markedly dilated but the left pupil is markedly constricted.

unless provided with an appropriate plus lens, and even then may claim an inability to read clearly. Indeed, it is the failure of a patient with normal distance vision and an inability to read despite an appropriate reading aid that should alert the physician to the possibility that the condition is nonorganic.

Nonorganic Disturbances of Eyelid Function

Nonorganic **ptosis** (pseudoptosis) is rare. In most cases, one can see or feel a fine spasm of the supposedly ptotic eyelid. There also tends to be elevation of the lower eyelid and variable relaxation of the elevators of the ipsilateral eyebrow, producing a mild brow ptosis. **Blepharospasm** may rarely be psychogenic in nature. Most cases of psychogenic blepharospasm occur in children and young adults and seem to be triggered by a particular emotionally traumatic event.

Nonorganic Disturbances of Ocular and Facial Sensation

Anesthesia of the skin of the eyelids and of one or both corneas may be nonorganic, as may hypersen-

sitivity, with the latter being associated with lacrimation, blepharospasm, photophobia, or a combination of these. Sensitive spots along the upper or lower margins of the orbits are common in patients with such complaints.

Nonorganic Disturbances of Lacrimation

Excessive secretion of tears may be nonorganic and may be associated with nonorganic blepharospasm. **Bloody tears** may be produced by depositing blood from self-induced nosebleeds into the conjunctival sacs.

Video List

The videos to accompany this text, listed below with their respective chapters, can be found in the online version.

Chapter 3: Congenital Anomalies of the Optic Disc

Video 3.1. Morning glory syndrome with contractile movements. (From Sawada Y, Fujiwara T, Yoshitomi T. Morning glory anomaly with contractile movements. *Graefes Arch Clin Exp Ophthalmol.* 2012;250: 1693–1695, with permission.)

Chapter 12: Topical Diagnosis of Optic Chiasmal and Retrochiasmal Lesions

Video 12.1. Seesaw nystagmus in a patient with a chiasmal syndrome.

Video 12.2. Asymmetric optokinetic nystagmus in a man with a left parietal lobe stroke.

Chapter 14: Examination of the Pupils and Accommodation

Video 14.1. Pupillary testing in an individual with dark irides demonstrates the improved visualization of the pupil with upgaze.

Video 14.2. Right RAPD in primary position and in upgaze in a patient with small pupils and dark irides. Defect is easier to appreciate in upgaze.

Chapter 15: Disorders of Pupillary Function and Accommodation

Video 15.1. Infrared pupillography in a patient with left Horner syndrome. Starting in darkness, anisocoria is present but of small magnitude. With light, both pupils show brisk constriction, and anisocoria is accentuated when the light is turned off because of dilation lag in the affected eye. (Courtesy of Randy H. Kardon, MD, PhD.)

Video 15.2. Light-near dissociation in a patient with Argyll Robertson pupils from syphilitic infection. Pupils are small bilaterally and show virtually no reaction to a bright light stimulus, but brisk bilateral constriction to a near target.

Video 15.3. **A:** Lack of pupillary light response in a patient with dorsal midbrain compression. Note larger pupils than seen in Video 15.2. **B:** Brisk pupillary constriction with near stimulus.

Chapter 17: Supranuclear and Internuclear Ocular Motor Disorders

Video 17.1. Dorsal midbrain (Parinaud) syndrome. Note symmetric limitation of upgaze as well mild bilateral deficit of abduction (pseudoabducens palsy), presumably due to increased convergence tone. On attempted upgaze, the patient develops marked convergence–retraction nystagmus.

Video 17.2. 54-year-old man with oculopalatal tremor that developed 8 months after a pontine hemorrhage from a cavernous malformation. Note undulating, rhythmic movements of the soft palate associated with vertical pendular nystagmus.

Chapter 19: Disorders of Neuromuscular Transmission

Video 19.1. Enhancement of ptosis in a 55-year-old man with myasthenia gravis. The patient also has thyroid eye disease.

Video 19.2. Cogan lid twitch in three patients with myasthenia gravis.

Video 19.3. Internal and external ophthalmoplegia from wound botulism. The patient was an 8-year-old girl who fell from a horse and sustained a compound open fracture of the left humerus. Clostridium botulinum was cultured from the wound. Note not only bilateral ptosis and ophthalmoplegia but also dilated, nonreactive pupils.

Chapter 21: Nystagmus and Related Ocular Motility Disorders

Video 21.1. The Heimann–Bielschowsky phenomenon demonstrated in a patient with poor vision in the right eye after cataract surgery. (From Jeong SH, Oh YM, Hwang JM, et al. Emergence of oscillopsia and diplopia due to Heimann-Bielschowsky phenomenon after cataract surgery. *Br J Ophthalmol.*2008;92:1402.)

Video 21.2. Acquired pendular nystagmus in a patient with multiple sclerosis. There is brief reduction of her nystagmus after attempted rightward saccades (which also demonstrates her left internuclear ophthalmoplegia).

Video 21.3. Oculomasticatory myoarrhythmia in a man with Whipple disease. The convergent-divergent nystagmus is not associated with globe retraction, unlike the nystagmus of Parinaud syndrome, and occurs in all horizontal gaze positions with accompanying rhythmic mastication. The final segment (in color) shows the same patient after treatment. (Courtesy of John B. Selhorst, MD.)

Video 21.4. Downbeat nystagmus in a patient with idiopathic disease of 12 months duration.

Amplitude increases on downgaze (Alexander law) and also upon lateral gaze.

Video 21.5. Upbeat nystagmus in a patient with new vertigo 3 months prior to his developing oscillopsia. Although he carried a diagnosis of pulmonary sarcoid, neuroimaging did not support this diagnosis and the underlying cause could not be identified with certainty. (Courtesy of Dr. Dan Gold.)

Video 21.6. A patient with torsional oscillopsia was initially thought to have superior oblique myokymia by her referring physician, but oscillation was present in both eyes. Periodic reversal of the nystagmus direction was seen, indicating a torsional PAN.

Video 21.7. Periodic alternating nystagmus in a patient with multiple sclerosis. An initially left-beating jerk nystagmus nearly stops and then becomes a right-beating nystagmus.

Video 21.8. Seesaw nystagmus, best appreciated in this case upon left gaze, in a patient with a suprasellar mass compressing the floor of the third ventricle.

Video 21.9. Bilateral internuclear ophthalmoplegia in a patient with acute brainstem stroke. During attempted lateral gaze in either direction, nystagmus of the abducting eye is observed.

Video 21.10. Dorsal midbrain syndrome in a 14-year-old girl with a pineal tumor showing convergence-retraction nystagmus during attempted upgaze. She also had pursuit-saccadic dissociation (not shown here).

Video 21.11. Spasmus nutans in a 2-year-old and an infant. The first child has the classic triad of head bobbing, anomalous head posture, and nystagmus. The nystagmus is essentially monocular in this child, while in the infant it is asymmetric. Both children were examined prior to routine availability of neuroimaging, and findings resolved by age 5.

Video 21.12. A spasmus nutans–like clinical presentation in a patient with an anterior visual pathway glioma found by magnetic resonance imaging. The clinical findings are indistinguishable from those of the previous patient, emphasizing the need for imaging in all patients with spasmus nutans.

Video 21.13. Saccadic intrusions (square-wave jerks) in the right eye of an asymptomatic patient with Parkinson disease.

Video 21.14. Ocular flutter in a young boy. Note that the involuntary eye movements are all in the horizontal plane.

Video 21.15. Opsoclonus in a young woman. Note that the involuntary eye movements are in multiple planes. Also note involuntary head movements.

Video 21.16. Voluntary nystagmus in a healthy young man.

Video 21.17. Superior oblique myokymia in the right eye of a patient with intermittent blurred vision. (Courtesy of David Newman-Toker, MD, PhD.)

Video 21.18. Ocular neuromyotonia in a patient with intermittent diplopia after sustained left gaze. At baseline, she has a mild partial right CN III palsy with ptosis and a slight exotropia. With sustained left gaze, there is progressive right upper eyelid elevation and right eye adduction, such that when she returns to primary position, she has a manifest esotropia. She had chronic compression of the right CN III by the posterior communicating artery. (From Cruz FM, Blitz AM, Subramanian PS. Partial third nerve palsy and ocular neuromyotonia from displacement of posterior communicating artery detected by high-resolution MRI. *J Neuroophthalmol.* 2013;33:263–265.)

Chapter 22: Normal and Abnormal Eyelid Function

Video 22.1. Cogan eyelid twitch phenomenon in a patient with myasthenia gravis. After looking down for 15 seconds, the patient is asked to look straight ahead. The more ptotic right upper lid in particular shows overelevation before settling into primary position.

Video 22.2. Enhancement of ptosis in a patient with myasthenia gravis (same patient as Video 22.1). The patient has bilateral ptosis, and elevation of either eyelid results in increased (enhanced) ptosis on the opposite side.

Video 22.3. Eyelid retraction associated with bilateral type II Duane syndrome. With attempted abduction of either eye, eyelid elevation occurs.

Video 22.4. Horizontal gaze paresis and bilateral facial nerve palsy in a patient after resection of a low-grade glial tumor abutting the floor of the fourth ventricle. Attempted blinks show facial weakness. Note preservation of vertical gaze and convergence.

Video 22.5. Benign essential blepharospasm. Note bilateral symmetric involuntary eyelid closure and spasms.

Video 22.6. This patient was referred for evaluation because of episodic blinking behaviors. While he does blink abnormally, the additional lip smacking, left-sided facial contraction, and sudden head movements are characteristic of motor tic and not benign essential blepharospasm.

Video 22.7. Right hemifacial spasm in a patient presenting for botulinum toxin injection. Note involvement of the right forehead, eyelids, cheek, and lips.

Note: Page numbers followed by *f* and *t* indicate figures and tables.

A

AAION. *See* Arteritic anterior ischemic optic neuropathy (AAION)
Abducens nerve palsies and nuclear horizontal gaze paralysis, 361–369
 acquired, 363–368
 congenital, 361
 evaluation and management of abducens nerve palsy, 368–369
Abducens nerve palsy
 evaluation and management of, 368
 left, 367f
Abducens nerve paralysis, 368
Abducens nuclei, pons at level of, 324f
Abducens nucleus, 364f
 lesions of, 324
Abduction, 302
 congenital absence of, 361
Abduction deficit, right, 367f
Aberrant regeneration of left facial nerve, 443f
Abetalipoproteinemia, 400
Abnormal eye movements and dementia, 336–337
Abnormalities
 of accommodation, 296–300
 afferent, 287–290
 efferent, 273–287
Accommodation
 disorders of, 296–300
 dynamic insufficiency, 297
 examination, 271–272
 insufficiency and paralysis, 296–298
 isolated insufficiency, 297
 nonorganic disturbances, 463
 range of, 271
 spasm and spasm of near reflex, 298–300
 static insufficiency, 297
Accommodation, convergence, and near response, 271–272
 examination, 271–272
 history, 271
Accommodation, disorders of, 296–300
 accommodation insufficiency and paralysis, 296–298
 accommodation spasm and spasm of near reflex, 298–300
Accommodation insufficiency and paralysis, 296–298
 acquired accommodation paresis, 297
 associated with focal or generalized neurologic disease, 297–298
 associated with neuromuscular disorders, 297

associated with primary ocular disease, 297
associated with systemic disease, 298
associated with trauma to head and neck, 298
congenital, 296–297
hereditary, 296–297
from pharmacologic agents, 298
sympathetic paralysis, 298
Accommodation spasm and spasm of near reflex, 298–300
 associated with organic disease, 298
 from pharmacologic agents, 300
 unassociated with organic disease, 298–300
Accommodative amplitude, 271
Accommodative convergence, 271
Achromatopsia
 cerebral, 246–247
 congenital, 29
Acquired accommodation paresis, 297
Acquired alexia, 249–252
Acquired Horner's syndrome in children, 279
Acquired ocular apraxia, 254
Acquired ocular motor apraxia, 336
Acquired oculomotor
 nerve palsy, 353
 synkinesis, 354
Acquired optic nerve disorders, topical diagnosis of
 appearance of disc, 91–102
 syndromes of prechiasmal optic nerve dysfunction, 102–108
Acquired myopathies, 401
Acute demyelinating optic neuritis, MRI of optic nerve in, 133f
Acute disseminated encephalomyelitis (ADEM), 140
Acute idiopathic demyelinating optic neuritis, 130–135
Acute ischemic hematoma, 297
Acute ischemic stroke, 297
Acute peripheral facial nerve paresis, 443f
Acute retinal necrosis (ARN), 143
Acute retrobulbar optic neuritis, optic atrophy after, 132f
Acute unilateral lesions, 332–333
Acute zonal occult outer retinopathy (AZOOR), 59
Adduction, 302
Adduction palsy, congenital right, 342f
ADEM. *See* Acute disseminated encephalomyelitis (ADEM)
Adenoma, pituitary, 215f
Adenosine triphosphate (ATP), 21

Adie's tonic pupil syndrome, 283f
ADOA. *See* Autosomal-dominant optic atrophy (ADOA)
Afferent abnormalities, 287–290
 paradoxical reaction of pupils to light and darkness, 290
 poorly reacting pupils from midbrain disease, 290
 relative afferent pupil defect (RAPD), 287–289
 Wernicke's pupil, 289
Afferent pathway, legions of, 291
Afferent pupillary defect macular lesions associated with relative, 57f
Afferent visual pathway
 decreased visual acuity, 453–457
 monocular diplopia, 459
 nonorganic disease affecting, 452–459
 visual field defects, 457–459, 460f
Afferent visual system, 452
Agnosia, visual, 247
Agrammatism, 251
Agraphia, alexia with, 251
AICA. *See* Anterior inferior cerebellar artery (AICA)
Aicardi syndrome, 86–88, 87f
 CNS anomalies in, 87
AION. *See* Anterior ischemic optic neuropathy (AION)
Akinetopsia, 252
Alexander's law, 408
Alexia
 acquired, 249–252
 with agraphia, 251
 lesions causing pure, 250f
 literal, 251
 pure, 250
Alexia without agraphia, 247, 250
Alignment
 alignment, disorders of ocular motility and, 459–463
 nonorganic disease affecting fixation, ocular motility and, 459–463
 ocular, 305–309
Allen Cards, 2f, 3
Allen, Henry, 2f
Alternate-cover test, 309
Alternating nystagmus, periodic, 411
Amacrine cells, 34f, 37
Amblyopia, 288
American Society of Anesthesiologists (ASA), 156
Amiodarone, 194
Amplitude, accommodative, 271

Amsler grid, 9, 10*f*
Amsler grid defect, 10*f*
Amyotrophic lateral sclerosis, 341
Ancillary information, 18
Ancillary testing
  electrophysiologic testing, 25–32
  of IIH, 125
  ocular imaging, 25, 26*f*–27*f*, 28*f*
Angioma
  endophytic capillary, 170*f*–171*f*
  exophytic capillary, 171*f*
  of optic disc, 162*f*
Angle kappa, 308
Anhidrosis, 275
Aniridia, 293
Anisocoria, 264, 273–287, 288
  causes of, 274*t*
  differentiating among causes of, 288*f*
  differentiation of, 287, 288*f*
  physiologic, 273, 274*f*
  simple, 273, 274*f*
Anisocoria in darkness, more, 273
Anisocoria in light, more, 281
Annular/ring scotomas, 58
Anomalies
  excavated optic disc, 74–84
  iris, 295*f*
  morning glory disc, 74–77, 75*f*
  of optic disc, 61–90
Anomalous disc elevation without
    drusen, 69, 70*f*
Anomalous optic disc elevation
    (pseudopapilledema), 61–69
  associated with buried drusen, 65*t*
  associated with optic disc drusen,
    62–69
  without drusen, 69
Anomia, color, 247
Anosognosia syndrome, 239
Anterior cerebral and middle cerebral
    arteries, infarct in left, 333*f*
Anterior compressive optic
    neuropathies, 161–164
Anterior inferior cerebellar artery
    (AICA), 316
Anterior ischemic optic neuropathy
    (AION), 94–95, 145–155
  arteritic anterior ischemic optic
    neuropathy (AAION), 145–151
  with associated cilioretinal artery
    occlusion, 150*f*
  automated quantitative perimetry
    in, 147*f*
  bilateral simultaneous, 149*f*
  development of optic atrophy after,
    153*f*
  fluorescein angiography in, 151*f*
  nonarteritic anterior ischemic optic
    neuropathy (NAION), 151–155
  occurrence of, 146*t*
  ophthalmoscopic appearance of
    NAION, 148*f*
  optic atrophy and
    pseudoglaucomatous cupping
    after attack of, 149*f*

optic disc swelling in, 94–95, 95*f*
  parapapillary retinal arteriolar
    narrowing in, 148*f*
  segmental optic disc edema in, 148*f*
Anterior occipital lobe, unilateral
    lesions of, 230–231
Anterior optic chiasmal syndrome, 212*f*
Anterior optic neuritis, 93, 130, 131*f*,
    132*f*, 140*f*
Anterior segment examination, visual
    sensory system, 24–25
Anterograde degeneration, 97
Anton syndrome, 239
Aphasia, nonfluent, 251
Aplasia, optic nerve, 88, 89*f*
Apparent enophthalmos, 274
Apperceptive prosopagnosia, 248
Apraclonidine, response of Horner's
    pupils to, 276*f*
Apraxia of eyelid opening (AEO), 426
Aquaporin-4, 136
Aqueductal stenosis, 122
Arcuate visual field defect, 57, 58*f*–59*f*
Argyll Robertson pupils, 290–291
  in patient with neurosyphilis, 290*f*
ARN. *See* Acute retinal necrosis (ARN)
Arnold-Chiari malformation, 319–320
Arteries
  cerebral, 333*f*
Arteritic anterior ischemic optic
    neuropathy (AAION), 145–151
  clinical manifestations, 145–146
  diagnostic confirmation, 146–151
  therapy, 151
Artery, internal carotid, 278
Artery occlusion, AAION with
    associated cilioretinal, 150*f*
ASA. *See* American Society of
    Anesthesiologists (ASA)
Associative prosopagnosia, 248
Astrocytes, 38
Astrocytic hamartomas, 168–169
  of optic disc, 169*f*
Astrocytomas
  cystic, 228*f*
  mulberry, 168–169
Asymmetric papilledema, 114–115,
    116*f*
Asymptomatic (subclinical) optic
    neuritis, 135
Ataxia, Friedreich, 207
Ataxias
  optic, 254
ATP. *See* Adenosine triphosphate (ATP)
Atrophy
  iris, 296
  postpapilledema, 113–114, 113*f*
Atrophy, optic, 97–102
  from chronic papilledema, 114
  differential diagnosis of, 100–102
  nonpathologic pallor of optic disc,
    97
  ophthalmoscopic features of, 98–100
  pathology and pathophysiology of,
    97–98

Attentional dyslexia, 252
Autoimmune optic neuropathy,
    141–142
Automated perimetry, 8
Automated visual field information,
    interpretation of, 13–18
  kinetic perimetry, 15
  probability plots, 15, 16*f*, 17*f*
  progression of visual field loss,
    16–18
  reliability indices, 13, 14*f*, 15
Autonomic function, general
    disturbances of, 300
Autosomal-dominant optic atrophy
    (ADOA), 202–204
Autosomal-dominant striatonigral
    degeneration, 446
Autosomal-recessive disorder, 389
Avascular zone, fovea, 43, 43*f*
Axes of rotation of eye, 303*f*
Axons, 40
  retinal ganglion cells, 40–41
  retinal nerve, 41*f*
  transport, 40–41
AZOOR. *See* Acute zonal occult outer
    retinopathy (AZOOR)

B
Bacille Calmette-Guérin (BCG), 141
Balint's syndrome, 252–255, 253*f*, 337*f*
Bartonella henselae, 143
Bassen–Kornzweig syndrome, 400
B-cell lymphoma, 174*f*–175*f*
BCG. *See* Bacille Calmette-Guérin
    (BCG)
Behr syndrome, 206–207
Bell phenomenon, 305
Benedikt syndrome, 345
Benign anisocoria. *See* physiologic
    anisocoria
Benign childhood epilepsy with
    occipital spike-waves, 258–259
Benign paroxysmal positional vertigo
    (BPPV), 408
Big blind spot syndrome, 59
Bilateral anterior optic neuritis, 140*f*
Bilateral anterior optic neuropathy, 194*f*
Bilateral central serous
    chorioretinopathy, bilateral
    visual field defects and, 54*f*
Bilateral eyelid retraction, 434*f*
Bilateral eyelid retraction in baby with
    communicating hydrocephalus,
    436
Bilateral hypoplasia, 70*f*, 72
Bilateral inferior altitudinal visual field
    defects, 106*f*
Bilateral lesions in three patients with
    prosopagnosia, location of, 249*f*
Bilateral lesions of riMLF, 329
Bilateral occipital lobe lesions, 233–237,
    238*f*
Bilateral optic disc drusen, bilateral
    visual field defects in patient
    with, 67*f*

Bilateral optic neuropathy, 286, 456
  hemifield slide phenomenon from, 107f
  multiple sclerosis, 213f
Bilateral orbicularis oculi weakness, 444f
Bilateral pseudo-internuclear
  ophthalmoplegia, 376f
Bilateral pupillary involved oculomotor
  pareses and neurofibromatosis,
  349f
Bilateral superior altitudinal visual field
  defects, 239f
Bilateral supranuclear oculopalpebral
  synkinesia, congenital, 427f
Bilateral toxic optic neuropathy
  caused by chloramphenicol, 189f
  from ethambutol, 188f
Bilateral trochlear nerve palsies, 357f
Bilateral visual dysfunction with optic
  neuropathies, 154f
Bilateral visual field defects
  in patient with bilateral central
    serous chorioretinopathy, 54f
  in patient with bilateral optic disc
    drusen, 67f
  in patient with occipital lobe infarct,
    23f
Bilateral visual loss, papilledema
  associated with, 119f–120f
Binasal hemianopia, 107
Binocular visual field, 216f
Bipolar cells, 34f, 37
Bitemporal field defects, 21f
Bitemporal hemianopias, 216f
Bitemporal hemianopic scotomas, 215f
Blepharoclonus, 445
Blepharospasm, 464
  associated with drug-induced tardive
    dyskinesia, 445
  associated with lesions of brainstem
    and basal ganglia, 445
  essential, 444f
  nonorganic, 446
Blepharospasm-oromandibular
  dystonia syndrome, 444–445
Blindness, 250
  cerebral, 238–239, 240f, 241t
  cortical, 238–239
Blindsight and residual vision, 245–246
Blind spot, 58–59
  in patient with papilledema, 59f
Blood supply
  to dorsal aspect of optic chiasm and
    intracranial optic nerves, 51f
  to intraocular optic nerve, 47f
  to proximal optic nerve and choroid,
    46f
  of retina, 43f
Blood vessels, retinal, 43
Blurred vision, 302–303
Bobbing, 338
Body of optic chiasm lesions, 210–211
  after severe head trauma, 214f
  bilateral optic neuropathy in
    sclerosis, 213f
  bitemporal hemianopia, 212f

Bonnet, Charles syndrome, 256–258, 257f
Borrelia burgdorferi, 141
Botulinum toxin treatment, 420–421
Botulism, 292, 296–297, 381, 384
Bradykinin, 183
Brainstem and cerebellum, nystagmus
  projections to, 405–408
Brainstem, blepharospasm associated
  with lesions of, 445
Brainstem tuberculoma, cysticercosis,
  446
Brightness comparison, color vision
  and, 24
Broca aphasia, 251
Buried drusen, pseudopapilledema
  associated with, 65t

C
Caloric testing, 304
Capillary hemangiomas, 170
Carbonic anhydrase inhibitors, 128
Carcinomatosis, meningeal, 173
Carcinomatous meningitis, 173
Carotid artery blood supply to orbit
  and eye, 46f
Carotid nerve, 277
Carotid plexus, 277
Cascade, phototransduction, 36f
Cataract, 288–289, 389–390
Cavernous hemangiomas, 170–171
Cecocentral scotoma, 57, 57f–58f
Cell layer, retina
  ganglion cell layer, 34f, 35t, 39
  inner nuclear layer, 34f, 35t
  outer nuclear layer, 34f, 35t
Cell layer, retinal ganglion, 34f, 35t, 39
Cells
  amacrine, 34f, 37
  bipolar cells, 34f, 37
  horizontal, 34f, 37
  interplexiform, 34f, 37–38
  magnocellular, 39
  Müller, 34f, 38
  parvocellular, 39
  photoreceptor, 35–37
  retinal ganglion, 38f
  of rod and cone pathways, 38f
Cell types and layers of retina, 33–43
Cellular organization, retina, 35t
Central anisocoria, 274f. See
  physiologic anisocoria
Central disorders of visual function,
  244–262
  acquired alexia, 249–252
  Balint's syndrome and related
    visuospatial disorders, 252–255
  blindsight and residual vision, 245–246
  cerebral achromatopsia, 246–247
  disorders of motion perception, 252
  glossary of cerebral visual deficits,
    261–262
  positive visual phenomena, 255–260
  prosopagnosia and related
    disturbances of object
    recognition, 247–249

  segregation of visual inputs,
    244–245
  tests of higher visual function,
    260–261
Central dyslexias, 252
Central Horner's syndromes, 276,
  277f
Central nervous system (CNS), 61
  anomalies in Aicardi syndrome, 87
  malformations, 71–72
Central retinal vein occlusion (CRVO),
  288
Central serous chorioretinopathy, 54,
  54f
Central syndrome, 292
Central vision, lose, 118–119
Central visual acuity, 53–54
Central visual loss, 66–67
Cerebellar cortex, inferior cerebellar
  peduncle (ICP) and, 320f
Cerebellar structures, clinical signs of
  damage to, 321f
Cerebellar tonsillar ectopia, 77
Cerebellum
  human, 319f
Cerebellum, ocular motor syndromes
  caused by lesions of, 317–322
  etiologies, 319–322
  location of lesions and their
    manifestations, 318–319
Cerebral achromatopsia, 246–247
Cerebral akinetopsia, 252
Cerebral arteries, infarct in left anterior
  cerebral and middle, 333f
Cerebral blindness, 238–239, 240f
  circumstances of, 241t
Cerebral cortex of nonhuman primate,
  visual function in, 245f
Cerebral disorders of vision. See
  Central disorders of visual
  function
Cerebral dyschromatopsia, 246, 246f
Cerebral hemispheres, ocular motor
  syndromes caused by lesions
  in, 332–339
  abnormal eye movements and
    dementia, 336–337
  acute unilateral lesions, 332–333
  eye movements in stupor and coma,
    338–339
  focal lesions, 334–336
  ocular motor apraxia, 336
  ocular motor manifestations of
    seizures, 337–338
  persistent deficits caused by large
    unilateral lesions, 333–334
Cerebral hemispheres upon ocular
  motor function, lesions of,
  334t
Cerebral micropsia, drawing, 260f
Cerebral polyopia, 256
Cerebral venous drainage
  obstruction/impairment of, 123t
Cerebral vision deficits, glossary of,
  261–262

Cerebrospinal fluid (CSF), 109
  examination for diagnosis of IIH, 125
  flow, 120–123
  rhinorrhea, 118
Charcot-Marie-tooth disease (CMTD), 208–209
CHARGE syndrome, 78
Chiari I malformation, 77
Chiari malformations, eye signs in, 321t
Chiasmal and retrochiasmal lesions, topical diagnosis of, 210–243
  topical diagnosis of optic chiasmal disorders, 210–217
  topical diagnosis of retrochiasmal visual field defects, 217–243
Chiasm and postchiasmal visual sensory system, 211f
Children
  acquired Horner's syndrome in, 279
  confrontation visual field testing in, 9f
  with optic nerve aplasia, 88
  with optic nerve hypoplasia, 72
  optic neuritis in, 142
Chloramphenicol, bilateral toxic neuropathy caused by, 189f
Chondrodystrophic myotonia, 395
Chorioretinopathy, 392f
Chronic progressive external ophthalmoplegia (CPEO), 390
Claude syndrome, 345
Choroid
  blood supply to proximal optic nerve and, 46f
Chronic demyelinating optic neuritis, 135
Chronic inflammatory demyelinating polyneuropathy (CIDP), 124
Chronic papilledema, 113, 113f
  optociliary shunt veins in patient with, 114f
Chronic progressive external ophthalmoplegia (CPEO), 206
CIDP. See Chronic inflammatory demyelinating polyneuropathy (CIDP)
Cilioretinal artery occlusion, AAION with associated, 150f
11-cis-retinol, 35
Claude syndrome, 345
Clinical office examination, visual sensory system, 4–32
  ancillary testing, 25–33
    electrophysiologic testing, 25–33
    ocular imaging, 25, 26f–27f
  anterior segment examination, 24–25
  brightness comparison, 24
  color vision, 4–7
    Farnsworth–Munsell 100 Hues test, 6–7
    Farnsworth Panel D-15 test, 6
    pseudoisochromatic plates, 5–6, 6f
  contrast sensitivity, 3–4, 4f

cranial nerves, 24–25
exophthalmometry, 24–25
external examination, 24–25
fundus examination, 25
photostress recovery test, 24
pupillary examination, 22, 24
stereoacuity, 4
visual acuity, 1–3, 2f
visual field, 7–22
  automated information, interpretation of, 13–18, 14f, 16f, 17f, 18f–19f
  five-step approach to visual field interpretation, 18, 19, 21f, 22, 22f, 23f
  general principles, 7–8
  testing techniques for, 8–13
Clostridium botulinum, 292, 384
Clostridium tetani, 384
CMTD. See Charcot-Marie-tooth disease (CMTD)
CNS. See Central nervous system (CNS)
Cocaine, response of Horner's pupils to, 275f
Cocaine test, 275
Colobomas, 77, 294
Color anomia, 247
Color comparison tests, 6–7, 7f
Color dysnomia, lesions causing, 250f
Color vision, 4–7, 55, 181
  Farnsworth–Munsell 100 Hues test, 6–7, 7f
  Farnsworth Panel D-15 test, 6
  pseudoisochromatic plates, 5–6, 6f
Coma
  disturbances in, 292
  eye movements in stupor and, 338–339
  metabolic, 292
Comitant strabismus, 305
Complementary techniques, 8. See also Visual field examination
Compression tests, color, 6–7, 7f
Compressive optic neuropathies, 161–166
  with optic disc swelling, 161–164
  visual recovery following decompression, 166
  without optic disc swelling, 164–166
Concentric sclerosis of Baló, 139
Cone pathways, neurotransmitters used by cells of rod and, 38f
Cone pedicles, 37
Cones, photoreceptor cells, 35–37
Cone through pathways, rod and, 43–44
Confrontation visual fields, 8–9
Confrontation visual field testing, 8–9, 8f
  in children, 9f
Confusion, visual, 302
Congenital Adduction Palsy, 341
Congenital adherence, 386

Congenital anomalies of optic disc, 61–90
Congenital Brown syndrome, 387, 387f
Congenital Bulbar Paralysis, 361
Congenital fibrosis of the extraocular muscles (CFEOM), 386
Congenital fibrosis syndrome, 387f
Congenital homonymous hemianopia, post-geniculate, 289
Congenital Horner's syndrome, 279, 279f
Congenital left oculomotor nerve palsy, 342f
Congenital miosis, 295
Congenital motor nystagmus, 414
Congenital muscular dystrophies, 388
Congenital myasthenic syndromes, 381
Congenital mydriasis, 296
Congenital optic disc pigmentation, 86, 87f
Congenital paradoxic gustolacrimal reflex, 300
Congenital recessive optic atrophy, 204
Congenital tilted optic disc syndrome, 84–86, 84f, 85f
Congruous homonymous horizontal sectoranopia, 224, 226f
Congruous homonymous quadruple sectoranopia, 224, 225f
Consciousness, loss of, 117–118
Consensual light response, 265
Contrapulsion of saccades, 315
Contrast sensitivity, 3–4, 4f
Contrast sensitivity chart Pelli-Robson, 4f
Convergence, 271, 272
  accommodative, 271
  assessment of, 271–272
  fusional, 272
  tonic, 271
  voluntary, 272
Convergence insufficiency, 461
Convergence–retraction nystagmus, 328, 413
Convergent-Divergent Pendular Oscillations, 408
Converse bobbing, 338
Conversion disorder, 452
"Conversion neurosis", 452
Cookie theft picture, 254f, 337f
Corneal light reflex, 307–308
Corneomandibular reflex, 446
Cortical blindness, 238–239
Cortical ptosis, 426
Corticosteroids, 134
Counter rolling, eye movement, 303
Countertorsion, eye movement, 303
Course, papilledema, 117
Cover tests, 308–309
Covert familiarity, 247
Covert semantic knowledge, 247
Cover–uncover test, 308f, 309
CPEO Plus Syndromes, 397
CPEO. See Chronic progressive external ophthalmoplegia (CPEO)

Cranial nerves examination, 24–25
Craniosynostoses, 123–124
C-reactive protein (CRP), 146
Criterion shift, 245
Crossed diplopia, 306
Crossed-quadrant hemianopia, 237f
CRP. *See* C-reactive protein (CRP)
CRVO. *See* Central retinal vein occlusion (CRVO)
CSF. *See* Cerebrospinal fluid (CSF)
Cystic astrocytoma, left temporal lobe, 228f

D

Dandy–Walker syndrome, 320
Darkness
    anisocoria in, 273
    paradoxical reactions of pupils to light and, 290
Decreased visual acuity, 453
Defects
    Amsler grid, 10f
    peripheral visual field, 66
Deficiency optic neuropathies, toxic and, 186–194
    clinical characteristics of nutritional and toxic optic neuropathies, 187
    differential diagnosis, 187–190
    etiologic criteria, 186–187
    specific nutritional optic neuropathies, 190–192
    specific toxic optic neuropathies, 192–194
Deficiency, vitamin E, 341
Degeneration
    anterograde, 97
    hepatolenticular, 341
    paraneoplastic cerebellar, 321
    retrograde, 97
    transsynaptic (transneuronal), 98
Delayed recovery, 166
Dementia, abnormal eye movements and, 336–337
de Morsier syndrome, 71
Demyelinating diseases, optic neuritis in other primary, 136–139
    concentric sclerosis of Baló, 139
    Devic's disease, 136–138
    encephalitis periaxialis concentrica, 139
    encephalitis periaxialis diffusa, 138–139
    myelinoclastic diffuse sclerosis, 138–139
    neuromyelitis optica, 136–138
    Schilder's disease, 138–139
Demyelinating optic neuritis, MRI of optic nerve in acute, 133f
Demyelination, causes of optic neuritis other than primary, 139–142
    infectious and parainfectious optic neuritis, 140–141
    inflammatory optic neuritis, 141–142
    miscellaneous causes, 142
    postvaccination optic neuritis, 141

Denervation supersensitivity test, 284
Depigmentation of ipsilateral iris, 275
Depression, eye movement, 302
Depth of field, 272
Detachment, retinal, 288
Developmental prosopagnosia, 248–249
Devic's disease. *See* Neuromyelitis optica (NMO)
Diabetes mellitus, 298
Diabetic papillopathy, 159, 160f
DIDMOAD, 205–206
Diencephalon, 292
Diffuse white-matter disease, 209
Dilated pupil, pharmacologically, 286f
Dilation
    intermittent unilateral pupillary, 287f
    of pupil, 286–287
    pupillary, 265–266
Dilation lag, 274–275
Diopters, 271
Diphtheria, 298
Diplopia, 119–120, 302
    crossed, 306
    principle of tests, 306f
    uncrossed, 306
Direct optic nerve injuries, 179
Direct vertical vestibulo-ocular projections, 340f
Disc anomalies, morning glory, 74–77, 75f
Disc at risk
    appearance of, 45f
    in nonarteritic ischemic optic neuropathy, 154f
Disc drusen
    buried, 63f
    buried optic, 64f
    visible, 64f
Disc syndrome, congenital tilted, 84–86, 84f, 85f
Disease-modifying antirheumatic drugs (DMARDs), 193
Diseases
    accommodation insufficiency associated with ocular, 297
    Devic's, 136–138
    generalized or focal neurologic, 297–298
    Hippel–Lindau, 170
    Huntington's, 332
    lipid storage, 339
    Lyme, 141
    macular, 288
    midbrain, 290
    occipital lobe disease, 241–242
    organic disease, 298–300
    Parkinson's, 331–332
    Pelizaeus-Merzbacher, 340–341
    Schilder's, 138–139
    thyroid eye, 162
    Whipple's, 331
    Wilson's, 297–298

Diseases, optic neuritis in other primary demyelinating, 136–139
    concentric sclerosis of Baló, 139
    Devic's disease, 136–138
    encephalitis periaxialis concentrica, 139
    encephalitis periaxialis diffusa, 138–139
    myelinoclastic diffuse sclerosis, 138–139
    neuromyelitis optica, 136–138
    neuromyelitis optica (Devic disease), 136–138
    Schilder's disease, 138–139
Disorders
    of neuromuscular junction, disturbances in, 292
    topical diagnosis of acquired optic, 91–108
    toxic and metabolic, 96
Disorders of neuromuscular junction, disturbances in, 292
Disorders of vision, higher. *See* Central disorders of visual function
Dissociation, light-near, 290–291
Distal optic nerve syndrome, 102, 104f
Distortions, visual, 260
Disturbances
    in coma, 292
    during seizures, 291
Divergence insufficiency, 119
Divergence nystagmus, 414
DMARDs. *See* Disease-modifying antirheumatic drugs (DMARDs)
DOA. *See* Dominant optic atrophy (DOA)
Doll's head maneuver, 304
Dominant optic atrophy (DOA), 202–204, 203f, 204f–205f
    optic disc with, 205f
Dorsal mesencephalon, 297
Dorsal midbrain syndrome, 328f
Dorsal vermis, 318
Double-ring sign, 69
Downbeat nystagmus, etiology of, 410, 410t
Drugs
    parasympatholytic (anticholinergic), 292, 293f
    parasympathomimetic (cholinergic), 293
    sympatholytic (antiadrenergic), 293
    sympathomimetic (adrenergic), 292, 294f
Drugs on eye movements, effects of, 341–342, 342t
D-15 scoring chart, 6
Duane's retraction syndrome (DRS), 361–363
Ductions, 302
Dural folds, optic nerves and falciform, 183f

Dursen
  anomalous disc elevation without, 69, 70f
  fluorescent characteristics of, 65f
  intrapapillary, 68f
  optic disc, 66f
  pseudopapilledema associated with optic disc, 62–69
Dynamic insufficiency, accommodation, 297
Dyschromatopsia, cerebral, 246, 246f
Dysfunction
  endocrine, 126, 126t
  metabolic, 126, 126t
  syndromes of prechiasmal optic nerve, 102–108
Dyslexias
  attentional, 252
  central, 252
  hemianopic, 251
Dysnomia, color, 250f
Dysplasia, optic disc, 86, 86f
Dystrophies
  retinal, 60f

E
Ectopia, posterior pituitary, 73f
Ectopic pupils, 294
Edema in AION, segmental optic disc, 148f
Edrophonium test, 377–380, 379f
Efferent abnormalities, 273–287
  anisocoria in darkness, 273
  anisocoria in light, more, 281
  damage to iris sphincter, 285
  Horner's syndrome, 273–280
  pharmacologic blockade with parasympatholytic agents, 285
  pharmacologic stimulation of iris dilator, 281
  pharmacologic stimulation of iris sphincter, 280–281
  sympathetic hyperactivity, 280
  tonic pupil, 281–285
  Tournay phenomenon, 285
"E game," 3
Eight-and-a-half syndrome, 324, 326f
Electrophysiologic tests, 3, 381
  full-field (Ganzfeld) electroretinogram (ERG), 25, 27–29, 29f
  multifocal electroretinogram (mfERG), 29–30, 30f
  pattern electroretinogram (PERG), 29, 29f
  visual-evoked potential, 30, 32, 32f
Electroretinogram (ERG), 25, 27–29, 29f
  components of, 27, 29f
  multifocal electroretinogram (mfERG), 29–30, 30f
  pattern electroretinogram (PERG), 29, 29f
Elevation, eye movement, 302
Ellipsoid, 36

Encephalitis, 122–123
Encephalitis periaxialis concentrica, 139
Encephalopathy, Wernicke's, 341
Encephalomyopathy with Ophthalmoplegia from Vitamin E Deficiency, 400–401
Endocrine dysfunction, 126, 126t
Endocrinologic deficiencies, associated, 71
Endophytic capillary angioma, 170f–171f
Enophthalmos, apparent, 274
Epidemic nutritional optic neuropathy, 190–191
Epilepsy
  benign childhood, 258–259
  occipital lobe, 258f
Episodic unilateral mydriasis, 280
ERG. See Electroretinogram (ERG)
Erythrocyte sedimentation rate (ESR), 146
ESR. See Erythrocyte sedimentation rate (ESR)
Ethambutol, 192–193
  bilateral toxic neuropathy from, 188f
Examination
  anterior segment, 24–25
  color vision, 4–7, 55
  fundus, 25, 181
  pupillary, 24
  pupillary size, assessing, 263–264
  visual field, 7–22
  visual sensory system, 1–32
Excessive lacrimation, 300
Exogenous substances, 126, 126t
Exophthalmometry, 24–25
Exophytic capillary angioma, 171f
External examination, visual sensory system, 24–25
Extinction, visual, 241
Extorsion, eye movement, 303
Extracranial lesions, 124
Extraocular muscles, 284f, 386
  actions of, 303t
  agenesis of, 386
  developmental disorders of, 386
Extrastriate cortex with defects in visual field, lesions of, 240
Eyelid fatigue, 375f
Eye closure, hallucinations with, 260
Eyelid
  anatomy of, 424
  examination of, 424t
Eyelid function, nonorganic disturbances of, 463
Eyelid myokymia, 446
Eyelid opening
  abnormalities of, 426
Eyelid retraction, 426
  in baby with communicating hydrocephalus, 436f
  bilateral, 434f, 444f
  oculomotor nerve dysfunction, 436–437
  unilateral, 435, 437

Eye movements
  control of, 325f
  effects of drugs on, 341–342, 342t
  horizontal, 331
  illustration of cortical regions in supranuclear, 335f
  range of, 302–305
  reflex, 339
  spontaneous, 338–339
  in stupor and coma, 338–339
Eyes
  axes of rotation of, 303f
  gaze deviations, 338
  intermittent deviation, 338
  macular lesions with unexplained vision loss in both, 55f
  primary position, 302
  secondary position, 302–303
  tertiary position, 303
  tonic downward deviation, 338
  tonic upward deviation, 338
Eyes-open coma, 338

F
Facial myokymia, 446
Facial sensation, nonorganic disturbances of, 464
Falciform dural folds, optic nerves and, 183f
False-negative errors, 13
False orientation, 305
False-positive errors, 13
Familial periodic paralysis, 394
Farnsworth–Munsell 100 Hues test, 6–7
  color comparison tests, 6–7, 7f
Farnsworth Panel D-15 test, 6
FEF. See Frontal eye field (FEF)
Fibrinogen, 150
Fibrosis syndromes, 386
Field defect, testing of patients with, 18f–19f, 20f, 21f, 23f
Five-step approach to visual field interpretation, 18, 19, 21f, 22, 22f, 23f
Flocculus, 318
Fluorescein angiogram, 43f
Fluorescein angiography, 64
Focal and multifocal electroretinogram, 29–30, 30f
Focal lesions, 334–336
Focal or generalized neurologic disease, accommodation insufficiency associated with, 297–298
Forced duction testing, 304, 304f
Foster Kennedy syndrome, 102, 104, 105f
Fovea, 41
  avascular zone, 43, 43f
  section through center of, 35f
Foveal avascular zone, 43, 43f
Foveal (macular) sparing, 231–233, 234f
Foveal (macular) splitting, 210, 212f
Foville syndrome, 363

Fractures, optic canal, 182f
Free radicals, oxygen, 183
Fresnel press-on prisms for homonymous hemianopia, 242f
Friedreich ataxia, 207, 207f
    mild bilateral optic atrophy in, 207f
Frisén grading system, papilledema, 110t
Frisén scale, 110t
Frontal eye field (FEF), 335
Frontal lobe lesions, 335–336, 335f, 336f
Fulminant IIH, 129
Fukuyama Congenital Muscular Dystrophy, 388–389
Fundus
    direct observation of, 309
    examination, 25, 181
    ocular, 218f, 310f
    photo, 65f
Fundus examination, 25, 181
Fusional convergence, 272

G
Ganglion cell complex (GCC), 135
Ganglion cell layer, 34f, 35t
Ganglion cells, retinal, 38f
Gauges, pupils, 264f
Gaze deviations, eyes, 338
Gaze-evoked nystagmus, 412
Gaze-holding ability, fixation and, 302
GBS. See Guillain–Barré syndrome (GBS)
GCA. See Giant cell arteritis (GCA)
GCC. See Ganglion cell complex (GCC)
Generalized or focal neurologic disease, accommodation insufficiency associated with, 297–298
General principles, visual field examination, 7–8
    abnormalities detection, 7
    differential diagnosis, 7
    monitoring progression and remission, 7
    revealing hidden visual loss, 7
Gerstmann syndrome, 251
Giant cell arteritis (GCA), 145, 150
    anterior ischemic optic neuropathy in, 145–151, 146t
    diagnosis of, 146–151
    therapy in, 151
Glaucoma, 288
Glaucomatous cupping, 100f
Gliomas
    malignant optic nerve, 168, 169f
    optic nerve, 167, 167f
GMP. See Guanidine monophosphate (GMP)
Goldmann perimeter, 7, 11, 11f, 15
Gradenigo's syndrome, 367
Grading system, papilledema, 110t
Grasping, reaching and, 254
Gravis, myasthenia, 297

Grid, Amsler, 9, 10f
Guanidine monophosphate (GMP), 36
Guillain–Barré syndrome (GBS), 124
Gustolacrimal reflex, congenital paradoxic, 300

H
Hallucinations
    with eye closure, 260
    migrainous, 259
    other types of, 259–260
    peduncular, 259
    release, 256–258, 257f
    visual, 256
Hallucinations, visual, 256
Hamartomas, astrocytic, 168–169
Haploscopic tests, 307
    principle of, 307f
Hardy–Rand–Rittler pseudoisochromatic color plate, 5, 6f
Headaches, 117
Head tilts, 305–306
    test, 309
Head turns, 305
Heijl, Anders, 11
Hemangioblastoma, 172
Hemangiomas
    capillary, 170
    cavernous, 170–171
Hematomas
    acute ischemic, 297
Hemi-alexia, 250–251
Hemianopias
    bilateral superior or inferior (altitudinal), 104–106, 106f
    bitemporal, 21f, 215f, 216f
    congruous right homonymous, 23f, 232f
    crossed-quadrant, 237f
    homonymous, 22f, 250f
    incongruous left homonymous, 23f
    nasal, 106–108, 108f
    right homonymous, 220f, 235f
Hemianopic dyslexia, 251
Hemianopic optic atrophy, 223f
Hemianopic scotomas
    bitemporal, 215f
Hemifield slide phenomenon, 106, 107f, 216, 216f
Hemiparalexia, 251, 251f
Hemodynamic compromise, ischemic optic neuropathy in settings of, 156–157
Hemorrhages
    nerve fiber layer, 111f, 112
    with papilledema, 112
    peripapillary, 67
    peripapillary subretinal, 68f
    prepapillary, 67
    spontaneous, 156
    subarachnoid, 122
Hepatolenticular degeneration, 341
Hereditary ataxias, 207–208

Hereditary optic atrophy with neurologic or systemic signs, 204–207
    complicated hereditary infantile optic atrophy, 206–207
    DIDMOAD, 205–206
    progressive optic atrophy with juvenile diabetes mellitus, 205–206, 206f
    Wolfram syndrome, 205–206, 206f
Hereditary optic neuropathies, 195–209
    degenerative/developmental diseases, 207–209
    hereditary optic atrophy with neurologic or systemic signs, 204–207
    miscellaneous isolated, 204
    monosymptomatic hereditary optic neuropathies, 195–204
Hereditary optic neuropathies, monosymptomatic, 195–204
    dominant optic atrophy (DOA), 202–204
    isolated hereditary optic neuropathies, 204
    Leber's hereditary optic neuropathy, 195–202
Hereditary polyneuropathies, 208–209
Hering law of motor correspondence, 303
Heterochromia iridis, 296
Heterophoria, 309
Heteroplasmy, 199
Heterotropia, 309
Higher visual function, tests of, 260–261, 261f
Hippel–Lindau disease, 170
Hirschberg test, 308
HIV. See Human immunodeficiency virus (HIV)
Holmes–Adie tonic pupil syndrome, 283–285
Homonymous hemianopia
    Fresnel press-on prisms for treatment of, 242f
    hemianopic optic atrophy in patient with left, 223f
    lesions causing, 250f
    right, 220f, 232f
    treatment and rehabilitation for, 242–243
Homonymous hemianopia, postgeniculate congenital, 289
Homonymous hemioptic hypoplasia, 74
Homoplasmy, 199
Hooper Visual Organization Test, 261f
Horizontal cells, 34f, 37
Horner's pupils
    to apraclonidine, response of, 276f
    to cocaine, response of, 275f
    response to hydroxyamphetamine, 278f

Horner's syndrome, 273–280, 274f, 428
  acquired Horner's syndrome in children, 279
  clinical features, 273–275
  congenital, 279, 279f
  diagnosis, 275–276
  differentiating localizations, 278–279
  facial coloration changes in, 280f
  localization, 276–278
"HOTV" test, 3
Human cerebellum, 319f
Human immunodeficiency virus (HIV), 140, 141
Human optic nerve, cross-section of, 48f
Humphrey visual field analyzer, 9, 10–11, 10f, 16f, 20f, 21f, 22f
  mean deviation (MD) on, 15
  pattern standard deviation (PSD) on, 15
Hydrocephalus
Hydrocephalus, suprasellar mass with, 222f
Hydroxyamphetamine
  response of Horner's pupils to, 278f
  tests, 278
Hyperactivity, sympathetic, 280
Hyperemic swelling, 95f
Hypochondriasis, 452
Hypoplasia
  homonymous hemioptic, 74
  optic nerves, 69–74, 70f, 71f
  segmental optic nerve, 73–74
  superior segmental optic, 73f
Hypotension, 157
Hypothalamus, 292
Hypovitaminosis A, 37
"Hysteria", 452

I
Ice test, 377, 378f
ICP. See Intracranial pressure (ICP)
Idiopathic demyelinating optic neuritis, 130–135
  acute idiopathic demyelinating optic neuritis, 130–135
  asymptomatic (subclinical) optic neuritis, 135
  chronic demyelinating optic neuritis, 135
Idiopathic demyelinating optic neuritis, acute, 130–135
  clinical presentation, 131–132
  demographics, 130–131
  diagnostic studies, 132–133
  management recommendations, 135
  neurologic prognosis, 134
  treatment, 134–135
  visual prognosis, 133–134
Idiopathic intracranial hypertension (IIH), 124–129
  complications, 127
  diagnosis of
    ancillary testing, 125
    clinical manifestations, 125
  endocrine dysfunction, 126, 126t

etiology of, 126–127, 126t
exogenous substances associated with, 126t
fulminant, 129
metabolic dysfunction, 126, 126t
overall incidence of, 124
pathophysiology of, 127
during pregnancy, 126, 129
special circumstances, 129
systemic illnesses associated with, 126t
treatment
  medical therapy, 127–128
  surgical procedures, 128–129
Idiopathic orbital inflammation, 161–162
IIH. See Idiopathic intracranial hypertension (IIH); Intracranial hypertension (IIH)
Illusory visual spread, 256
INC. See Interstitial nucleus of Cajal (INC)
Incomitant strabismus, 305
Indices
  reliability, 13, 14f
  visual field, 15
Indirect optic nerve injuries, 179
Infections, 140
Infectious and parainfectious optic neuritis, 140–141
Infectious disorders, 178
Inferior arcuate defect, 20f
Inferior cerebellar peduncle (ICP) and cerebellar cortex, 320f
Inferior olivary nucleus (ION), 312
Infiltration, optic disc, 96–97
Infiltrative optic neuropathies, 166–178
  inflammatory and, 176–178
    infectious disorders, 178
    sarcoidosis, 176–178, 177f–178f
  tumors, 166–176
    primary, 166–172
    secondary, 172–176
Inflammation, 183
Inflammatory optic neuritis, 141–142
Information, ancillary, 18
Infranuclear ocular motility disorders, nuclear and, 341–371
Inhibitors, carbonic anhydrase, 128
Injuries
  direct optic nerve, 179
  indirect optic nerve, 179
Inner nuclear layer, 34f, 35t
Inner plexiform layer (IPL), 34f, 37, 38
INO. See Internuclear ophthalmoplegia (INO)
Intermittent deviation, eyes, 338
Intermittent unilateral pupillary dilation, 287f
Internal capsule, lesions of, 225–227, 227f
Internal carotid artery, dissections of, 278
Internal ophthalmoplegia, 281
International Optic Nerve Trauma Study, 184, 185

Internuclear ocular motor disorders, supranuclear and, 312–342
Internuclear ophthalmoplegia (INO), 317, 322–324, 363
  etiologies, 323–324, 324t
  manifestations, 322–323
  neuroimaging of patient with left, 323f
  unilateral conjugate gaze palsy and, 325–326
  unilateral, right, 323f
Interplexiform cells, 34f, 37–38
Interstitial nucleus of Cajal (INC), 312, 329, 330f
Intorsion, eye movement, 303
Intracanalicular (intraosseous) optic nerve, 48–50
Intracranial hypertension (IIH), 109
Intracranial masses, 122
Intracranial optic nerves, 50–52
  appearance, 50f
  blood supply to dorsal aspect of optic chiasm and, 51f
Intracranial pressure (ICP), 109
  causes of increased, 122t
  measurements of, 109–110
Intraocular optic nerve, blood supply to, 47f
Intrapapillary drusen
  peripapillary subretinal hemorrhage in patient with, 68f
  subretinal neovascularization in patient with, 68f
Intrinsically photosensitive RGCs (ipRGCs), 39–40, 40f
Inverse bobbing, 338
Ion channel disorders, 394
ION. See Inferior olivary nucleus (ION)
IONDT. See Ischemic Optic Neuropathy Decompression Trial (IONDT)
IPL. See Inner plexiform layer (IPL)
ipRGCs. See Intrinsically photosensitive RGCs (ipRGCs)
Ipsilateral iris, depigmentation of, 275
Ipsipulsion of saccades, 315
Iridis, heterochromia, 296
Iridocyclitis, 296
Iris
  acquired structural defects of, 296
  anomalies, 295f
  atrophy, 296
  congenital structural defects of, 293–296
  parasympathetic innervation of, 293f
  structural defects of, 293–296
  sympathetic innervation of, 294f
Iris dilator
  pharmacologic stimulation of, 281
Iris sphincter
  after damage to innervation of, 291
  damage to, 285
  pharmacologic stimulation of, 280–281
Iritis, 296
Ischemia, 183, 296, 349

Ischemic optic disc edema with minimal dysfunction, 158–160
Ischemic optic neuropathies (ION), 145–160, 152t
  anterior ischemic optic neuropathy (AION), 145–155
  ischemic optic disc edema with minimal dysfunction, 158–160
  posterior ischemic optic neuropathy (PION), 155–156
  radiation optic neuropathy (RON), 158, 159f
  in settings of hemodynamic compromise, 156–157
Ischemic Optic Neuropathy Decompression Trial (IONDT), 151
Ishihara pseudoisochromatic color plate, 5, 6f
Isolated accommodation insufficiency, 297
Isolated nutritional optic neuropathy, 191–192
Isopter, 11, 13, 15

J
Junctional scotoma, 102, 210

K
Kearns-Sayre syndrome (KSS), 395, 397, 398f
  Bilateral orbicularis oculi weakness, 444f
Kinetic perimetry, 7, 11, 11f, 13, 15
  demonstrates supertemporal visual field defect, 85f
  scotomas mapped by, 189f
Kjer/juvenile optic atrophy. See Autosomal-dominant optic atrophy (ADOA)
Knowledge, covert semantic, 247
Krabbe disease, bilateral optic atrophy with, 208f
Krimsky test, 308
KSS, See Kearns-Sayre syndrome (KSS)

L
Lacrimation
  disorders of, 300
  excessive, 300
  nonorganic disturbances of, 464
Lacrimation, disorders of, 300
Lambert–Eaton myasthenic syndrome, 381–382
Lamina cribrosa, 44f, 45, 45f, 46f
Langerhans cell histiocytosis, 174
Lateral geniculate body (LGB)
  anatomy and visual field representation, 224f
  magnocellular and parvocellular pathways from, 245f
  topical diagnosis of lesions of, 224–225
Lateral geniculate nucleus (LGN), 39, 52

Lateral medullary infarction, 314–316
Late recovery, 166
Lateropulsion, 314–315
  of saccades, 315f
Leber plus syndromes, 198
Leber's hereditary optic neuropathy (LHON), 187, 195–202, 197f
  associated findings, 196, 197f, 198, 198f–199f
  clinical features, 195–196
  genetics, 199–201
  inheritance, 199–201
  mutations associated with, 199, 200f, 201
  natural history, 201
  treatment, 202
  unanswered questions, 201–202
  visual loss in patients with, 196
Left anterior cerebral and middle cerebral arteries, infarct in, 333f
Left homonymous hemianopia, hemianopic optic atrophy in patient with, 223f
Left temporal lobe cystic astrocytoma, 228f
Leigh's syndrome, 341
Lesions
  of abducens nucleus, 324
  of afferent pathway, 291
  anterior occipital lobe, 230–231, 232f
  bilateral, 248
  bilateral occipital lobe, 233–237, 238f
  causing color dysnomia, 250f
  causing homonymous hemianopia, 250f
  causing pure alexia, 250f
  central and posterior occipital lobe, 230
  of cerebellum, 317–322
  of cerebral hemispheres upon ocular motor function, 334t
  extracranial, 124
  of extrastriate cortex with defects in visual field, 240
  focal, 334–336
  frontal lobe, 335–336
  infiltrate optic nerve, 167t
  of internal capsule, 225–227, 227f
  of lateral geniculate body (LGB), 224–225
  macular, 54f, 55f, 56f, 57f
  mass, 321–322
  of medulla, 312–317
  mesencephalic, 291
  of mesencephalon, 327–331
  occipital lobe, 334
  of occipital lobe and visual cortex, 229–243
  of optic radiation, 225–229
  optic tract, 219–223
  in papillomacular bundles, 57f–58f
  of paramedian pontine reticular formation (PPRF), 325
  parietal lobe, 334–335
  of parietal lobe, 229

pons, 322–327
  slow saccades from pontine, 326–327
  temporal lobe, 335
  of temporal lobe, 227–229
  that damage anterior angle of optic chiasm, 210
  that damage body of optic chiasm, 210–211, 212f
  that damage posterior angle of optic chiasm, 211–214
  in three patients with prosopagnosia, 249f
  tonic pupil, 281–285
  unilateral, 333–334
  visual field defects caused by, 214–216
Lesions in cerebral hemispheres, ocular motor syndromes caused by, 332–339
  abnormal eye movements and dementia, 336–337
  acute unilateral lesions, 332–333
  eye movements in stupor and coma, 338–339
  focal lesions, 334–336
  ocular motor apraxia, 336
  ocular motor manifestations of seizures, 337–338
  persistent deficits caused by large unilateral lesions, 333–334
Lesions of optic chiasm, topical diagnosis of, 210–217
  neuro-ophthalmologic signs and symptoms, 216–217
  visual field defects, 210–216
Lesions, topical diagnosis of chiasmal and retrochiasmal, 210–243
  topical diagnosis of optic chiasmal disorders, 210–217
  topical diagnosis of retrochiasmal visual field defects, 217–243
Leukemia, 174
Levator palpebrae superioris, 424
LGB. See Lateral geniculate body (LGB)
LGN. See Lateral geniculate nucleus (LGN)
LHON. See Leber's hereditary optic neuropathy
Lid-Triggered Synkinesias, 446
Light
  more anisocoria in, 281
  testing pupillary reaction to, 264–265
Light and darkness, paradoxical reaction of pupils to, 290
Light-near dissociation, 290–291
  aberrant regeneration after damage to innervation of iris sphincter, 291
  Argyll Robertson pupils, 290–291, 290f
  lesions of afferent pathway, 291
  mesencephalic lesions, 291
  pupillary, 291f
  testing for, 266

Light reflex, pupillary, 289f
Light response, consensual, 265
Lipid storage diseases, 339
Literal alexia, 251
Localized deviations, 15
Local tonic pupil, 282
Locked-in syndrome, 339
Longitudinal Optic Neuritis Study
    (LONS), 134, 135f
LONS. See Longitudinal Optic Neuritis
    Study (LONS)
Loss of temporal crescent, 232f
Low-Contrast Sloan Letter Charts,
    3–4, 4f
LP. See Lumbar puncture (LP)
Lumbar puncture (LP), 109
Lumboperitoneal shunting, 128
Lyme borreliosis, 141
Lyme disease, 94f, 141
Lymphoma, infiltration of right optic
    nerve, chiasm, and tract by,
    174f
Lymphomatoid granulomatosis, 174
Lymphoreticular malignancies,
    173–174

M
Machado–Joseph disease, 446
Macropsia, 260
Macrosaccadic oscillations, 416
Macrosquare-wave jerks, 416
Macular disease, 288
Macular lesions
    causing visual loss, 54f
    pupillary defect, 57f
    with unexplained vision loss in both
        eyes, 55f
    unexplained visual loss from, 56f
Macula, sparing of, 231–233, 234f
Macula, splitting of, 210, 212f
Maculopathies vs. optic neuropathies,
    54t
Magnetic resonance imaging (MRI)
    of brain of patient with isolated
        optic neuritis, 133f
    of optic nerve in acute
        demyelinating optic neuritis,
        133f
    of optic nerve sheath meningioma
        (ONSM), 164f
Magnocellular, 244
Magnocellular cells, 39
Major pretectal nuclei, drawing of, 327f
Malignancies, lymphoreticular,
    173–174
Malignant optic nerve gliomas, 168,
    169f
Malingering, 452
Marcus Gunn jaw-winking
    phenomenon, 436
Marcus Gunn phenomenon, 427
MAR. See Melanoma-associated
    retinopathy (MAR)
Marcus Gunn jaw-winking
    phenomenon, 436

Marcus Gunn pupil, 266
Masses, intracranial, 122
Mass lesions, 321–322
MD. See Mean deviation (MD)
Mean deviation (MD)
    on Humphrey field analyzer, 15
Mechanisms
    primary, 183
    secondary, 183
Medial inferior pontine syndrome,
    363
Medial vestibular nucleus (MVN), 312
Medulla oblongata, schematic drawing
    of, 313f
Medulla, ocular motor syndromes
    caused by lesions of, 312–317
    skew deviation and ocular tilt
        reaction, 317
    syndrome of anterior inferior
        cerebellar artery (AICA), 316
    syndrome of superior cerebellar
        artery, 316–317, 317f
    Wallenberg's syndrome, 314–316
Megalopapilla, 80–81, 81f
Meige syndrome, 445
Melanocytomas, 172, 172f
Melanoma-associated retinopathy
    (MAR), 37
Melanopsin, 4, 39
Membrane remnants, persistent
    pupillary, 294
Meningeal carcinomatosis, 173
Meningitis, 122–123
    carcinomatous, 173
Mesencephalic lesions, 291
Mesencephalon, 292
    dorsal, 297
    neurologic disorders that primarily
        affect, 329–331
Mesencephalon, ocular motor
    syndromes caused by lesions
    of, 327–331
    neurologic disorders that primarily
        affect mesencephalon, 329–331
    sites and manifestations of lesions,
        327–329
Metabolic coma, 292
Metabolic disorders ocular motor
    manifestations of, 339–341
Metabolic disorders, toxic and, 96
Metabolic dysfunction, 126
Metamorphopsia, 1, 9, 10f, 54, 260
Metastases, 172–173
Methylprednisolone, 183–184
MEWDS. See Multiple evanescent
    white dot syndrome (MEWDS)
Meyer loop, 227
mfERG. See Multifocal
    electroretinogram (mfERG)
Micropsia, 1, 260
    cerebral, 260f
Midbrain disease, poorly reacting
    pupils from, 290
Midbrain syndrome, dorsal, 328f, 328t
Midget system, 37

Migraine phosphene protocol,
    photographic negative of
    259f
Migrainous hallucinations, 259
Millard–Gubler syndrome, 363, 3
Miosis, 272, 299
    congenital, 295
Miotic pupil, 281
Misregeneration theory, tonic pu
    syndrome, 286f
Mitochondrial myopathies, 395
Mitochondrial neurogastrointesti
    encephalomyopathy synd
    398
Möbius Syndrome, 361
MOG. See Myelin-oligodendrocyt
    glycoprotein (MOG)
Monocular bobbing movements,
Monocular diplopia, 459
Monocular field defects, 20f
Monosymptomatic hereditary op
    neuropathies, 195–204
    dominant optic atrophy (DOA
        202–204
    isolated hereditary optic
        neuropathies, 204
    Leber's hereditary optic neuro
        195–202
Morning glory disc anomalies, 74
    75f, 76f
    with contractile movements, 7
    CT scan of, 76f
    and optic disc colobomas, 79t
    peripapillary staphylomas and
        80t
Motion perception
    disorders of, 252
    PET study of, 253f
Motor nerves, ocular, 284f
Motor rigidity, generalized,
    117–118
MRI. See Magnetic resonance im
    (MRI)
MS. See Multiple sclerosis (MS)
Mulberry astrocytomas, 168–169
Müller cells, 34f, 38
Müller muscle, 424
Multifocal electroretinogram (m
    29–30, 30f
Multifocal visual-evoked potenti
Multiple evanescent white dot
    syndrome (MEWDS), 59
Multiple myeloma, 174
Multiple sclerosis (MS)
    cumulative probability of, 135
    one-and-a-half syndrome in m
    with, 324f
Munchausen syndrome, 452
Muscle–Eye–Brain Disease, 389
Muscular dystrophies, 388
Muscles, extraocular, 284f
MVN. See Medial vestibular nucl
    (MVN)
Myasthenia gravis (MG), 292, 29
    372–385

bilateral pseudo-internuclear ophthalmoplegia in patient with, 376f
clinical tests, 376
diagnostic testing, 376–379
disorders of neuromuscular transmission other than, 382–383
electrophysiologic tests, 381
epidemiology, 372
neostigmine test, 380–381, 380f
nonocular signs, 376
ocular, 382
ocular signs, 373–376
ocular versus generalized, 372–373
ophthalmoparesis and other eye movements, 374–376
orbicularis oculi involvement, 376
orbicularis oculi involvement, 376, 376f
pharmacologic test, 377
pupillary function, 376
repetitive nerve stimulation, 381
single-fiber electromyography, 381
sleep test, 377, 377f
specific autoantibody assays, 377
treatment, 381
Mydriasis
congenital, 296
episodic unilateral, 280
postoperative, 296
Myelinated (medullated) nerve fibers, 88–90, 89f
Myelinoclastic diffuse sclerosis, 138–139
Myelin-oligodendrocyte glycoprotein (MOG), 136
Myeloma, multiple, 174
Myoid, 36
Myopathic Eyelid Retraction, 438
Myotonia congenita, 394
Myotonic dystrophy, 297, 389
appearance of cataracts, 390f
Myotonic muscular dystrophies, 389

N
NAION. See Nonarteritic anterior ischemic optic neuropathy (NAION)
Naloxone, 183
Nasal hemianopia, 106–108, 108f
NASCIS II. See National Acute Spinal Cord Injury Study (NASCIS II)
National Acute Spinal Cord Injury Study (NASCIS II), 183
Nausea, 117
Near point of accommodation (NPA), 271
Near point of convergence (NPC), 272
Near reflex, 461, 462f
Near reflex. See Near response spasm of, 298–300
Near reflex, spasm of, 461, 462f
Near response, 271
assessment of, 271–272
testing pupillary, 265

Negative phenomena, visual fields, 255
Negative scotoma, 1
Neostigmine test, 380–381, 380f
Nerve axons, retinal, 41f
Nerve fascicle, oculomotor, 282f
Nerve fiber layer (NFL), 37, 41–42
atrophy of peripapillary retinal, 101f
three-dimensional organization, 42f
Nerve fibers
myelinated, 88–90, 89f
preganglionic autonomic, 283f
Nerve palsies
abducens, 368
abducens gaze paralysis, 361–368
congenital left oculomotor, 342f
neuroimaging, 367f
nuclear oculomotor, 344f
oculomotor, 341–355
right oculomotor, 348, 348f
trochlear, 355–361, 367f, 360–361
Nerves
ocular motor, 284f
peripheral oculomotor, 292
preganglionic oculomotor, 291
Neuritis, anterior optic, 93
Neuritis, optic, 5, 10f, 32f
anterior, 93
causes of optic neuritis other than primary demyelination, 139–142
in children, 142
chronic demyelinating optic neuritis, 134
idiopathic demyelinating optic neuritis, 130–136
neuroretinitis, 93–94, 142–144
optic perineuritis, 144
in other primary demyelinating diseases, 136–139
Neurofibromatosis type 1 (NF-1), 167–168, 168f
Neuroimaging studies, IIH, 125
Neurologic disease, generalized or focal, 297–298
Neurologic disorders that primarily affect mesencephalon, 329–331
Neuromuscular junction disorders of, 292
Neuromuscular ptosis, 431
Neuromuscular transmission, normal, 372
Neuromuscular transmission
normal, 372
other than MG, 382–383
toxins that damage both pre- and postsynaptic, 384–385
Neuromuscular transmission, disorders of, 372–385
acquired disorders of neuromuscular transmission other than MG, 382–385
congenital myasthenic syndromes, 381
myasthenia gravis (MG), 372–381
normal neuromuscular transmission, 372

Neuromuscular transmission other than MG, acquired disorders of
Lambert-Eaton myasthenic syndrome, 382
neuromuscular disorders caused by drugs or toxins, 383–385
ocular manifestations, 382
pathophysiology, 382
therapy, 383
Neuromyelitis optica (NMO)
clinical manifestations, 136, 138
diagnosis, 138
pathology, 136
treatment, 138
Neuromyelitis optic spectrum disorder (NMOSD), 137f
Neuro-ophthalmologic signs and symptoms, 216–217
Neuropathic tonic pupil, 282
Neuropathies
anterior compressive optic, 161–164
autoimmune optic, 141–142
bilateral anterior optic, 194f
compressive optic, 161–166
hemifield slide phenomenon from bilateral optic, 107f
hereditary optic, 195–209
infiltrative optic, 166–178
ischemic optic, 145–160, 152t
isolated hereditary optic, 204
nutritional optic, 186
retrobulbar compressive optic, 164–166
toxic optic, 186–187
traumatic optic, 179–185
Neuroretinitis, 93–94, 94f, 140, 143f
Neurotransmitters used by cells of rod and cone pathways, 38f
Neurotransmitters, retinal neurons and, 42t
NFL. See Nerve fiber layer (NFL)
NHL. See Non-Hodgkin lymphoma (NHL)
NMO. See Neuromyelitis optica (NMO)
NMO-IgG, 136, 138
NMOSD. See Neuromyelitis optic spectrum disorder (NMOSD)
Nodulus, 318
Nonarteritic anterior ischemic optic neuropathy (NAION), 95f, 148f, 151–155
clinical course, 154–155
clinical presentation, 151–152
diagnosis, 155
disc swelling from, 158–159
histopathology, 152–154
pathophysiology, 152–154
sectoral optic atrophy after, 154f
therapy, 155
vision loss due to, 150f
Noncomitant strabismus, 305
Nonfluent aphasia, 251
Nonglaucomatous cupping, 100f
Non-Hodgkin lymphoma (NHL), 173–174

Nonhuman primate, visual function in cerebral cortex of, 245f
Nonorganic blepharospasm, 446
Nonorganic monocular hemianopias, 458
Nonorganic ptosis, 463
Nonorganic visual loss, testing, 454f
Nonpathologic pallor of optic disc, 97
Normal optic nerves
  axial section of, 48f
  sagittal section of, 47f
  topographic sections of, 44f
Nothnagel syndrome, 345
NPA. *See* Near point of accommodation (NPA)
NPC. *See* Near point of convergence (NPC)
NPH. *See* Nucleus prepositus hypoglossi (NPH)
Nucleus prepositus hypoglossi (NPH), 312
Nuclear oculomotor nerve palsy, 344f, 345t
Nutritional and toxic optic neuropathies, clinical characteristics of, 187
Nutritional optic neuropathies, 186
Nutritional optic neuropathies, specific, 190–192
  epidemic nutritional optic neuropathy, 190–191
  isolated nutritional optic neuropathy, 191–192
Nutritional optic neuropathy, isolated, 190–191
Nyctalopia, 36–37
Nystagmus, 315
Nystagmus waveform, 404
  slow-phase of, 404f

O

Object recognition face and prosopagnosia and related disturbances of, 247–249
Oblique illumination *vs.* upgaze pupil testing technique, 265f
Occipital head trauma, 237f
Occipital lobe and visual cortex, lesions of, 229–243
  bilateral occipital lobe lesions, 233–237
  cerebral blindness, 238–239
  cortical blindness, 238–239
  dissociation of visual perceptions, 240–241
  extrastriate cortex with defects in visual field, 240
  homonymous hemianopia, treatment and rehabilitation for, 242–243
  macular sparing, 231–233, 234f
  nonvisual symptoms and signs of, 240–241
  other visual features of occipital lobe damage, 239–240

unilateral lesions of anterior occipital lobe, 230–231
unilateral lesions of central and posterior occipital lobe, 230
Occipital lobe disease, nonvisual symptoms and signs of, 241–242
Occipital lobe epilepsy, visual illusions of, 258f
Occipital lobe infarct, bilateral visual field defects in patient with, 23f
Occipital lobe lesions, 334
  bilateral, 233–237
Occipital lobes
  bilateral lesions, 233–237
  unilateral lesions of anterior, 230–231
  unilateral lesions of posterior, 230
Occipital spike-waves, benign childhood epilepsy with, 258–259
Occlusions, retinal vascular, 67–68
OCT. *See* Optical coherence tomography (OCT)
Octopus perimeter, 9
Ocular alignment, 305–309
  disturbances of egocentric localization, 305
  head tilts, 305–306
  head turns, 305–306
  objective testing, 307–309
  past-pointing, 305
  primary deviations, 305, 306f
  principles, 305
  secondary deviations, 305, 306f
  subjective testing, 306–307
  techniques, 306
Ocular bobbing, 338, 418
Ocular colobomas, 78
Ocular dipping, 338
Ocular disease
  accommodation insufficiency associated with, 297
Ocular fundus, torsion of, 310f
Ocular Flutter, 417, 417t
Ocular motility and alignment, disorders of, 461
Ocular imaging, 25, 26f–27f, 28f
Ocular manifestations
  diagnosis, 392
  pathology, 392
  treatment, 392
Ocular motility disorders, nuclear and infranuclear, 341–371
  abducens nerve palsies and nuclear horizontal gaze paralysis, 361–369
  hyperactivity of ocular motor nerves, 369–370
  oculomotor nerve palsies, 341–355
  synkineses involving ocular motor and other cranial nerve, 371
  trochlear nerve palsies, 355–358
Ocular motility and alignment, examination of, 301–311

blurred vision, 302–303
corneal light reflex, 307–308
cover tests, 307–308
diplopia, 302
direct observation of fundus, 309
examination, 302–311
fixation and gaze-holding ability, 302
head tilt test, 309
history, 301–302
ocular alignment, 305–309
performance of versions, 309–311
range of eye movements, 302–305
vertigo, oscillopsia, and tilt, 302
vestibular symptoms, 302
visual confusion, 302
Ocular motor abnormalities and disease of basal ganglia, 331–332
  Huntington's disease, 332
  Parkinson's disease, 331–332
Ocular motor apraxia, acquired, 336
Ocular motor disorders, supranuclear and internuclear, 312–342
Ocular motor function, lesions of cerebral hemispheres upon, 334t
Ocular motor manifestations of metabolic disorders, 339–341
Ocular motor manifestations of seizures, 337–338
Ocular motor nerves, 284f
  hyperactivity of, 369
Ocular motor syndromes, caused by lesions in cerebral hemispheres, 332–339
  abnormal eye movements and dementia, 336–337
  acute unilateral lesions, 332–333
  eye movements in stupor and coma, 338–339
  focal lesions, 334–336
  ocular motor apraxia, 336
  ocular motor manifestations of seizures, 337–338
  persistent deficits caused by large unilateral lesions, 333–334
Ocular motor syndromes caused by lesions of cerebellum, 317–322
  etiologies, 319–322
  location of lesions and their manifestations, 318–319
Ocular motor syndromes caused by lesions of medulla, 312–317
  skew deviation and ocular tilt reaction, 317
  syndrome of anterior inferior cerebellar artery (AICA), 316
  syndrome of superior cerebellar artery, 316–317, 317f
  Wallenberg's syndrome, 314–316
Ocular motor syndromes caused by lesions of mesencephalon, 327–331
  neurologic disorders that primarily affect mesencephalon, 329–331

sites and manifestations of lesions, 327–329
Ocular motor syndromes caused by lesions of pons, 322–327
internuclear ophthalmoplegia, 322–324
lesions of abducens nucleus, 324
lesions of paramedian pontine reticular formation (PPRF), 325
one-and-a-half syndrome, 325–326
slow saccades from pontine lesions, 326–327
unilateral conjugate gaze palsy, 325–326
Ocular neuromyotonia, 369–370, 370f
Ocular tilt reaction (OTR), 315, 316f, 330f
Ocular tilt reaction, skew deviation and, 317
Oculocephalic testing, 304
Oculogyric crises, 331
with postencephalitic Parkinsonism, 332f
Oculogyric crisis in patients with postencephalitic parkinsonism, 332f
Oculomotor nerve
aberrant reinnervation of, 298
peripheral, 292
preganglionic, 291
Oculomotor nerve fascicle, 282f
Oculomotor nerve palsy, 348f
Oculomotor nerve paralysis, 353
Oculomotor nerve palsies, 341–355
acquired, 358–360
congenital, 341
congenital left, 342f
management of patients with, 368–369
nuclear, 344f, 345t
right, 349f
Oculomotor nerve to intracranial arteries, relationship of, 347f
Oculomotor nucleus
lesions of, 434
Warwick schema of, 343f
Oculomotor palsies/risk of compressive lesion, evaluation of, 351t
Oculopalpebral synkinesia
congenital bilateral supranuclear, 427f
congenital unilateral supranuclear, 427f
Oculopalatal myoclonus syndrome, 312
Oculopalatal tremor, 312, 313f
Oculopharyngeal muscular dystrophy (OPMD), 393–394, 393, 393f
Oculosympathetic pathway, 275f, 428
ODOA Plus syndrome, 203–204
OFF-center cells, 37, 39
ON-center cells, 37, 39
One-and-a-half syndrome, 325–326

ONSD. *See* Optic nerve sheath decompression (ONSD)
ONSF. *See* Optic nerve sheath fenestration (ONSF)
ONSM. *See* Optic nerve sheath meningioma (ONSM)
ONTT. *See* Optic Neuritis Treatment Trial (ONTT)
Ophthalmic artery, anatomy of proximal portion of, 52f
Ophthalmoparesis, asymmetric, 391f
Ophthalmoplegia
autosomal dominant optic atrophy, deafness and, 203–204, 228
etiology of Internuclear, 322t
internal, 281
from vitamin E deficiency, 400–401
OPL. *See* Outer plexiform layer (OPL)
Ophthalmoparesis and other abnormalities of eye movements, 374–376
Opsoclonus, 417, 417t
Optokinetic drum, use of, 453f
Orbicularis oculi, anatomy of, 425f
Optical coherence tomography (OCT), 25, 83f, 98, 217
of maculae, 27f
of peripapillary retinal nerve fiber layer, 26f, 28f
visual field defects, 26f
Optic ataxia, 254, 255
Optic atrophy
after acute retrobulbar optic neuritis, 132f
after NAION, 154f
congenital recessive, 204
development after AION, 153f
differential diagnosis of, 100–102
with Krabbe disease, 208f
nonpathologic pallor of optic disc, 97
ophthalmoscopic features of, 98–100
pathology and pathophysiology of, 97–98
and pseudoglaucomatous cupping after attack of AAION, 149f
retinal arteries in, 101f
in retinal dystrophy, 60f
in vitamin A deficiency, 60f
X-linked, 204
Optic canal fracture, 182f
Optic chiasm
and intracranial optic nerves, 51f
lesions that damage anterior angle of, 210
lesions that damage body of, 210–211, 212f
lesions that damage posterior angle of, 211–214
of macaque monkey, 52f
relationships of optic nerves and, 211f
visual field defects caused by lesions that damage, 214–216
Optic chiasmal, anterior, 212f

Optic chiasm lesions, body of, 210–211
after severe head trauma, 214f
bilateral optic neuropathy in sclerosis, 213f
bitemporal hemianopia, 212f
Optic chiasm, topical diagnosis of lesions of, 210–217
neuro-ophthalmologic signs and symptoms, 216–217
visual field defects, 210–216
Optic disc, 45
appearance of tilted, 45f
astrocytic hamartoma, 169f
band or bow-tie atrophy of right, 102f
cavernous angioma of, 162f, 171f
cupping, 100f, 165f
with dominant optic atrophy "plus," 205f
doubling of, 88, 88f
drusen *vs.* astrocytic hamartoma, 170f
infiltration of, 96–97, 173f
melanocytomas of, 172f
nonpathologic pallor of, 97
in patient with longstanding bilateral optic neuropathy, 190f
sarcoid granulomas infiltrating, 176f
sarcoidosis, 177f–178f
sectoral and diffuse pallor of, 99f
traumatic avulsion of, 180f
with Wolfram syndrome, 206f
Optic disc anomalies, excavated, 74–84
megalopapilla, 80–81, 81f
morning glory disc anomaly, 74–77, 75f
optic disc coloboma, 77–80
optic pit, 81–82, 82f
papillorenal syndrome, 82–84, 83f
peripapillary staphyloma, 80
Optic disc, appearance of, 91–102
infiltration of optic disc, 96–97
optic atrophy, 97–102
optic discs swelling, 91–96
Optic disc colobomas, 77–80, 78f
bilateral, 79f
morning glory disc anomaly and, 79t, 80t
unilateral, 79f
Optic disc, congenital anomalies of, 61–90
Aicardi syndrome, 86–88
anomalous optic disc elevation (pseudopapilledema), 61–69
congenital optic disc pigmentation, 86
congenital tilted optic disc syndrome, 84–86
doubling of the optic discs, 88
excavated optic disc anomalies, 74–84
myelinated (medullated) nerve fibers, 88–90
optic disc dysplasia, 86
optic nerve aplasia, 88
optic nerve hypoplasia, 69–74

Optic disc drusen, 288
  bilateral visual field defects in
      patient with bilateral, 67f
  buried, 63f, 64f, 65f
  calcifications, 66f
  in patient with retinitis pigmentosa,
      69f
  pseudopapilledema associated with,
      62–69
  visible, 64f
Optic disc dysplasia, 86, 86f
Optic disc edema
  in AION, 148f
  with minimal dysfunction, 158–160
Optic disc elevation, 96f
Optic disc pigmentation, congenital,
    86, 87f
Optic disc swelling, 92f, 93t, 95f, 96f
  in anterior ischemic optic
      neuropathy, 95f
  in anterior ischemic optic
      neuropathy (AION), 94–95, 95f
  appearance, 91–92
  in patient with optic nerve sheath
      meningioma (ONSM), 164f
  in patient with orbital cavernous
      angioma, 162f
  in patient with pars planitis, 142f
  in patient with thyroid eye disease,
      163f
  specific etiologies, 92–96
  vs. pseudopapilledema with buried
      drusen, 65t
Optic foramen, 48
Optic hypoplasia, superior segmental,
    73f
Optic nerve and choroid, blood supply
    to proximal, 46f
Optic nerve aplasia, 88, 89f
Optic nerve disorders, topical diagnosis
    of acquired, 91–108
  appearance of disc, 91–102
  syndromes of prechiasmal optic
      nerve dysfunction, 102–108
Optic nerve dysfunction, syndromes of
    pre-chiasmal, 102–108
  bilateral superior or inferior
      (altitudinal) hemianopia,
      104–106, 106f
  distal optic nerve syndrome, 102,
      104f
  Foster Kennedy syndrome, 102,
      104, 105f
  nasal hemianopia, 106–108, 108f
  optociliary shunts, 102
  syndromes of optic nerve
      compression, 102
Optic nerve glioma, 167, 167f
  pseudo-CSF sign in patient with,
      168f
Optic nerve gliomas, malignant, 168,
    169f
Optic nerve head (intraocular optic
    nerve), 44–47, 44f
Optic nerve hypoplasia, 74

associated central nervous system
    malformations, 71–72
associated endocrinologic
    deficiencies, 71
  in children, 72
  clinical features, 69, 71
  magnetic resonance imaging (MRI)
      in, 72f
  pathogenesis, 74
  segmental, 73–74
  systemic and teratogenic
      associations, 72–73
Optic nerve in acute demyelinating
    optic neuritis, MRI of, 133f
Optic nerve injuries
  direct, 179
  indirect, 179
Optic nerve physiology, 52
Optic nerves, 44
  axial section of normal, 48f
  blood supply, 47f
  blood supply to dorsal aspect of optic
      chiasm and intracranial, 51f
  compression, 95–96, 96f, 102
  cross-section of human, 48f
  and falciform dural folds, 183f
  fiber arrangement in, 53f
  glioma, 167f
  gliomas, 167f
  hypoplasia, 70f, 71f
  intracanalicular, 48–50
  intracranial, 50–52
  intracranial portions of, 47f, 163f
  intraorbital, 47f
  lesions infiltrate, 167t
  normal, 44f
  orbital, 47–48
  orbit showing, 47f
  in patient with neurofibromatosis
      type 1, 168f
  physiology, 52
  relationship to ocular motor nerves,
      284f
  sarcoidosis, 177f–178f
  topographic anatomy of, 52–53
  traumatic avulsion of, 180f
Optic nerves, anatomy and physiology
    of, 44–53
  intracanalicular (intraosseous) optic
      nerve, 48–50
  intracranial optic nerve, 50–52
  optic nerve head (intraocular optic
      nerve), 44–47, 44f
  optic nerve physiology, 52
  orbital optic nerve, 47–48
  topographic anatomy of optic
      nerve, 52–53
Optic nerves and optic chiasm,
    relationships of, 211f
Optic nerve sheath decompression
    (ONSD), 114
Optic nerve sheath fenestration
    (ONSF), 128
Optic nerve sheath meningioma
    (ONSM), 162

magnetic resonance imaging of, 164f
optic disc swelling in patient with,
    164f
Optic nerve sheaths, schematic
    drawing of, 50f
Optic nerve syndrome, distal, 102,
    104f
Optic neuritis, 5, 10f, 32f
  anterior, 93, 131f
  bilateral anterior, 140f
  causes of optic neuritis other
      than primary demyelination,
      139–142
  in children, 142
  idiopathic demyelinating optic
      neuritis, 130–136
  infectious and parainfectious,
      140–141
  inflammatory, 141–142
  MRI of brain of patient with
      isolated, 133f
  MRI of optic nerve in acute
      demyelinating, 133f
  neuroretinitis, 93–94, 142–144, 143f
  optic atrophy after acute
      retrobulbar, 132f
  optic perineuritis, 144
  in other primary demyelinating
      diseases, 136–139
  postvaccination, 141
  severe anterior, 132f
Optic neuritis, causes other than
    primary demyelination,
    139–142
  infectious and parainfectious optic
      neuritis, 140–141
  inflammatory optic neuritis, 141–142
  miscellaneous causes, 142
  postvaccination optic neuritis, 141
Optic neuritis, idiopathic
    demyelinating, 130–135
  acute idiopathic demyelinating optic
      neuritis, 130–135
  asymptomatic (subclinical) optic
      neuritis, 135
  chronic demyelinating optic neuritis,
      135
Optic neuritis in other primary
    demyelinating diseases,
    136–139
  concentric sclerosis of Baló, 139
  encephalitis periaxialis concentrica,
      139
  myelinoclastic diffuse sclerosis,
      138–139
  neuromyelitis optica (Devic disease),
      136–138
Optic Neuritis Treatment Trial
    (ONTT), 130, 135f
Optic neuropathies
  anterior compressive, 161–164
  bilateral anterior, 194f
  bilateral toxic, 188f, 189f
  bilateral visual dysfunction with,
      154f

clinical characteristics of nutritional and toxic, 187
compressive, 161–166
distinguishing retinal disease by clinical examination, 53–59
distinguishing retinal disease by visual field, 56–59
epidemic nutritional, 190–191
hemifield slide phenomenon from bilateral, 107f
hemodynamic compromise, ischemic optic neuropathy in settings of, 156–157
infiltrative, 166–178
isolated hereditary, 204
isolated nutritional, 190–191
Leber's hereditary, 187, 195–202, 197f
miscellaneous isolated hereditary, 204
nonglaucomatous, 98
nutritional, 186
retrobulbar compressive, 164–166
specific toxic, 192–194
toxic, 186–187
vs. maculopathies, 54t
Optic neuropathies, hereditary, 195–209
degenerative/developmental diseases, 207–209
hereditary optic atrophy with neurologic or systemic signs, 204–207
miscellaneous isolated, 204
monosymptomatic hereditary optic neuropathies, 195–204
Optic neuropathies, monosymptomatic hereditary, 195–204
dominant optic atrophy (DOA), 202–204
isolated hereditary optic neuropathies, 204
Leber's hereditary optic neuropathy, 195–202
Optic neuropathies, toxic and deficiency, 186–194
clinical characteristics of nutritional and toxic optic neuropathies, 187
differential diagnosis, 187–190
etiologic criteria, 186–187
specific nutritional optic neuropathies, 190–192
specific toxic optic neuropathies, 192–194
Optic neuropathies, traumatic, 179–185
classification, 179
clinical assessment, 181–182
epidemiology, 179–181
management, 184–185
pathogenesis, 183
pathology, 182–183
pharmacology, 183–184
Optic neuropathy and hereditary degenerative/developmental diseases, 207–209

diffuse white-matter disease, 209
hereditary ataxias, 207–208
hereditary polyneuropathies, 208–209
Optic perineuritis, 140
Optic pit, 81–82, 82f, 83f
Optic radiation, lesions of, 225–229
internal capsule, 225–227, 227f
parietal lobe, 229
pathway, 229f
temporal lobe, 227–229
Optic strut, 49
Optic tract, 289
Optic tract lesions, topical diagnosis of, 219–223
Optociliary shunts and syndromes of optic nerve compression, 102
Optociliary shunt veins, 102, 103f
Optokinetic nystagmus, 3
Optokinetic system, 311
Orbit
posterior, 49f
showing optic nerve, 47f
Orbital cavernous angioma of optic disc, 162f
Orbital emphysema, 181
Orbital optic nerve, 47–48
Orbital pseudotumor, 161–162
Oscillopsia, 302
OTR. See Ocular tilt reaction (OTR)
Outer nuclear layer, 34f, 35t
Outer plexiform layer (OPL), 34f, 37
Oxygen free radicals, 183

P

PACAP. See Pituitary adenylate cyclase-activating polypeptide (PACAP)
Palinopsia, 255
Pallid swelling, 95f
Palpebromandibular synkinesia, 446
PAN. See Periodic alternating nystagmus (PAN)
Papilledema, 64, 92, 93f–94f. See also Pseudopapilledema
associated with bilateral visual loss, 119f–120f
chronic, 113, 113f, 114f
course, 117
diagnosis of, 115–117
differential diagnosis of, 116
etiology of, 120–124
fiber layer in, 110, 111f
Frisén grading system, 110t
idiopathic intracranial hypertension (pseudotumor cerebri), 124–129
macular star figure in fully developed, 112f
measurements of intracranial pressure (ICP), 109–110
miscellaneous signs of, 112–113
ophthalmoscopic appearance of, 110–115
optociliary shunt veins in patient with chronic, 114f

stages of, 110, 111f, 112
subhyaloid hemorrhage with, 113f
symptoms and signs of, 117–120
unilateral/asymmetric, 114–115
visual field defects in, 121f
Papilledema, etiology of, 120–124
craniosynostoses, 123–124
disorders of CSF flow, 122–123
extracranial lesions, 124
intracranial masses, 122
syndromes of elevated venous pressure, 123, 123t
trauma, 123
Papilledema, ophthalmoscopic appearance of, 110–115
chronic papilledema, 113, 113f
grading system, 110t
miscellaneous signs of papilledema, 112–113
postpapilledema atrophy, 113–114, 113f, 115f
stages of papilledema, 110, 111f, 112
unilateral/asymmetric papilledema, 114–115
Papilledema, symptoms and signs of, 117–120
nonvisual manifestations, 117–118
visual manifestations, 118–120
Papillitis, 93, 130
Papillomacular bundle, 41
cecocentral scotoma caused by lesion in, 57f
Papillopathy, diabetic, 159, 160f
Papillorenal syndrome, 82–84, 83f
Paraflocculus, 318
Parainfectious optic neuritis, infectious and, 140–141
Paramyotonia Congenita, 394
Paralysis, 461
horizontal gaze, 462
sympathetic, 298
vertical gaze, 462
Paralytic pontine exotropia, 326
Paramedian pontine reticular formation (PPRF), 305
lesions of, 325
Paramyotonia congenital, 394
Paraneoplastic cerebellar degeneration, 321
Parapapillary retinal arteriolar narrowing in AION, 148f
Parasympatholytic agents, pharmacologic blockade with, 285
Parasympatholytic (anticholinergic) drugs, 292, 293f
Parasympathomimetic (cholinergic) drugs, 293
Paretic (deviated) eye, image from, 307f
Parietal lobe lesions, 229, 334–335
Parinaud syndrome, 328f, 328t, 329f
Parkinsonism, postencephalitic, 332f
Parkinson's disease, 331–332
saccades in, 331

Pars planitis, optic disc swelling in patient with, 142f
Parvocellular cells, 39
Past-pointing, 305
Pattern Deviation Plot, 15, 17f
Pattern electroretinogram (PERG), 29, 29f
Pattern standard deviation (PSD) on Humphrey field analyzer, 15
Peduncular hallucinations, 259
Pelizaeus–Merzbacher disease, 340–341
Pelli–Robson chart, 3, 4f
Pendular Nystagmus, etiology of, 406t
PERG. See Pattern electroretinogram (PERG)
Periodic alternating gaze deviation, 418
Perimetry, 7
    automated, 8
    diagnostic functions, 7
    kinetic, 7
    static, 9–11, 10f, 16f
    suprathreshold static, 11, 15
Perimetry and visual field testing
    Amsler grid, 9, 10f
    ancillary testing, 25–32, 26f–27f, 28f–32f
    confrontation visual field testing, 8–9, 8f
    five-step approach to visual field interpretation, 18, 19, 21f, 22, 22f, 23f
    general principles, 7–8
    Goldmann manual projection perimeter, 7, 11, 11f, 15
    graphic representation of visual field data, 15
    kinetic perimetry, 15
    probability plots, 15, 16f, 17f
    progression of visual field loss, 16–18
    reliability indices, 13, 14f, 15
    static perimetry, 9–11, 10f
    tangent screen, 15
    techniques for, 8–13
    visual field indices, 15
Periodic alternating nystagmus (PAN), 317, 411
Perioperative ION, 156
Perioptic neuritis, 140, 144
Peripapillary hemorrhages, 67
Peripapillary retinal nerve fiber layer (PRNFL), 25, 98–99, 217
    atrophy of, 101f
    OCT of, 26f, 28f
Peripapillary staphyloma, 80, 80f
    and morning glory disc anomaly, 80t
Peripapillary subretinal hemorrhage, 68f
Peripapillary subretinal neovascularization, 68–69, 68f
Peripheral oculomotor nerve, 292
Peripheral visual field defects, 66
PHACE syndrome, 75
Pharmacologically dilated pupil, 286f

Pharmacologic blockade with parasympatholytic agents, 285
Pharmacologic tests, 377
Phenomena, hemifield slide, 216, 216f
Phenomenon
    Bell, 305
    Riddoch, 240
    Tournay, 285
    visual extinction, 241
Photophobia, 54
Photopsias, 1, 131
Photoreceptor cells, 35–37
    cones, 35–36
    rods, 35–36
Photoreceptors cells, 33, 34
Photoreceptors, ultrastructure of, 36f
Photostress recovery test, 24
Photostress recovery time (PSRT), 24
Phototransduction cascade, 36f
Physiologic anisocoria, 264, 273, 274f
PICA. See Posterior inferior cerebellar artery (PICA)
Picture, cookie theft, 254f, 337f
Pigmentation, congenital optic disc, 86, 87f
Pigmentosa, retinitis, 29
Ping-pong gaze, 339, 418
Pituitary adenoma
    bitemporal hemianopic scotomas in patient with, 215f
Pituitary adenylate cyclase-activating polypeptide (PACAP), 40
Pituitary ectopia, posterior, 73f
Plates, pseudoisochromatic, 5–6
Plots, probability, 15, 16f, 17f
PMR. See Polymyalgia rheumatica (PMR)
Pneumosinus dilatans, 50
POEMS syndrome, 124
Polyarteritis nodosa, 141
Polycoria, 294. See also Pseudopolycoria
Polymyalgia rheumatica (PMR), 145
Polyneuropathies, hereditary, 208–209
Polyopia, cerebral, 256
Pons, 292
Pons at level of abducens nuclei, 324f
Pons, ocular motor syndromes caused by lesions of, 322–327
    internuclear ophthalmoplegia, 322–324
    lesions of abducens nucleus, 324
    lesions of paramedian pontine reticular formation (PPRF), 325
    one-and-a-half syndrome, 325–326
    slow saccades from pontine lesions, 326–327
    unilateral conjugate gaze palsy, 325–326
Pontine astrocytoma, 447f
Pontine lesions, slow saccades from, 326–327
Positive phenomena, visual fields, 255
Positive scotoma, 1
Positive visual phenomena, 255–260
    migrainous hallucinations, 259

other types of hallucinations, 259–260
    release hallucinations, 256–258
    visual distortions, 260
    visual hallucinations, 256
    visual perseveration, 255–256
    visual seizures, 258–259
Postchiasmal visual sensory system, chiasm and, 211f
Postencephalitic parkinsonism, oculogyric crisis in patients with, 332f
Posterior commissure, 327–328
Posterior inferior cerebellar artery (PICA), 314
Posterior ischemic optic neuropathy (PION), 155–156
    DWI in, 157f
Posterior occipital lobe, unilateral lesions of, 230
Posterior optic chiasmal syndrome, 211–214
    bitemporal hemianopic scotomas, 215f
    bitemporal inferior quadrantic scotomas, 215f
    in patient with craniopharyngioma, 214f
Posterior orbit, view of, 49f
Posterior pituitary ectopia, 73f
Postganglionic Horner's syndromes, 277–278
Postganglionic neuron, 277–278
Postganglionic supersensitivity in tonic pupil syndrome, 285f
Post-geniculate congenital homonymous hemianopia, 289
Postoperative mydriasis, 296
Postoperative Visual Loss (POVL), 156
Postpapilledema atrophy, 113–114, 113f
Postvaccination optic neuritis, 141
Pourfour du Petit syndrome, 437, 437f
POVL. See Postoperative Visual Loss (POVL)
P100 peak, 32, 32f
PPRF. See Paramedian pontine reticular formation
Pre-chiasmal optic nerve dysfunction, syndromes of, 102–108
    bilateral superior or inferior (altitudinal) hemianopia, 104–106, 106f
    distal optic nerve syndrome, 102, 104f
    Foster Kennedy syndrome, 102, 104, 105f
    nasal hemianopia, 106–108, 108f
    optociliary shunts, 102
    syndromes of optic nerve compression, 102
"Preferential-looking" techniques, 3
Preganglionic autonomic nerve fibers, course of, 283f
Preganglionic Horner's syndromes, 276–277, 277f

Preganglionic neuron, 276–277, 277f
Preganglionic oculomotor nerve, 291
Pregnancy, 126, 129
Prepapillary hemorrhages, 67
Pretectal nuclei, drawing of major, 327f
Pretectal nucleus or in brachium of superior colliculus, 289
Primary deviation, eye, 305, 306f
Primary mechanisms, 183
Primary oculomotor nerve synkinesis, 354–355
Primary tumors, 166–172
Primate retina, cellular component of fully developed, 34f
Primate, visual function in cerebral cortex of nonhuman, 245f
Principle of diplopia tests, 306f
Prism dissociation tests, 455
PRNFL. See Peripapillary retinal nerve fiber layer (PRNFL)
Probability plots, 15, 16f, 17f
Progression of visual field loss, 16–18, 18f–19f
Progressive supranuclear palsy (PSP), 327, 329, 331
Projection perimeter, Goldmann manual, 7, 11, 11f, 15
Prosopagnosia, 247
  apperceptive, 248
  associative, 248
  developmental, 248–249
  location of bilateral lesions in three patients with, 249f
  and related disturbances of object recognition, 247–249
Proximal myotonic myopathy, 392
PSD. See Pattern standard deviation (PSD)
Pseudoabducens palsy, 328
Pseudo-CSF sign, 167, 168f
Pseudo-Foster Kennedy syndrome, 155
Pseudo-Graefe sign, 354
Pseudoglaucomatous cupping after attack of AAION, 149f
Pseudo-internuclear ophthalmoplegia, Bilateral, 376f
Pseudoisochromatic plates, 5–6, 6f
Pseudopapilledema, 61–69
  associated with buried drusen, 65t
  associated with optic disc drusen, 62–69
  fiber layer in, 111f
  without drusen, 69
Pseudopapilledema associated with optic disc drusen, 62–69
Pseudopapilledema with buried drusen vs. optic disc swelling, 65t
Pseudopolycoria, 294–295
Pseudoptosis, 432
Pseudotumor cerebri, 116f, 124–129
  CT angiogram of head in patient with, 126f
PSP. See Progressive supranuclear palsy (PSP)

PSRT. See Photostress recovery time (PSRT)
Psychic paralysis of gaze, 254
Psychogenic disturbance, 452
Psychomotor epilepsy, 228
Ptosis, 12f, 13, 273
  bilateral, 393
Pupil conditions, testing in diagnosing common, 270t
Pupillary capture, 264
Pupillary defect. See also Relative afferent pupillary defect (RAPD)
  macular lesions associated with ipsilateral relative afferent, 57f
Pupillary dilation, 117–118
  assessment of, 265–266
  intermittent unilateral, 287f
Pupillary escape, 264
Pupillary examination, 24
Pupillary function, disorders of, 273–296
  afferent abnormalities, 287–290
  anisocoria, 273–287
  disturbances during seizures, 291
  disturbances in coma, 292
  disturbances in disorders of neuromuscular junction, 292
  drug effects, 292–293
  efferent abnormalities, 273–287
  light-near dissociation, 290–291
  structural defects of iris, 293–296
Pupillary light-near dissociation, 291f
Pupillary light reflex, path of, 289f
Pupillary membrane remnants, persistent, 294
Pupillary near response, testing, 265
Pupillary reaction to light, testing, 264–265
Pupillary size, assessing, 263–264
Pupillary size, shape, and function, assessment of, 263–271
  examination, 263–270
  history, 263
  pharmacologic testing, 270–271
Pupils, 12f
  Argyll Robertson, 290–291, 290f
  drugs that constrict, 293
  drugs that dilate, 292–293
  ectopic, 294
  gauges, 264f
  from midbrain disease, 290
  miotic, 281
  paradoxical reactions to light and darkness, 290
  pharmacologically dilated, 286f
  size, 266f
  tadpole, 280
  tonic, 281–285
  transient unilateral dilation of, 286–287
  Wernicke's, 289
Pupils, examination of, 263–271
  examination, 263–270
  history, 263
  pharmacologic testing, 270–271

Pupil-sparing oculomotor nerve palsies, 350
Pure alexia, 247, 250

Q
Quadrantanopia, 247

R
Radiation optic neuropathy (RON), 158, 159f
"Ragged red" muscle fibers, 395
Range of eye movements, 302–305
  principles, 302–303
  techniques, 303–305
RAPD. See Relative afferent pupillary defect (RAPD)
Rapid recovery, 166
Reaching and grasping, 254
Recovery
  delayed, 166
  late, 166
  rapid, 166
Reference cap, 6
Reflexes
  corneal light, 307–308
  pupillary light, 289f
Reflex eye movements, 339
Relative afferent pupillary defect (RAPD), 24, 55–56, 181, 219, 221f, 268f, 269f, 287–289
  macular lesions associated with, 57f
  testing for, 266–268, 266f, 267f
  in various situations, 270t
Release hallucinations, 256–258, 257f
Reliability indices, 13, 14f, 15
Renal-coloboma syndrome. See Papillorenal syndrome
Residual vision, blindsight and, 245–246
Retina, anatomy and physiology of, 33–44
  blood supply, 43f
  blood vessels, 43
  cell types and layers of, 33–43
  cellular organization, 35t
  rod and cone through pathways, 43–44
Retina and optic nerve, anatomy and physiology of, 33–60
  cell types and layers of retina, 33–43
  intracanalicular (intraosseous) optic nerve, 48–50
  intracranial optic nerve, 50–52
  optic nerve head (intraocular optic nerve), 44–47
  optic nerve physiology, 52
  orbital optic nerve, 47–48
  retinal blood vessels, 43
  rod and cone through pathways, 43–44
  topographic anatomy of optic nerve, 52–53
  topographic diagnosis of retinal lesions, 53–60

Retinal abnormalities, 391
Retinal arteries in optic atrophy, 101*f*
Retinal arteriolar narrowing in AION,
    parapapillary, 148*f*
Retinal blood vessels, 43
Retinal detachment, 288
Retinal disease, 53–60
    appearance of optic disc in, 59–60
    distinguishing from optic
        neuropathy by clinical
        examination, 53–56
    distinguishing from optic
        neuropathy by visual field,
        56–59
Retinal dystrophy, optic atrophy in,
    60, 60*f*
Retinal ganglion cells (RGCs), 33
    axon of, 40–41
    layers, 39
    pathways to, 38*f*
    receptive fields, 39
Retinal lesions, topographic diagnosis
    of, 53–60
    appearance of the optic disc in
        retinal disease, 59–60
    distinguishing retinal disease from
        optic neuropathy by clinical
        examination, 53–56
    distinguishing retinal disease from
        optic neuropathy by visual
        field, 56–59
Retinal nerve axons, drawing of, 41*f*
Retinal nerve fiber layer (RNFL),
    atrophy of peripapillary, 101*f*
Retinal neurons and neurotransmitters,
    42*t*
Retinal pigment epithelium (RPE), 33,
    34*f*, 35
    functions, 33, 35
Retinal vascular occlusions, 67–68
Retinitis pigmentosa, 69
    optic disc drusen in patient with, 69*f*
Retrobulbar compressive optic
    neuropathies, 164–166
Retrobulbar optic neuritis, optic
    atrophy after acute, 132*f*
Retrochiasmal lesions, topical diagnosis
    of chiasmal and, 210–243
    topical diagnosis of optic chiasmal
        disorders, 210–217
    topical diagnosis of retrochiasmal
        visual field defects, 217–243
Retrochiasmal visual field defects,
    topical diagnosis of, 217–243
    lesions of occipital lobe and visual
        cortex, 229–243
    topical diagnosis of lesions of lateral
        geniculate body, 224–225
    topical diagnosis of lesions of optic
        radiation, 225–229
    topical diagnosis of optic tract
        lesions, 219–223
Retrograde degeneration, 97
Reverse bobbing, 338
Reverse dipping, 338

RGCs. *See* Retinal ganglion cells
    (RGCs)
Rhinorrhea, CSF, 118
Rhodopsin, 36
Riddoch phenomenon, 240
Right homonymous hemianopia, 220*f*,
    232*f*
    visual fields, 235*f*
Riley–Smith syndrome, 69
riMLF. *See* Rostral interstitial nucleus
    of medial longitudinal
    fasciculus (riMLF)
Ring scotomas, 58
Rod and cone pathways,
    neurotransmitters used by cells
    of, 38*f*
Rod and cone through pathways, 43–44
Rods, photoreceptor cells, 35–37
RON. *See* Radiation optic neuropathy
    (RON)
Rostral interstitial nucleus of medial
    longitudinal fasciculus (riMLF),
    328–329
    bilateral lesions of, 329
    unilateral lesions of, 329
RPE. *See* Retinal pigment epithelium
    (RPE)

S
Saccades
    clinical examination of, 309
    contrapulsion of, 315
    ipsipulsion of, 315
    lateropulsion of, 315*f*
    in Parkinson's disease, 331
Saccadic and vestibular eye movement
    control, 325*f*
Saccadic dysmetria, 309
Saccadic pulses, 417
Sarcoid granulomas infiltrating optic
    disc, 176*f*
Sarcoidosis, 141, 176–178, 177*f*–178*f*
Sarcoidosis lupus erythematosus, 127
SCA. *See* Spinocerebellar ataxia (SCA);
    Superior cerebellar artery
    (SCA)
Scale, Frisén, 110*t*
Schilder's disease, 138–139
Schwartz–Jampel Syndrome, 395*f*
Scotomas, 9, 10*f*, 12*f*, 20*f*, 102
    annular/ring, 58
    cecocentral, 57, 57*f*–58*f*
    junctional, 102, 210
    mapped by kinetic perimetry, 189*f*
Screen, tangent, 15
Secondary deviation, eye, 305, 306*f*
Secondary mechanisms, 183
Secondary oculomotor nerve
    synkinesis, 354
Secondary tumors, 172–176
Sectoranopia
    congruous homonymous
        horizontal, 224, 226*f*
    congruous homonymous
        quadruple, 224, 225*f*

Seesaw nystagmus, 217
    etiology of, 412, 412*t*
SEF. *See* Supplementary eye fields (SEF)
Segmental optic nerve hypoplasia,
    73–74
Seizures
    disturbances during, 291
    ocular motor manifestations of,
        337–338
    visual, 258–259
Seizures, visual, 258–259
Sensitivity, contrast, 3–4, 4*f*
Septo-optic dysplasia, 71–72, 72*f*
Single-Fiber Electromyography, 381
Sherrington law of reciprocal
    innervation, 303
Shift, criterion, 245
Schwartz–Jampel Syndrome, 395
Simultanagnosia, 252, 254
Single-cover test, 308–309, 308*f*
Single-fiber electromyography, 381
Sinusitis, 141
SITA. *See* Swedish interactive threshold
    algorithm (SITA)
Skew deviation and ocular tilt reaction,
    317
Sleep test, 377, 412, 412*f*
SLE. *See* Systemic lupus erythematosus
    (SLE)
Slit lamp examination, 24–25, 132
Slow saccades, etiology of, 326*t*
Slow saccades from pontine lesions,
    326–327
Snellen notation, 2. *See also* Visual
    acuity
Somatization disorder, 452
Spasm
    accommodation, 298–300
    of near reflex, 298–300, 299*f*
Spasm of fixation, 254
Spasmus nutans, 415
Spastic-paretic facial contracture, 446
Specific autoantibody assays, 377
Sphenocavernous syndrome, 351
Spinal canal, tumors in, 124
Spinocerebellar ataxia (SCA), 208
Spontaneous eye movements, 338–339
Spontaneous hemorrhage, 156
Spontaneous venous pulsations (SVPs),
    110
Square-wave jerks, 416
Stages of Papilledema, 110–112
    early papilledema (Frisén stage 1),
        110, 111*f*
    early papilledema (Frisén stage 2),
        110, 111*f*
    marked papilledema (Frisén stage 4),
        111*f*, 112
    moderate papilledema (Frisén stage
        3), 110, 111*f*, 112
    normal optic disc (Frisén stage 0),
        110, 111*f*
    severe papilledema (Frisén stage 5),
        111*f*, 112
Standard eye chart for visual acuity, 2*f*

Staphyloma, peripapillary, 80, 80f
Static countertorsion, 303
Static insufficiency, accommodation, 297
Static perimetry, 9–11, 10f, 16f
    suprathreshold, 11, 15
Static perimetry, suprathreshold, 11, 15
Stenosis, aqueductal, 122
Stereoacuity, 4
Stilling-Turk-Duane syndrome, 361–363, 397–398
Strabismus, 305
Structural defects of iris, 293–296
    acquired, 296
    congenital, 293–296
Stupor and coma, eye movements in, 338–339
Subarachnoid hemorrhage, 122
Subarachnoid oculomotor nerve palsy
    dilated pupil, 348
    isolated fixed, 348
    pupillary involvement, 348
    with pupillary sparing, 349
Subclinical optic neuritis, 135
Subretinal hemorrhage, peripapillary, 68f
Substances, exogenous, 126, 126t
Superior altitudinal defect, 20f
Superior cerebellar artery (SCA), 316, 317f
Superior colliculus, pretectal nucleus or in brachium of, 289
Superior oblique microtremor, 370
Superior oblique myokymia (SOM), 370, 418
Superior orbital fissure, 351–352, 360
Super sensitivity test, denervation, 284
Supplementary eye fields (SEF), 335
Supranuclear and internuclear ocular motor disorders, 312–342
Supranuclear oculopalpebral synkinesia, 426
Supranuclear ptosis, 426
Suprasellar mass with hydrocephalus, 222f
Suprathreshold static perimetry, 11, 15
SVPs. See Spontaneous venous pulsations (SVPs)
Swedish interactive threshold algorithm (SITA), 10–11
Swelling, optic disc, 92f, 93t, 95f, 96f
    appearance, 91–92
    specific etiologies, 92–96
Swinging flashlight test, 266–268, 267f
Swollen disc, differential diagnosis of, 93t
Sympathetic hyperactivity, 280
Sympathetic paralysis, 298
Sympatholytic (antiadrenergic) drugs, 293
Sympathomimetic (adrenergic) drugs, 292, 294f
Syndromes
    acute retinal necrosis (ARN), 143
    Adie's, 283f

Adie's tonic pupil, 283–285, 283f
Aicardi, 86–88, 87f
anosognosia, 239
of anterior inferior cerebellar artery (AICA), 316
anterior optic chiasmal, 212f
Anton, 239
Balint's, 252–255, 253f, 337f
Behr, 206–207
Benedikt, 345
Bonnet, Charles, 256–258, 257f
central, 292
central Horner's, 276, 277f
CHARGE, 78
chronic progressive external ophthalmoplegia (CPEO), 206
congenital tilted optic disc, 84–86, 84f, 85f
CPEO Plus, 397
Dandy-Walker, 320
de Morsier, 71
distal optic nerve, 102, 104f
dorsal midbrain, 328f, 328t
Duane's retraction, 361–363
eight-and-a-half, 324, 326f
of elevated venous pressure, 123
Foster Kennedy, 102, 104, 105f
Foville, 363
Gerstmann, 251
Gradenigo, 367
Guillain-Barré, 124
half-moon, 231, 232f
Holmes-Adie tonic pupil, 283–285
Horner's, 273–280
Kearns–Sayre, 397
Leber plus, 198
Leigh's, 341
locked-in, 339
medial inferior pontine, 363
Millard–Gubler, 363, 365f
MNGIE, 398
Möbius, 361
morning glory, 76f
oculopalatal myoclonus, 312
ODOA Plus, 203–204
one-and-a-half, 325–326, 363
optic chiasmal, 216–217
papillorenal, 82–84, 83f
Parinaud, 328f, 328t, 329f
PHACE, 75
POEMS, 124
postganglionic Horner's, 277–278
of pre-chiasmal optic nerve dysfunction, 102–108
preganglionic Horner's, 277f
Raymond Céstan, 363
Riley–Smith, 69
Schwartz–Jampel, 395
Stilling–Turk–Duane, 361–363
of superior cerebellar artery, 316–317
temporal crescent, 231, 232f
tonic pupil, 283–285, 283f, 298
uncal, 292

Wallenberg's, 276, 314–316, 314f, 315f
Wolfram, 205–206, 206f
Synkinesis, 371
Syphilis, 140–141
Systemic and teratogenic associations, 72–73
Systemic illnesses, IIH, 126t, 127
Systemic lupus erythematosus (SLE), 127, 133, 141
System, visual sensory, 1–32

T
Tadpole pupil, 280
Tangent screen, 11, 15
Telative afferent pupillary defect, testing for, 266–268, 266f, 267f
Temporal conus, 97
Temporal crescent
    loss of, 232f
    sparing of, 233f
    syndromes, 231
Temporal lobe
    cystic astrocytoma, 228f
    lesions of, 227–229, 335
    visual field defect, 228f
Temporal raphe, 41
Tenon capsule, 386
Tensilon (Edrophonium chloride) test, 379f
Teratogenic associations, systemic and, 72–73
Testing
    caloric, 304
    in children, 9f
    color comparison, 6–7, 7f
    confrontation visual field, 9f
    corneal light reflex, 307–308
    in diagnosing common pupil conditions, 270t
    electrophysiologic testing, 25–32
    forced duction, 304, 304f
    for light-near dissociation, 266
    ocular imaging, 25
    oculocephalic, 304
    pupillary near response, 265
    pupillary reaction to light, 264–265
    for relative afferent pupillary defect, 266–268, 266f, 267f
    standard eye chart for visual acuity, 2f
    techniques for visual field, 8–13
    visual field, 8f
Tests
    alternate-cover, 309
    cocaine, 275
    color comparison, 6–7, 7f
    cover, 308–309
    cover–uncover, 308f, 309
    denervation supersensitivity, 284
    diplopia, 306f
    electrophysiologic, 25–32
    Farnsworth–Munsell 100 Hues test, 6–7
    Farnsworth Panel D-15 test, 6

Tests (*continued*)
head tilt, 309
higher visual function, 260–261, 261*f*
Hirschberg, 308
Hooper Visual Organization Test, 261*f*
Krimsky, 308
photostress recovery, 24
principle of diplopia, 306*f*
principle of haploscopic, 307*f*
single-cover, 308–309, 308*f*
swinging flashlight, 266–268, 267*f*
Tests, prism dissociation, 455
Tetanus, 297, 384
Threshold, 3
Thyroid eye disease, 162, 163*f*
Tilt, 302
Titmus/Randot Stereo Testers, 4
TNF-a. *See* Tumor necrosis factor-
alpha (TNF-a) inhibitors
Tonic convergence, 271
Tonic downward deviation, eyes, 338
Tonic pupil, 281–285
local, 282
neuropathic, 282
Tonic pupil syndrome, 283*f*
Adie's, 283*f*
Holmes–Adie, 283–285
misregeneration theory, 286*f*
Postganglionic supersensitivity in, 285*f*
Tonic pupil syndromes, 298
Tonic upward deviation, eyes, 338
Topographagnosia, 247
Topographic anatomy of optic nerve, 52–53
Torsional nystagmus, etiology of, 411, 411*t*
Total Deviation Plot, 15, 17*f*
Tournay phenomenon, 285
Toxic and deficiency optic
neuropathies, 186–194
clinical characteristics of nutritional
and toxic optic neuropathies, 187
differential diagnosis, 187–190
etiologic criteria, 186–187
specific nutritional optic
neuropathies, 190–192
specific toxic optic neuropathies, 192–194
Toxic and metabolic disorders, 96
Toxic optic neuropathies, 186–187
bilateral, 188*f*, 189*f*
clinical characteristics of nutritional
and, 187
Toxic optic neuropathies, specific, 192*t*
amiodarone, 194
ethambutol, 192–193
substances to cause, 192*t*
tumor necrosis factor-alpha (TNF-a)
inhibitors, 193–194, 193*f*
Toxins
damage both pre- and postsynaptic
neuromuscular transmission, 384

damage presynaptic neuromuscular
transmission, 383–384
neuromuscular disorders caused by
drugs or, 383–384
Tract, optic, 289
Transient visual loss, 68
Transient visual obscurations, 118
trans-Retinol, 36*f*
Transsphenoidal encephalocele, 76*f*, 77
Transsynaptic (transneuronal)
degeneration, 98
Trauma, 123, 296
Traumatic optic neuropathies, 179–185, 180*f*
classification, 179
clinical assessment, 181–182
epidemiology, 179–181
management, 184–185
pathogenesis, 183
pathology, 182–183
pharmacology, 183–184
Trochlear nerve nucleus, lesions of, 358–359
Trochlear nerve palsies, 355–361
acquired, 358
congenital, 358
evaluation and management of, 360–361
Trochlear nerve paresis, 359*f*
True monocular diplopia, 459
"Tumbling E Cube," 2*f*, 3
Tullio's phenomenon, 409
Tumor necrosis factor-alpha (TNF-a)
inhibitors, 193–194, 193*f*
Tumors, 166–176, 296
primary, 166–172
secondary, 172–176
in spinal canal, 124
Tunnel vision, visual fields, 236*f*

U
Uhthoff symptom, 134
Uncal syndrome, 292
Uncrossed diplopia, 306
Unilateral/asymmetric papilledema, 114–115
Unilateral conjugate gaze palsy and
internuclear ophthalmoplegia
(INO), 325–326
Unilateral dilation of pupil, transient, 286–287
Unilateral hypoplasia, 70*f*, 72*f*
Unilateral lesions
of anterior occipital lobe, 230–231
central and posterior occipital lobe
of, 230, 231*f*
persistent deficits caused by large, 333–334
Unilateral lesions of riMLF, 329, 330*f*
Unilateral ptosis, 426
Unilateral pupillary dilation,
intermittent, 287*f*
Unilateral tilted optic disc, 84*f*
Unilateral visual loss, sudden onset
of, 166

Upbeat nystagmus
etiology of, 410*t*
one cause of, 410*f*
Upper eyelid retraction, contralateral, 435*f*

V
Vascular occlusions, retinal, 67–68
Vascular processes, 353
Vasculitides, miscellaneous, 141
Veins, optociliary shunt, 102
Venous drainage, cerebral, 123*t*
Venous pressure, syndromes of
elevated, 123
Venous sinus stenting, 128–129
Ventriculoperitoneal shunting, 128
VEP. *See* Visual-evoked potential (VEP)
Vergence, eye movement, 303
Vermis, dorsal, 318
Versions, eye movement, 303
Versions, performance of, 309–311
clinical examination of pursuit, 309–310
clinical examination of saccades, 309
optokinetic system, 311
vestibular and optokinetic systems,
clinical examination of, 311
vestibulo-ocular reflex, 311
Vertical retraction syndrome, 342
Vertical semicircular canals, 340*f*
Vertical vestibulo-ocular projections, 340*f*
Vertigo, 302
oscillopsia, and tilt, 302
Vestibular eye movement control,
saccadic and, 325*f*
Vestibular symptoms, 302
Vestibular nystagmus, 419
Vestibulo-ocular projections, direct
vertical, 340*f*
Vestibulo-ocular reflex, 311
Visible optic disc drusen, 64, 64*f*
Vision
blindsight and residual, 245–246
blurred, 302–303
brief, transient obscurations of, 118
color, 4–7, 55, 181
Vision deficits, glossary of cerebral, 261–262
Visual acuity, 1–3, 2*f*
central, 53–54
Visual agnosia, 247
Visual angle, 2, 9
Visual confusion, 302
Visual cortex
lesions of occipital lobe and, 229–243
Visual distortions, 260
Visual-evoked potential (VEP), 3, 30
method for generating and
recording, 30, 32*f*
multifocal, 32
waveform, 30, 32, 32*f*
Visual extinction, 241
Visual field defects, 118, 210–216

arcuate, 57
bilateral superior altitudinal, 239f
caused by lesions that damage optic
    chiasm, 214–216
from damage to anterior angle of
    optic chiasm, 210
from damage to body of optic
    chiasm, 210–211, 212f
from damage to posterior angle of
    optic chiasm, 211–214
fabricated, 460f–461f
glaucomatous, 98
kinetic perimetry demonstrates
    supertemporal, 85f
in papilledema, 121f
in patients with lesions of parietal
    lobe, 230f
in patient with bilateral central
    serous chorioretinopathy, 54f
in patient with bilateral optic disc
    drusen, 67f
peripheral, 66
temporal lobe, 228f
visual loss, 239f
Visual field defects, retrochiasmal,
    217–243
lesions of occipital lobe and visual
    cortex, 229–243
topical diagnosis of lesions of lateral
    geniculate body, 224–225
topical diagnosis of lesions of optic
    radiation, 225–229
topical diagnosis of optic tract
    lesions, 219–223
Visual field examination, 7–22
automated visual field information,
    interpretation of
    kinetic perimetry, 15
    probability plots, 15, 16f, 17f
    progression of visual field loss,
        16–18, 18f–19f
    reliability indices, 13, 14f, 15
    visual field indices, 15
five-step approach to visual field
    interpretation, 18, 19, 21f, 22,
        22f, 23f
general principles, 7–8
techniques for
    Amsler grids, 9, 10f
    confrontation testing, 8–9, 8f, 9f
    kinetic perimetry, 11, 11f, 13
    static perimetry, 9–11, 10f
Visual field indices, 15
Visual fields
binocular, 216f
with hypertension, 235f
lesion, left lateral geniculate body,
    226f
lesion, right lateral geniculate body,
    226f
lesions of extrastriate cortex with
    defects in, 240
negative phenomena, 255
positive phenomena, 255

right homonymous hemianopia,
    235f
tunnel vision, 236f
Visual field testing, 182
in children, 8f
confrontation testing, 8–9, 9f
Visual function
in cerebral cortex of nonhuman
    primate, 245f
test of higher, 260–261, 261f
Visual function, central disorders
glossary of cerebral vision deficits,
    261–262
Visual function, central disorders of,
    244–262
acquired alexia, 249–252
Balint's syndrome and related
    visuospatial disorders, 252–255
blindsight and residual vision,
    245–246
cerebral achromatopsia, 246–247
disorders of motion perception, 252
glossary of cerebral visual deficits,
    261–262
positive visual phenomena, 255–260
prosopagnosia and related
    disturbances of object
    recognition, 247–249
segregation of visual inputs, 244–245
tests of higher visual function,
    260–261
Visual hallucinations, 256
Visual illusions of occipital lobe
    epilepsy, 258f
Visual inputs, segregation of, 244–245
Visual loss
central, 66–67
macular lesions causing, 54f, 55f,
    56f, 57f
papilledema associated with
    bilateral, 119f–120f
in patients with LHON, 196
sudden onset of unilateral, 166
transient, 68
visual field defects, 239f
Visual pathway, afferent, 452–459
decreased visual acuity, 453–457
monocular diplopia, 459–461
visual field defects, 457–459
Visual pathways
acquired pendular nystagmus and
    disease of, 406–408
nystagmus with lesions affecting,
    405–406
Visual perceptions, dissociation of,
    240–241
Visual perseveration, 255–256
Visual restoration therapy (VRT),
    242
Visual seizures, 258–259
Visual sensory system, chiasm and
    postchiasmal, 211f
Visual sensory system examination,
    1–32

clinical office examination
ancillary testing, 25–32, 26f–27f,
    28f–32f
anterior segment examination,
    24–25
brightness comparison, 24
color vision, 4–7, 6f, 7f
contrast sensitivity, 3–4, 4f
cranial nerves, 24–25
exophthalmometry, 24–25
external examination, 24–25
fundus examination, 25
photostress recovery test, 24
pupillary examination, 22, 24
stereoacuity, 4
visual acuity, 1–3, 2f
visual field, 7–22, 8f–12f, 14f,
    16f–23f
history, 1
Visual spread, illusory, 256
Visual system, nystagmus associated
    with disease of, 405–406
Visuospatial disorders, Balint's
    syndrome and, 252–255
Vitamin A, 36
deficiency, optic atrophy in, 60f
Vitamin E deficiency, 341
encephalomyopathy with
    ophthalmoplegia from,
        400–401
Voluntary convergence, 272
Voluntary nystagmus, 417, 459
Voluntary saccadic oscillations, 417,
    459
Vomiting, 117
VRT. See Visual restoration therapy
    (VRT)

W
Wallenberg's syndrome, 276, 314–316
neuroimaging of, 314f, 315f
Walker–Warburg Syndrome, 389
Waveform, visual-evoked potential
    (VEP), 30, 32f
Weber syndrome, 345, 346, 346f
Weight loss, 127
Wernicke–Korsakoff syndrome, 442
Wernicke's encephalopathy, 341
Wernicke's pupil, 289
Whipple disease, 331
Whitnall ligament, 424
Wilbrand's knee, 52f, 53, 210
Wilson's disease, 297–298
Wolfram syndrome, 205–206
optic disc with, 206f

X
X-linked optic atrophy, 204

Y
Yoke pair, 303

Z
Zinn–Haller circle, 47